Urgent Care Dermatology

SYMPTOM-BASED DIAGNOSIS

Urgent Care Dermatology

SYMPTOM-BASED DIAGNOSIS

JAMES E. FITZPATRICK, MD
Professor of Dermatology and Pathology (retired)
University of Colorado School of Medicine
Aurora, Colorado

WHITNEY A. HIGH, MD, JD, MEng
Associate Professor, Dermatology and Pathology
Director of Dermatopathology (Dermatology)
University of Colorado School of Medicine
Aurora, Colorado

W. LAMAR KYLE, MD
Private Practice
Urgent Care
Fort Smith, Arkansas

ELSEVIER

ELSEVIER

1600 John F. Kennedy Blvd.
Ste 1800
Philadelphia, PA 19103-2899

URGENT CARE DERMATOLOGY: SYMPTOM-BASED DIAGNOSIS   ISBN: 978-0-323-48553-1

Library of Congress Cataloging-in-Publication Data

Names: Fitzpatrick, James E., 1948- author. | High, Whitney A., author. | Kyle, W. Lamar, author.
Title: Urgent care dermatology : symptom-based diagnosis / James E. Fitzpatrick, Whitney A. High, W. Lamar Kyle.
Description: Philadelphia, PA : Elsevier, [2018] | Includes bibliographical references and index.
Identifiers: LCCN 2017019068 | ISBN 9780323485531 (pbk. : alk. paper)
Subjects: | MESH: Skin Diseases—diagnosis | Skin Diseases—etiology
Classification: LCC RL74 | NLM WR 141 | DDC 616.5—dc23 LC record available at
    https://lccn.loc.gov/2017019068

Senior Content Strategist: Charlotta Kryhl
Director, Content Development: Rebecca Gruliow
Publishing Services Manager: Patricia Tannian
Senior Project Manager: Sharon Corell
Book Designer: Bryan Salisbury

Working together
to grow libraries in
developing countries

www.elsevier.com • www.bookaid.org

Printed in the United States of America.
Last digit is the print number: 10   9   8

This book is dedicated to
my sons, Jeff and Josh
-JEF
and
Misha, Madison, and Morgan – "my three M's"
-WAH

Preface

Urgent Care Dermatology: Symptom-Based Diagnosis had its genesis on a bass fishing trip on the Arkansas River in 2000. Lamar Kyle, a private practice physician, who had worked in an emergency room and urgent care clinic environment for decades, complained to me, an academic dermatologist, that dermatology textbooks were not organized in a useful fashion. He opined that dermatology books for a primary care provider needed to be organized by physical findings and not grouped by pathogenesis, needed copious photographs, and needed written text to be short and to the point. From this pivotal conversation, this textbook was born.

We caught very few fish, but when I returned home, I started outlining the book and experimenting with formats. For years, the book was something that I worked on early in the morning before the family woke up and on planes when traveling. After 7 years, the book had begun to take shape and was about two-thirds finished when a simultaneous computer disaster on two different computers containing the original and backup versions of the book brought the project to a halt. An older version of the manuscript on a third computer was found, but more than 100 completed pages of the manuscript were absent in this dated version. Disheartened, my interest in returning to work on the manuscript lagged, and the venture lay in limbo. The project was brought back to life by my energetic colleague, Whitney High, who worked with me in the Department of Dermatology at the University of Colorado. He offered to help write portions of the book and bring the book into a publishable state.

The concept of the book was simple. First, the dermatologic diseases needed to be organized by physical findings and not by pathogenesis. Whereas this would on the surface appear to be easy to do, it was difficult because we were using a morphologic model that is rarely utilized in dermatology textbooks. Second, cutaneous disorders that had a significant mortality rate or that were more likely to present urgently to a primary care provider were emphasized, and many trivial or genetic disorders were excluded. Third, the provided text, with very few exceptions, had to be kept to a single page. Finally, the book had to have numerous quality photographic examples of each entity.

We hope that we have succeeded in our objectives and that this will be a book that is actually used in the clinical setting while the practitioner is actively seeing patients, and not a book that sits on the shelf gathering dust.

James E. Fitzpatrick, MD
Aurora, Colorado

Acknowledgments

The authors would like to thank the outstanding team at Elsevier for their continued effort, support, and patience. Whereas there were many contributors from Elsevier, we would like to especially acknowledge Jim Merritt, Executive Content Strategist, and Suzanne Toppy, Senior Content Strategist, who were critical in getting the initial approval for this textbook. Once the textbook was started, we principally worked with Sarah Barth, Senior Content Strategist, and especially Rebecca "Becca" Gruliow, Director, Content Development. Becca was fantastic in guiding us through the editorial process and deserves special recognition for her patience, diligence, and promptness, and for just being a great individual to work with. In the final stages of this book, we would like to especially acknowledge the crucial role of of Sharon Corell, our Senior Project Manager, who we worked with on an almost daily basis.

The senior author (JEF) would especially like to acknowledge Linda Belfus, Senior Vice President of Content, for her role in not just this book but for other projects and for bringing us into the Elsevier family. I have worked with Linda for more than 20 years. Linda retired near the end of the editorial process, and I wish her happiness in her retirement.

Contents

1 Introduction to Clinical Dermatology   1

2 Diagnostic Techniques   7

3 Morbilliform Eruptions   31

4 Diffuse or Reticulated Erythema   51

5 Urticarial and Indurated Eruptions   63

6 Papular Eruptions: No Scale   83

7 Scaly Papular Lesions   97

8 Plaques With Scale   113

9 Scaly Disorders   123

10 Dermatitis (Eczematoid Reactions)   135

11 Blisters and Vesicles   163

12 Pustular Eruptions, Nonfollicular   205

13 Abscesses   217

14 Necrotic and Ulcerative Skin Disorders   231

15 Subcutaneous Diseases   253

16 Annular and Targetoid Lesions   269

17 Linear and Serpiginous Lesions   289

18 Sporotrichoid Disorders   301

19 Photosensitive Disorders   307

20 Purpuric and Hemorrhagic Disorders   327

21 Sclerosing and Fibrosing Disorders   353

22 Atrophic Disorders   367

23 Follicular Disorders   375

24 Alopecia   385

25 Nail Disorders   403

26 Infestations, Stings, and Bites   429

27 Discolorations of the Skin   441

28 Papillomatous and Verrucous Lesions   461

29 Tumors With Scale   477

30 Papular and Nodular Growths Without Scale   489

31 Pigmented Lesions   507

32 Vascular Tumors   535

33 Yellow Lesions   553

34 Cysts and Sinuses   565

35 Subcutaneous Lumps   579

36 Cutaneous Diseases of Travelers   587

37 Topical Treatment Pearls   597

Chapter 1

Introduction to Clinical Dermatology

"THINKING" LIKE A DERMATOLOGIST

The skin represents the largest organ of the human body. It consists of the epithelium, dermis, subcutaneous fat, and adnexal structures (hair follicles and glands), as well as supportive structures (blood vessels and nerves), all of which function to protect and maintain homeostasis.

Dermatology is a field of medicine that focuses on the skin, adjacent mucosa (oral and genital), and other adnexal structures (e.g., hair, nails, and sweat glands). Undoubtedly, dermatologists are the most adroit diagnosticians with regard to skin disease. However, much of their acumen comes from pattern recognition, a cultivated appreciation for diagnostic subtleties, and trained recognition of historical factors that make one particular disease more likely than another.

Thus, any clinician may improve when diagnosing and treating skin ailments simply by learning to think like a dermatologist. This includes fostering an appreciation for the classification schemes used in dermatology and for learning descriptive terminologies used by dermatologists.

ETIOLOGIC PREMISES

With regard to etiology, one of the most basic branch points in dermatology is to decide if a skin condition is neoplastic (benign or malignant) or inflammatory (e.g., rash, infection, autoimmune condition). Although it is likely that inflammatory conditions will prevail in urgent care and emergency settings, one must realize that a patient may present to these types of clinics with a neoplasm that has been ignored too long, until it can no longer be neglected.

Moreover, on occasion, there is visual and conceptual overlap with regard to inflammatory versus neoplastic conditions. For example, mycosis fungoides, the most common form of cutaneous T cell lymphoma, is a clonal lymphoproliferative disorder (a neoplasm), yet its clinical presentation resembles that of an inflammatory disorder. Conversely, sarcoidosis is an inflammatory condition that may present with discrete nodular lesions that mimic those of a neoplasm.

MORPHOLOGY

In dermatology, the term *morphology* refers to the appearance of a skin lesion(s), irrespective of the underlying pathophysiology. For example, a small blister is referred to as a *vesicle*, whether it is due to

an infection (e.g., herpes simplex) or autoimmune condition (e.g., bullous pemphigoid).

Therefore, it is important to use correct morphologic terms to classify skin diseases. This is because these terms represent a native language, or lexicon, that allows professionals to describe skin disease in a consistent manner.

There are primary morphologic terms (Table 1.1), which refer to the characteristic appearance of skin lesions (e.g., *papule*), and secondary morphologic terms (Table 1.2), which are used in addition to primary morphologic terms. These secondary morphologic terms reflect exogenous factors or temporal changes that evolve during the course of a skin disease.

PALPATION AND APPRECIATION OF TEXTURE

Textural changes are appreciated by palpating the skin; doing so may provide diagnostic clues. For example, macules and patches are flush with the surrounding skin, whereas papules and plaques are palpable. Some forms of connective tissue disease, such as morphea and scleroderma, may cause induration (firmness) of the skin, even when visual findings are limited. Finally, purpura (hemorrhage into the skin) may be palpable or nonpalpable, which implies a different underlying pathology. Small-vessel vasculitis causes palpable purpura, whereas simple bruising causes macular nonpalpable purpura.

COLOR

Skin color provides important clues about the nature of a disease process. For example, many skin lesions appear erythematous (red). However, it is important to ascertain whether the erythema is blanching, which disappears with pressure, because this suggests that the erythema is due to vasodilation, or whether it is nonblanching erythema (purpura), which implies hemorrhage into the skin. Other causes of pigment in the skin include hypoxia, topical medications, oral drugs, other ingestants, or even infections.

Also, there is variation in normal skin tones, even in the general population. These variations in skin color are due to differences in the amount and distribution of melanin in the epidermis. Sometimes, the term *skin of color* is used to describe any skin tone darker than white skin, but dermatologists more often use the Fitzpatrick scale (see "Fitzpatrick Skin Types"

TABLE 1.1 Primary Morphologic Terms

Morphologic Term	Salient Features	Classic Disease Image	Classic Diagnoses
Macule (or patch)	• Flat lesion <1 cm in diameter (macule) >1 cm in diameter (patch) • Circumscribed • Color change that cannot be appreciated by tactile sensation alone		• Vitiligo (photo) • Café-au-lait spot • Flat component of exanthems (measles) • Freckle • Lentigo
Papule	• Elevated lesion • Usually <1 cm in diameter • Often with other secondary features (e.g., scale, crust)		• Lichen nitidus (photo) • Elevated component of exanthems (measles) • Melanocytic nevi • Verruca or molluscum • Lichen planus • Guttate psoriasis
Plaque	• Elevated lesion • Usually >1 cm in diameter • Nonvesicular • Often with other secondary features (e.g., scale, crust)		• Psoriasis vulgaris (photo) • Lichen simplex chronicus • Eczematous plaques • Granuloma annulare • Sarcoidosis
Nodule	• Large elevated lesion • Usually ≥2 cm in diameter • Involves the dermis and may extend into the subcutis		• Neurofibromata (photo) • Basal cell carcinoma • Cutaneous lymphoma • Erythema nodosum • Lipoma
Vesicle	• Small elevated lesion • <1 cm in diameter • Filled with clear fluid • Circumscribed		• Herpes simplex infection (photo) • Varicella zoster infection • Dermatitis herpetiformis

TABLE 1.1	Primary Morphologic Terms—cont'd		
Morphologic Term	**Salient Features**	**Classic Disease Image**	**Classic Diagnoses**
Bulla	• Elevated lesion • Usually >1 cm in diameter • Filled with clear fluid • Circumscribed		• Epidermolysis bullosa (photo) • Bullous drug eruption • Bullous pemphigoid • Linear immunoglobulin A disease • Pemphigus • Porphyria
Pustule	• Elevated lesion • Usually <1 cm in diameter • Filled mainly with purulent fluid • Circumscribed		• Pustular psoriasis (photo) • Acute generalized exanthematous pustulosis • Candidiasis • Folliculitis • Subcorneal pustular dermatosis
Wheal	• Firm edematous papule or plaque • Evanescent • Pruritic		• Urticaria (photo) • Dermatographism • Urticaria pigmentosa

Fitzpatrick Skin Types

Type I	Always burns, never tans
Type II	Usually burns, then tans
Type III	May burn, tans well
Type IV	Rarely burns, tans well
Type V	Very rarely burns, tans well, brown skin
Type VI	Very rarely burns, tans well, dark brown skin

box), which describes skin color based on a response to sun exposure.

Baseline pigmentation also affects cutaneous findings in skin disorders. For example, erythema may be difficult to appreciate in darker skin. Keloids (aberrant scarring) are more common in those with darker skin types. Even after a disease process has resolved, postinflammatory hypopigmentation and postinflammatory hyperpigmentation are more marked (or more evident) in those with darker skin types.

Cyanosis is also more difficult to appreciate when the skin is more darkly pigmented.

CONFIGURATION AND DISTRIBUTION

A dermatologist must always analyze two closely related properties—configuration and distribution—to find the correct diagnosis. The configuration, or arrangement of skin lesions, includes descriptors such as linear, annular, arciform, clustered, reticulated, dermatomal, and retiform. For example, pruritic and fragile vesicles, arranged in clusters on the elbows and knees, should prompt consideration of dermatitis herpetiformis. Grouped vesicles on an erythematous base, but confined to a single dermatome, mandates consideration of herpes zoster.

Assessment of distribution includes stepping back and observing the anatomic pattern of skin lesions on the body. For example, plaques of psoriasis often favor extensor surfaces—elbows and knees; atopic dermatitis often favors flexural surfaces in older children and adults (antecubital and popliteal fossae), and lichen planus favors other flexural surfaces (wrists and

TABLE 1.2 Morphologic Terms for Secondary Skin Lesions

Morphologic Term	Salient Features	Classic Disease Image	Classic Diagnoses
Crust	• Collection of dried serum, cellular debris • Antecedent primary lesion (e.g., dermatitis, vesicle)		• Impetigo (photo) • Resolving dermatitis • Resolving vesiculobullous disorders
Erosion	• Partial loss of the epidermis • Variable size • Often red, oozing base		• Secondary finding in many bullous lesions that have broken (photo depicts pemphigus) • Superficial trauma
Ulcer	• Full-thickness loss of the epidermis and dermis • Heals with scarring		• Ulcerated necrobiosis lipoidica (photo) • Arterial ulcer • Chancroid • Primary syphilis • Stasis ulcers
Excoriation	• Partial loss of the epidermis and superficial dermis • Often linear • May be associated with scars from old excoriations		• Neurotic excoriation (photo) • Pruritic vesiculobullous disorders (e.g., dermatitis herpetiformis) • Pruritic dermatitis
Fissure	• Vertical loss of epidermis and dermis • Sharply defined walls (crack)		• Many forms of dermatitis (photo) • Xerosis

ankles). It is also important simply to notice if the condition is focal or generalized, unilateral or bilateral, and sharply circumscribed or more difficult to perceive. These factors will ultimately shape the final differential diagnosis.

Terminology that is encountered frequently in dermatology includes discussion of a seborrheic distribution, which includes the head, neck, and upper trunk, areas with a high density of sebaceous oil glands, and use of the term *photodistributed,* which describes an accentuation in areas exposed to ultraviolet light (e.g., the face, parts of the neck outside of the natural shadow beneath the chin, upper chest, forearms, dorsal hands). Connective tissue disease and some drug-induced processes may show a photodistributed pattern.

TEMPORAL COURSE

The temporal course is central to any medical history, and dermatology is no exception. All patients presenting with skin lesions should be queried about duration and any change in intensity or distribution over time. For example, some inflammatory conditions, such as measles, pityriasis rubra pilaris, and dermatomyositis, have a notorious cephalocaudal progression over time.

However, the examiner is always at an advantage because the skin is so readily accessible. Any information provided by the patient can be readily compared to observations made on physical examination.

Armed with some basic knowledge of the skin, the clinician can usually determine whether cutaneous lesions are acute, subacute, or chronic by observation. For example, because of the relative transit times of proliferating skin, true scale (not to be confused with crust) requires 2 weeks to develop. Similarly, lichenification, or thickening of the skin, with accentuation of normal skin markings, takes weeks or even months to develop. Therefore, if scale or lichenification is apparent, then the skin problem has been present for more than a few days, no matter what the patient may believe or has noticed.

OTHER HISTORICAL INFORMATION

A complete discourse on the pertinent aspects of history cannot be adequately addressed in this short introduction. Moreover, the finer details are better learned in association with specific diseases. Suffice it to say that there is always a need to take a good history regarding when, where, what, who, and how. The patient may be asked the following questions:

When did the rash (or lesion) develop, or for how long do you remember having the condition?
- When have you had similar eruptions in the past?
- When have you sought care in the past?

Where were the first lesions on your body?
- Where did the condition progress to next on the body?
- Where were you when you first noticed the condition (e.g., traveling, at home, at work)?
- Where have you sought care in the past (for records or phone consultation)?

What has been done about the condition to date?
- What makes the problem better?
- What makes the problem worse?
- What were you told about the condition by other professionals in the past?

- What was the plan for any follow-up (if it is a known condition)?
- What other relevant past medical history do you have?
- What kinds of medical conditions do you see a physician for regularly or take medications for on a regular basis?

Who has weighed in on this problem in the past (e.g., primary care provider, other urgent care or emergency care provider, dermatologist)?
- Who is in charge of your general health care?
- Who would have other information about your skin condition that you would like me to speak with, given your explicit permission? Who can you follow up with regarding this condition (is there a primary care physician [PCP] or dermatologist you have seen, now or in the past)?

How sick is the patient? This is a question an urgent care or emergency provider is uniquely equipped to answer. Perhaps the patient has other issues that take precedence over his or her long-term, non-critical, non–life-threatening skin complaint(s). If so, it may be necessary to acknowledge this skin complaint but defer work until another visit or the patient sees another clinician.

CONCLUSION

In summary, dermatology is a discipline that can definitely be learned. Although one cannot expect to master the entire domain of dermatology to the same degree as a dermatologist, who has completed an entire residency in the subject, any clinician can improve in the approach to patients with skin complaints simply by focusing on the following:

- Etiologic premise. Is this an inflammatory or neoplastic condition?
- Morphology. What morphologic term can be applied to the native lesion(s) of the condition (macular, maculopapular, papulosquamous, vesiculobullous, etc.)? Are there secondary morphologies (excoriated, lichenified, crusted, impetiginized, etc.)?
- Palpation. Are there any textural features, detected by palpation, which may be useful in refining the morphologic descriptors of the lesion(s), such as scaling, crusting, induration, and palpable or nonpalpable purpura?
- Color. What colors are identifiable in association with the condition? If there is erythema present, is it blanching or nonblanching (purpura)? Is the patient's own background skin tone such that the color of the lesion may be altered or more difficult to perceive?
- Configuration and distribution. What is the configuration of the lesions (linear, annular, reticulated,

retiform, etc.), and how is the condition distributed upon the body (flexural areas, extensor surfaces, photodistributed, etc.)? Is it focal or generalized? Is it unilateral or bilateral? Does it involve mucosal surfaces or not?

- Temporal course. Has the condition evolved over days, weeks, months, or even years?
  - Has it changed in its appearance (or its primary morphology) during that time?
  - Was it initially macular or maculopapular and then became bullous?
  - Is it waxing and waning over time?
  - Is it worsening or improving?
- Other historical information. Clearly, any final questioning and discourse will be affected by the specific disease categories under consideration. However, it is always important to focus on questioning that is broad enough to describe any items in the general medical history more fully, such as determining when, where, what, who, and how.

Simply thinking like a dermatologist, without learning any additional dermatologic information, will not meaningfully affect the care rendered. If the information in this chapter is kept in mind, particularly as one reads the rest of this text—which will fill in the gaps with regard to basic skin disease—there is little doubt that treating dermatologic ailments will be easier for you, as a clinician, and more rewarding for the patients under your care.

Chapter 2
Diagnostic Techniques

EQUIPMENT NEEDED

This chapter, on diagnostic techniques, not only discusses how to perform the procedures, but also lists the type of equipment needed to perform these techniques.

Purchase of Equipment

There are numerous medical supply houses that supply surgical and diagnostic equipment that can equip an emergency room or an office adequately. Although we do not have any financial interest in this company, we can recommend Delasco, which has a complete line of equipment directed for dermatologists, including anything mentioned in this text.

Core cutaneous surgical equipment

- Scalpel, no. 14 blade
- Scalpel handle
- 3-mm disposable punch
- 4-mm disposable punch
- Curved iris scissors
- Suture scissors
- Tissue forceps (e.g., 4-inch iris with teeth)
- Needle holders

Optional cutaneous surgical equipment

- 2-mm disposable punch
- 5-mm disposable punch

- 6-mm disposable punch
- 8-mm disposable punch
- Flexible, double-edged razor blades

Core diagnostic equipment

- Microscope
- Mineral oil
- Mycologic media—Sabouraud agar (plates, tubes or slants)
- 10% to 20% potassium hydroxide (KOH) solution, with or without dimethyl sulfoxide (DMSO)
- Glass slides and coverslips

Optional diagnostic equipment

- Antifungal stains (as alternatives to KOH)
  - Chlorazol black fungal stain
  - PMS fungal stain
  - Swartz Lamkins fungal stain
  - Methylene blue Triton X (for *Malassezia* yeast)
- Dermatophyte test medium (DTM)
- Tzanck stains
  - PMS Tzanck stain
  - Wright-Giemsa stain
- Wood light (Wood lamp)

WOOD LIGHT

Introduction

The Wood light or Wood lamp emits long-wave UV light (black light) that is filtered by a Wood filter (barium silicate and nickel oxide) that only allows a band of UV light between 320 and 400 nm (peak, 365 nm) to be emitted.

Applications

- Diagnosis of fluorescent species of tinea capitis
- Diagnosis of erythrasma
- Examination of porphyrins in urine in porphyrias, such as porphyria cutanea tarda (Fig. 2.1)
- Examination for *Propionibacterium acnes* in patients with acne vulgaris (Fig. 2.2)
- Demonstration of hypopigmentation and depigmentation in light-skinned individuals
- *Pseudomonas aeruginosa* infection (e.g., burns, ulcers)
- Detection of tetracycline deposition in children's teeth

Supplies

- Wood light (Wood lamp)
- Wood lights are available as small, portable, battery-powered units or as larger units with a cord

Technique

- Completely darken the examination room and allow your eye to accommodate.
- Turn on the lamp and allow it to warm up for 30 to 60 seconds.
- Hold the lamp approximately 4 to 6 inches from examination site.

Interpretation

- A positive examination result for tinea capitis consists of yellow-green or blue-green fluorescence of the broken hair shafts caused by the production of a compound called *pteridine*. Care must be taken

not to confuse this with fibers and lint from clothing that may fluoresce a white color (due to optical brightening agents) or scale mixed with sebum that may demonstrate a dull yellow color.
- A positive test for erythrasma demonstrates a coral red fluorescence confined to the areas of infection. The color is due to a water-soluble porphyrin (coproporphyrin III) produced by the bacteria *Corynebacterium minutissimum*. The porphyrins are water-soluble and, if the patient has recently bathed, the test will be negative because the fluorescent porphyrins will be washed out.
- In acne vulgaris, untreated patients will demonstrate follicular coral red fluorescence. In treated patients, if fluorescence is still present, the patient is not using the medication or the *Propionibacterium acnes* is now resistant to the antibiotics.
- A positive test for urinary porphyrins is the demonstration of coral red fluorescence in the urine. If the amount of uroporphyrins is low, only the meniscus will demonstrate the color, but if the quantitative porphyrin level is high, the entire sample will demonstrate coral red fluorescence.
- *Pseudomonas* infections show a greenish fluorescence due to the pigment pyoverdin.
- Hypopigmented or depigmented skin in fair-skinned individuals is accentuated with a Wood light.
- False-negative results may occur in acne vulgaris and erythrasma if the patient has recently bathed.
- False-positive fluorescent substances include some cosmetics, deodorants, soaps, lint, and petrolatum.

Comments

The Wood light has severe limitations in the diagnosis of tinea capitis because most infections in the United States are due to nonfluorescent species, especially *Trichophyton tonsurans*. The only species that is commonly fluorescent in the United States is *Microsporum canis*, which only accounts for about 5% to 10% of cases.

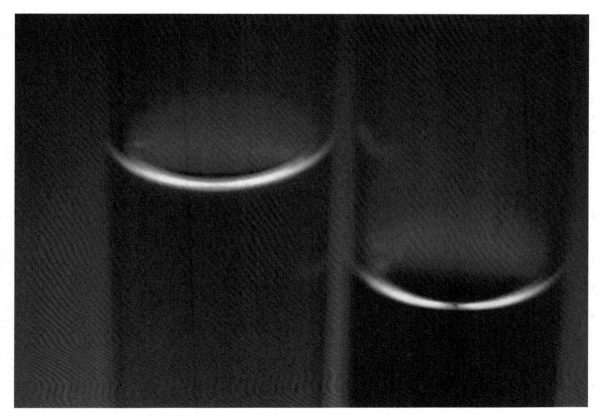

Fig. 2.1. Wood light examination of urine demonstrating coral red fluorescence in a patient with porphyria cutanea tarda. Fluorescence can be accentuated by adding dilute hydrochloric acid. *Left,* Positive. *Right,* Negative. (From the Fitzsimons Army Medical Center Collection, Aurora, CO.)

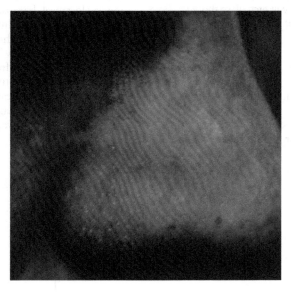

Fig. 2.2. Wood light examination of a patient's nose demonstrating coral red porphyrins produced by *Propionibacterium acnes*. Because this patient is under treatment for acne, this finding indicates that the patient is not taking the antibiotic or the organism is resistant to the antibiotic. (From the Fitzsimons Army Medical Center Collection, Aurora, CO.)

POTASSIUM HYDROXIDE PREPARATION

Applications

- Diagnosis of dermatophytes and yeast infections of the skin and mucous membranes

Supplies

- Microscope glass slide
- Coverslip (any size)
- No. 14 or 15 scalpel blade
- KOH, 10% to 20% concentration (Fig. 2.3). Variants include the following:
  - KOH, 10% to 20%, with DMSO
  - KOH, 10%, with DMSO and chlorazol black
- Access to a microscope

Technique

- For **tinea corporis,** the best samples are from annular edges with scale.
- Wet the area with an alcohol pad or, if in a sensitive area, with water.
- Gently scrape the site (you should not draw blood) and gather as much scale on the edge of the scalpel blade as possible. It is best to do this on more than one site to ensure that you have enough material (Fig. 2.4).
- Transfer the material on the edge of the scalp to the glass slide and spread it across the slide.

> ### Warning!
> Be very careful not to get the KOH on the microscope objectives because KOH can permanently etch the lens. Obviously, anything that will etch glass should not come into contact with the skin of patients, the staff, or yourself.

- Apply one or two drops of KOH to the slide (Fig. 2.5) and coverslip.
- If the coverslip is not even, gently press with your finger.
- Blot any excess KOH at the edges of the coverslip.
- If DMSO is used, wait for 1 minute to examine.

- If DMSO is not used, gently heat (do not boil) the glass slide to enhance clearing of the keratinocytes (Fig. 2.6).
- The hyphae are easier to visualize if the condenser is dropped. The amount that it needs to be dropped is variable and depends on the amount of light used and thickness of the specimen.

Interpretation

- A positive examination consists of demonstrating hyphae (dermatophyte infections), short hyphae and yeast (tinea versicolor), or yeast (candidiasis; Figs. 2.7 and 2.8). Other fungal species are only rarely seen on the skin or skin appendages.
- Fragments of clothing fibers and refractile material between the keratinocyte walls may lead to confusion. The false hyphae-like structures seen between keratinocytes can be differentiated by their angulated appearance, lack of linear shape for long distances, and tendency to break up. They also do not demonstrate nuclei that can sometimes be seen in hyphae.
- Epithelial lipids and exogenous lipids (e.g., moisturizers) may be difficult to differentiate from yeast. In general, they are more irregular in shape and lack nuclei. In some cases, there is so much exogenous lipid that it is almost impossible to interpret the specimen.

Comments

- Performing KOH examinations of the skin and mucous membrane samples is increasingly becoming a lost art because of Clinical Laboratory Improvement Amendments (CLIA) regulations. However, for those who carry out a KOH examination, or learn how to do it, it is frequently the quickest and is often the more sensitive test when compared to cultures. KOH examinations of mucosal scrapings are easier to interpret than scrapings from skin, hair, and nails, and some health care providers may want to limit this study for mucosal lesions.

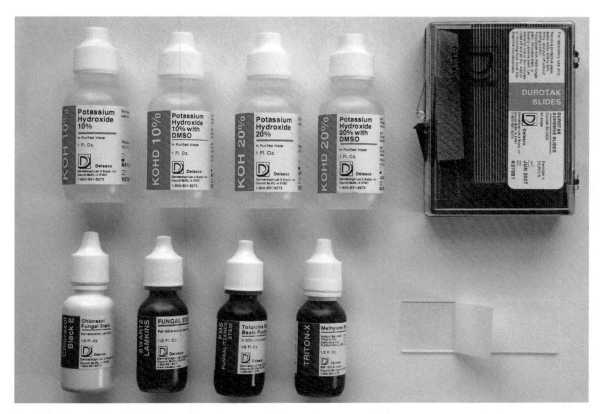

Fig. 2.3. *Top row,* Fungal KOH (with and without DMSO). *Bottom row,* Four different types of fungal stains. *Far right,* Special glass slides with adhesive tape used for the diagnosis of tinea versicolor.

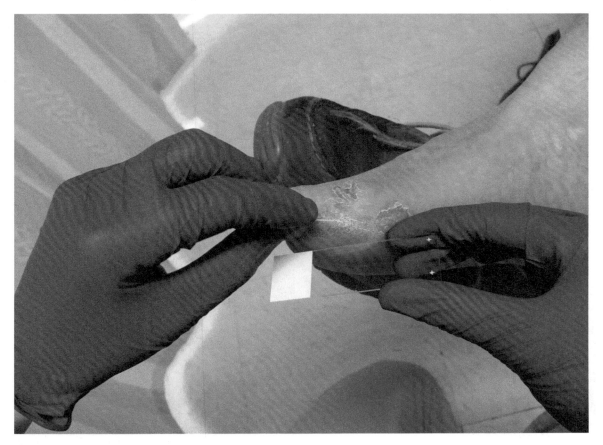

Fig. 2.4. After wetting the skin of a patient with suspected tinea pedis, the area is gently scraped with a no. 15 scalpel blade. Because the stratum corneum (scale) is the material of interest, the procedure should not draw blood.

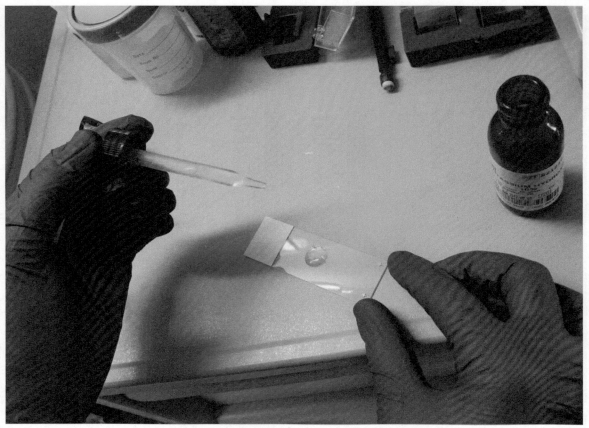

Fig. 2.5. A single drop of KOH is placed on the scale and then cover-slipped. Note that the physician is wearing gloves—remember that KOH is toxic to the skin.

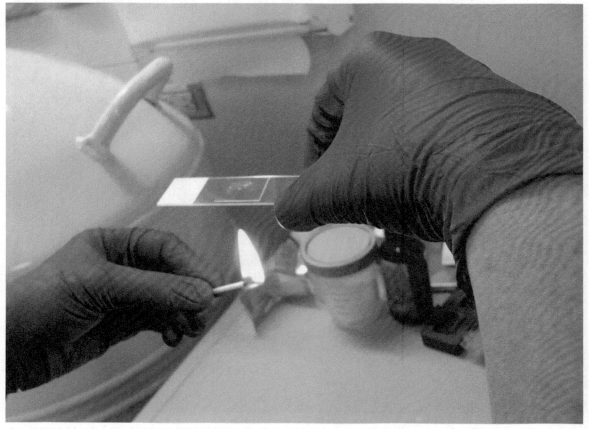

Fig. 2.6. After being cover-slipped, the KOH preparation is gently heated over a flame. If the KOH contains DMSO, this step can often be omitted. After heating, the slide is ready to be examined under the microscope.

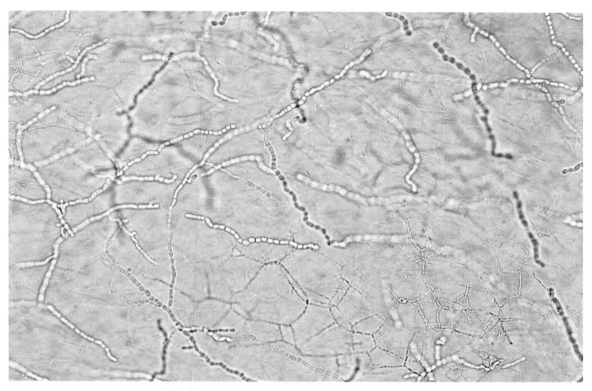

Fig. 2.7. Positive KOH finding of patient with tinea pedis demonstrating numerous linear segmented hyphae. The thin lines represent the cell walls of the keratinocytes (KOH, 400×).

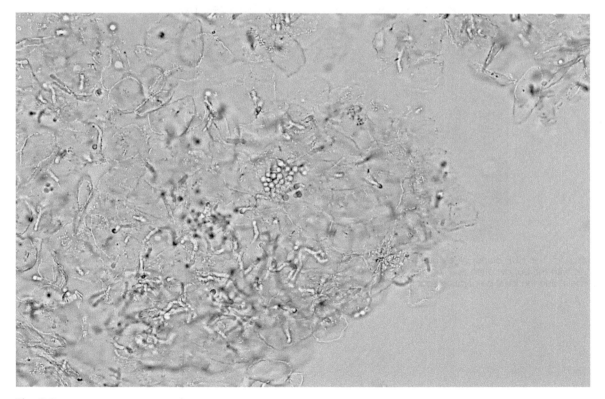

Fig. 2.8. Positive KOH finding of patient with tinea versicolor demonstrating numerous refractile, clumped yeast and short hyphae (so-called spaghetti and meatballs) (KOH, 400×).

MINERAL OIL PREPARATION

Application
- Diagnosis of scabies

Supplies
- Microscope glass slide
- Coverslip
- No. 14 scalpel blade (handle is not needed)
- Mineral oil is generally used, although any clear oil can be used (e.g., vegetable oil).
- Access to a microscope

Technique
- Place one drop of oil on one or more suspected burrows.
- If no suspected burrows are seen, place one drop of oil on multiple small papules.
- The scraping should be superficial enough so that no blood is produced because the level of the burrow is just below the cornified layer of skin. It is important to understand where the mite lives (Fig. 2.9).

- Gently scrape with a no. 15 scalpel blade that is held at an approximately 45- to 80-degree angle (Fig. 2.10) or use a disposable curette.
- As you scrape, the oil and superficial layer of skin will transfer to the blade (Fig. 2.11).
- Transfer the scraping to a microscope glass slide (Fig. 2.12).
- Use a coverslip.
- Examine at a low power (40×) to intermediate power (100×) for mites, eggs, or feces (Figs. 2.13–2.15).

Interpretation
- A positive test result is the unequivocal demonstration of the mite, egg, or feces (scybala).

Comments
Although some texts state that the scraping needs to be done vigorously, this does not mean that you should be scraping deep enough to draw blood. The photograph of an H&E stained slide clearly demonstrates the very superficial location of the mite (see Fig. 2.9).

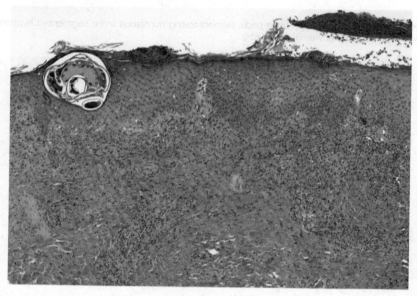

Fig. 2.9. This H&E biopsy nicely demonstrates the level of the mites. They are typically in a burrow below the cornified layer, with the burrow often pushing into the epidermis. The scraping does not need to be down to the level of the blood vessels, and the ideal preparation should be bloodless and thus painless to the patient (H&E, 100×).

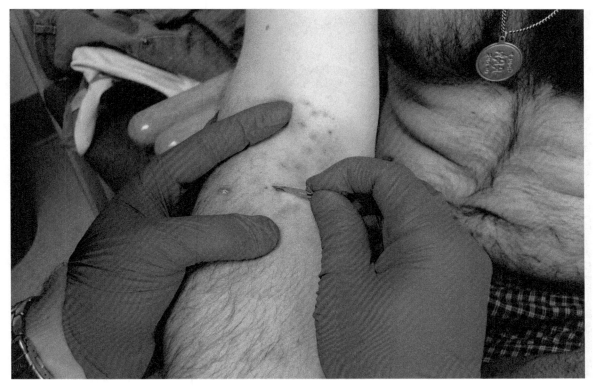

Fig. 2.10. After placing mineral oil on a patient with suspected scabies, one or more sites are gently scraped with a no. 15 scalpel blade.

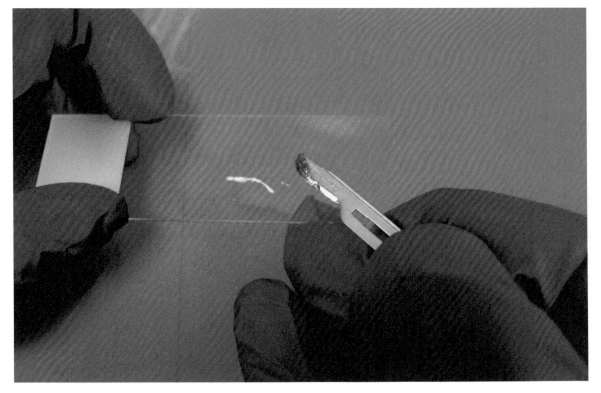

Fig. 2.11. Collected mineral oil and debris are transferred using the scalpel blade. This scraping contains blood, suggesting that the scraping was unnecessarily aggressive.

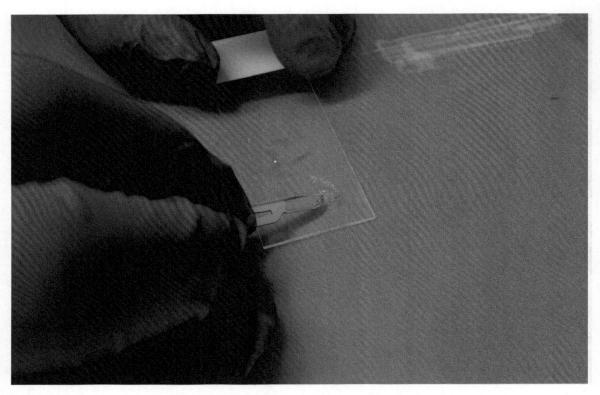

Fig. 2.12. The collected scraping is transferred to a glass slide, which is then cover-slipped. Additional oil can be added if necessary.

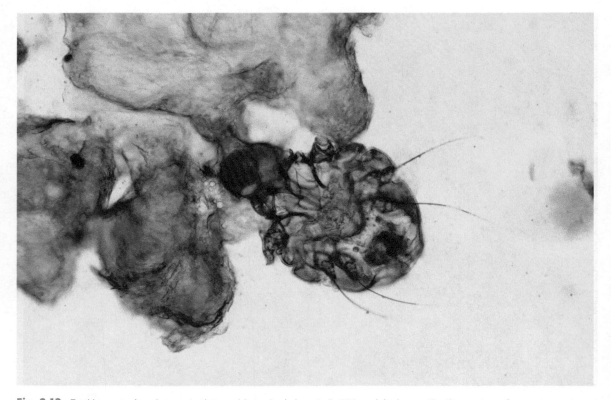

Fig. 2.13. Positive scraping demonstrating scabies mite (mineral oil, 200× original magnification, cropped).

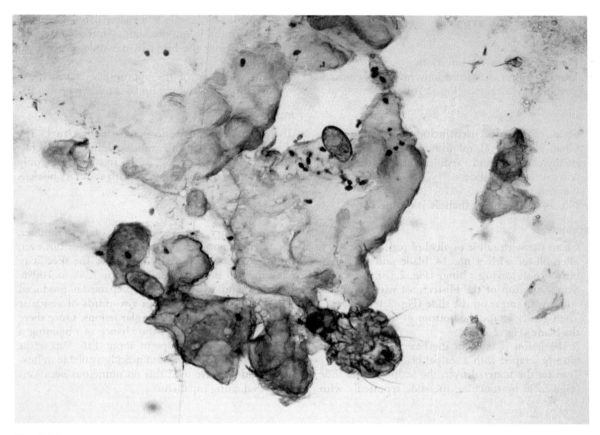

Fig. 2.14. Positive mineral preparation for scabies demonstrating mite, eggs, and scybala (mineral oil, 200×).

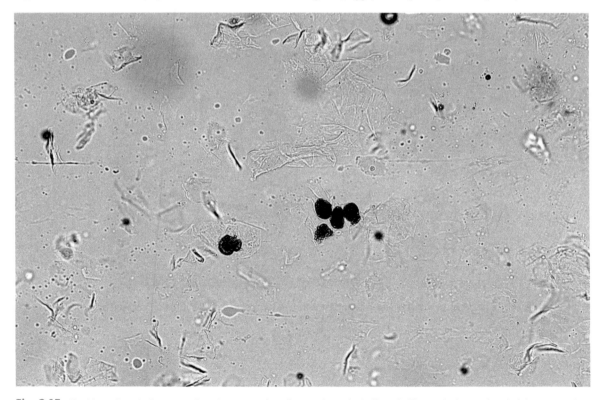

Fig. 2.15. Positive mineral oil preparation demonstrating diagnostic scybala (feces). The scybala are the dark brown oval structures in the center of the field (mineral oil, 400×).

TZANCK PREPARATION

Applications

- Herpes simplex virus infections
- Varicella-zoster virus infections, including chicken-pox and herpes zoster (Fig. 2.16)

Supplies

- Stains that can be used include Giemsa, Wright-Giemsa (Fig. 2.17), toluidine blue (see Fig. 2.17), methylene blue, and Papanicolauo (Pap) stains.
- Microscope glass slide
- Coverslip
- No. 14 scalpel blade (handle is not needed)

Technique

- Clean site with saline or alcohol pad.
- Slice blister with a no. 14 blade and fold back blister roof, leaving a hinge (Fig. 2.18).
- Scrape the top of the blister roof with the blade and gently smear on the slide (Fig. 2.19).
- Then gently scrape the bottom of the blister with the blade (Fig. 2.20).
- If the lesion is crusted, the base of the lesion is bluntly scraped with a scalpel blade.
- Transfer the material from the scalpel to the slide (Fig. 2.21) by touching the slide repeatedly with the blade. If there is still material on the blade, gently smear it on the slide. Thus, transfer the material from the blade to the slide as gently as possible.
- Stain with one of the appropriate stains, use a coverslip, and examine under a microscope.

Interpretation

There are two diagnostic cytopathic variants. The classic finding is that of a multinucleated giant keratinocyte (Fig. 2.22; see Fig. 2.21). In some cases, only enlarged rounded keratinocytes with a solitary nucleus are present.

Comments

The results vary with the expertise of the examiner, age of the lesion, and quality of the stain; however, in one study, the sensitivity was 80%. The specificity has varied in different studies, from 73% to 100%. In other studies, the Tzanck preparation produced a diagnostic sample in about two-thirds of vesicular lesions and about half of pustular lesions. Once there is an ulcer or scale crust, the chance of obtaining a diagnostic specimen drops to about 1:6. Pap stains are almost always readily and quickly available in hospitals, and we have used this on numerous occasions when evaluating inpatients.

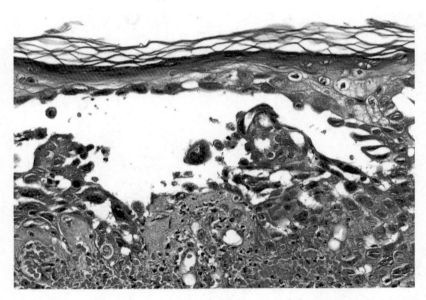

Fig. 2.16. This H&E-stained biopsy of a blister in a patient with herpes zoster demonstrates an intraepidermal split that is very near the dermis. Although a gentle scraping of the lesion is desired, some specimens will be contaminated with blood (H&E, 400×).

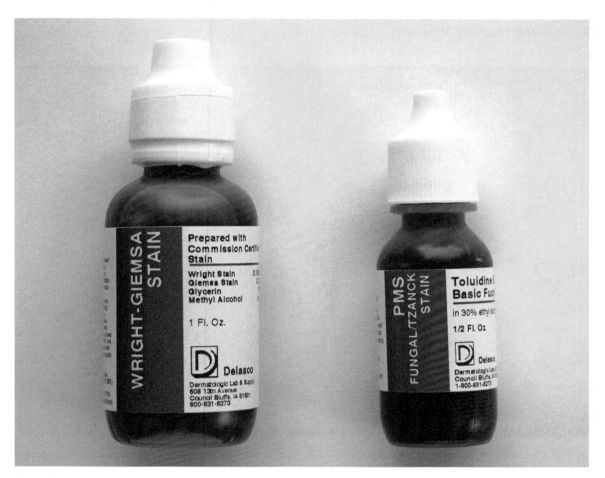

Fig. 2.17. Examples of stains used for Tzanck preparations. These include a Wright-Giemsa stain and PMS fungal Tzanck stain (toluidine blue–based stain).

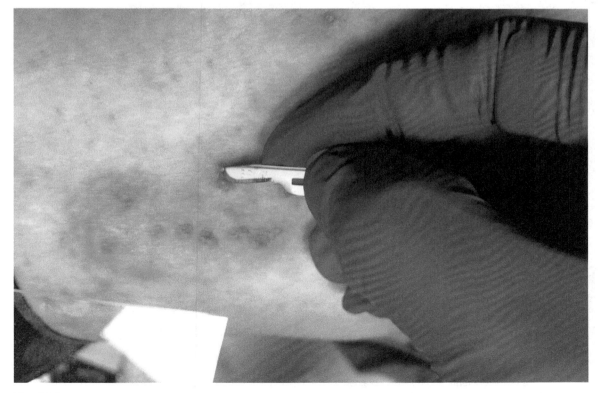

Fig. 2.18. An intact blister in a patient with suspected herpes zoster is horizontally sliced so that the contents of the blister cavity are exposed.

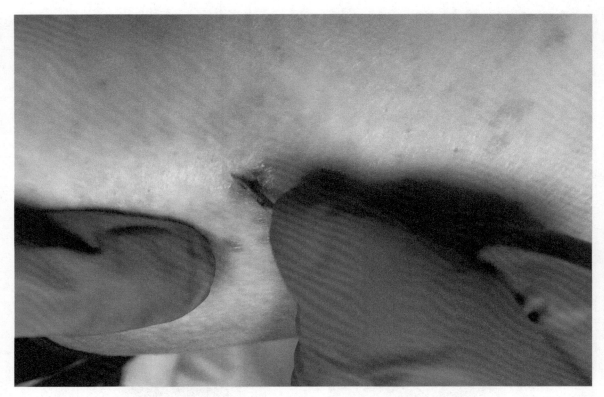

Fig. 2.19. The blister is now opened and reflected on a hinge of epidermis. The base and roof of the blister are now gently scraped while attempting to transfer the contents of the blister cavity to the top of the scalpel blade.

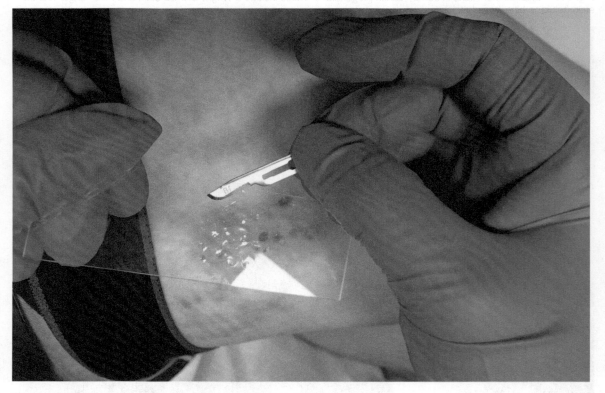

Fig. 2.20. The blister contents and material obtained from scraping the base and roof of the blister have been transferred to a glass slide. The specimen is now ready for staining.

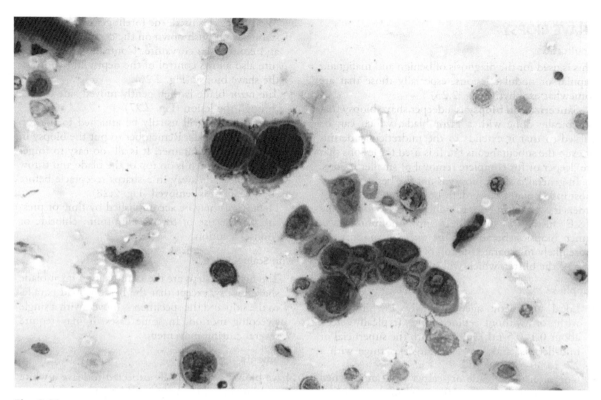

Fig. 2.21. Wright-Giemsa–stained specimen of a patient with herpes zoster demonstrating numerous multinucleated keratinocytes with swollen nuclei (400×).

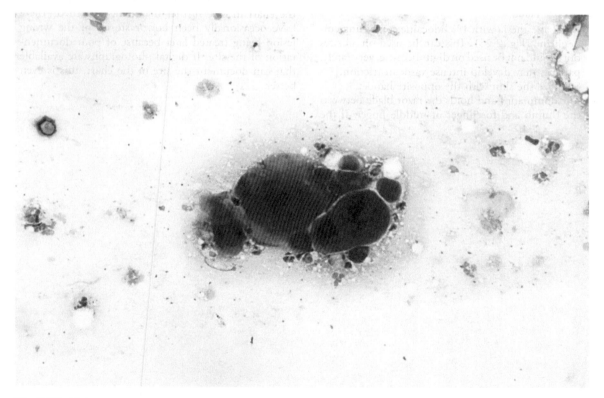

Fig. 2.22. High-power view (400× original magnification, cropped) of a Tzanck preparation taken from a patient with herpes zoster infection. The preparation nicely demonstrates a diagnostic aggregate of multinucleated keratinocytes and swollen nuclei.

SHAVE BIOPSY

Applications

This is used for the diagnosis of benign and malignant papular or nodular lesions, especially those that are somewhat exophytic (Fig. 2.23).

Saucerization biopsy is a deeper shave biopsy that is typically done with a razor blade, which can be curved so that it extends to the midreticular dermis or even the subcutaneous fat. It is used for lesions that are deeper or for complete removal of smaller lesions.

In general, a shave biopsy is not the best choice for most inflammatory disorders; however, in bullous disorders it is often superior to punch biopsies for routine H&E histology and direct immunofluorescence. Punch biopsies, because of the twisting motion, are more likely to separate the top of the blister from the base of the blister, which will hinder interpretation.

Supplies

- Local anesthetic agent, usually 1% lidocaine, with or without epinephrine (typically need about 0.1–0.5 mL) injected into the superficial or mid-dermis, and 1-mL (or larger) syringe with a 27- to 30-gauge needle
- Common razor blade or scalpel with an attached no. 14 scalpel or a no. 10 scalpel for large lesions (Fig. 2.24)

Technique

With Razor Blade

- Local anesthesia with 1% lidocaine containing epinephrine (Fig. 2.25). This can be used on all sites but should not be used on digits because, very rarely, patients may develop intense vasoconstriction.
- Stabilize the skin with the opposite hand.
- The dominant hand holds the razor blade between the thumb and forefinger or middle finger. If the middle finger is used, the forefinger can be used to stabilize and push down on the center of the blade and control the curvature. Controlling the curvature also allows control of the depth and width of the shave biopsy (Fig. 2.26).

- The razor blade is then gently moved side to side through the lesion (Fig. 2.27).
- The specimen will usually be attached to the top of the razor blade. Remember to put the biopsy in the specimen container! It is all too easy to forget that the specimen is on top of the blade and throw the razor blade away in a sharps receptacle before the specimen is removed (Fig. 2.28).
- Hemostasis may be accomplished by time or pressure or the use of topical aluminum chloride or Monsel solution.

With Scalpel Blade

- The first two steps are the same as for a razor blade shave biopsy, except that the blade is held parallel to the skin and the specimen is moved with a single sweeping motion. In some cases, it may require several cutting movements.

Comments

Shave biopsies are typically expected to leave a white scar, although occasionally, in older patients, the scar may be so minimal that it is not visible. The site of a shave biopsy done for all benign, premalignant, and malignant neoplasms should always be diagrammed in the chart in case further treatment is needed. There have occasionally been horror stories of the wrong lesion being treated later because of poor documentation of the site. If digital photographs are available that can document the site in the chart, this is even better.

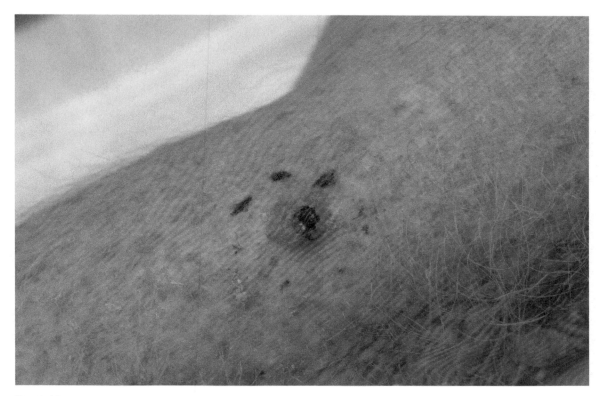

Fig. 2.23. Suspected squamous cell carcinoma partially outlined by ink. Note the background of numerous actinic keratoses.

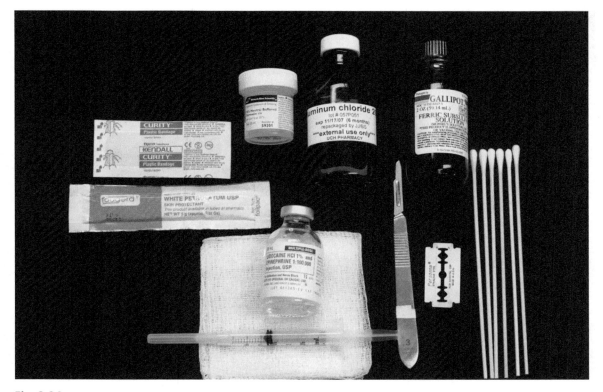

Fig. 2.24. Typical shave biopsy setup with a razor blade or no. 14 scalpel. The setup also includes aluminum chloride and Monsel solution for hemostasis.

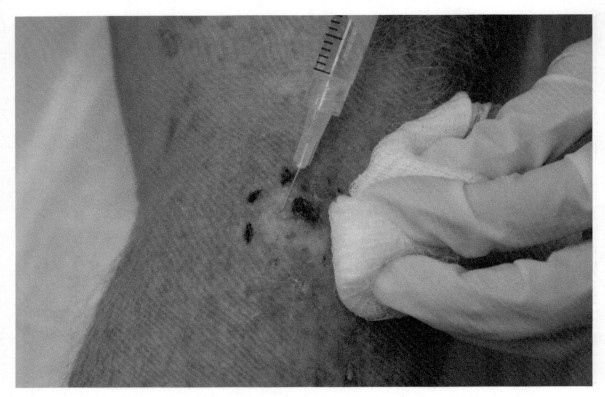

Fig. 2.25. 1% lidocaine with epinephrine is injected around and under the tumor. Ideally, the entire lesion should blanch before proceeding with the biopsy.

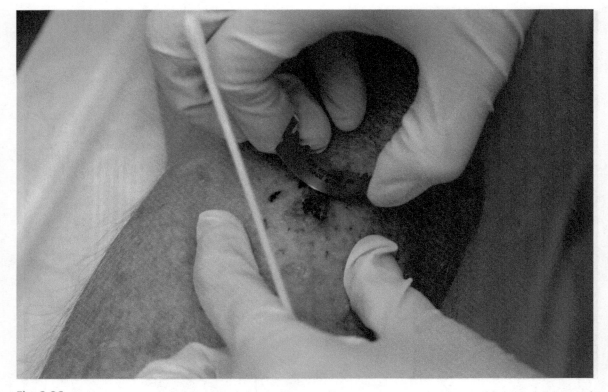

Fig. 2.26. Razor blades can be broken in half, as in this case, or can be used intact. Note that the blade has been curved with lateral pressure so that the deeper portions of the lesion can be removed.

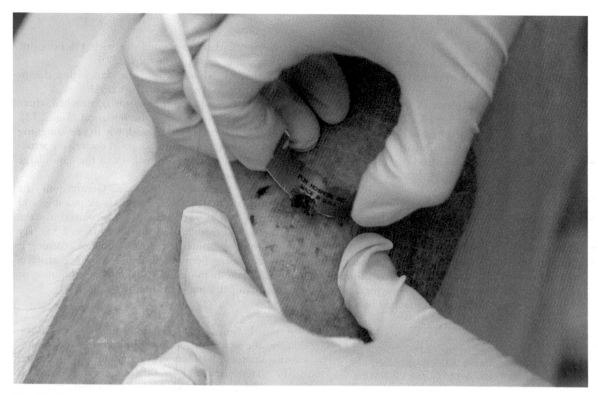

Fig. 2.27. The lesion is removed with a slow back and forth motion.

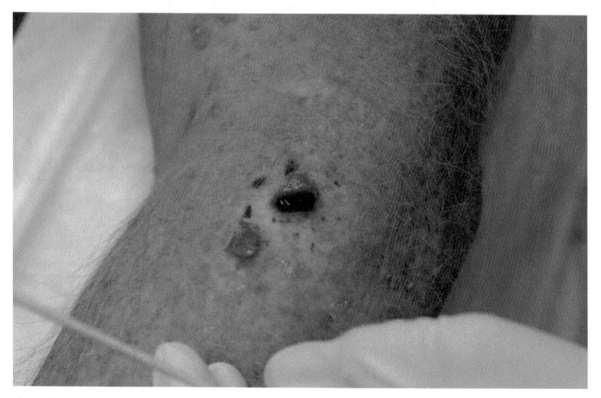

Fig. 2.28. The removed lesion is ready for placement in a formalin-containing specimen bottle. The base of the lesion is now ready for hemostasis with 20% aluminum chloride, petrolatum, and a dressing.

PUNCH BIOPSY

Applications

- Punch is the preferred sampling technique for the assessment of most inflammatory skin conditions. The one potential exception involves blisters that are larger than the diameter of the punch biopsy. The rotating motion of a punch biopsy will often separate the roof from the base of the blister, which may hinder microscopic examination.
- It is useful for the diagnosis and complete removal of some skin tumors.

Supplies

- Local anesthetic agent and 1-mL syringe with a 27- to 30-gauge needle
- Disposable 3-, 4-, 5-, 6-, and 8-mm punch biopsy
- In the past, reusable all-metal punch biopsies were used. However, most facilities now have disposable punch biopsies consisting of a hollow metal cylinder with a sharp cutting edge attached to a plastic handle (Fig. 2.29).

To Suture or Not to Suture

A prospective randomized trial has compared the outcomes of 4- and 8-mm biopsies that were randomized to heal by secondary intention or with closure with interrupted 4-0 nylon sutures. At 9 months, there were no differences in the clinical appearance, as evaluated blindly by three physicians. Even though there were no cosmetic differences, patients still preferred closure of the 8 mm wounds with sutures.

From Christenson LJ, Phillips PK, Weaver AL, Otley CC: Primary closure vs second-intention treatment of skin punch biopsy sties. A randomized trial. *Arch Dermatol* 141:1093-1099, 2005.

Technique

- Local anesthesia is carried out with 1% lidocaine containing epinephrine (Fig. 2.30).
- The punch is pushed into the skin with a downward twisting movement (Fig. 2.31).
- In most cases, once the dermis is breached, there will be a distinct give to the sensation (Fig. 2.32). At this point, proceed more slowly to prevent going too deeply in areas with potential underlying structures (e.g., tendons on the back of the hand, large nerves, large blood vessels).
- Handle the tissue with care. Gently pull the punched-out specimen as much as possible and cut the base as far down as possible to maximize the amount of tissue that is submitted (Fig. 2.33). Try to avoid spearing the biopsy sample or crushing it with forceps because these may produce artifacts that make it more difficult for the pathologist or dermatopathologist to interpret (Fig. 2.34).

Comments

A punch biopsy is easily done and is one of the most important diagnostic techniques for diagnosing inflammatory disorders and removing small tumors. The diagnostic yield in inflammatory disorders is improved if specimens are taken from more than one site and if specimens are taken from lesions at different stages of evolution. When possible, avoid secondarily infected lesions and lesions that are not intact (e.g., ruptured blister or excoriated lesion).

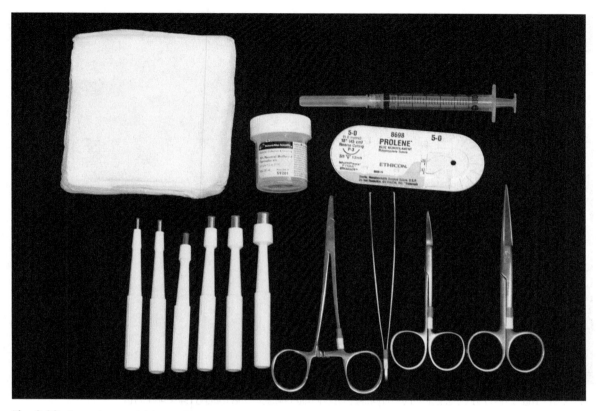

Fig. 2.29. Setup for punch biopsy. *Bottom row, left to right,* 2-, 3-, 4-, 5-, 6-, and 8-mm punch biopsies are shown.

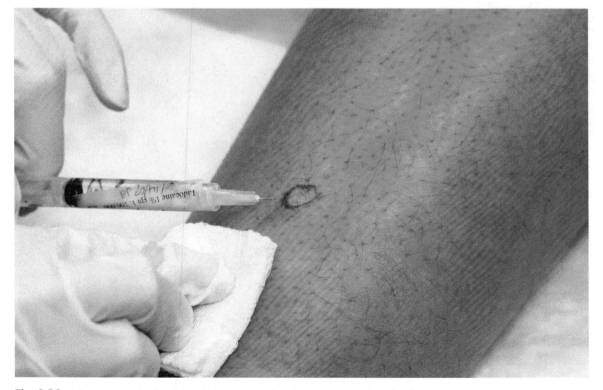

Fig. 2.30. After marking the location, 1% lidocaine with epinephrine is used to blanch the biopsy site.

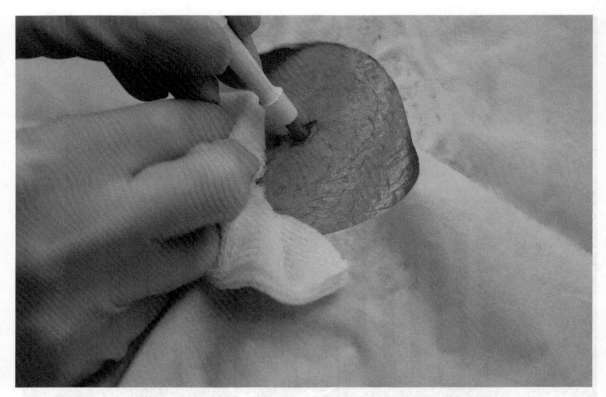

Fig. 2.31. The punch biopsy is started with gentle to moderate pressure and rotated back and forth.

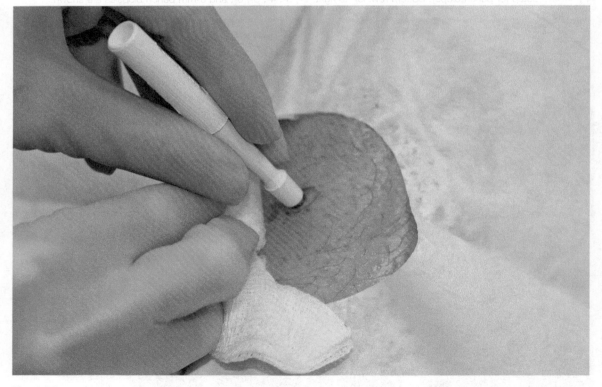

Fig. 2.32. The punch biopsy is slowly twisted until the desired depth is reached. On some areas, such as the trunk, the biopsies are carried to the hub, as seen here, but in other areas, such as the back of the hand, where there are tendons, the depth is more superficial.

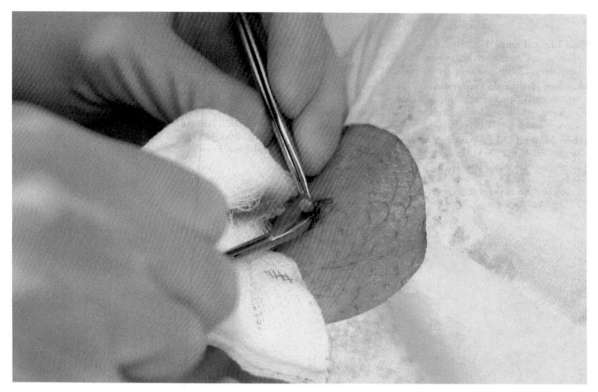

Fig. 2.33. The punch biopsy is gently pulled up with a forceps, and the base is released with an iris scissor.

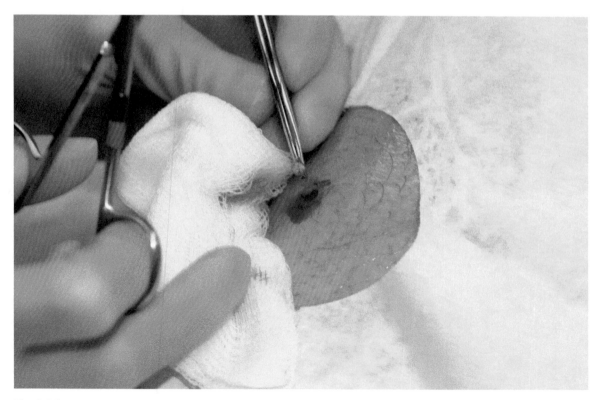

Fig. 2.34. After release of the base, the specimen is removed and placed in a formalin-containing specimen jar. After hemostasis is achieved, the defect can be left open to heal secondarily or sutured (see "To Suture or Not to Suture" box).

References

Wood Light (Lamp)

1. Klatte JL, van der Beek N, Kemperman PM. 100 years of Wood's lamp revised. *J Eur Acad Dermatol Venereol.* 2015;29:842-847.

Potassium Hydroxide Preparation

1. Wilkison BD, Sperling LC, Spillane AP, Meyerle JH. How to teach the potassium hydroxide preparation: a disappearing clinical art form. *Cutis.* 2015;96:109-112.

Scabies Mineral Oil Preparation

1. Brodell RT, Helms SE. Office dermatologic testing: the scabies preparation. *Am Fam Physician.* 1991;44:505-558.
2. Jacks SK, Lewis EA, Witman PM. The curette prep: a modification of the traditional scabies preparation. *Pediatr Dermatol.* 2012;29:544-545.

Tzanck Preparation

1. Ozxan A, Senol M, Saglam H, et al. Comparison of the Tzanck test and polymerase chain reaction in the diagnosis of cutaneous herpes simplex and varicella zoster virus infections. *Int J Dermatol.* 2007;46:1177-1179.

Shave and Punch Biopsy

1. Schmidt DKT, Wentzell M. Fundamentals of cutaneous surgery. In: Fitzpatrick JE, Morelli JG, eds. *Dermatology Secrets Plus.* Philadelphia: Elsevier; 2016:454-461.

Chapter 3
Morbilliform Eruptions

Morbilliform eruptions are eruptions that resemble measles. The term is derived from the Latin word for measles, *morbilli*. Morbilliform reactions are never due to external factors and always indicate an internal problem; the most important are viral and drug reactions, and connective tissue disorders are a distant third.

IMPORTANT HISTORY QUESTIONS

How long have your spots been present?

Most morbilliform eruptions present acutely (e.g., morbilliform drug eruptions, morbilliform viral eruptions, rickettsial infections), whereas some disorders, such as lupus erythematosus, are more likely to be chronic or recurrent.

> **Differential Diagnosis of Morbilliform Reactions**
> Common
> * Morbilliform drug eruptions
> * Morbilliform viral eruptions (many)
>
> Uncommon
> * Severe drug hypersensitivity reaction
> * Lupus erythematosus
> * Rickettsial infections
> * Serum sickness
> * Roseola vaccinatum

Have you started any new medications in the last 10 days?

This is a very important question, because a morbilliform drug eruption is a common cause of this pattern. Oral antibiotics are the most common cause of morbilliform reactions.

Have you had any fever?

This question is directed toward determining a potential infectious cause, such as a viral or rickettsial infection.

Do you have any other medical problems?

This question can produce an abundance of important clinical information, including a history of a connective tissue disorder or mononucleosis. Mononucleosis is notorious for producing morbilliform reactions when the patient has been given ampicillin.

IMPORTANT PHYSICAL FINDINGS

What is the distribution of the lesions?

Most morbilliform eruptions do not have a characteristic distribution; however, some, such as Rocky Mountain spotted fever, tend to start acrally, whereas unilateral thoracic exanthem, as the name implies, typically is predominantly unilateral at its initial presentation.

Presence or absence of lesions in the oral mucosa

Oral lesions are more frequently seen in some but not all morbilliform viral eruptions and are usually absent in morbilliform drug eruptions and rickettsial infections.

Are any blisters present?

Morbilliform eruptions, by definition, do not have blisters; however, it is important to remember that some eruptions may initially appear to be morbilliform (e.g., very early erythema multiforme) before they blister. Obviously, if blisters are present, the differential diagnosis and thought process change.

Do any of the lesions demonstrate hemorrhage?

Focal hemorrhage, especially minute areas of hemorrhage on the lower extremities, can occur in morbilliform viral and drug eruptions. The presence of hemorrhage obviously raises the possibility of Rocky Mountain spotted fever or even a very early leukocytoclastic vasculitis.

Do any of the lesions demonstrate a reticulated (netlike) appearance?

A morbilliform eruption with a reticulated appearance should raise the possibility of erythema infectiosum; however, reticulated patterns are not specific and may occasionally be seen in other morbilliform eruptions.

Pathogenesis

The pathogenesis of a morbilliform drug eruption is not understood, and very little research has been directed toward resolving the mechanism(s) involved. The frequent development of morbilliform drug eruptions precipitated by ampicillin in a patient with Epstein-Barr virus infection and by sulfonamides in a patient with HIV infection suggests that an altered immune system may be important in some cases. This might explain why not all patients develop a morbilliform reaction when rechallenged later. An older study has demonstrated antipenicillin antibodies, an interesting finding, but one that has not been verified by other studies.

Common Offending Drugs

- Ampicillin
- Allopurinol
- Penicillin
- Phenytoin (Dilantin)
- Sulfonamides

Clinical Features

- Morbilliform drug eruptions typically begin 3 to 10 days after administering the offending drug.
- In most cases, lesions are primarily located on the trunk.
- The primary lesion is a 1- to 10-mm blanchable macule that can demonstrate coalescence into large patches of erythema (Figs. 3.1–3.3).
- Symptoms range from absent to significant pruritus.
- Lower extremity lesions may demonstrate focal hemorrhage.

Serum Sickness

Morbilliform reactions may also be a component of serum sickness. Serum sickness is characterized by a cutaneous eruption (urticaria, morbilliform dermatitis, and purpura or erythema multiforme), fever, joint involvement (arthritis or arthralgias), edema, and lymphadenopathy.

Diagnosis

- Drug exposure history is critical. The exposure period of interest is usually 3 to 10 days, but occasional cases may fall outside of this range.
- Skin biopsies typically demonstrate a superficial perivascular lymphocytic dermatitis. This pattern is not diagnostic and can be seen in other morbilliform reactions, including viral morbilliform exanthems, which can be clinically identical. Most cases do not require a biopsy. If a biopsy is needed, always do a 3- or 4-mm punch biopsy, never a shave biopsy.
- Check a complete blood count (CBC). An elevated eosinophil count favors a drug eruption, and a very high eosinophil count may suggest a severe drug hypersensitivity reaction, a drug reaction with eosinophilia and systemic symptoms (DRESS).
- Liver function tests (LFTs) should be ordered when DRESS is a clinical consideration.

Treatment

- Discontinue the offending medication. Although cases may resolve with continuation of the drug, occasional cases demonstrate continued progression to full body erythema.
- Use symptomatic treatment measures, such as sedating antihistamines (e.g., diphenhydramine), in patients who are markedly pruritic. There is no evidence to suggest that the clinical course is altered or shortened by antihistamines.
- Rare cases may require topical corticosteroids or a brief course of oral corticosteroids.

Clinical Course

In most cases, the reaction will start to subside within 1 to 3 days and be completely resolved in 7 to 10 days.

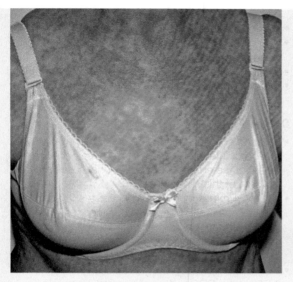

Fig. 3.1. Morbilliform drug eruption due to a sulfonamide antibiotic. (From the Fitzsimons Army Medical Center Collection, Aurora, CO.)

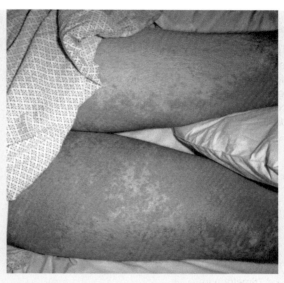

Fig. 3.2. Morbilliform drug eruption secondary to penicillin. (From the William Weston Collection, Aurora, CO.)

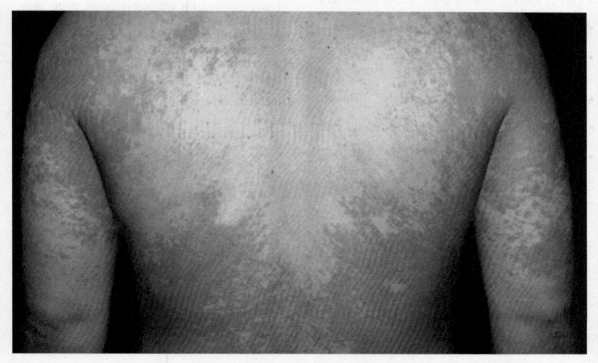

Fig. 3.3. Morbilliform drug eruption due to oral penicillin. Note the focal confluence of macules into the patches of erythema. (From the Fitzsimons Army Medical Center Collection, Aurora, CO.)

Pathogenesis

The pathogenesis of DRESS is not understood, but it is clearly an immunologically mediated hypersensitivity syndrome. The eosinophils are thought to be related to interleukin-5 released by stimulated T cells. This constellation of findings has also been referred to as *drug hypersensitivity syndrome*.

Drugs Implicated in DRESS
- Allopurinol
- Carbamazepine (Tegretol)
- Lamotrigine
- Minocycline
- Phenobarbital
- Phenytoin (Dilantin)
- Piperacillin-tazobactam
- Salazopyrin
- Sulfasalazine
- Trimethoprim
- Valproic acid

Clinical Features

- Clinical features typically begin 1 to 8 weeks after starting the drug.
- Lesions are located on the face, trunk, and extremities, primarily on the trunk in many cases.
- Early primary lesions are 1- to 10-mm blanchable macules that quickly coalesce into large patches of erythema (Figs. 3.4–3.6).
- Facial (hallmark of the disease) and limb edema are frequently present (see Fig. 3.4).
- Symptoms range from being absent to significant pruritus.
- Clinical variations include primary lesions that are pustular, bullous, or purpuric.

- Lymphadenopathy is frequently present.
- On the CBC, eosinophilia may be profound, with variable numbers of atypical lymphocytes.
- Hepatitis may be mild to severe and potentially fatal.
- Other organ systems that may be involved include the brain, lungs, heart, and kidneys.

Diagnosis

- A drug exposure history is critical. The exposure period of interest is usually 2 to 6 weeks before the onset of the eruption, but occasional cases may fall outside of this range.
- A 3 or 4 mm punch biopsy (never a shave biopsy) will demonstrate nonspecific findings. It typically demonstrates a superficial perivascular lymphocytic dermatitis, with variable numbers of eosinophils. A biopsy may help exclude other diseases.
- A minimal initial laboratory evaluation would include LFTs and a CBC, with a differential diagnosis.

Treatment

- The offending or suspected offending medications should be discontinued immediately. Although cases may resolve with continuation of the drug, occasional cases demonstrate continued progression to full body erythema and a fatal outcome.
- Oral corticosteroids, at a dose of 40 to 60 mg/day, is the treatment of choice. Therapy may need to be maintained for weeks or even 1 month or longer.

Clinical Course

The mortality rate has been reported to be as high as 10% in untreated patients.

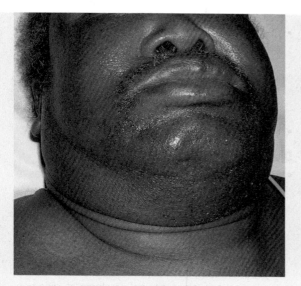

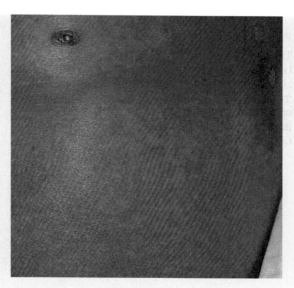

Fig. 3.4. Patient with DRESS demonstrating characteristic facial erythema and edema. (Courtesy Dr. Tim Chang.)

Fig. 3.5. Patient with DRESS demonstrating macular erythema of the trunk. (Courtesy Dr. Tim Chang.)

Fig. 3.6. Patient with DRESS with confluent truncal macular erythema. (Courtesy Dr. Tim Chang.)

Pathogenesis

There are many different viruses that produce morbilliform (measles-like) viral exanthems. Most are not clinically distinct, although some are distinct enough that they can be discussed separately (e.g., roseola, erythema infectiosum). Morbilliform reactions may be produced by viral infections of the host cells or may be due to the host response.

Morbilliform Viral Eruptions
- Adenovirus
- Coxsackie virus
- Erythema infectiosum
- Measles
- Respiratory syncytial virus
- Roseola
- Rubella virus
- West Nile virus (morbilliform eruption in 50%)

Clinical Features

- Viral exanthems most commonly affect infants and children but can affect those at any age, including geriatric patients.
- Viral exanthems are frequently but not always associated with other findings of a viral syndrome, such as a prodrome of malaise and fever or active oral mucosal infection (sore throat, rhinorrhea) or gastrointestinal infection (abdominal pain, diarrhea). Measles is typically associated with coryza, conjunctivitis, and cough.
- The primary lesion—pink to red macules or subtle papules—may vary in size from 1 mm to more than 1 cm.
- Variations include petechial or vesicular lesions.
- Rubella lesions are often rose pink rather than erythematous.
- The distribution is typically generalized and often spares the palms and soles (Figs. 3.7–3.10).
- Patients may be asymptomatic or demonstrate variable pruritus.
- Some patients may also demonstrate malar erythema (so-called slapped cheeks).

- Oral involvement commonly occurs (enanthem).
  - Koplik spots (blue-white spots on an erythematous base) are distinctive lesions, often seen in measles, that appear before the exanthem.
  - Oral ulcerative lesions are common in herpangina.
  - Palatal petechiae are more common in mononucleosis.
- Lymphadenopathy is often present.

Diagnosis

- The differential diagnosis usually also includes a morbilliform drug eruption; the onset of the exanthem needs to be correlated with any new medications. Physical findings that favor a viral rather than a drug cause include the presence of other findings of a viral infection (e.g. prodrome, coryza, diarrhea), the presence of lymphadenopathy, or the presence of an enanthem.
- Acute and convalescent viral serologic studies can be done but are of little help in the acute management of the viral infection, which will have resolved by the time results are available.
- Rubella immunoglobulin G (IgG) antibodies can be determined in 1 day at some institutions by the chemiluminescent immunoassay (ChLIA) on any serum red-top tube.
- A 3 or 4 mm punch biopsy (never a shave biopsy) can be done in atypical cases. However, the findings are consistent with the diagnosis and are not diagnostic by themselves. In most cases, viral and drug morbilliform reactions are histologically identical.

Treatment

- No treatment is required because most cases resolve in 3 to 10 days.
- Weak to moderate-strength topical corticosteroids can be used for pruritic lesions.
- Sedating antihistamines (e.g., diphenhydramine) can be used in patients who are markedly pruritic.

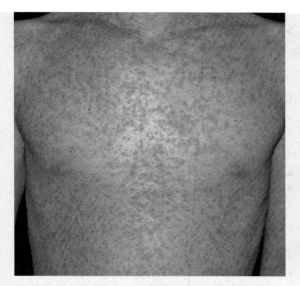

Fig. 3.7. Patient with papular viral exanthema of an unknown viral type affecting the trunk and extremities.

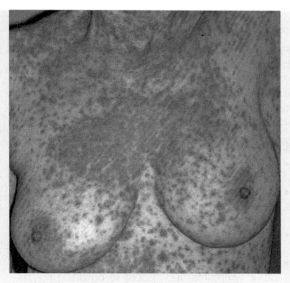

Fig. 3.8. Patient with papular and morbilliform viral exanthema of an unknown viral type, with focal confluence of lesions. (From the Fitzsimons Army Medical Center Collection, Aurora, CO.)

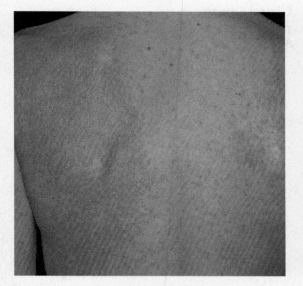

Fig. 3.9. Patient with papular viral exanthema of an unknown viral type demonstrating confluence on the lateral aspects of the back.

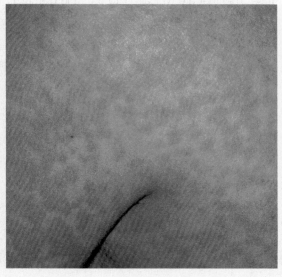

Fig. 3.10. Close-up of the morbilliform lesions in viral exanthem in a child.

Roseola (Infantum; Exanthem Subitum, Sixth Disease) ICD10 code B08.20

Pathogenesis

Roseola is caused by two closely related viruses, human herpesvirus-6 (HHV-6) and human herpesvirus-7 (HHV-7), both of which are tropic viruses for CD4+ (helper) T cells. How this produces a morbilliform reaction is not entirely understood. It is the most common infectious exanthem during the first two years of life.

Clinical Features

- The incubation period from time of exposure to fever is typically 7 to 14 days.
- Roseola typically affects infants and young children, with most cases occurring between the ages of 4 months and 3 years.
- Patients typically have 2 to 5 days of high fever (102–105°F [39–41°C]).
- Despite the high fever, the infants are devoid of other symptoms and appear to be doing surprisingly well, although some patients may have febrile seizures or mild upper respiratory symptoms.
- Lymphadenopathy (usually cervical and occipital) is variably present.
- As the patients defervesce, they develop faint pink to erythematous macules (classically described as rose pink) that are typically 1 to 5 mm in diameter. They most commonly affect the trunk and proximal extremities. Rarely, there is an admixture of macules and subtle papules (Figs. 3.11 and 3.12). The face is only occasionally affected.

- The oral mucosa may also demonstrate red papules of the soft palate and uvula, called *Nagayama spots,* and/or ulcers at the uvulopalatoglossal junction. These typically occur 2 days before the exanthem.

Diagnosis

- The clinical presentation is that of a young infant with high fever, followed by defervescence and a faint morbilliform eruption, which is a clinical pattern, characteristic if not diagnostic.
- Skin biopsies are not specific and are not indicated.
- Specific diagnostic tests (e.g., serologic studies, culture) are currently only available in research facilities, and the results are not generally available until after the infection has resolved.

Treatment

- Supportive therapy includes antipyretics during the febrile phase and hydration, which are all that is needed for most patients.
- Various antiviral therapies, including ganciclovir, foscarnet, and cidofovir, have demonstrated promise but have not been systematically studied and are not indicated at this time.

Clinical Course

The cutaneous eruption may last for hours or up to 3 days.

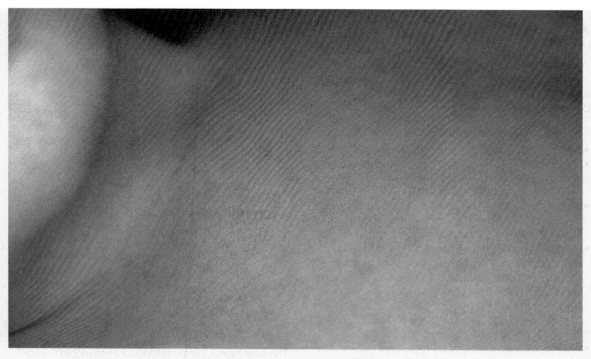

Fig. 3.11. Faint pink to red macular eruption on the upper chest of an infant. (From the Fitzsimons Army Medical Center Collection, Aurora, CO.)

Fig. 3.12. Infant with roseola demonstrating an admixture of macular erythema and subtle erythematous papules. (From the William Weston Collection, Aurora, CO.)

Pathogenesis

Unilateral thoracic exanthem is an uncommon but very distinct eruption thought to be due to an unidentified virus. This is supported by occasional cases that have found more than one sibling with the disease and the presence of a viral prodrome in many patients.

Clinical Features

- Most cases occur in the spring months.
- It almost exclusively affects infants and children, with most infections occurring in those between 6 months and 10 years of age.
- About 50% of patients have a viral prodrome consisting of low-grade fever, diarrhea, and/or upper respiratory symptoms.
- The skin lesions begin distinctly with a partial or complete unilateral thoracic distribution of morbilliform (less commonly, papular or eczematous) lesions, with the axillary area being the most common site of initial involvement (Figs. 3.13 and 3.14). Less commonly, it may localize to the proximal extremities (Fig. 3.15).
- As the cutaneous eruption progresses over several days, it typically becomes more bilateral and symmetric.
- The face and palms are always spared.
- Regional lymphadenopathy (usually axillary) is variably present.
- Pruritus may be present or absent.

Diagnosis

- The clinical presentation of a predominantly unilateral truncal (or, less commonly, proximal extremity) exanthem in a child is essentially diagnostic. The frequent involvement of the axillary area is a useful clinical clue.
- A biopsy is not typically indicated. If done, it should be a 3 or 4 mm punch biopsy that will at most be consistent with the diagnosis but not specific.

Treatment

- No treatment is an option in asymptomatic patients.
- Mild topical corticosteroids (e.g., hydrocortisone, desonide) can be used for pruritic lesions, although there is no evidence to suggest that this shortens the course of the disease.

Clinical Course

The exanthem typically disappears within 2 to 6 weeks.

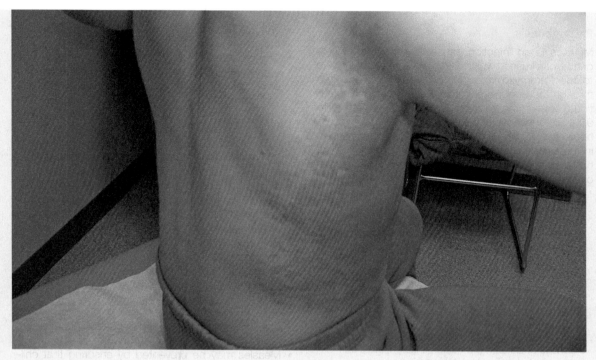

Fig. 3.13. Unilateral thoracic exanthem. This is a dramatic example of morbilliform lesions in a boy. (Courtesy Dr. Gavin Powell.)

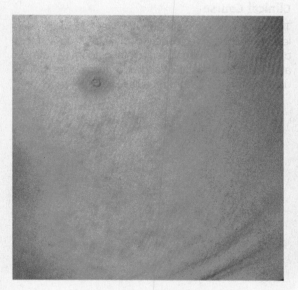

Fig. 3.14. Left side of chest of a child demonstrating subtle macular lesions.

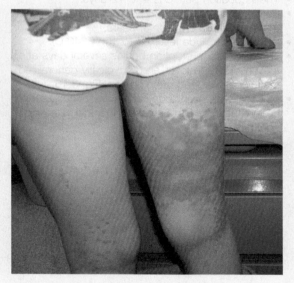

Fig. 3.15. Less commonly, the eruption involves an extremity. Note some extension to the contralateral lower extremity.

Pathogenesis

Measles is an infection caused by the *Morbillivirus* genus of viruses, which is an RNA virus belonging to the Paramyxoviridae family. Measles is acquired through the upper respiratory tract. It is highly infectious, with some studies demonstrating that up to 90% of susceptible individuals living in the same home will acquire the infection. Indigenous measles in the United States has been essentially eliminated; however, miniepidemics continue to occur because of cases imported from other countries.

Measles and Vaccination

Although measles was declared to be eliminated in the United States in 2000, it remains a global problem, and new cases continue to be imported into the United States. In 2014, the Centers for Disease Control and Prevention (CDC) documented 667 new cases. Worldwide, there are about 20,000,000 new cases every year. In 2015, there was a highly publicized outbreak in Disneyland, with 147 documented cases.

Measles will continue to be an issue because more than 12% of children (>8 million children) are either not vaccinated or incompletely vaccinated.

Clinical Features

- The incubation period is 4 to 12 days.
- Patients can transmit the disease up to 5 days after the morbilliform eruption appears.
- Symptoms include fever up to 104°F (40°C).
- The morbilliform eruption begins several days after the onset of the fever and is typically generalized, maculopapular, and often pruritic (Fig. 3.16).
- Mucosal findings include conjunctivitis, coryza, and cough (the three Cs of measles) in addition to Koplik spots (Fig. 3.17).

- The maculopapular lesions often become brown as they resolve (Fig. 3.18).
- Complications include pneumonia, encephalitis, and, rarely, death (1/1000 cases). Worldwide, approximately 134,200 (2015) individuals still die every year from measles.

Diagnosis

- Laboratory studies include the demonstration of IgM antibodies in serum or isolation of the measles virus RNA from the respiratory system.
- If the patient has previously been vaccinated, or the patient is a vaccine failure, IgM antibodies may not be detectable. In this scenario, the diagnosis can still be established by isolation of the measles virus RNA from respiratory secretions or by demonstrating increased IgG antibody levels.
- Exposure to a patient known to have measles is strong epidemiologic evidence.

Treatment

- This includes hydration and paracetamol or ibuprofen for the management of fever.
- Measles may be prevented by ensuring that children are immunized against measles with the MMR vaccine, which covers measles, mumps, and rubella.

Clinical Course

The fever typically lasts about 1 week, and the skin lesions resolve over a period of 7 to 9 days. Most cases are benign; however, a fatal outcome occurs in about 0.2% of cases. Worldwide, there were still 15 deaths every hour from measles.

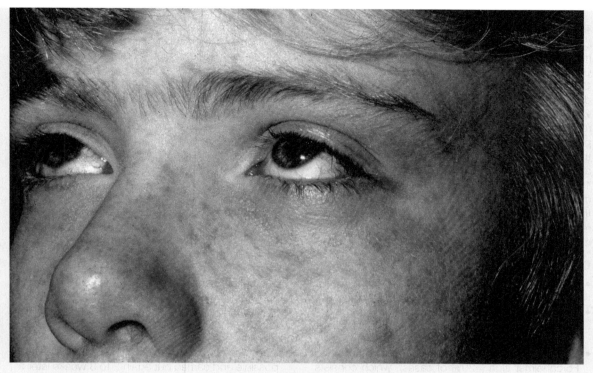

Fig. 3.16. Measles—conjunctivitis and macular eruption of the face. (From the William Weston Collection, Aurora, CO.)

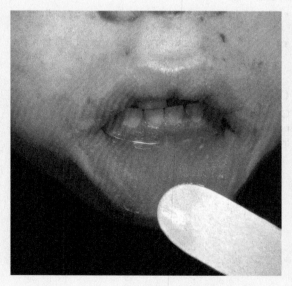

Fig. 3.17. Koplik spots. Shown are three characteristic whitish spots surrounded by a rim of erythema. These are most common on the buccal mucosa.

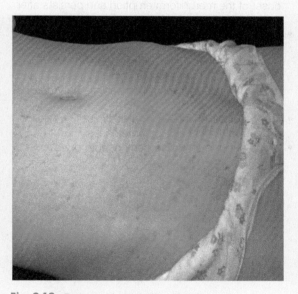

Fig. 3.18. Patient with morbilliform lesions on the abdomen, with a slightly brownish color. (From the William Weston Collection, Aurora, CO.)

The name *rubella* is derived from the Latin word *rubellus*, meaning reddish. It is also known as German measles or 3-day measles. It is usually called German measles because it was first described in the German medical literature in 1814. Rubella is produced by a togavirus belonging to the genus *Rubivirus*. The virus enters the body through the upper respiratory tract and primarily replicates in the nasopharynx and regional lymph nodes before entering the viremic phase. The use of rubella vaccination has almost eliminated rubella in the United States. In the 1964–1965 epidemic, there were an estimated 12.5 million cases; however, between 2005 and 2011, there were an average of only 11 cases/year. Most reported cases in the United States occur in nonimmunized foreign born Hispanic adults.

Clinical Features

- The incubation period is typically about 2 weeks (range, 12–23 days; mean, 18 days).
- A prodrome of low-grade fever (usually <100.4°F [38°C]) is often seen in adults but is often absent in children.
- Mucosal manifestations include conjunctivitis and Forchheimer sign (≈20% of cases), which consists of small red papules localized to the soft palate.
- Variable lymphadenopathy is present before the onset of the morbilliform eruption and persists after the eruption has faded.
- Cutaneous manifestations include a discrete morbilliform eruption that initially appears on the face (Fig. 3.19) and then spreads to the trunk and extremities (Fig. 3.20). The macules are typically less red and pinker than those seen in measles, but there is considerable overlap.
- The macules of rubella do not typically coalesce, except on the cheeks in some cases.
- Some patients may also demonstrate dry skin.

- Extracutaneous manifestations include arthralgia and arthritis (particularly in adults), eye pain, sore throat, headache, cough, and chills.
- Complications are rare but include encephalitis (1/6000 cases), orchitis, hemorrhagic lesions in the skin and internal organs, and neuritis.
- During the first 20 weeks of pregnancy, pregnant patients are at risk for **congenital rubella syndrome,** which consists of numerous congenital defects, including fetal death, blindness, and mental retardation.

Diagnosis

- If lymphadenopathy is found in someone who has not had the MMR vaccination, the clinical presentation of a morbilliform eruption should raise the suspicion of rubella.
- A viral culture is usually done from the nasopharynx, but cultures from the blood, urine, and cerebrospinal fluid can also be used. However, very few laboratories perform this test. Details on how to perform it can be found at https://www.cdc.gov/rubella/lab/serology.html.
- Ideally, serologic studies should be done as early as possible and carried out again 2 to 3 weeks later to confirm acute and convalescent titer levels.

Treatment

- This includes hydration and paracetamol or ibuprofen for the management of fever.
- This may be prevented by ensuring that children are immunized against measles with the MMR vaccine, which covers measles, mumps, and rubella.

Clinical Course

Cutaneous manifestations are short lived—hence the name *3-day measles.* However, the duration can vary from 1 to 5 days.

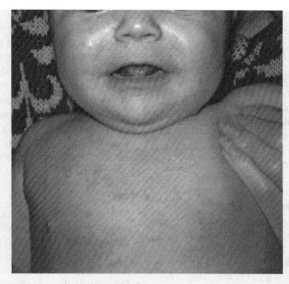

Fig. 3.19. Rubella. Shown are faint, pinkish-red macules on the face and trunk of an infant. (From the William Weston Collection, Aurora, CO.)

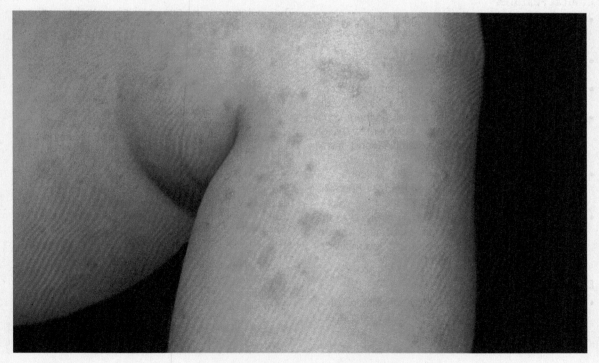

Fig. 3.20. Patient with rubella. This is a close-up of faint, pinkish-red macules of the trunk and proximal upper arm. (From the William Weston Collection, Aurora, CO.)

Roseola Vaccinatum ICD10 code T88.1

Pathogenesis

The term *roseola vaccinatum* (benign hypersensitivity reaction to smallpox vaccine) is used here as a universal term to describe patients receiving smallpox vaccination who develop a hypersensitivity reaction. Although the most common presentation is a morbilliform eruption, in some cases it may resemble urticaria or erythema multiforme. This reaction is included here because of the 2002 initiative by the US government to restart mass smallpox vaccinations of active duty military personnel. Between 2002 and 2014, 2.4 million service members and other personnel were vaccinated. There are four known different formulations of the live virus vaccine, and all produce these reactions. The vaccinations now continue in a more limited fashion. In a study of more than 16,000 soldiers at one military base, the incidence for the erythematous (morbilliform) reaction was 0.054%, with an urticarial reaction occurring in 0.018% and erythema multiforme–like reactions occurring in 0.009%.

Clinical Features

- Typically, the patient is a young adult in the military, because most of the patients receiving the vaccines are on active duty.
- Eruptions typically develop 7 to 11 days after vaccination.
- Morbilliform reactions may surround and be accentuated around the vaccination site (Figs. 3.21–3.23).
- Morbilliform lesions vary from small erythematous maculopapular lesions to large confluent areas of erythema, with the upper extremities and trunk being most severely affected.
- Urticarial lesions typically resemble urticaria, although they often persist longer than 24 hours at the same spot.
- Erythema multiforme–like lesions usually demonstrate an annular red margin associated with a dusky center. The classic targetoid lesions with central blisters are not present.

Diagnosis

- The diagnosis is established by the history of a smallpox vaccination being given to the patient within the last 7 to 11 days. The accentuation of the reaction around the vaccination site, which will typically be crusted at this stage, is characteristic.
- Viral cultures are not needed because these represent hypersensitivity reactions, and no virus is present in the lesional areas.
- A 3.4-mm punch biopsy can be done to exclude other possibilities (e.g., erythema multiforme). However, the histologic findings are not diagnostic and are generally only consistent with roseola vaccinatum.

Treatment

- No treatment is an option because these are self-limited reactions that resolve spontaneously.
- Patients who are pruritic can be treated with topical emollients and topical anesthetic agents, such as pramoxine.
- Patients with an urticarial tissue reaction can be treated with oral antihistamines.

Clinical Course

The cutaneous lesions typically resolve without sequelae over 3 to 7 days.

The Monster in the Freezer

Why does the military still vaccinate against smallpox when it has been eradicated? In theory, the live *Variola* virus only exists in one secure laboratory in the United States (the CDC) and a similar secure one in Russia (VECTOR). However, it is highly likely that not all the virus is confined to these sites. In 2014, six apparently lost vials of the virus were found in a cold storage unit in a US Food and Drug Administration laboratory, and there have been a number of controversial reports of vials of live smallpox virus at one (or more) Russian military bases. There is also concern that live virus might have found its way into North Korea.

Of all the known biologic agents, smallpox is the most wildly infectious and easily aerosolized; it has a mortality rate of about 30% in those who are not immunized.

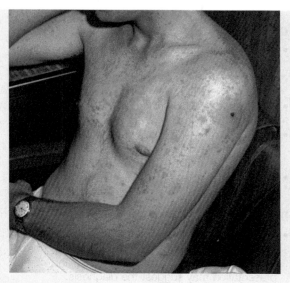

Fig. 3.21. Patient with roseola vaccinatum demonstrating marked erythema surrounding the vaccination site and a morbilliform reaction.

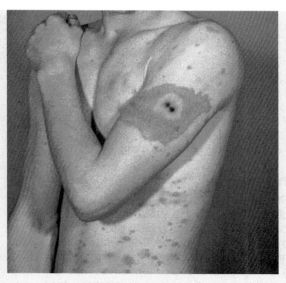

Fig. 3.22. This figure demonstrates a severe reaction around the vaccination site. (From the Walter Reed Army Medical Center Collection, Washington, DC.)

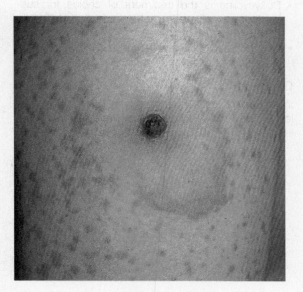

Fig. 3.23. Patient with morbilliform morphology of roseola vaccinatum. (From the Fitzsimons Army Medical Center Collection, Aurora, CO.)

Rickettsial Infections (Partial List)

Typhus Group
- Epidemic typhus *(Rickettsia prowazekii)*
- Murine typhus *(Rickettsia typhi)*
- Scrub typhus *(Orientia tsutsugamushi)*

Spotted Fever Group
- Rocky mountain spotted fever *(Rickettsia rickettsii)*
- Boutonneuse fever *(Rickettsia conorii)*
- Rickettsialpox *(Rickettsia akari)*

Pathogenesis

Rickettsial diseases are the result of infection by obligate intracellular bacteria transmitted to humans by arthropod vectors, including ticks, lice, chiggers, mites, and other species. The bacteria primarily but not exclusively attack endothelial cells and produce a morbilliform eruption that mimics viral and drug morbilliform eruptions. In some infections, the vascular damage is more severe, resulting in hemorrhagic lesions or ulcers. There are numerous species in the genus; however, the infections are usually broken up into the typhus and spotted fever groups.

Important Clues
- Morbilliform eruption plus fever. Always consider rickettsial infection, especially if there is a history of foreign travel.
- Morbilliform eruption plus fever plus necrotic papule (eschar at the tick bite site). This classic triad is seen in a specific subset of rickettsial infections, such as rickettsialpox, boutonneuse fever, African tick bite fever, Queensland tick typhus, and others.
- Morbilliform eruption that starts to become purpuric plus fever. This combination is suspicious for Rocky Mountain spotted fever (see Chapter 20).

Clinical Features

- Following the arthropod introduction of the rickettsial organisms, the incubation period is usually 5 to 17 days but can be as short as 2 days and as long as 24 days.
- The classic triad of rickettsial infections is fever, headache, and rash.
- The morbilliform eruption is not specific and consistent with erythematous macules, with some lesions being more papular (Figs. 3.24 and 3.25).
- Many of the rickettsial infections will demonstrate an eschar (Fig. 3.26) at the bite site (tache noir).

Diagnosis

- The appearance of cutaneous rickettial infection is not specific; however, a constellation of findings from the history, arthropod exposure, and clinical presentation may suggest the diagnosis.
- Serologic studies include testing of acute and convalescent sera.

Treatment

- Doxycycline is the treatment of choice for suspected or confirmed rickettsial infections in adults and children.
- Chloramphenicol is an alternative choice if doxycycline is contraindicated.

Comment

In suspected cases, patients should be treated empirically. The CDC Rickettsial Zoonoses Branch (Tel. +001-404-639-1075) is an invaluable resource.

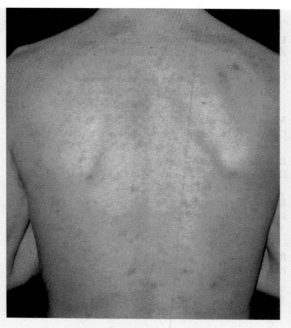

Fig. 3.25. Close-up of the morbilliform eruption in the same patient as in Fig. 3.24.

Fig. 3.24. Patient with boutonneuse fever demonstrating morbilliform eruption of the trunk. The infection was acquired from a tick bite in southern Europe. (From the Walter Reed Army Medical Center Collection, Washington, DC.)

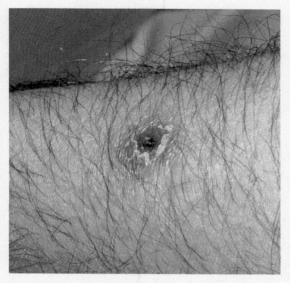

Fig. 3.26. Necrotic papule at the tick bite site in a different patient with boutonneuse fever. (From the Fitzsimons Army Medical Center Collection, Aurora, CO.)

References

Morbilliform Drug Eruptions

Gerson D, Srigansehan V, Alexis JB. Cutaneous drug eruptions: a 5-year experience. *J Am Acad Dermatol.* 2008;59:995-999.

Drug Eruption With Eosinophilia and Systemic Symptoms (DRESS)

Fahim S, Jain V, Victor G, Pierscianowski T. Piperacillin-tazobactam–induced drug hypersensitivity syndrome. *Cutis.* 2006;77:353-357.

Maoz KB, Brenner S. Drug rash with eosinophilia and systemic symptoms syndrome: sex and the causative agent. *Skinmed.* 2007;6:271-273.

Salem SB, Slim R, Denguezili M, et al. A recurrent drug rash with eosinophilia and systemic symptoms. *Pediatr Dermatol.* 2007;24:666-668.

Morbilliform Viral Exanthems

Bialecki C, Feder HM Jr, Grant-Kels JM. The six classic childhood exanthems: a review and update. *J Am Acad Dermatol.* 1989;21:891-903.

Roseola Infantum

Stone RC, Micali GA, Schwartz RA. Roseola infantum and its causal human herpesviruses. *Int J Dermatol.* 2014;53:397-403.

Unilateral Laterothoracic Exanthem

Bodemer C, de Prost Y. Unilateral laterothoracic exanthem in children: a new disease? *J Am Acad Dermatol.* 1992;27:693-696.

Duarte AF, Cruz MJ, Baudrier T, Mota A, Azevedo F. Unilateral laterothoracic exanthem and primary Epstein-Barr virus infection: case report. *Pediatr Infect Dis J.* 2009;28:549-550.

Measles (Rubeola)

Goodson JL, Seward JF. Measles 50 years after use of measles vaccine. *Infect Dis Clin North Am.* 2015;29:725-743.

Rubella (German Measles)

Lambert N, Strebel P, Orenstein W, Icenogle J, Poland GA. Rubella. *Lancet.* 2015;385:2297-2307.

Roseola Vaccinatum

Bessinger GT, Smith SB, Olivere JW, James BL. Benign hypersensitivity reactions to smallpox vaccine. *Int J Dermatol.* 2007;46:460-465.

Rickettsiosis

Faccini-Martinez AA, Garcia-Alvarez L, Hidalgo M, Oteo JA. Syndromic classification of rickettsioses: an approach for clinical practice. *Int J Infect Dis.* 2014;28:126-139.

Chapter 4
Diffuse or Reticulated Erythema

Key Term

Mucocutaneous lymph node
  syndrome

Erythema is defined as cutaneous diseases that present with large patches of red skin, without overlying changes in the epidermis. Included in this group are disorders that have a netlike or reticulated pattern of redness. Notably absent in this pattern are blisters, targetoid lesions, scale, or erythema that is photodistributed. As one would expect, as the lesions age, they may become scaly or peel. A classic example of this is a first-degree sunburn in which there is erythema confined to the site of sun exposure, with no primary epidermal changes that can be seen grossly. However, as the erythema resolves, the skin becomes scaly or even peels in sheets. Photodistributed erythema is discussed in Chapter 19.

Differential Diagnosis of Erythema

Nonphotodistributed
- Erythema infectiosum
- Kawasaki disease
- Rosacea
- Scarlet fever
- Toxic shock syndrome

Photodistributed (see Chapter 19)
- Dermatomyositis
- Lupus erythematosus
- Phototoxic drug eruptions
- Sunburn

Reticulated Erythemas
- Erythema infectiosum
- Erythema ab igne

IMPORTANT HISTORY QUESTIONS

How long has your redness been present?

Most causes of erythema are of recent duration because many, but not all of them, are due to a bacterial or viral toxin or a medication.

Have you started any new medications in the last 10 days?

This is a critical question because some erythemas may be drug-induced. The classic example would be doxycycline, which produces a photodistributed erythema.

Have you had any fever?

This question is directed toward determining a potential infectious cause, such as a viral or bacterial infection.

Do you have any other medical problems?

This question can elicit much important clinical information, including a history of a connective tissue disorder or history of rosacea.

IMPORTANT PHYSICAL FINDINGS

What is the distribution of the lesions?

Although not discussed in this chapter, some erythemas are photodistributed, including dermatomyositis, lupus erythematosus, phototoxic drug eruptions, and sunburn. Other erythemas, such as chemotherapy-induced acral erythema, demonstrate a predominantly acral distribution, and erythema secondary to rosacea is usually confined to the face.

Are lesions present in the oral mucosa?

Erythema associated with mucosal lesions are more likely to be due to infections, lupus erythematosus, or drug eruptions.

Are vesicles or blisters present?

Although a so-called pure erythema should not demonstrate blisters, some severe erythemas may at some time in their development develop vesicles or blisters. For example, a severe sunburn (second-degree sunburn) may develop blistering, which may be very focal, and although most cytoxic chemotherapy reactions present as erythema, severe reactions can develop focal blister formation.

Presence or absence of lesions with a reticulated (netlike) appearance

Although most variants of erythema do not demonstrate a reticulated appearance, some erythemas, including erythema infectiosum and erythema ab igne, frequently demonstrate a reticulated appearance.

Pathogenesis

Scarlet fever (scarlatina) is a toxic reaction to toxins (erythrogenic toxins A, B, and C) produced by group A β-hemolytic streptococci *(Streptococcus pyogenes)*. Once patients acquire antibodies against these toxins, scarlet fever does not develop. This accounts for why most patients affected are children between the ages of 1 to 10 years, because they are less likely to have these antibodies. In the antibiotic era, scarlet fever has become much less common than it was formerly.

Clinical Features

- Scarlet fever typically affects infants and children between the ages of 1 and 10 years.
- Most patients have streptococcal pharyngitis, with symptoms that include sore throat, headache, fever (102–105° F [39–40.5°C]), malaise, or tonsillitis and, less commonly, streptococcal wound or pelvic infections.
- Erythema typically begins 12 to 48 hours after the development of the primary infection.
- Erythema most commonly begins on the neck, chest, and axillae, with rapid spread to the remainder of the body (Fig. 4.1).
- On the face, there is marked erythema, with a slapped cheek appearance and circumoral pallor.
- Punctate erythematous papules rapidly develop on areas with erythema, typically described as sunburn with goose bumps (Fig. 4.2).
- Linear petechial streaks may be seen in the flexures (e.g., axillae, antecubital, inguinal).
- Patients may demonstrate a positive Rumpel-Leede tourniquet test result.
- The tongue is initially white with prominent papillae, but as the illness progresses, the entire tongue becomes red, with prominent papillae classically described as a red strawberry tongue (Fig. 4.3).
- Rarely, clusters of small vesicles may appear on the trunk and/or extremities.
- Desquamation that is most prominent on the hands and feet typically begins 7 to 10 days later.

Diagnosis

- The clinical presentation of a child with pharyngitis or tonsillitis and systemic symptoms, which include fever and rapidly spreading erythema, should initially suggest the diagnosis. As the disease progresses, numerous physical findings further support the diagnosis.
- The complete blood count (CBC) reveals a leukocytosis with a left shift (~85%–95% polymorphonuclear leukocytes).
- A throat culture should be done.
- The antistreptolysin O (ASO) titer or streptozyme level is typically elevated.

Treatment

- Oral penicillin VK or oral erythromycin for 10 days is the treatment of choice.

Clinical Course

- In the preantibiotic era, this disease often resulted in a fatal outcome (≈3%–20%). Complications of scarlet fever include acute glomerulonephritis and rheumatic fever (2%–3% of patients). With recognition and antibiotic treatment, the mortality rate is less than 1%. It is important to note that patients may continue to desquamate for as long as 6 weeks.

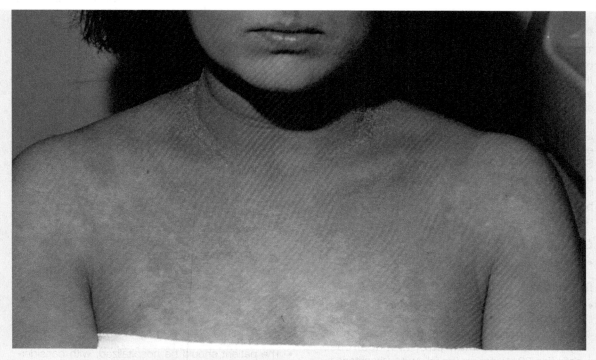

Fig. 4.1. Scarlet fever. Shown here is marked diffuse erythema of the neck, upper chest, and arms. Note early desquamation of the neck. (From the Fitzsimons Army Medical Center Collection, Aurora, CO.)

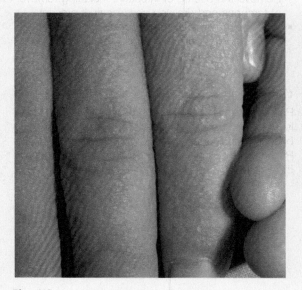

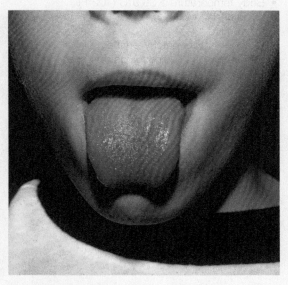

Fig. 4.2. Punctate papules on a background of erythema, a pattern known as sunburn with goose bumps. (From the Fitzsimons Army Medical Center Collection, Aurora, CO.)

Fig. 4.3. Strawberry tongue in a patient with scarlet fever. (From the Fitzsimons Army Medical Center Collection, Aurora, CO.)

⚠ Toxic Shock Syndrome ICD10 code A48.3

Pathogenesis

Toxic shock syndrome (TSS) is a rare complication of infection by strains of *Staphylococcus aureus* that produce TSS toxin-1 (TSST-1). Less commonly a similar disorder, sometimes referred to as toxic shock–like syndrome (TSLS), is produced by a streptococcal pyrogenic exotoxin produced by strains of *Streptococcus pyogenes*. In the 1980s, there was an epidemic associated with superabsorbent tampons. Since the withdrawal of these products, the number of reported cases has decreased. The source of the infection can still be a tampon; however, it also can be produced by infections of other mucosal and cutaneous sites.

Clinical Features

- See diagnostic criteria below.

Diagnosis

- The 2011 Centers for Disease Control and Prevention (CDC) criteria for the diagnosis of TSS (http://www.cdc.gov/nndss/conditions/toxic-shock-syndrome-other-than-streptococcal/case-definition/2011) include the following (six criteria are needed for confirmed infection and five criteria are needed for presumed infection; see the CDC site for more information):
- Body temperature ≥ 38.9°C (102°F)
- Hypotension with systolic blood pressure ≤ 90 mm Hg
- Diffuse macular-patchy erythema, with nonspecific cutaneous findings (Figs. 4.4 and 4.5)
- Evidence of involvement of three or more organ systems:
  - Gastrointestinal tract—vomiting or diarrhea
  - Muscular system—severe myalgia or more than twice the creatine phosphokinase level
  - Mucous membrane hyperemia—vaginal, oral, conjunctival (Fig. 4.6)
  - Kidney failure—creatinine level more than twice normal

- Liver inflammation—bilirubin, aspartate aminotransferase (AST), or alanine aminotransferase (ALT) level of twice the normal level or higher
- Low platelet count, $<100,000/mm^3$
- Central nervous system—confusion without focal neurologic findings
- Negative workup up for other potential causes, including other bacterial infections and negative serologic studies for rickettsial infection, leptospirosis, and measles
- Desquamation (usually of the palms and soles)—typically 1 to 2 weeks after the onset (Fig. 4.7). Note that this criteria does not help in the evaluation of patients in the early stages of the disease.
- Mucocutaneous findings that should suggest the possibility of this diagnosis include conjunctival erythema (in addition to toxic shock syndrome, this finding can be seen in leptospirosis, Colorado tick fever, Kawasaki disease, Rocky Mountain spotted fever, and some viral syndromes) and edema of the hands and feet.

Treatment

- The patient should be hospitalized, with consideration for admission into an intensive care unit for supportive care (e.g., fluid management, management of renal disease).
- Remove the source of infection, including removal of tampons and draining abscesses, if present.
- Antibiotic treatment should cover *S. aureus* and *S. pyogenes,* typically penicillins, cephalosporins, or vancomycin, with consideration for the addition of clindamycin or gentamycin.

Clinical Course

Patients with TSS may progress rapidly, and there is urgency in establishing a presumptive diagnosis, because the mortality rate ranges from 5% to 15%. Patients with TSS may also develop a recurrence of their disease with a subsequent infection.

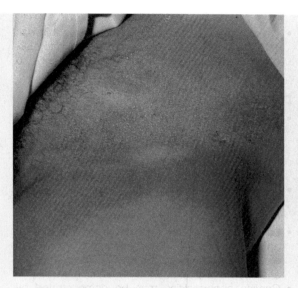

Fig. 4.4. Woman with culture-positive *S. aureus* infection of the groin and marked erythema extending to the thigh and abdomen. The patient's tampon was also culture-positive.

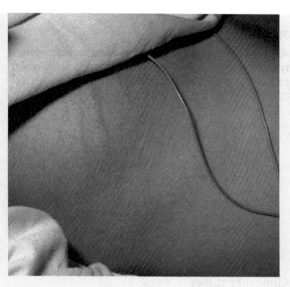

Fig. 4.5. Marked erythema of the same patient in Fig. 4.4 involving the breast and abdomen. This erythema also extended into the axillae.

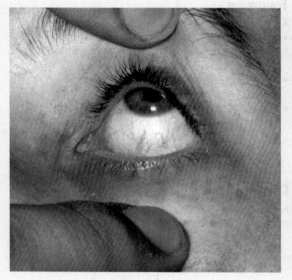

Fig. 4.6. Same patient as in Fig. 4.4, with mild conjunctival hyperemia. The patient also had involvement of the oral pharynx in addition to fever (104.3°F [40.2 °C]), profound hypotension (80/20 mm Hg), vomiting, low platelet count, renal failure, and abnormal liver enzymes.

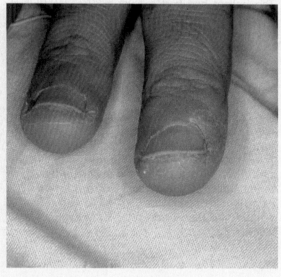

Fig. 4.7. Desquamation of the fingertips 1 week later in the same patient as in Fig. 4.4. (Tripler Army Medical Center, Honolulu, HI.)

🛡 Kawasaki Disease ICD10 code M30.3

Pathogenesis

Kawasaki disease, also known as **mucocutaneous lymph node syndrome,** is a disease of unknown cause that is presumed to be due to an unknown toxin or antigenic substance.

Diagnosis of Kawasaki Disease
- Five days of fever (required), plus four of the five remaining criteria:
  - Oropharyngeal changes to include erythema, strawberry tongue, or cracking or fissuring of the lips
  - Bilateral nonpurulent conjunctivitis
  - Erythema of skin that does not vesiculate
  - Erythema or swelling of the hands or feet
  - Cervical lymphadenopathy (≥1.5 cm)

Clinical Features

- It typically affects children (frequently of Asian descent) between the ages of 3 months and 10 years, with most cases occurring in children younger than 5 years.
- It is more common in the winter.
- The patient has had a fever (>39°C [102°F]) of more than 5 days' duration that is not responsive to antibiotics.
- Mucosal changes include bilateral nonpurulent conjunctivitis, oral erythema, strawberry tongue, and fissured tongue (Figs. 4.8 and 4.9).
- Nonsuppurative cervical lymphadenopathy is present in most but not all cases.
- The hands and feet typically demonstrate variable edema and palmoplantar erythema, which frequently desquamates (Fig. 4.10).
- The cutaneous changes of the trunk are nonspecific. They consist of variable erythema that may be morbilliform, scarlatiniform, or erythema multiforme–like in appearance (Fig. 4.11).
- Variable features include irritability, arthralgias, and tachycardia.

- Complications include vasculitic changes that can lead to coronary artery aneurysms, with up to 18% of children developing coronary involvement and rare cases being fatal (<1%).

Diagnosis

- The diagnosis is established by the criteria listed above—namely, fever of 5 days' duration, plus four of the five remaining criteria. Some clinicians establish a presumptive diagnosis after only 3 days of fever if all the other criteria are met.
- If a coronary artery disease or aneurysm is detected, a presumptive diagnosis can be made, even if all the necessary criteria are present.
- Laboratory tests that may be abnormal include an elevated erythrocyte sedimentation rate (ESR), elevated C-reactive protein (CRP) level, normocytic anemia, sterile pyuria, and liver function studies.
- Cardiac abnormalities may be demonstrated by an abnormal electrocardiogram (e.g., arrhythmia, ventricular dysfunction), echocardiogram (e.g., aneurysm or more subtle changes), or coronary angiogram.

Treatment

- Hospitalization is recommended in all cases.
- The standard of care treatment is intravenous immunoglobulin (IVIG), with most patients improving in 24 hours.
- Aspirin is usually begun immediately and then slowly tapered as the fever resolves.
- Corticosteroids were formerly used, but the failure to show benefit in a randomized controlled trial has diminished their popularity, although they are still occasionally added to IVIG and aspirin in severe cases.

Clinical Course

Most patients quickly respond to therapy, and the mortality rate is well under 1%.

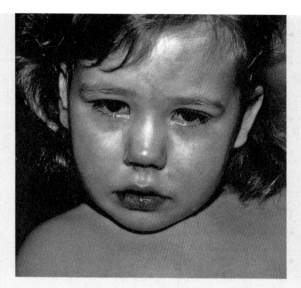

Fig. 4.8. Facial erythema, conjunctivitis, and fissured lips in a patient with Kawasaki disease. (From the William Weston Collection, Aurora, CO.)

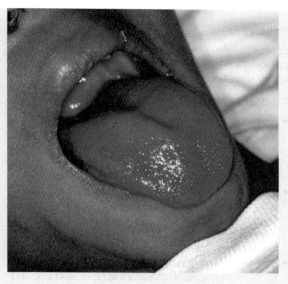

Fig. 4.9. Strawberry tongue and fissured lips in a patient with Kawasaki disease. (From the William Weston Collection, Aurora, CO.)

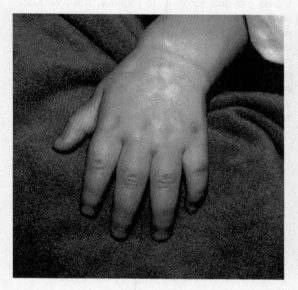

Fig. 4.10. Marked erythema and edema of the hands in a child with Kawasaki disease.

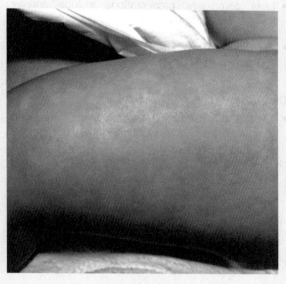

Fig. 4.11. Large patches of erythema on the upper thigh of a young child with Kawasaki disease. (From the William Weston Collection, Aurora, CO.)

Erythema Infectiosum

Pathogenesis

Erythema infectiosum is due to infection by the human parvovirus B19 (B19V). The virus is found in the respiratory secretions and spread by aerosolization.

Clinical Features

- Based on inoculation studies of volunteers, the incubation period from the time of exposure to the prodrome is 6 days, with another 10 to 14 days needed for the onset of the cutaneous eruption. Some patients may not experience a prodrome.
- There is a variable prodrome of fever, chills, myalgias, sore throat, and gastrointestinal symptoms. It is generally more severe in adults and may include symmetric polyarthritis of the peripheral joints—hands, feet, wrists, knees.
- The facial exanthem consists of erythema that is most pronounced on malar areas (so-called slapped cheeks); this usually appears first (Fig. 4.12A).
- Truncal and extremity lesions initially consist of erythematous macules that may eventually connect to form a reticulated or netlike appearance (Fig. 4.12B). This exanthem may come and go.
- Less commonly, presentations include annular lesions, hemorrhagic macules, and confluent erythema.
- Patients may be pruritic during the prodromal phase and occasionally demonstrate mild pruritus associated with the exanthem.

Diagnosis

- The clinical presentation is usually all that is required to make a presumptive diagnosis.

- A CBC may demonstrate neutropenia, lymphocytopenia, or thrombocytopenia.
- Skin biopsies are not specific and are not indicated, although some laboratories have stains directed against HPV B19 and can demonstrate viral antigens in tissue.
- Specific diagnostic testing is available in many areas. It consists of the detection of immunoglobulin G (IgM) anti-HPV B19 antibodies in the early phase (by week 2 after inoculation) and the development of IgG anti-HPV B19 antibodies later in the course of the illness (several weeks into the infection).

Treatment

- Supportive therapy includes antipyretics as needed during the prodromal phase.
- No specific treatment of the exanthem is needed; antihistamines can be used in patients complaining of pruritus.

Clinical Course

The facial erythema typically lasts for 1 to 5 days and then disappears, whereas the reticulated erythema may last for days to months. The reticulated erythema frequently disappears and then reappears with anything that flushes the skin (e.g., fever, exercise, sunlight exposure). The arthralgias and arthritis may be short lived or persist for years in adults. Rare patients may develop a transient aplastic crisis. It is important to note that pregnant women may pass the virus to the fetus, resulting in fetal hydrops, but this is uncommon.

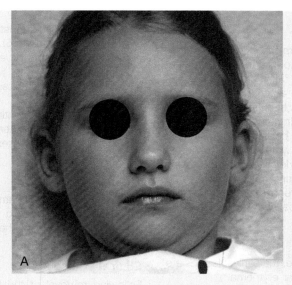

Fig. 4.12A. Young girl with characteristic diffuse bilateral edema of the face (slapped cheek appearance). (Courtesy Dr. Amanda Tauscher.)

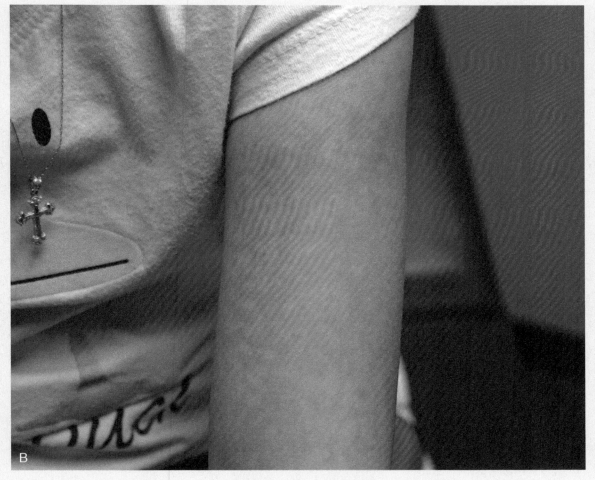

Fig. 4.12B. Same patient as in Fig. 4.12A with areas of diffuse and reticulated erythema of the arm. (Courtesy Dr. Amanda Tauscher.)

Erythema Ab Igne ICD10 code L59.0

Pathogenesis

Erythema ab igne results from the skin being chronically or repeatedly exposed to mild to moderate heat (typically, 43–47°C [109–117°F]). Formerly, this was most commonly seen on the anterior legs of women who were exposed to chronic heat from sitting in front of hearths or heating stoves. In recent years, the most common causes are heating pads, heating blankets, heated car seats, and hot water bottles, although laptop exposure on the anterior aspect of the thighs has become increasingly common. It can also be an occupational hazard in jobs requiring repeated exposure to high heat, such as bakers, cooks, smelters, glassblowers, and jewelers.

Clinical Features

- During the very acute phase, the earliest lesions are transient patches of reticular erythema.
- With continued exposure, the reticular erythema becomes increasingly fixed and will eventually not resolve (Figs. 4.13 and 4.14).
- Mature lesions demonstrate tan to brown reticulated patches (Fig. 4.15).
- Very rarely, patients have demonstrated reticulated blistering.
- Symptoms may be absent or present, with variable itching and burning.
- Complications with continued exposure to the heat source include actinic keratoses and squamous cell carcinoma. In most cases, this requires decades of exposure.

Treatment

- The cornerstone of treatment is removal of the heat source that is inducing the reaction. There is no specific treatment of the skin changes once they develop.

Clinical Course

Following removal of the heat source, most cases demonstrate gradual resolution over a period of 1 month to several months.

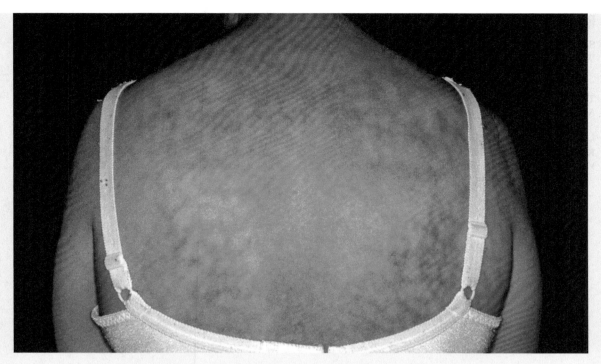

Fig. 4.13. Patient with acute erythema ab igne demonstrating a dramatic reticular erythema of the back. This was due to sleeping on a heated blanket. (From the Fitzsimons Army Medical Center Collection, Aurora, CO.)

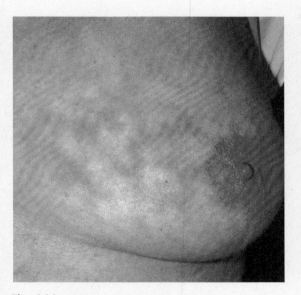

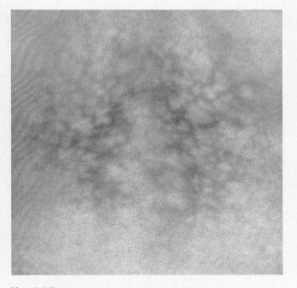

Fig. 4.14. Patient with acute erythema ab igne of the breast from an electric heating pad. (From the Fitzsimons Army Medical Center Collection, Aurora, CO.)

Fig. 4.15. Patient with chronic erythema ab igne of the lower back from an electric heating pad. (From the Fitzsimons Army Medical Center Collection, Aurora, CO.)

References

Scarlet Fever

Wong SS, Yeun KY. Streptococcus pyogenes and re-emergence of scarlet fever as a public health problem. *Emerg Microbes Infect.* 2012;7:e2.

Toxic Shock Syndrome

Andrey DO, Ferry T, Siegenthaler N, et al. Unusual staphylococcal toxic shock syndrome presenting as a scarlet-like fever. *New Microbes New Infect.* 2015;18:10-13.

Kawasaki Disease

Velez-Torres R, Callen JP. Acute febrile mucocutaneous lymph node (Kawasaki) syndrome. An analysis of 24 cases. *Int J Dermatol.* 1987;26:96-102.

Yu JJ. Use of corticosteroids during acute phase of Kawasaki disease. *World J Clin Pediatr.* 2015;8:135-142.

Erythema Infectiosum

Valentin MN, Cohen PJ. Pediatric parvovirus B19: spectrum of clinical manifestations. *Cutis.* 2013;92:179-184.

Erythema Ab Igne

Ladizinski B, Sankey C. Erythema ab igne. *J Emerg Med.* 2015;49:e29-e30.

Levinbrook WS, Mallett J, Grant-Kels JM. Laptop computer–associated erythema ab igne. *Cutis.* 2007;80:319-320.

Chapter 5
Urticarial and Indurated Eruptions

Urticarial eruptions yield, as a primary lesion, a wheal (hivelike) or something that resembles a wheal, creating a fixed indurated papule or plaque, without scale. This pattern may be produced by internal and external causes. Most lesions are erythematous (red).

IMPORTANT HISTORY QUESTIONS FOR URTICARIAL ERUPTIONS

How long have you had these lesions?

Attempt to establish the duration of illness. Some urticarial processes are acute (e.g., acute urticaria, Sweet syndrome), whereas others are present for weeks, months, or even years (e.g., chronic urticaria).

How long do individual lesions last?

In simple urticaria (hives), the individual lesions lasts less than 24 hours, although the rash may last longer. This differs from urticarial vasculitis, in which individual lesions last longer than 24 hours. As a separate question, it is important to query the patient about how long individual lesions last, distinct from how long the overall condition has been present. This information is often overlooked in emergency department (ED) and urgent care settings.

What medications do you take?

Most urticarial eruptions represent a hypersensitivity process. These conditions, including urticaria, angioedema, serum sickness, and Sweet syndrome, may be induced by drugs.

Do the lesions itch or are they painful?

Simple urticaria (hives) is usually pruritic, whereas urticarial vasculitis, Sweet syndrome, cellulitis, and especially necrotizing fasciitis may be described as burning or painful.

Have you had any difficulty breathing?

This is a critical question to ask and document in the medical record. Sinopulmonary involvement distinguishes angioedema and anaphylaxis from simple urticaria, which is without mucosal or sinopulmonary involvement.

IMPORTANT PHYSICAL FINDINGS FOR URTICARIAL ERUPTIONS

Are any of the lesions annular?

Some urticarial eruptions may be annular, or vaguely annular, and this is an important pattern to observe. Simple urticaria (hives) may present with annular and nonannular lesions.

Are any of the lesions linear?

Linear lesions suggest dermatographism, which can be tested by stroking the skin with a firm object and waiting 3 to 6 minutes to identify an erythematous line. The line should disappear in 15 to 30 minutes.

Do any of the lesions demonstrate focal hemorrhage?

Simple urticaria does not demonstrate associated hemorrhage unless the hemorrhage is simply due to increased hydrostatic pressure in the lower extremities. Urticarial vasculitis and hemorrhagic edema of infancy often demonstrate associated hemorrhage.

How large are the lesions?

Small papular wheals (1–4 mm) often suggests cholinergic urticaria, which is related to heat or sweating.

What is the distribution of the lesions?

Some forms of physical urticaria may demonstrate a distinct distribution. For example, solar urticaria is photoaccentuated, whereas pressure urticaria occurs in areas of pressure, such as the hands, feet, trunk, buttocks, and legs.

Is any fever present?

A fever should prompt consideration of an infectious cause of urticaria (e.g., reaction to streptococcal pharyngitis or a viral infection). Also, some mimics of urticaria may be caused by infection, such as erythema migrans, the cutaneous manifestation of Lyme disease.

Drugs Often Implicated in Iatrogenic Urticaria
- Ampicillin
- Amoxicillin
- Penicillin
- Sulfonamides

Pathogenesis

Urticaria (hives) is ubiquitous, with about 20% of the world's population experiencing at least one episode of urticaria in a lifetime. A cause is identified in about 50% of cases of acute urticaria (<6 weeks' duration). Common instigators include food (e.g., seafood, nuts), wasp and bee stings, blood products, viral infections, radiocontrast media, and drugs. It is believed that many cases of chronic urticaria (>6 weeks) are due to autoantibodies directed against the high-affinity immunoglobulin E (IgE) receptor and/or IgE itself. Hence, even extensive and detailed patient workups in chronic urticaria often fail to demonstrate a cause.

Clinical Features

- Acute urticaria (<6 weeks' duration)—pruritic wheals, of variable size, which may be annular. Although the condition may last for a prolonged duration, individual lesions last less than 24 hours (Figs. 5.1–5.3).
- Chronic urticaria (>6 weeks' duration, with nearly daily eruptions)—a cause is less often identified.

Diagnosis

- A drug exposure history is critical. Most causative drugs were initiated in the last 8 to 14 days, but occasionally an eruption may be caused by a drug used for a longer period. The query should include also drugs used on an occasional basis, as well as any vitamins or supplements that the patient may have taken.
- Skin biopsies are not usually diagnostic but may exclude other disorders. The findings may suggest urticaria or another hypersensitivity process. Moreover, a biopsy does not discriminate among different causes of urticaria (e.g., drug-induced, pressure-induced, cholinergic urticaria).
- Sometimes, direct immunofluorescent studies may be useful to exclude urticarial vasculitis.
- Blind laboratory evaluations are usually not helpful. Laboratory studies are more significant when directed by a pertinent medical history, review of systems, or physical examination. Studies may include a complete blood count (CBC), erythrocyte sedimentation rate (ESR), thyroid antibodies (present in ~25% of patients with chronic urticaria), determination of cryoglobulin levels, and tests for hepatitis B, hepatitis C, and antinuclear antibody (ANA) and extractable nuclear antigen antibodies (ENA) (connective tissue disease can be associated with urticaria).

Treatment

- Acute urticaria
  - Discontinue potentially offending medications when possible.
  - Classic histamine-1 (H1) nonsedating antihistamines represent first-line therapy; the most common treatments are cetirizine, fexofenadine, loratadine, and desloratadine.
  - Patients who fail nonsedating antihistamines might consider a sedating antihistamine in the evening (e.g., hydroxyzine, diphenhydramine).
  - For patients failing H_1 antihistamines, an H2 antagonist (e.g., cimetidine, ranitidine) may be added.
  - Oral prednisone may be used for severe cases. A typical adult dose is 40 mg/day for 3 days, tapering to 20 mg/day for 3 days and then 10 mg/day for 3 days.
- Chronic urticaria
  - Classic H1 antihistamines (as above)
  - Doxepin (potent H1 and H2 receptor antagonist)—typical doses are 10 to 30 mg at night.
  - Leukotriene inhibitors (zafirlukast, montelukast sodium)—anecdotal success
  - Omalizumab is a monoclonal antibody that inhibits IgE binding to high-affinity IgE receptors on mast cells.

Strongest Antihistamine?
Studies comparing inhibition of the wheal and flare response of injected histamine have demonstrated that of the nonsedating antihistamines such as cetirizine is more effective than terfenadine, epinastine, ebastine, fexofenadine, and loratadine. Despite the evidence provided by the experimental model, the clinical relevance of the findings was challenged.

Note that the term *nonsedating* is not always accurate, because some patients will note variable sedation with these drugs. The weaker sedation observed in this class of drugs is due to lowered crossing of the blood-brain barrier, at least relative to classic sedating antihistamines.

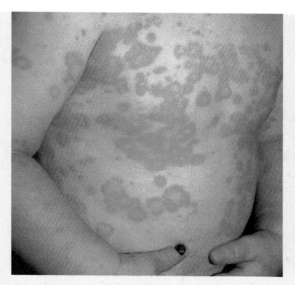

Fig. 5.1. Acute urticaria in a child from an unknown cause. Some lesions maintain an annular appearance. (From the Fitzsimons Army Medical Center Collection, Aurora, CO.)

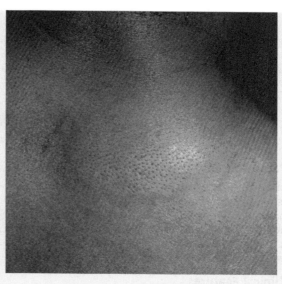

Fig. 5.2. Large lesion of urticaria demonstrating a dimpled appearance due to dermal edema *(peau d'orange)*.

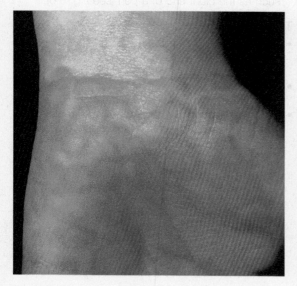

Fig. 5.3. Patient with acute urticaria of the palm from an unknown cause. The location suggests possible pressure urticaria. (From the Fitzsimons Army Medical Center Collection, Aurora, CO.)

The Physical Urticarias
- Aquagenic urticaria: L50.8
- Cholinergic urticaria: L50.5
- Cold urticaria: L50.2
- Dermatographism: L50.3
- Pressure urticaria: L50.8
- Solar urticaria: L50.8
- Vibratory urticaria: L50.6

Pathogenesis

In physical urticarias (see box), the wheal and flare response is a result of cutaneous physical stimuli (e.g., pressure, heat, cold). Physical urticaria accounts for about 15% to 20% of all cases. Dermatographism and cholinergic urticaria are the most common physical urticarias.

Clinical Features

- Clinical features depend on the type of physical urticaria:
  - Aquagenic urticaria is a rare variant confined to sites of water exposure.
  - Cholinergic urticaria is relatively common and is caused by heat and sweating. It results in small (1- to 4-mm) papules on the trunk and proximal extremities (Fig. 5.4). Patients often report that the condition is precipitated by warm showers, exercise, and emotional stress.
  - Cold urticaria is an uncommon variant caused by cold exposure (Fig. 5.5). In some cases, angioedema may be associated. In extreme circumstances, anaphylaxis may ensue. The condition is present in 1 in 2000 adults.
  - Dermatographism (Fig. 5.6) is characterized by red linear indurated streaks with stroking of the skin.
  - Solar urticaria occurs on photoexposed skin. It usually occurs within minutes to 1 hour of sun exposure, which differs from other photosensitive conditions, such as polymorphous light eruption, which is more delayed (Fig. 5.7).

Diagnosis

- The diagnosis of cholinergic urticaria, the most common form of physical urticaria, requires clinical correlation about precipitating factors with the small size of the lesions. In addition to pruritus, cholinergic urticaria typically produces a subtle stinging sensation.
- Cold urticaria is diagnosed by the ice cube test, in which an ice cube is applied to the skin for 2 to 5 minutes, with re-examination at 10-minute intervals (Fig. 5.5). Test sensitivity is about 85%, but the specificity is nearly 100%.
- Dermatographism is easily diagnosed by wheals produced by firmly stroking the skin with an object such as the blunt end of a pen (see Fig. 5.6).

Treatment

- Cold urticaria is treated with avoidance of exposure. Remember that angioedema and anaphylaxis can occur and can even be fatal.
- Cholinergic urticaria is treated with avoidance of activities that cause undue overheating.
- All forms of physical urticaria may be treated with antihistamines, as discussed for simple urticaria.

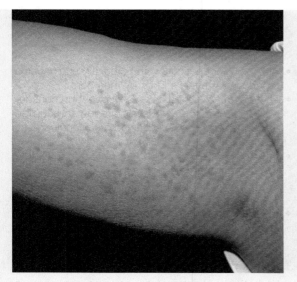

Fig. 5.4. Patient with small urticarial uniform papules characteristic of cholinergic urticaria. (From the Fitzsimons Army Medical Center Collection, Aurora, CO.)

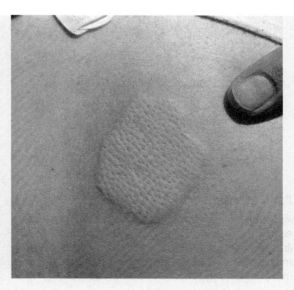

Fig. 5.5. Wheal produced by an ice cube in a patient with cold urticaria. (From the Fitzsimons Army Medical Center Collection, Aurora, CO.)

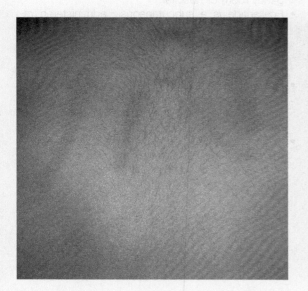

Fig. 5.6. Patient with dermatographism. Linear wheals of the back are created by stroking the skin with a pen.

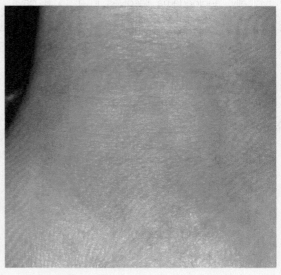

Fig. 5.7. Patient with solar urticaria on the back of the hand. (From the Fitzsimons Army Medical Center Collection, Aurora, CO.)

Classification of Angioedema

Hereditary
Acquired
- Acquired C1 esterase inhibitor (C1-INH) deficiency
- Allergic
- Drug-induced
  - Angiotensin-converting enzyme (ACE) inhibitors
  - Penicillin
  - Nonsteroidal antiinflammatory drugs (NSAIDs)
- Malignancy

Pathogenesis

Angioedema is characterized by deeply situated edema of the lower dermis and/or subcutaneous tissue (including the submucosa). Although some patients may present with both urticaria and angioedema, in many cases angioedema occurs in isolation.

Clinical Features

- Sudden localized swelling of skin and/or mucosal surfaces is seen, usually without a wheal and flare reaction (Figs. 5.8 and 5.9).
- Typically, angioedema resolves in 1 to 3 days, without permanent sequelae.
- Involvement of the respiratory tract can be fatal, but this is more common in hereditary angioedema (see below).
- Abdominal pain due to edema of the bowel wall can be severe, but this is also more common in hereditary angioedema (see below).

Diagnosis

- The presence of coexisting urticaria is an important finding. Nearly all patients with hereditary angioedema have the condition in isolation. Patients with acquired disease often have both angioedema and urticaria at the same time.
- About 80% of patients with hereditary angioedema report similar attacks in family members.
- The serum C4 level is a sensitive but nonspecific screening tool. C4 levels are low in acquired angioedema and in hereditary forms of angioedema caused by C1-INH deficiency.
- Therefore, if a low level of C4 is detected, quantitative (type I) and functional (type II) C1-INH studies should be commissioned to refine the diagnosis further.
- Mast cell tryptase levels are usually normal in hereditary angioedema but may be elevated in acquired forms.

Treatment

- Intubation or tracheostomy may be necessary in patients with severe laryngeal edema and respiratory distress.
- Severe attacks need to be observed in the emergency room or hospital.
- Ecallantide is a subcutaneously administered recombinant plasma kallikrein inhibitor. However, it must be administered in a controlled environment because anaphylactic reactions to the drug have been reported.
- Icatibant is a bradykinin B2 receptor antagonist that is given subcutaneously and may even be self-administered by the patient during an acute attack.
- Danazol was used as a prophylactic treatment in the past, but it has now largely been replaced by more effective and safer treatments.

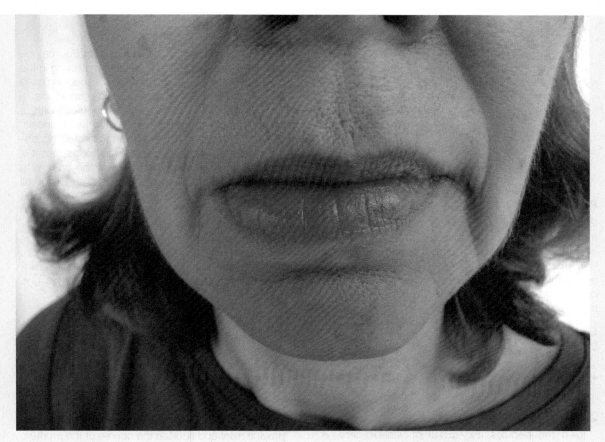

Fig. 5.8. Patient with mild acquired angioedema of the lips that was unassociated with urticaria. The cause was never identified.

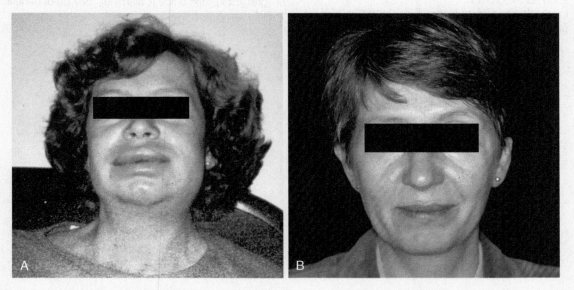

Fig. 5.9 A, Hereditary angioedema in a patient during an acute attack. The photograph was taken by the patient at home. B, Same patient as seen between attacks. (From the Fitzsimons Army Medical Center Collection, Aurora, CO.)

Arthropods That Frequently Cause Papular Urticaria

- Bedbugs
- Black flies *(Simulium)*
- Chiggers
- Deerflies
- Fleas
- Lice
- Midges
- Mites
- Mosquitoes

Pathogenesis

Papular urticaria is defined as an urticarial reaction that persists for longer than 24 hours at the site of an insect or arthropod bite. If a papule lasts for less than 24 hours at the site, it is simply insect- or arthropod-induced urticaria. Papular urticaria and bullous insect—arthropod—bite reactions differ only in the intensity of the reaction.

Clinical Features

- Lesions may be single or multiple and are usually located on exposed skin.
- Typically, lesions consist of 2- to 10-mm erythematous red papules (Fig. 5.10). Less often, the lesions are larger (Fig. 5.11).
- Lesions may resolve within hours or may become fixed red papules (Fig. 5.12) of variable size. A central punctum may sometimes be identified.
- Papular urticaria often demonstrates a tendency to become more pruritic and urticate with trauma, such as excoriation.
- Later changes include scaling, central erosion or ulceration, and a brown-red color (Fig. 5.13).

Diagnosis

- Patients may suspect the diagnosis and/or may be aware of the source. Some patients may bring in the insect or arthropod. In the last decade, bedbug bites in particular have reached epidemic proportions.
- The presence of erythematous papules, with a central punctum, are consistent with the diagnosis.
- In some situations, other similarly affected household members may support the diagnosis, but it is important to realize that this is not the case with all insects and arthropods. For example, not all persons react to bedbug bites, and two people, both living in an infested environment, may not each demonstrate bite reactions.
- A 3- or 4-mm punch biopsy that extends to the subcutaneous fat may provide strong evidence, because bite reactions very often manifest eosinophils in the deepest aspects of the dermis and subcutis.

Treatment

- Most lesions are self-limited, but in the case of ongoing exposure (e.g., bedbug infestation), professional extermination services will be necessary.
- For some infestations (e.g., fleas), destruction of infested fomites or treatment of family pets may be necessary.
- Potent topical corticosteroids to affected areas may provide relief and shorten the course of the pruritus.
- Antihistamines may be used for pruritus.
- Other topical medications containing antipruritic agents (e.g., menthol and camphor [Sarna], prasugrel [Prax], zinc oxide [Calamine]) may be of benefit.

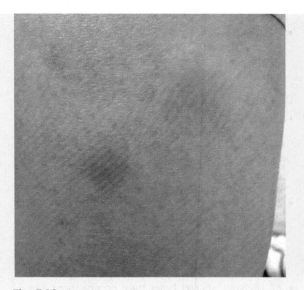

Fig. 5.10. Papular urticaria in an adult due to mosquito bites.

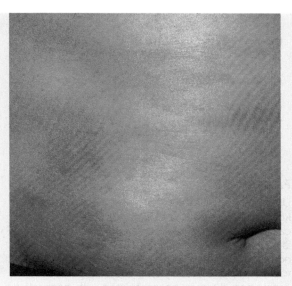

Fig. 5.11. Papular urticaria with large wheals occurring in a child and with an unknown cause. (From the William Weston Collection, Aurora, CO.)

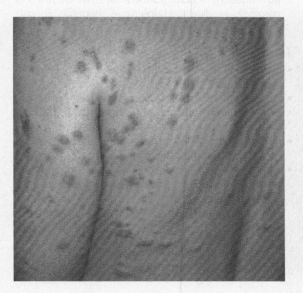

Fig. 5.12. Patient with older lesions of papular urticaria, with some lesions in lines, as is typically seen in some bite reactions. (From the Fitzsimons Army Medical Center Collection, Aurora, CO.)

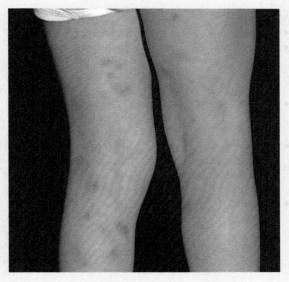

Fig. 5.13. Patient with resolving lesions of papular urticaria, with brownish color and focal scaling. (From the William Weston Collection, Aurora, CO.)

Drugs Reported to Cause Urticarial Vasculitis
- Chewing gum preservative
- Enalapril
- Fluoxetine (Prozac)
- Glimepiride
- Paroxetine (Paxil)
- Procainamide
- Trimethoprim-sulfamethoxazole

Pathogenesis

Urticarial vasculitis is a low-grade, small-vessel, leukocytoclastic (neutrophil-mediated) vasculitis. Clinically, the condition resembles urticaria. The disease is subdivided into patients with urticarial vasculitis and normal complement levels and patients with urticarial vasculitis and low complement levels. Cases of urticarial vasculitis may be associated with connective tissue disease (e.g., systemic lupus erythematosus [SLE], Sjögren syndrome), infections (e.g., hepatitis B and C), malignancies (e.g., multiple myeloma) and drugs (see box).

Clinical Features

- Urticarial vasculitis is more common in women.
- Patients may demonstrate three types of primary lesions, including classic urticaria (Fig. 5.14) lesions, angioedema, and fixed urticarial plaques that last longer than 24 hours.
- Patients frequently complain of burning or a combination of burning and itching rather than itching alone.
- Primary lesions are often fixed erythematous plaques (lasting >24 hours at a specific location), with central clearing, focal hemorrhage, or central discoloration (Fig. 5.15).
- Individual lesions usually last 3 to 7 days, but some may persist longer.

- Systemic findings often include malaise, low-grade fever, arthralgias, and arthritis. Less often, there is lymphadenopathy, hepatosplenomegaly, gastrointestinal disturbances, and upper airway symptoms.

Diagnosis

- Fixed urticarial plaques, lasting longer than 24 hours, should arouse suspicion for urticarial vasculitis. Moreover, if the patient relates a burning sensation, this also supports that diagnosis. In some cases, lesions demonstrate a focal hemorrhage or red-brown or yellow color due to hemosiderin.
- A 3- or 4-mm punch biopsy should be performed to determine the diagnosis. However, the diagnostic features may be missed in a single biopsy. Sometimes, more than one biopsy will be necessary to establish the diagnosis. In some cases, direct immunofluorescence studies may be helpful.
- All patients should have their complement levels determined because this is a major branch point in disease classification.
- If no cause is immediately apparent, laboratory investigations should include ANA-ENA studies and serologic studies for hepatitis A, hepatitis B, and Epstein-Barr virus infections.

Treatment

- Withdraw any drugs that may cause urticarial vasculitis.
- Antihistamines are often used, particularly in patients with coexisting urticaria and angioedema, but this treatment is not useful for fixed plaques.
- Oral prednisone, 20 to 80 mg/day (depending on severity), is used for acute management.
- Steroid-sparing medications used in chronic management include hydroxychloroquine, dapsone, azathioprine, colchicine, and sometimes indomethacin, although NSAIDs sometimes cause simple urticaria.

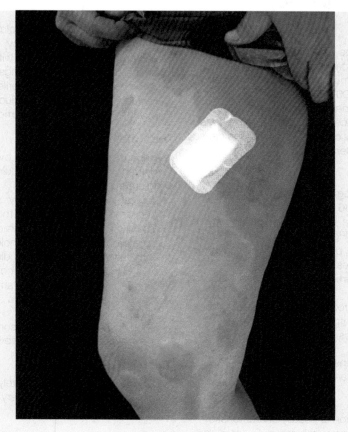

Fig. 5.14. Large urticarial wheals on the leg in a patient with urticarial vasculitis. These wheals are indistinguishable from those of urticaria, and the diagnosis was established by biopsy.

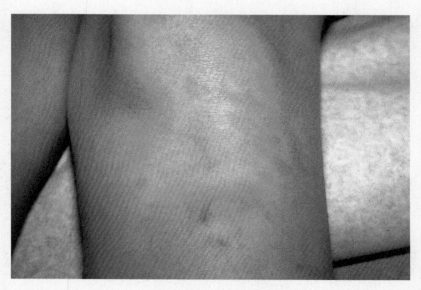

Fig. 5.15. Patient with urticarial vasculitis. In this case, in addition to the wheals, there were several areas of yellow-brown dyspigmentation, which suggests hemorrhage. This finding is suspicious for urticarial vasculitis.

INTERNAL ETIOLOGY

Pathogenesis

Pruritic urticarial papules and plaques of pregnancy (PUPPP), also called *polymorphic eruption of pregnancy,* is the most common dermatosis of pregnancy. It occurs in about 1 in 200 pregnancies. The condition is more common in women with a male fetus, women with rapid and pronounced weight gain, and women who ultimately deliver by cesarean section. The cause of PUPPP is poorly understood.

Clinical Features

- Typically, PUPPP begins in the third trimester (average onset is at 36 weeks gestation).
- Often, PUPPP begins in the striae gravidarum of the lower abdomen (Fig. 5.16) and over time may spread to the thighs, proximal arms, low back, or even more distant sites.
- Primary lesions are urticarial papules and plaques (Figs. 5.17–5.19).
- Less often, there are focal vesicular or eczematous features or even targetoid lesions.
- Unusual morphologies are observed later in the course of disease.
- PUPPP is usually intensely pruritic.
- Mucous membranes are not involved.

Diagnosis

- The clinical presentation is usually characteristic.
- Occasional patients may require a 3- or 4-mm punch biopsy to exclude herpes gestationis, a variant of bullous pemphigoid occurring during or immediately after pregnancy. Typically, the biopsy shows features consistent with PUPPP, but there are no pathognomonic findings of only that disorder.
- A biopsy of uninvolved perilesional skin may be needed for direct immunofluorescence studies to exclude herpes gestationis more definitively.

Treatment

- Because the lesions resolve over 1 to 3 weeks after delivery, no treatment is required if the patient can tolerate the condition.
- Topical corticosteroids may reduce pruritus and erythema but do not alter the course of disease. Usually, a moderate-strength or strong topical corticosteroid is used (triamcinolone or fluocinolone), with patients typically responding within 2 to 4 days.
- Oral H1 antihistamines are considered safe during pregnancy, and diphenhydramine is often used to relieve pruritus and provide a sedative effect before bed.
- Short courses of oral prednisone (10–40 mg/day for 3–7 days) are reserved for severe cases.

Clinical Course

Most cases resolve completely, without sequelae, within 1 to 3 weeks after delivery. There are no known harmful effects on the fetus.

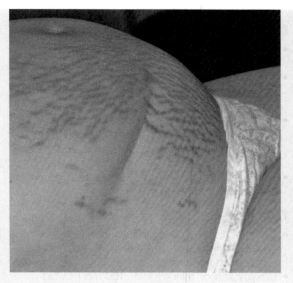

Fig. 5.16. Early PUPPP in a primigravida woman with involvement of the striae. (From the John Aeling Collection, Aurora, CO.)

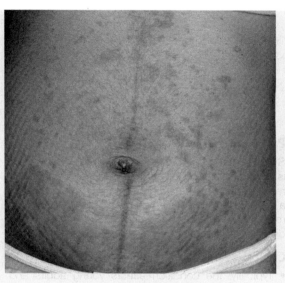

Fig. 5.17. Patient with PUPPP demonstrating urticarial papules and plaques. Note accentuation in the striae. (From the William Weston Collection, Aurora, CO.)

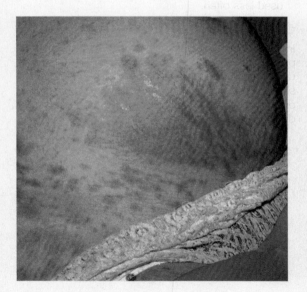

Fig. 5.18. Patient with urticarial plaques developing in the striae, associated with smaller papular lesions. (From the Fitzsimons Army Medical Center Collection, Aurora, CO.)

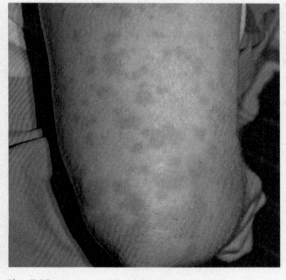

Fig. 5.19. Patient with urticarial papules and plaques on the arm and elbow. (From the Fitzsimons Army Medical Center Collection, Aurora, CO.)

Drugs Frequently Implicated in Sweet Syndrome
- Abacavir
- Granulocyte colony-stimulating factor (G-CSF)
- Lenalidomide
- Minocycline
- Trimethoprim-sulfamethoxazole

Pathogenesis

Sweet syndrome (acute febrile neutrophilic dermatosis) is a neutrophilic condition that yields an urticaria-like reaction pattern. The condition may be precipitated by a variety of insults, including medications, underlying malignancy (myeloid and solid tumors), autoimmune disorders, inflammatory bowel disease, and infection.

Clinical Features

- Typically, the condition affects young adults and geriatric patients; children are rarely affected.
- The condition is more common in women than men.
- Symptoms of an upper respiratory syndrome or malignancy are present in many patients.
- The primary lesion is a tender, round to oval, erythematous papule or plaque (Figs. 5.20–5.22).
- The condition usually affects the distal extremities and acral areas.
- Some patients may demonstrate a pseudovesicular (juicy) edge, frank pustules, or even ulceration (Fig. 5.23).
- Systemic findings include fever, malaise, arthralgias and/or arthritis, conjunctivitis, and oral lesions that resemble aphthous ulcers.

Diagnosis

- Because the clinical findings are rather nonspecific, a biopsy is usually recommended.
- A CBC may demonstrate neutrophilia, and neutropenia in the setting of Sweet syndrome is more concerning for an associated lymphoid malignancy.
- Antibodies to neutrophil cytoplasmic antigens, antineutrophil cytoplasmic antibodies (ANCAs), are demonstrated in about 80% of cases, and the ESR can also be elevated.
- A 3- or 4-mm punch biopsy is often suggestive or even diagnostic of the condition.

Treatment

- Oral prednisone, with an initial dose of 20 to 60 mg/day, tapering over 2 to 4 weeks, is the most commonly used treatment.
- Doxycycline or minocycline, 100 mg PO bid for 2 to 6 weeks, can also be used.
- Indomethacin, 100 to 150 mg/day for 1 to 3 weeks, can also be used.
- Colchicine and dapsone are alternatives that are used less often.

Clinical Course

In most cases, Sweet syndrome resolves over a period of weeks, without sequelae. Patients who do not respond to therapy or who have neutropenia should be evaluated for an underlying systemic disorder (e.g., myelogenous leukemia, connective tissue disorder, inflammatory bowel disease).

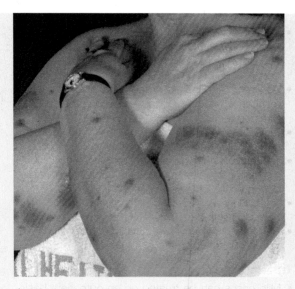

Fig. 5.20. Patient with numerous erythematous papules and plaques affecting the upper extremities. (From the Fitzsimons Army Medical Center Collection, Aurora, CO.)

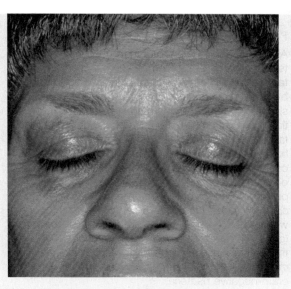

Fig. 5.21. Patient with Sweet syndrome, with urticarial lesions secondary to acute myelogenous leukemia. (From the Fitzsimons Army Medical Center Collection, Aurora, CO.)

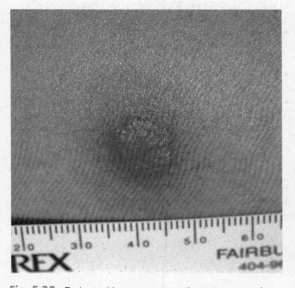

Fig. 5.22. Patient with numerous erythematous papules and plaques affecting the upper extremities. (From the William Weston Collection, Aurora, CO.)

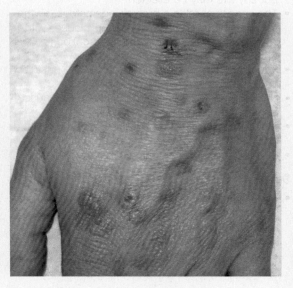

Fig. 5.23. Patient with numerous erythematous papules and small plaques, with some lesions demonstrating central crusting.

Pathogenesis

Although *cellulitis* is a broad term used for many bacterial infections of the dermis and subcutis, **erysipelas** is a specific clinical variant of facial cellulitis caused by *Streptococcus* spp. Erysipelas is characterized by sharply indurated, erythematous plaques with a distinct edge that results from lymphatic drainage of the face. Most cases are the result of the inoculation of bacteria through miniscule breaks in the skin. Rare cases are due to seeding of the skin from another distant nidus of infection (e.g., a dental abscess). The primary cause of erysipelas in adults is *Streptococcus pyogenes* (group A β-hemolytic streptococci), whereas in newborns it is *Streptococcus agalactiae* (group B streptococcus). Nonstreptococcal species that can produce erysipelas-like infection include *Haemophilus* spp., *Staphylococcus aureus,* and, rarely, gram-negative bacteria.

Clinical Features

- Erysipelas most often affects children or older adults, but those in any age group may be affected.
- Most erysipelas involves the central face (Fig. 5.24), but any site may be affected.
- The condition yields a brawny, edematous, erythematous, *peau d'orange*–appearing plaque, with a sharply demarcated (so-called cliff drop) edge (Figs. 5.25–5.27).
- Edema of the eyelids, vesicles, bullae, pustules, and/or petechiae may be present.
- Regional tender lymphadenopathy (i.e., preauricular) is often present.
- Systemic symptoms, including fever, chills, and prostration, are commonly present.
- Streptococcal cellulitis may be recurrent.

Diagnosis

- The diagnosis is usually based on the clinical presentation of an area of red tender induration that is often unilateral. The presence of tender regional lymphadenopathy is also supportive.

- A 3- or 4-mm punch biopsy is typically more sensitive than aspirations or blood cultures. The biopsy should be divided, with half being cultured and half undergoing routine histologic examination.
- Aspiration and culture of the edge yields a positive result in 4% to 50% of cases, whereas blood cultures are positive in only 10% of cases.
- A CBC may often demonstrate leukocytosis of more than 10,000 cells/mm^3 or a left shift.
- Serologic tests (e.g., antistreptolysin O titer [ASOT]) are of limited value because antibodies are not produced early in the course of the infection.
- Anti-DNase B assays are superior to the ASOT in detecting skin streptococcal infection.
- Response to appropriate antibiotic therapy is rapid, with rapid improvement in 48 hours.

Treatment

- Mild cases can be treated on an outpatient basis, but severe cases, especially those with central facial involvement, may require hospitalization. Diabetic or immunocompromised patients may also require admission.
- Mild cases may be managed on an outpatient basis with oral cephalexin (Keflex), dicloxacillin, erythromycin, clarithromycin, or azithromycin.
- Intravenous (IV) alternatives include cefazolin, 250 mg to 1 g IV or IM every 6 to 8 hours, depending severity of infection.
- Severe cases should be treated with IV nafcillin or oxacillin (1–2 g IV q 4h).
- Penicillin, often listed in the older literature, is no longer a wise choice because some cases of cellulitis caused by staphylococcal species have been noted. However, it may be used once culture and sensitivity studies have returned.

Clinical Course

In the preantibiotic era, the mortality rate was reported to be as high as 40%.

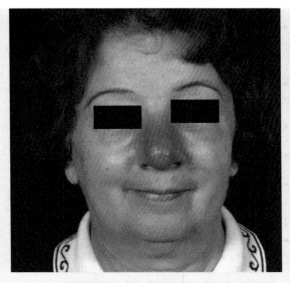

Fig. 5.24. Patient with erysipelas. Shown is a painful central, tender, red indurated plaque affecting the nose on the left nasolabial fold. (From the Fitzsimons Army Medical Center Collection, Aurora, CO.)

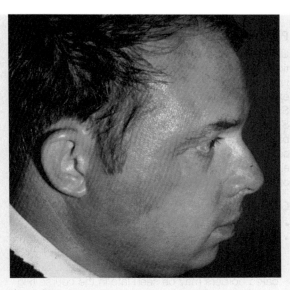

Fig. 5.25. Patient with erysipelas. Shown is a unilateral red, tender, edematous plaque. The patient also had a tender, enlarged, right preauricular lymph node. (From the Fitzsimons Army Medical Center Collection, Aurora, CO.)

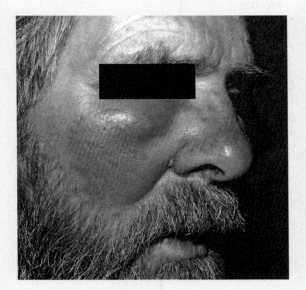

Fig. 5.26. Patient with erysipelas demonstrating a sharply demarcated red tender plaque of the nose and left cheek.

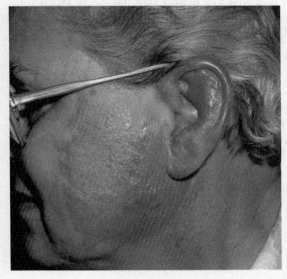

Fig. 5.27. Patient with erysipelas demonstrating a sharply demarcated tender plaque of the left side of the face, with involvement of the ear. (From the Fitzsimons Army Medical Center Collection, Aurora, CO.)

Pathogenesis

Cellulitis is a broad term that includes bacterial infections (rarely, fungal infections may mimic this pattern), which primarily affect the dermis and, to a lesser extent, the subcutis. The most common causes are *S. pyogenes* (group A β-hemolytic streptococci), *S. aureus,* and several species of gram-negative bacteria. Lymphangitis is a frequent component of cellulitis—hence the lay term *blood poisoning.* Erysipelas, facial streptococcal cellulitis, is a clinical subset of cellulitis that has been discussed earlier.

Clinical Features

- It may affect any age group.
- The primary lesion is a tender area of erythematous induration that usually demonstrates an indistinct border early on (Fig. 5.28); however, sharply demarcated borders may be seen late in the course (Fig. 5.29).
- In some cases, the site of introduction due to the break in the skin may be evident; it may vary from a small pustule (see Fig. 5.28) to an abscess or even an ulcer.
- Lymphangitis presents as linear ill-defined areas of erythema that extend from the site of infection to the regional lymph nodes (Fig. 5.30).
- Edema may be a prominent feature when an extremity or the genitalia are involved (Fig. 5.31).
- The regional lymph nodes may be enlarged and tender.
- Systemic symptoms may include malaise, fever, and anorexia.

Diagnosis

- The diagnosis is usually based on the clinical presentation of an area of red tender induration, which is often unilateral. The presence of lymphangitis and tender regional lymphadenopathy is also supportive.

- A 3- or 4-mm punch biopsy is typically more sensitive than aspirations or blood cultures. The biopsy should be divided, with half being cultured and half undergoing routine histologic examination.
- Aspiration and culture of the edge yields a positive result in 4% to 50% of cases, whereas blood cultures are positive in only 10% of cases.
- A CBC may often demonstrate leukocytosis of more than 10,000 cells/mm^3 or a left shift.
- Serologic tests are of limited value because many infections are not streptococcal.
- Response to appropriate antibiotic therapy is rapid, with improvement in 48 hours.

Treatment

- Mild cases can be treated on an outpatient basis; however, many cases will require hospitalization. Diabetic or immunocompromised patients are especially strong candidates for admission.
- Mild cases may be managed on an outpatient basis with oral cephalexin (Keflex), dicloxacillin, erythromycin, clarithromycin, or azithromycin.
- IV alternatives include cefazolin, 250 mg to 1 g every 6 hours, depending on the severity of the infection.
- Severe cases should be treated with IV nafcillin or oxacillin (1–2 ga q4h).
- As always, the culture and sensitivity results may dictate a change in therapy.

Clinical Course

The mortality rate in the antibiotic era is difficult to calculate; however, it has been estimated that there are about 30,000 deaths from cellulitis worldwide every year.

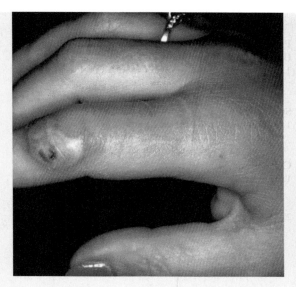

Fig. 5.28. Patient with staphylococcal cellulitis, with a large pustule at the site of injury, ill-defined painful erythema, and induration.

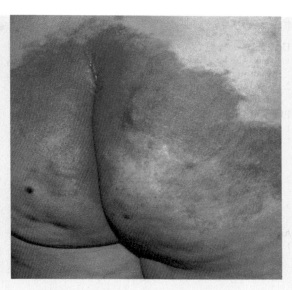

Fig. 5.29. Sharply defined cellulitis of the buttock region in a hospitalized patient. A biopsy failed to identify an organism; however, the patient responded to IV antibiotics.

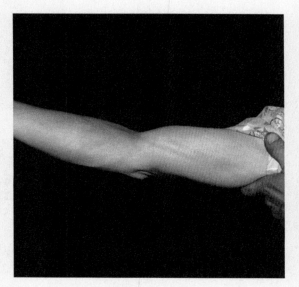

Fig. 5.30. Patient with streptococcal cellulitis of the finger and hand demonstrating lymphangitis extending into the axilla. (From the Fitzsimons Army Medical Center Collection, Aurora, CO.)

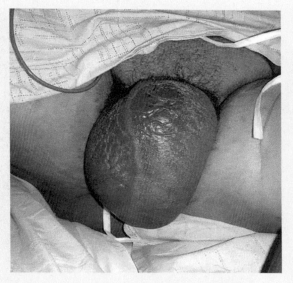

Fig. 5.31. Patient with cellulitis of the anogenital region due to *Escherichia coli*. This patient demonstrated significant systemic symptoms and required a biopsy for culture and sensitivities in addition to hospitalization.

References

Urticaria
1. Guldbakke KK, Khachemoune A. Etiology, classification, and treatment of urticaria. *Cutis*. 2007;79:41-49.
2. Soter NA. Treatment of chronic spontaneous urticaria. *J Drugs Dermatol*. 2015;14:332-334.

Physical Urticarias
1. Borzova E, Rutherford A, Konstantinou N, et al. Narrowband ultraviolet B phototherapy is beneficial for antihistamine-resistant symptomatic dermographism. A pilot study. *J Am Acad Dermatol*. 2008;59:752-757.
2. Botto NC, Warshaw EM. Solar urticaria. *J Am Acad Dermatol*. 2008;59:909-920.
3. Singleton R, Halverstam CP. Diagnosis and management of cold urticaria. *Cutis*. 2016;97:59-62.

Angioedema
1. Parish LC. Hereditary angioedema: diagnosis and management—a perspective for the dermatologist. *J Am Acad Dermatol*. 2011; 65:843-850.

Pruritic Urticarial Papules and Plaques of Pregnancy (Polymorphic Eruption of Pregnancy)
1. Regnier S, Fermand V, Levy P, et al. A case-control study of polymorphic eruption of pregnancy. *J Am Acad Dermatol*. 2008;58:63-67.

Sweet Syndrome
1. Rochet NM, Chavan RN, Cappel MA, et al. Sweet syndrome: clinical presentation, associations, and response to treatment in 77 patients. *J Am Acad Dermatol*. 2013;69:557-564.

Cellulitis and Erysipelas
1. Hirschmann JV, Raugi GJ. Lower limb cellulitis and its mimics. Part I. Lower limb cellulitis. *J Am Acad Dermatol*. 2012;67:163-174.
2. Morris AD. Cellulitis and erysipelas. *BMJ Clin Evid*. 2008 Jan2;2008.

Chapter 6
Papular Eruptions: No Scale

Differential Diagnosis of Papular Eruptions
- Bedbug bites
- Chiggers
- Fox-Fordyce disease
- Gianotti-Crosti syndrome
- Miliaria
- Mite bites (or bites of other insects or arthropods)
- Papular eczema (see atopic dermatitis)
- Papular drug eruptions
- Scabies

Although papular eruptions are not always listed as a separate clinical category in dermatology texts, there are some diseases that present with a decidedly papular quality. Moreover, whereas some diseases remain papular over time (e.g., insect and arthropod bite reactions), other skin conditions may present in a polymorphic fashion, with papules that coalesce into plaques.

IMPORTANT HISTORY QUESTIONS

How long have the papules (bumps) been present?
Acute presentations are typical of viral exanthems, id reactions, and acute drug eruptions, whereas a more chronic course favors papular atopic dermatitis, repetitive or chronic insect or arthropod bite reactions, or a prolonged or chronic drug reaction.

Did all the papules (bumps) start at the same time?
Some papular conditions present as a single wave of lesions (e.g., Gianotti-Crosti syndrome), whereas others present as crops of lesions in different phases (insect, arthropod reactions), and yet others present as continuous or seemingly random eruptions (e.g., papular atopic dermatitis).

Have you had a similar rash in the past?
An affirmative response favors exacerbation of a chronic condition (e.g., atopic dermatitis) or a repeat exposure to an exogenous agent or external trigger (e.g., insect or arthropod bite reactions, miliaria).

Where did the rash start?
Determining the area that was first involved may suggest a cause. The involvement of extremities that protrude from the bedsheets may suggest bedbugs, and involvement of the lower extremities after outdoor activities may suggest chiggers; a photodistribution may suggest polymorphous light eruption.

Have you or your immediate relatives had eczema, asthma, or hay fever (seasonal allergies)?
An affirmative response may suggest an atopic diathesis, leading to the consideration of papular atopic dermatitis.

What sort of work do you do?
Certain occupations predispose a person to insect or arthropod bite reactions (e.g., grocers, animal handlers or groomers, veterinarians, hotel and hospitality industry workers).

How do you feel?
Systemic symptoms such as fever, malaise, sore throat, or others may suggest a viral infection.

Have you started any new medications in the last month?
Papular drug eruptions are uncommon but are reversible with discontinuance.

How are you treating this rash?
Over-the-counter treatments, home remedies, or even some prescription medications may improve or worsen a papular dermatitis. This important information will guide the diagnosis and immediate care.

What do you think caused your rash?
This is an obvious question that is often overlooked—some patients may have keen insight into their condition.

IMPORTANT PHYSICAL FINDINGS

What is the distribution of the papules?
Some papular lesions have distinct distributions. Scabies preferentially affects the wrist, intertriginous areas, and genitalia, whereas chiggers preferentially occurs beneath areas of the skin where clothing is in close contact. Gianotti-Crosti, on the other hand, tends to affect acral areas.

Are any linear lesions present?
Scabies burrows are short linear lesions that can be a diagnostic clue in an otherwise enigmatic pruritic papular dermatitis.

Pathogenesis

Scabies is caused by the human scabies mite, *Sarcoptes scabiei* var. *hominis*. It is acquired chiefly by skin to skin contact, usually between family members and sexual partners. Although mites remain viable in bed linens for up to 96 hours, most infestations are not acquired from fomites. The pruritus of a scabies infestation is caused by an allergic response to mite antigens in their saliva, eggs, and feces (scybala).

Clinical Features

- Symptoms occur within 1 to 6 weeks after a first infestation and 1 to 3 days after a repeat infestation.
- Patients typically complain of marked generalized pruritus that is more pronounced at night.
- Primary lesions are usually found in the axillae, wrists, interdigital spaces, and groin. It has been found that 80% of all cases present with evidence on the wrists and interdigital webs of the hands.
- Other commonly affected areas include the nipples, beltline, umbilicus, and buttocks.
- The lesions of scabies often appear as follows:
  - Papules—1- to 3-mm erythematous papules; these are typically numerous (Figs. 6.1 and 6.2).
  - Nodules—5- to 10-mm red or red-brown nodules that are often found on the penis (Fig. 6.3)
  - Burrows—1- to 5-mm threadlike linear or serpiginous forms, with varying erythema and scale. The adult mite may appear as a gray fleck at the end of the burrow (Fig. 6.4).
  - Atypical lesions—pustules may occur on the acral surfaces of infants and toddlers or as psoriasiform hyperkeratotic plaques in immunocompromised and/or mentally impaired individuals (crusted, Norwegian scabies).

Diagnosis

- Scabies should be in the differential diagnosis for any patient with pruritus and numerous papules.
- The diagnosis is substantiated by recognition of a burrow and performance of a scabies prep (see

Chapter 2) to identify the mite, eggs, or scybala. A skin biopsy (usually a shave) can be performed in an attempt to recognize the same structures, but the results will be delayed by days.
- Even though a patient may have hundreds of papular lesions, in a typical case there are only 10 to 15 adult mites on the entire body, and a skin scraping or biopsy may not encapture diagnostic evidence.
- If microscopic evidence cannot be demonstrated by a skin scraping or skin biopsy, a response to appropriate empiric treatment may be diagnostic.

Treatment

- Topical permethrin, 5% cream, is a first-line agent for treating scabies. It is applied to the whole body, from the neck down, left on the skin for 8 hours (overnight), and then washed off in the shower. A second treatment a week later may be needed to eradicate all mites.
- Precipitated sulfur (10%) may be applied to the whole body, from the neck down, for 3 consecutive days. The use of sulfur was once advocated for pregnant women, although many literature reviews on the subject have expressed no reservations regarding the use of permethrin, 5% cream.
- Topical 1% lindane lotion is now a second- or third-line agent but should not be used in children or pregnant women. It is banned entirely in California.
- Crotamiton, 10% cream, is not as effective as other therapies, with resistance reported.
- Oral ivermectin use has been increasing, with 200 µg/kg of body weight given as a single dose. Because it is not an ovicide, many experts advocate giving a second dose 1 week later. Oral ivermectin may be used with topical permethrin 5% cream in recalcitrant cases. The safety of oral ivermectin use during pregnancy has not been established.
- Although there are little data to support it, all clothing and linens should be decontaminated by machine washing in hot water and drying using a hot cycle.

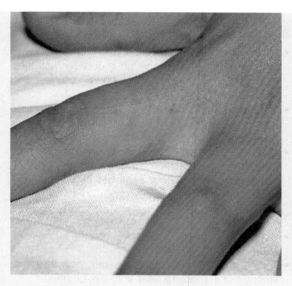

Fig. 6.1. Hand of a patient with scabies. There are small erythematous papules of the intertriginous space, a characteristic location. (From the William Weston Collection, Aurora, CO.)

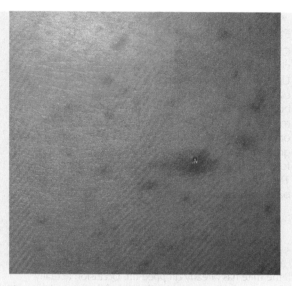

Fig. 6.2. Patient with scabies. There are small erythematous papules of the trunk, with one lesion demonstrating an excoriation.

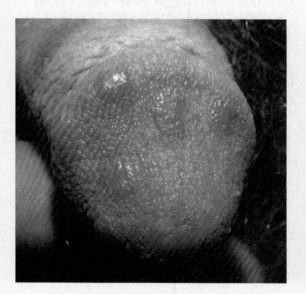

Fig. 6.3. Patient with so-called nodular scabies. The name is somewhat of a misnomer because most lesions are large papules. These diagnostic lesions are almost exclusively seen on the head of the penis.

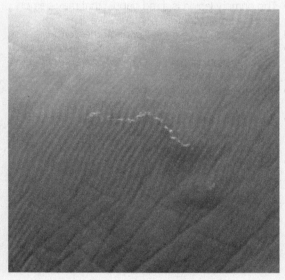

Fig. 6.4. Scabies burrows. There is a small, new linear burrow on the bottom and an older burrow on the top. (From the Fitzsimons Army Medical Center Collection, Aurora, CO.)

Chiggers (Trombiculosis) ICD10 code B88.0

Pathogenesis

Chigger bites are caused by the larval stage of certain species of trombiculid mites (Fig. 6.5). In the United States, the predominant species is *Trombicula alfreddugesi,* and chiggers occur chiefly in the humid portions of the Midwest and Southeast. The red six-legged larvae lie in ambush on blades of grass or other short vegetation (typically, <15 inches off the ground), leap onto a passing host, and attach and feed for 3 to 4 days before dropping to the ground. The chigger is smaller than 1 mm in size and can barely be seen by the human eye.

Patient Myth

Many patients have been taught by their families and friends to treat chigger bites with nail polish or various glues to suffocate the mite. In many cases, the mite has already dropped off. Occlusion actually increases heat retention at the site of the bite, which will increase pruritus. The only potential benefit is that the polish or glue will reduce skin damage from excoriations.

Clinical Features

- The primary lesion is a red papule that may demonstrate a small, central, punctum-like area.
- Marked pruritus is a near-constant feature.
- Lesions occur in crops and are notoriously grouped on the ankles, behind the knees, or along points of pressure or contact of clothing (Figs. 6.6–6.8).
- Patients with considerable sensitivity to chigger bites may develop bullous lesions, but this is uncommon.
- Secondary excoriation may be more impressive than the primary lesion and may lead to persistent papules or superimposed prurigo nodules.
- Secondary bacterial infection may also occur.

Diagnosis

- A clinical history of discrete erythematous papules, in appropriate areas, and after outdoor activities in an endemic area, should strongly suggest the diagnosis.
- Chiggers are found chiefly in the southeastern and south central United States and are not present in the Rocky Mountains.
- Skin scrapings may demonstrate the mite on rare occasion, but because the organism is only present transiently and does not complete its life cycle on humans, this is not typically used.

Treatment

- No treatment is reasonable because the lesions are self-limited.
- Topical products with pramoxine may provide some limited but immediate relief from the pruritus.
- Potent topical corticosteroids applied bid provide modest relief in 24 to 48 hours.
- For exceptional cases only, intralesional triamcinolone (2.5 mg/mL) may be used to reduce inflammation and decrease pruritus.
- The prevention of chigger bites is helpful, typically by applying *N,N*-diethyl-3methyulbenzamide (DEET) to the skin, using DEET-impregnated clothing, wearing long pants, and tucking pant legs into boots when hiking.

Clinical Course

The lesions resolve over 5 to 14 days.

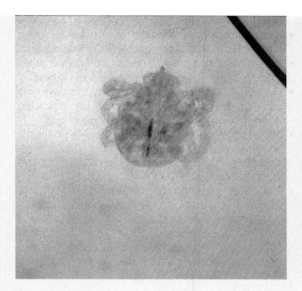

Fig. 6.5. Under the microscope, chigger mites demonstrate six legs and a reddish color. They are redder by gross examination (400× original magnification, cropped).

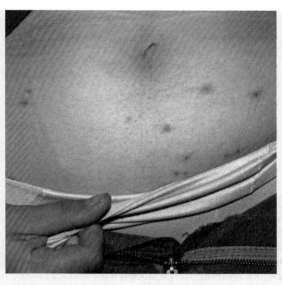

Fig. 6.6. Patient with typical papular lesion of chigger bites acquired in Georgia (United States), with accentuation under the elastic of the underwear. (From the Fitzsimons Army Medical Center Collection, Aurora, CO.)

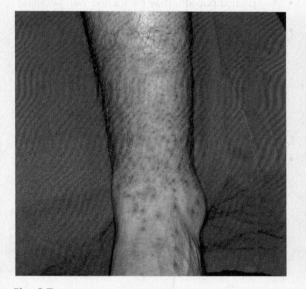

Fig. 6.7. Patient with innumerable pruritic papular lesions of chiggers, with marked accentuation under the elastic of the sock. (From the William Weston Collection, Aurora, CO.)

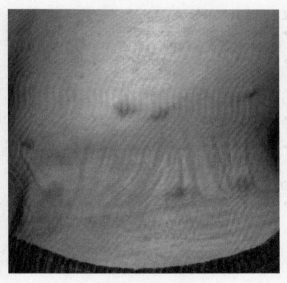

Fig. 6.8. Patient with unusually large pruritic papules, with accentuation under the elastic of the underwear. (From the Fitzsimons Army Medical Center Collection, Aurora, CO.)

Mite Bites (Ascarine Dermatitis) ICD10 code B88.0

Selected Mites That Produce Mysterious Papular Dermatitis

- *Acarus* (grains, flour)—baker's itch
- *Tyrolichus* (cheese)—grocer's itch
- *Cheyletiella* (dogs, cats)—pet itch
- *Dermanyssus* (birds)—poultry itch
- *Liponyssoides* (mouse)
- *Ophionyssus* (snakes)—snake mite itch
- *Ornithonyssus* (birds)—poultry itch
- *Pyemotes tritici* (straw)—straw itch
- *Pyemotes herfsi* (oak leaf itch)

Pathogenesis

In addition to scabies and chiggers, other mites found in the environment, on pets, on wild animals, and even on foods can yield a bite reaction. In these cases, the human is an accidental host, and the mite feeds and quickly drops off, producing a mysterious papular eruption that is self-limited.

The source of ascarine dermatitis can be difficult to establish. For example, in 2004, there were more than 300 cases of a mysterious itchy papular dermatitis in Kansas, Nebraska, and Missouri that required a team of health care providers and entomologists to identify the cause—the oak leaf itch mite.

Clinical Features

- There is a sudden onset of pruritic small papules (Figs. 6.9A and 6.10A).
- In some cases, the papular dermatitis may have a background of macular or patchy erythema or may demonstrate a microscopic focus of hemorrhage at the bite site.
- Typically, the eruptions last 3 to 7 days and are self-limited.
- The distribution is variable and is not particularly characteristic.

Diagnosis

- Ascarine dermatitis should be considered with any outbreak of a cryptic, pruritic, papular dermatitis.

- Scabies or chiggers should always be excluded through a medical history and physical examination.
- Suspicious lesions should be scraped for a scabies prep to include or exclude a scabies infestation.
- A 3- or 4-mm biopsy may support the diagnosis and exclude other diagnoses, but the histologic findings of ascarine dermatitis are nonspecific.
- Important factors to consider include the patient's home environment (especially any pets), work environment and occupation, leisure hobbies, and outdoor activities.
- The most common causes include *Cheyletiella yasguri* (found on dogs, especially puppies), *Cheyletiella blakei* (found on cats; see Fig. 6.9B), and *Cheyletiella parasitovorax* (found on rabbits). In animals, the organisms are often visible and are described as looking like so-called walking dandruff.

Treatment

- No treatment is a reasonable course of action because the lesions are self-limited.
- Topical products with pramoxine may provide some limited but immediate relief from the pruritus.
- Potent topical corticosteroids, applied twice daily, provide modest relief in 24 to 48 hours.
- Very pruritic patients may be treated with sedating antihistamines (diphenhydramine) at night.
- The exposure must be identified and eliminated. All pets should be examined by a veterinarian. A veterinarian specializing in animal dermatology is preferred because mites on animals can be difficult to identify. Even when animal mites cannot be identified, empiric treatment of pets is often a reasonable consideration.

Clinical Course

- The lesions typically resolve over 3 to 14 days without treatment.

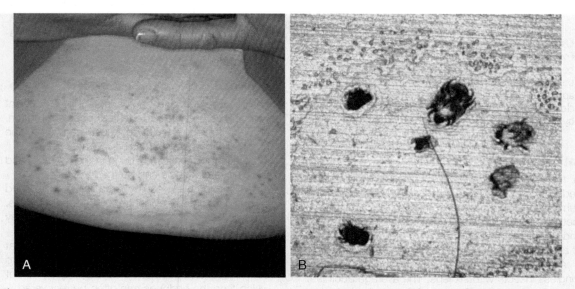

Fig. 6.9 A, *Cheyletiella* mite bite acquired from a cat that was often kept on the patient's lap. It is important to note that the cat was examined by a veterinarian and declared to be free of mites. B, Tape preparation prepared on the cat, which was brought in as requested. Multiple mites are clearly present. (From the Fitzsimons Army Medical Center Collection, Aurora, CO.)

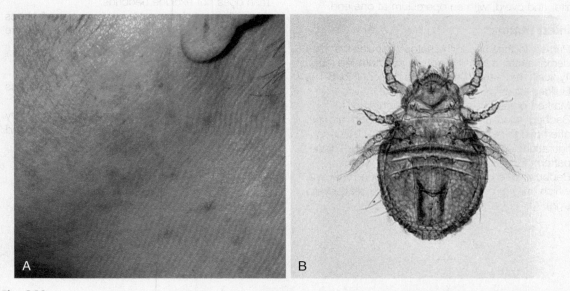

Fig. 6.10 A, Patient with a cryptic pruritic papular eruption, with a focal background of macular erythema. A careful history revealed that the patient slept on a tatami mat. B, Examination of the patient's rice straw from his tatami mat revealed numerous tatami mites, which are also known as *dani*. (From the Fitzsimons Army Medical Center Collection, Aurora, CO.)

Bedbug Bites ICD10 code S30.860

Online Tip

For travelers, there is a user-reported database of bedbug infestations in hotels and apartments that may be accessed on the Internet or via a free smartphone app (http://www.bedbugregistry.com). However, it is clearly a forum where postings cannot be substantiated by any third party.

Pathogenesis

In the past 2 decades, papular reactions due to bedbug bites (Cimex lectularius) have reached epidemic proportions. Evidence has suggested that this meteoric rise is due to increased international travel and lesser use of pesticides with long residual times of action.

Adult bedbugs are flattened, chestnut brown, wingless insects with six legs. The average adult is 4 to 5.5 mm in length (Fig. 6.11). The bedbug requires at least five blood meals to reach maturity. Adults are capable of elaborating an odor, and heavily infested rooms have a distinct smell, likened to that of coriander. Adult females lay eggs that are 1 mm in size, white, and ovoid, with an operculum at one end.

Clinical Features

- Primary lesions are erythematous papules that may demonstrate a small, central, punctum-like area. Typically, more than one lesion is present (Fig. 6.12). Bullous lesions are rare.
- Marked pruritus is a consistent feature.
- Bedbug bites are notoriously present in groups, often two to four papules, with a slightly linear configuration (so-called breakfast, lunch, and dinner pattern; Figs. 6.13 and 6.14).
- Bedbugs often bite the thin skin around the eye, which may produce edema (the so-called eyelid sign).

- Secondary features include excoriation or even features of a superimposed prurigo nodule.
- A secondary bacterial infection may also occur.

Diagnosis

- The diagnosis should be suspected in any patient who wakes up with a mysterious papular eruption, and the patient should be questioned about the home environment, particularly a travel history.
- The patient or family may bring in the bedbug, and a definitive diagnosis can be made.
- Inspection of the sleeping area is requisite, and in 80% of cases, evidence of bedbugs (adults, nymphs, eggs, or stains from blood or feces) may be found within 3 feet of the bed.
- It may be useful to have the patient go to bed at the normal time, turn off the lights, wait for 15 to 30 minutes, and then turn on the light suddenly, at which time the bedbugs can often be recovered.
- Examination of bedsheets may demonstrate red-brown bloodstains or small fragments of excrement.
- Not all persons react to bedbug bites, so the fact that only one person in the household has a papular rash does not exclude bedbugs.
- A small punch biopsy may demonstrate features consistent with a bite reaction, but the results are not diagnostic of only that entity.

Treatment

- Eradication of the infestation, which often requires professional assistance, is the only lasting cure.
- The bedbug bites may be treated symptomatically with topical pramoxine, topical corticosteroids, and antihistamines.

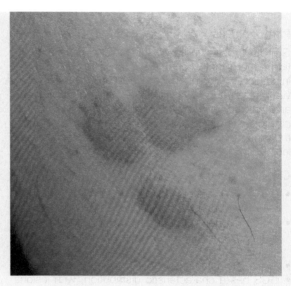

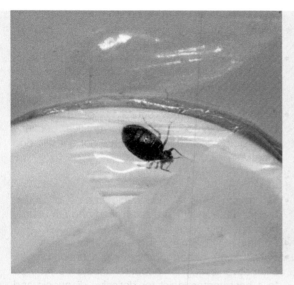

Fig. 6.11. Adult bedbug brought in a plastic baggie by a patient.

Fig. 6.12. Patient with grouped red edematous papules, without an identifiable punctum. (From the William Weston Collection, Aurora, CO.)

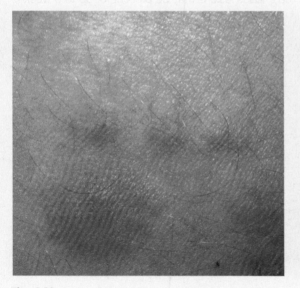

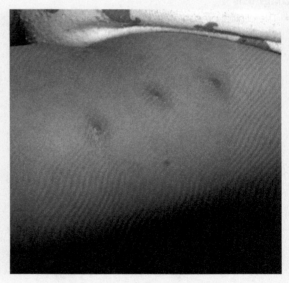

Fig. 6.13. Patient with grouped red papules of variable size, with a central punctum, with three of them demonstrating a linear arrangement. These bedbug bites were acquired in a college sorority house.

Fig. 6.14. Patient with three papules with central punctum in a line, the so-called breakfast, lunch, and dinner pattern.

Gianotti-Crosti Syndrome (Papular Acrodermatitis of Childhood)

ICD10 code L44.4

Pathogenesis

Gianotti-Crosti syndrome (GCS) is a distinct reaction pattern that occurs in response to different viral infections, including hepatitis B virus, Epstein-Barr virus, respiratory syncytial virus, various echoviruses and coxsackieviruses, and milker's nodules. Immunizations (e.g., polio, diphtheria-pertussis-tetanus, measles-mumps-rubella) and bacterial infections are less often associated with GCS.

Clinical Features

- GCS usually affects infants and young children, but the child appears otherwise well and is not febrile.
- Monomorphous papules begin abruptly and may be edematous (Fig. 6.15) or erythematous (Figs. 6.16 and 6.17).
- Pruritus is a variable feature.
- GCS has a characteristic distribution, with lesions on the face and extremities (even the proximal extremities), but with sparing of the trunk.
- On occasion, the lesions may be flat-topped (Fig. 6.18).

Diagnosis

- The clinical presentation of a monomorphic papular eruption or, less often, a flat-topped papular eruption, with involvement of the face and extremities and with sparing of the trunk, is diagnostic.
- Laboratory tests that include liver function tests (LFTs) and viral serologies for hepatitis B, hepatitis A, hepatitis C, and Epstein-Barr virus should be considered.
- Occasional cases may require a 3- or 4-mm punch biopsy, mostly to exclude other entities, because the histologic findings of GCS are not specific and merely support the diagnosis.

Treatment

- No treatment is a reasonable course of action because the lesions are self-limited and are usually not especially pruritic.
- Pruritus may be managed with antihistamines.
- Patients with abnormalities in liver function or with affirmative testing for hepatitis should be referred to a gastroenterologist for definitive diagnosis and management.

Clinical Course

The patient and/or parents should be informed that cutaneous lesions may be present for up to 6 weeks.

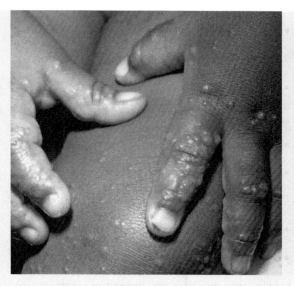

Fig. 6.15. Patient with monomorphic markedly edematous papules of the hands and legs. (From the Fitzsimons Army Medical Center Collection, Aurora, CO.)

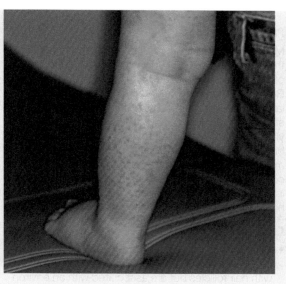

Fig. 6.16. Erythematous papular lesions without significant edema on the lower leg of a young child. (From the Joanna Burch Collection, Aurora, CO.)

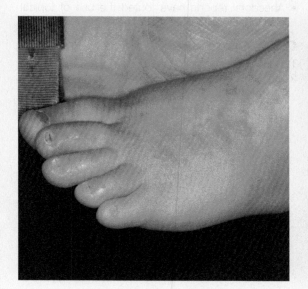

Fig. 6.17. Erythematous mildly edematous papules on the dorsum of a child's foot. (From the William Weston Collection, Aurora, CO.)

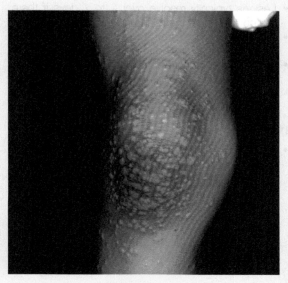

Fig. 6.18 Patient with flat-topped papular lesions of Gianotti-Crosti syndrome. In our experience, flat-topped lesions are a far less common clinical presentation.

Pathogenesis

Miliaria is a papular eruption produced by blockage of the eccrine sweat duct, with resultant extravasation of sweat into the skin and an inflammatory response. Research on human volunteers has revealed that miliaria can be produced by a combination of thermal stimulation, occlusion, and coagulase-negative staphylococci. Further studies have shown that antimicrobial agents prevent the development of experimental miliaria. Additional studies have implicated *Staphylococcus epidermidis* as the bacterial species involved in the development of miliaria. Miliaria is common in hot humid climates and during infancy and childhood.

Clinical Features

- Miliaria usually causes the acute onset of monomorphous erythematous papules that are unassociated with hair follicles but are associated with an environment that causes increased sweating (Fig. 6.19).
- Areas of the skin that are covered by clothing or under occlusion are predisposed.
- The palms and soles are uninvolved, and the face is rarely involved (Fig. 6.20).
- Symptoms vary from pruritus to stinging to burning.
- Lesions typically resolve over 2 to 7 days if there are no additional thermal insults to the skin.
- With repeated episodes, the eccrine sweat duct may become permanently damaged with anhidrosis.
- Clinical variants include malaria rubra, miliaria pustulosa (see Fig. 6.20), and miliaria profunda (Fig. 6.21). Often, more than one variant may be present in the same patient.

Diagnosis

- In most cases, the diagnosis may be made on clinical grounds based on a characteristic appearance and on the relevant environmental circumstances.

- Rare cases or atypical presentations may require a 3- or 4-mm punch biopsy that can be supportive or even diagnostic (if the correct tissue plane is present).
- In cases with a pustular component, bacterial culture of the purulent debris should be considered.

Treatment

- Reassurance is adequate in most cases because the lesions are self-limited.
- It is important to keep the patient cool and the area dry and well-ventilated. However, sometimes this is not possible due to the patient's occupation or other environmental circumstances
- Lightweight loose-fitting clothing is helpful; occlusive clothing should be avoided (see Fig. 6.21).
- In patients with unpreventable heat exposure (e.g., soldiers in the field) and recurring episodes of miliaria, oral antibiotics may prevent or ameliorate the development of lesions. One of the authors (JEF) has met with variable anedotal success using oral erythromycin or tetracyclines, but many strains of *S. epidermidis* are resistant to these antibiotics, and culture and sensitivity testing may be required.
- Anecdotal reports have touted the use of topical skin lubricants, but controlled trials are lacking.

Clinical Course

The lesions spontaneously resolve over a period of 2 to 7 days.

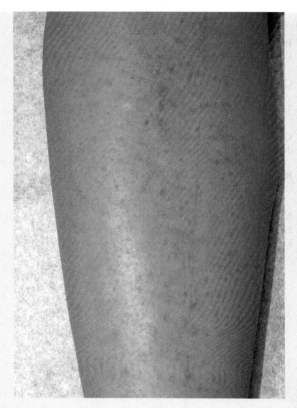

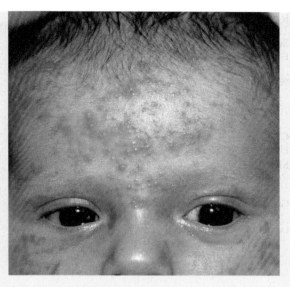

Fig. 6.20 Miliaria rubra on the face of an infant, including some lesions that are pustular (miliaria pustulosa). The face is an unusual location of miliaria. (From the William Weston Collection, Aurora, CO.)

Fig. 6.19 Typical lesions of miliaria rubra on the leg. Of importance is that they do not demonstrate an association with hair follicles.

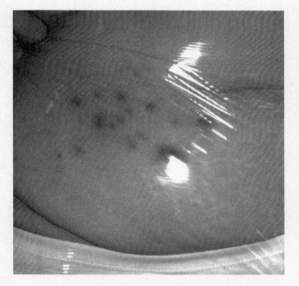

Fig. 6.21 A mixture of smaller lesions (miliaria rubra) and larger, more indurated lesions (miliaria profunda) in a patient who was using elastic wraps in an attempt to lose weight around the waist. (From the Fitzsimons Army Medical Center Collection, Aurora, CO.)

References

Scabies

Hicks MI, Elston DM. Scabies. *Dermatol Ther.* 2009;22:279-292.

Walter B, Heukelbach J, Fengler G, et al. Comparison of dermoscopy, skin scraping, and the adhesive tape test for the diagnosis of scabies in a resource-poor setting. *Arch Dermatol.* 2011;147:468-473.

Chiggers

Elston DM. What's eating you? Chiggers. *Cutis.* 2006;77:350-352.

Mite Bites

Creel NB, Crowe MA, Mullen GR. Pet hamsters as a source of rat mite dermatitis. *Cutis.* 2003;71:457-461.

Green B, Sparling J, Sparling MB. What's eating you? Pigeon mite (*Dermanyssus gallinae*). *Cutis.* 2007;80:461-462.

Lucky AW, Sayers CP, Argus JD, Lucky A. Avian mite bites acquired from a new source—pet gerbils: report of 2 cases and review of the literature. *Arch Dermatol.* 2001;1376:167-170.

Bedbugs

Kolb A, Needham GR, Neyman KM, High WA. Bedbugs. *Dermatol Ther.* 2009;22:347-352.

Quach KA, Zaenglein AL. The eyelid sign: a clue to bed bug bites. *Pediatr Dermatol.* 2014;31:353-355.

Ter Poorten MC, Prose NS. The return of the common bedbug. *Pediatr Dermatol.* 2005;22:183-187.

Gianotti-Crosti Syndrome

de la Torre C. Gianotti-Crosti syndrome following milker's nodules. *Cutis.* 2004;74:316-318.

Retrouvey M, Koch LH, Williams JV. Gianotti-Crosti syndrome following childhood vaccinations. *Pediatr Dermatol.* 2013;30:137-138.

Milaria

Feng E, Janniger CK. Miliaria. *Cutis.* 1995;55:213-216.

Kirk JF, Wilson BB, Chun W, Cooper PH. Miliaria profunda. *J Am Acad Dermatol.* 1996;35:854-856.

Chapter 7
Scaly Papular Lesions

Key Terms

Lichen Planus
  Annular lichen planus
  Bullous lichen planus
  Hypertrophic lichen planus

Grover Disease
  Transient acantholytic
    dermatosis

Actinic Keratosis
  Atrophic actinic keratosis
  Hypertrophic actinic keratosis
  Pigmented actinic keratosis

Scaly papular disorders include an unrelated admixture of neoplastic and inflammatory disorders characterized by small palpable lesions with variable scale, which are usually smaller than 1 cm in their greatest diameter. Some disorders, such as guttate psoriasis, may contain some lesions larger than 1 cm and would technically be classified as scaly plaques. Some lesions that are typically papular may become exuberant enough (e.g., actinic keratosis) that they are morphologically scaly nodules.

IMPORTANT HISTORY QUESTIONS

How long has the lesion(s) been present?

Some of the disorders in this group may appear acutely (e.g., guttate psoriasis, lichen planus); other disorders (e.g., actinic keratoses) appear gradually.

Have you had a similar lesion(s) in the past?

A "yes" answer favors some disorders with a genetic basis, such as psoriasis or actinic keratoses, that tend to occur in the background of chronic sun damage.

Do any of your immediate relatives have psoriasis?

A "yes" answer indicates a genetic predisposition for the development of psoriasis.

Have you had any previous pre–skin cancers or skin cancers?

A positive history of a previous pre–skin cancer or skin cancer indicates that the patient has had enough sun damage to promote the development of pre–skin cancers (e.g., actinic keratoses), squamous cell carcinoma in situ, and squamous cell carcinoma.

How are you treating your skin condition?

Many patients use home-based, over-the-counter (OTC), or prescription remedies that can alter the appearance of the condition.

Are you taking any medications?

Some medications may precipitate or aggravate some of the disorders discussed in this chapter. For example,

psoriasis can be worsened by beta blockers, lithium, and terbinafine. Lichen planus can be mimicked by numerous medications (e.g., thiazide diuretics).

Have you had a recent illness?

This is important because streptococcal infections frequently precipitate episodes of guttate psoriasis, and lichen planus can be associated with virus-induced hepatitis.

IMPORTANT PHYSICAL FINDINGS

How many lesions are present?

Some of the disorders in this section can be solitary or multiple (e.g., actinic keratosis) or are characteristically multiple (e.g., psoriasis, lichen planus, lichen nitidus).

What is the distribution of the lesions?

Some of the disorders demonstrate a characteristic location. For example, guttate psoriasis usually affects the trunk and proximal extremities.

Is the oral mucosa involved?

Lichen planus frequently involves the oral mucosa, and finding characteristic involvement can be useful in establishing the diagnosis. In contrast, psoriasis only rarely involves the oral cavity and, if present, it is usually confined to the tongue. Actinic keratoses may involve the sun-exposed mucosa of the lower lip (actinic cheilitis) but do not involve the protected oral mucosa.

Are the nails normal or abnormal?

The nails are frequently involved in psoriasis, Darier disease, and occasionally lichen planus, but most of the remaining disorders typically demonstrate normal nails.

Pathogenesis

Psoriasis is a common hereditary disease with a chronic course that primarily affects the skin, with variable involvement of the joints and oral mucosa. The cutaneous manifestations are protean; these include classic plaques (see Chapter 8), pustular psoriasis (see Chapter 12), erythrodermic psoriasis, and the guttate pattern of psoriasis. Although psoriasis is a genetic disorder, it is generally preceded by a trigger; guttate psoriasis is often the initial manifestation of the psoriatic diathesis. The most common trigger in the guttate variant is streptococcal pharyngitis (63%). Less commonly implicated triggers include a recent life crisis (46%), skin injury, drugs, and exposure to ultraviolet (UV) light.

Drugs Implicated in Triggering Guttate Psoriasis
- Beta blockers (most common)
- Biologic agents (e.g., infliximab)
- Lithium
- Terbinafine

Clinical Features

- Guttate psoriasis can affect any portion of the body; however, it demonstrates a marked predilection for the trunk and proximal extremities (Fig. 7.1).
- The primary lesion is manifested by small, pink to reddish papules that typically vary from 2 to 10 mm in size; however, larger lesions can be present. Very early lesions may not yet demonstrate scale (Fig. 7.2), with mature lesions demonstrating variable scale (Fig. 7.3).
- The Koebner phenomenon—psoriasis developing at sites of superficial trauma—occurs in about 5% of patients with psoriasis and is especially common during acute flares of guttate psoriasis (see Fig. 7.3).
- Nail involvement (see Chapter 25) can be present but usually does not occur in early guttate psoriasis, when patients are most likely to present to an urgent care or emergency room setting. If present, it is usually seen as distinct nail pits. Less commonly in guttate psoriasis, the patient may demonstrate yellowish-brown areas of discoloration below the nail (oil spots).

Diagnosis

- There is a clinical presentation of uniform papules with scale that is of an acute onset.
- The presence of the Koebner phenomenon is strongly supportive of the diagnosis.
- The presence of significant nail pitting or oil spots in the nail bed is strongly suggestive of psoriasis.
- There may be a family history; first-degree relatives with psoriasis can be identified in about one-third of patients.
- Some cases may require a 3- or 4-mm punch biopsy of a well-developed lesion, which is more likely diagnostic.

Treatment

The selection of therapy depends on the patient's age and general health, cost, local availability of specialized treatment facilities, distribution and extent of the lesions, and motivation of the patient.

- In most cases, the treatment of choice is light therapy; the best options are natural sunlight (cheapest), UVB phototherapy, which includes narrow-band UVB, or methoxsalen plus UVA.
- The primary topical option is once- or twice-daily application of topical corticosteroids of varying strengths, depending on the location, severity of disease, and response to therapy.
- For severe or resistant cases, acitretin is a consideration.
- In patients with guttate psoriasis, strongly consider empiric oral antibiotics to eliminate infectious triggers, and carefully review the patient's medications for potential triggering drugs.

Guttate Psoriasis Outcomes
- In the largest study to date (79 patients), 25% of patients went on to develop chronic plaque psoriasis, but the remaining patients did not. There were no known clinical or laboratory findings that could predict the outcome for a given individual.
- Of patients with guttate psoriasis, only 65% were clear or improved at 3 months, and 99% were clear or improved at 12 months.
- Although not evaluated in this study, some patients will have more than one episode of guttate psoriasis.

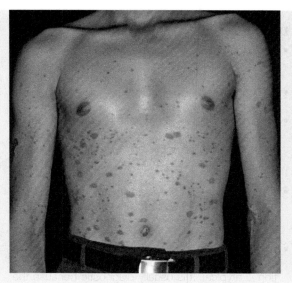

Fig. 7.1. Typical trunk and proximal extremity distribution of guttate psoriasis. Note the koebnerized lesions on the left upper arm. (From the Fitzsimons Army Medical Center Collection, Aurora, CO.)

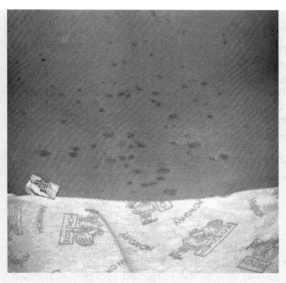

Fig. 7.2. Early guttate psoriasis in a young child. In early lesions, the scale is not present or minimal; however, the prominent red color and uniform appearance is strongly suggestive. (From the William Weston Collection, Aurora, CO.)

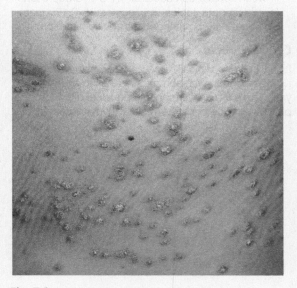

Fig. 7.3. Close-up of a patient with developed lesions of guttate psoriasis demonstrating abundant white scale. These lesions are diagnostic and do not require a biopsy. (From the William Weston Collection, Aurora, CO.)

Pathogenesis

This is a relatively uncommon, self-limited dermatosis of unknown cause that is usually discussed as a papulosquamous disorder in most texts. Although the pathogenesis is understood, occasional patients have associated lichen planus. This association, plus the finding of dead keratinocytes, suggests a host autoimmune response against keratinocytes.

Clinical Features

- Lichen nitidus usually affects children, adolescents, and young adults, but any age group can be affected. It can be found in any ethnic group, but black patients are most commonly affected.
- Patients are typically asymptomatic, but rare patients may complain of mild pruritus.
- Typically, there is a symmetric diffuse eruption that usually affects the trunk and proximal extremities (Fig. 7.4). In males, the genitalia are frequently involved (Fig. 7.5).
- The primary lesion consists of a 1- to 3-mm round papule, with no scale or a small amount of detectable scale. The papules can be skin-colored but are often lighter than the surrounding skin due to the scale.
- Lesions may focally have linear configurations due to superficial minor trauma (Koebner phenomenon; Fig. 7.6).
- Lichen nitidus with focal hemorrhage is a very rare clinical variant.

Diagnosis

- The differential diagnosis includes atypical lichen planus, papular secondary syphilis, papular sarcoidosis, and atypical Langerhans cell histiocytosis.
- Clinical appearance is usually diagnostic, and further testing is not required.
- If secondary syphilis is a clinical consideration (i.e., atypical presentation in a sexually active adolescent or young adult), a rapid plasma reagin (RPR) test or venereal disease research laboratory (VDRL) test is appropriate.
- If papular sarcoidosis is a clinical consideration—that is, the patient has clinical features such as larger lesions, facial lesions, or systemic symptoms—a screening chest x-ray may be indicated.
- A skin biopsy (e.g., shave biopsy, 3-mm punch biopsy) is not usually indicated, but if the presentation is atypical, it is usually diagnostic because the histologic findings are specific.

Treatment

- Reassurance should be given to the patient because this a self-limited, harmless skin disorder.
- A weak topical corticosteroid (1% hydrocortisone) to midstrength topical corticosteroid (0.1% triamcinolone) is recommended if the lesions are pruritic.

Clinical Course

Lichen nitidus typically goes away within weeks but usually months, with some cases lasting as long as 1 year. There are no permanent sequelae, although rare patients may demonstrate residual hyperpigmentation.

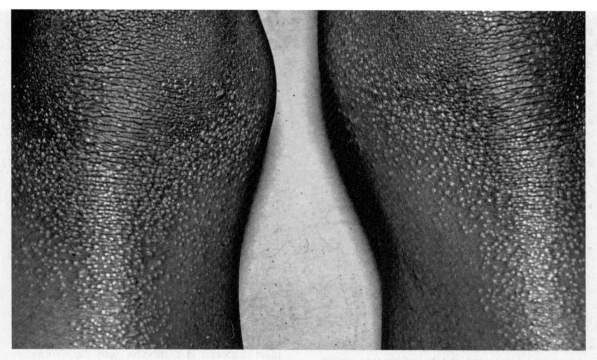

Fig. 7.4. Patient with lichen nitidus. Shown are the characteristic uniform symmetric papules, with white scale on the extremities. The large number of lesions is unusual. (From the Walter Reed Army Medical Center Collection, Washington, DC.)

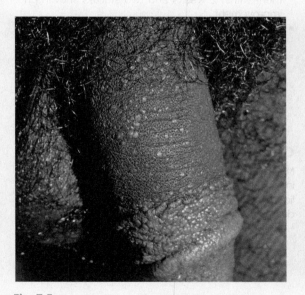

Fig. 7.5. In males, the genitalia is frequently affected in lichen nitidus. (From the Fitzsimons Army Medical Center Collection, Aurora, CO.)

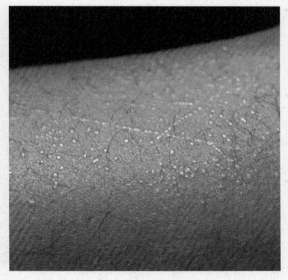

Fig. 7.6. Close-up of lesions demonstrating the Koebner phenomenon. This is a helpful feature for the diagnosis of lichen nitidus.

Lichen Planus ICD10 code L43

Pathogenesis

Lichen planus is relatively common, with one epidemiologic study reporting a prevalence of 0.4% in the United States. The cause is not entirely understood, although studies have suggested that it is an autoimmune disease based on histologic findings, immunologic data, and association with other autoimmune diseases. Of interest is the weak association of chronic, ulcerative lichen planus with hepatitis C infection.

Clinical Features

- Lichen planus may occur at any age (average age of onset, 52 years); pediatric cases only account for 2% of cases.
- The primary lesions are intensely pruritic, violaceous, polygonal papules that may demonstrate a fine white lacy appearance on the surface; these are called *Wickham striae* (Figs. 7.7 and 7.8). Although classified as a papulosquamous disease, the amount of scale is variable and may even be absent.
- In patients with a darker skin color, the lesions may be heavily pigmented due to pigmentary incontinence (see Fig. 7.7). The Koebner phenomenon (isomorphic response), consisting of linear lesions at the site of trauma, is commonly present and usually occurs in active disease.
- In regard to distribution, any cutaneous site can be affected, although the most common locations are the arms (especially the wrists) and legs. Rare patients may demonstrate an inverse distribution affecting the axillae and groin. Very rarely, the lesions may be unilateral and linear.
- Other mucocutaneous findings include lacy white lesions of the buccal mucosa (Fig. 7.9), oral ulcerations, scarring alopecia (lichen planopilaris), and nail dystrophy. Approximately two-thirds of patients with cutaneous lichen planus will demonstrate oral involvement.
- Clinical variants include **annular lichen planus,** in which there is a central area of clearing that is often hyperpigmented, **hypertrophic lichen planus,** characterized by thick, hyperkeratotic pruritic papules on the anterior aspect of the lower legs, and **bullous lichen planus,** which is very rare.

Diagnosis

- In regard to the clinical presentation, beware of lichenoid tissue reactions that are photodistributed because these are, without fail, lichenoid drug eruptions.
- A 3- or 4-mm punch biopsy is better than a shave biopsy for distinguishing lichen planus from lichenoid drug eruptions.

Treatment

The following therapeutic options may be considered:
- Topical corticosteroids (betamethasone inhalers useful in diffuse oral disease)
- Intralesional corticosteroids
- Oral corticosteroids, with the dose and duration dependent on the extent of disease and response
- Topical isotretinoin, 0.1% gel, for oral lesions
- Oral hydroxychloroquine, 200 to 400 mg/day. Expect that about 50% of patients will show a complete response in 6 months, with the remainder demonstrating a partial or no response.
- Oral griseofulvin, 500 mg/day, is a controversial treatment, with two studies demonstrating improvement within 2 weeks and two studies showing no improvement.
- Psoralen and UVA—in one study of 35 patients, 86% of patients were improved or cleared.
- Patients with what appears to be oral lichen planus, with no involvement elsewhere, should have patch testing performed to exclude amalgam filling sensitivity. More than 95% of patients with a positive patch test can expect complete or partial resolution with removal of their amalgam fillings.

Clinical Course

Most cases of lichen planus spontaneously resolve in 1 to 2 years, but it can persist for decades. Oral lichen planus has a slightly increased incidence for the development of squamous cell carcinoma.

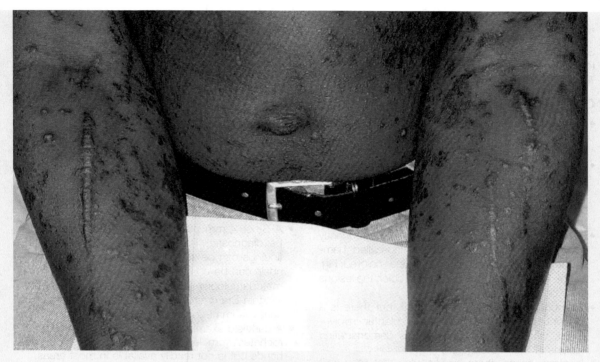

Fig. 7.7. Lichen planus. Numerous hyperkeratotic papules have focally coalesced into small plaques in a patient of color. This patient has prominent koebnerization.

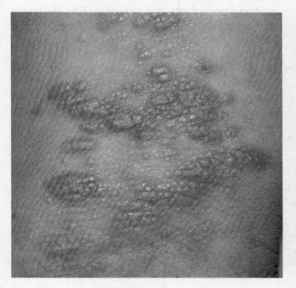

Fig. 7.8. Close-up of characteristic violaceous polygonal papules on the wrist and volar forearm, which is a characteristic site for lesions.

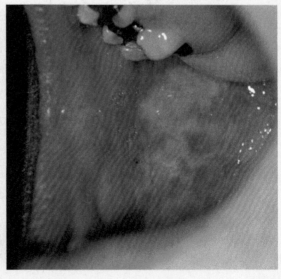

Fig. 7.9. Patient with oral lichen planus. Shown are superficial erosions and lacy white lesions on the buccal mucosa. (From the John Aeling Collection, Aurora, CO.)

Pathogenesis

Secondary syphilis is due to the lymphatic and hematogenous spread of the sexually acquired spirochete *Treponema pallidum*.

Clinical Features

- It typically starts 6 to 12 weeks after the chancre of primary syphilis. There may be no history of a chancre, or the chancre may still be present.
- The most common primary lesions are maculopapular lesions of variable size, with variable scale. However, the primary lesions can also be macular only, papular (may even appear acneiform), or nodular. Some cases may also be annular.
- The lesions are typically red but also frequently demonstrate a red-brown color (so-called ham-colored) or yellow-brown color (copper-colored; Fig. 7.10). In patients with a darker skin color, the lesions may be pigmented.
- Distribution is typically generalized, but there is a distinct tendency for palmar and plantar involvement, with about 50% of patients demonstrating lesions at these sites (Fig. 7.11).
- In some cases, there are papules that may split at the angle of the mouth; these are appropriately called *split papules,* and they strongly support the diagnosis (Fig. 7.12).
- The oral mucosa may demonstrate mucous patches that can be white or red, with some patients demonstrating linear white patches reminiscent of snail tracks.
- The genital mucosa may demonstrate condyloma lata, which are papules that vary from being moist and eroded to scaly and eroded (Fig. 7.13). These lesions have a distinct tendency to be flat-topped.
- Alopecia is often present; it varies from being subtle to demonstrating modest hair loss. Although patchy alopecia (moth-eaten alopecia) is most characteristic, diffuse alopecia that is indistinguishable from telogen effluvium is more common. Less commonly, discrete areas of hair loss that may mimic those of alopecia areata are present.

Diagnosis

- The clinical presentation can be strongly suggestive; however, confirmation is always needed.
- For serologic testing, an RPR or VDRL test should be done as a screening test. If positive, the diagnosis can be confirmed with a more specific test, such as the fluorescent treponemal antibody absorption (FTA-ABS) test.
- A 3- or 4-mm punch biopsy of lesional skin can be diagnostic. The hematoxylin and eosin (H&E) findings can be strongly suggestive, and the diagnosis can be confirmed by the pathologist or dermatopathologist with the use of a silver stain (e.g., Warthin-Starry or modified Steiner) or with a more sensitive immunoperoxidase stain.
- A darkfield examination of serous exudates for spirochetes from lesional skin is sensitive in skilled hands but is not readily available in most areas.

Treatment

- The treatment of secondary syphilis is dependent on a number of factors and is in constant flux. Before treating a patient with any form of syphilis, the latest Centers for Disease Control and Prevention (CDC) treatment guidelines should be consulted (http://www.cdc.gov/std/tg2015/syphilis.htm).
- The requirements for reporting a patient with syphilis vary from state to state; however, given that this disease is transmitted from person to person, all cases should be reported to the appropriate local health authorities.

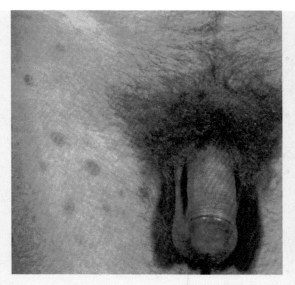

Fig. 7.10. Patient with secondary syphilis presenting with yellow-brown scaly papules on the trunk, extremities, and head of the penis (Fitzsimons Army Medical Center Collection, Aurora, CO).

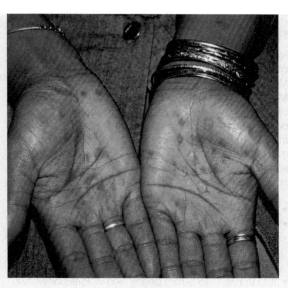

Fig. 7.11. Patient with secondary syphilis presenting as hyperpigmented maculopapules, with subtle scales on the palms.

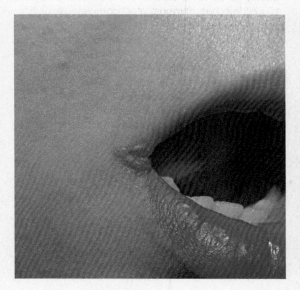

Fig. 7.12. Characteristic split papule at the corner of the mouth in a patient with secondary syphilis.

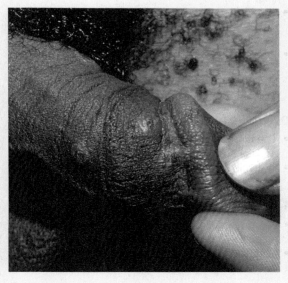

Fig. 7.13. Patient with condyloma lata. There are flat-topped crusted and scaly papules on the distal penis. (From the Fitzsimons Army Medical Center Collection, Aurora, CO.)

Pathogenesis

Molluscum contagiosum is caused by four serotypes of the molluscum contagiosum virus (MCV-1 through MCV-4). MCV-1 predominantly affects children, and MCV-2 is primarily a sexually transmitted disease of young adults—that is highly contagious (40% of patients can identify an infected relative or close friend). Epidemiologic studies have suggested that most cases are due to close physical contact (e.g., sexual activity); however, it is clear that fomites (e.g., shared towels) can transmit infection.

Clinical Features

- It predominantly affects children, young adults, and immunocompromised patients, with up to 18% of all HIV-infected individuals reported to be infected in one study.
- It features 1- to 5-mm pearly skin-colored or whitish papules (occasionally larger), with central keratotic umbilication that resembles small volcanoes (Fig. 7.14).
- The number of lesions varies from one to hundreds (Fig. 7.15).
- Atypical presentations include lesions with hyperkeratotic spicules (Fig. 7.16) and lesions that become inflamed (Fig. 7.17).
- In regard to distribution, it may affect any area of the skin that normally has hair follicles (spares palms and soles). It has a genital predilection in sexually active adolescents and young adults.

Diagnosis

- The clinical presentation is usually diagnostic, and additional testing is not required.
- In atypical cases (inflamed lesions), the lesions can be biopsied with a shave or punch biopsy.

Treatment

- Benign neglect is an option because spontaneous resolution is normal.
- Curettage is time-consuming, is difficult to carry out in young children, and may require the use of a local anesthetic; however, it is the most efficacious therapy in skilled hands.
- Cryotherapy with liquid nitrogen by spray, probe, or cotton-tipped applicator is the most commonly used provider therapy. Freeze for about 6 to 8 seconds and repeat in 3 weeks if needed.
- Tunable dye laser use is limited to clinicians that have this in their facility.

Topical Application

- When using topical cantharidin (0.7% in a flexible collodion base), applied to the top of lesions, patients should be instructed to wash it off in 2 to 6 hours. Warn patients about blisters that may become painful. It is recommended that no more than 20 lesions be treated in a single session with this modality.
- Topical 0.05% podophyllotoxin, applied once daily for up to 2 weeks
- Topical 12% salicylic acid gel, applied twice weekly for up to 12 weeks
- Topical 5% imiquimod cream—apply three times weekly for up to 16 weeks. An open label study on 15 children has demonstrated complete resolution or a partial response in 9 of 13 children (69%) who completed the study. In a second randomized trial of 23 patients, in which the patients applied imiquimod for 12 weeks, there was a 46% reduction in the number of lesions compared to the vehicle group, in which there was a 27% increase in the number of lesions. This treatment has also been used as adjunctive therapy following other therapies (e.g., topical cantharidin).

Clinical Course

- The course is highly variable, although most untreated lesions resolve within 2 to 4 years in immunocompetent patients. As one would expect, the number and duration of lesions is greater in immunocompromised patients.

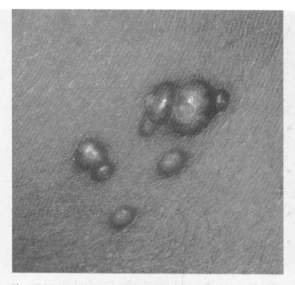

Fig. 7.14. Patient with molluscum contagiosum. Multiple papules of variable size demonstrate the characteristic central keratotic core.

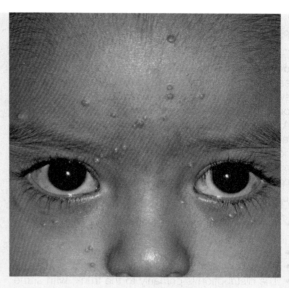

Fig. 7.15. Patient with numerous smaller, umbilicated, keratotic papules of the face. The treatment of young children with lesions near the eyes with a destructive or caustic substance is often not possible.

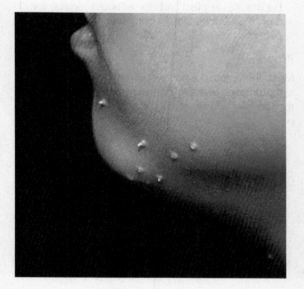

Fig. 7.16. Patient with an uncommon presentation of molluscum contagiosum, with unusually prominent keratotic cores. (From the William Weston Collection, Aurora, CO.)

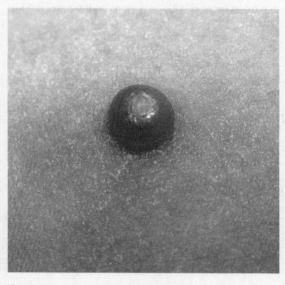

Fig. 7.17. Patient with inflamed molluscum contagiosum, with some resemblance to an eroded pyogenic granuloma. Inflamed lesions are more frequently biopsied.

Grover Disease ICD10 code L11.1

Pathogenesis

Grover disease, also called **transient acantholytic dermatosis,** is a disease of uncertain pathogenesis that demonstrates an association with altered sweating, including frequent hot tub use, sauna use, bedridden patients, and sweat-inducing exercise. A respected dermatologist has noted that he can induce lesions on himself by just taking a prolonged hot shower that has a sauna function. In some but not all patients, the keratotic papules have shown a connection to the opening of eccrine sweat glands.

Clinical Features

- Typically, it affects middle-aged and older patients (>45 years).
- It is more common in men than women.
- There is an abrupt or gradual onset of lesions.
- The distribution is primarily to the trunk, with some patients demonstrating involvement of the proximal extremities (Figs. 7.18 and 7.19). In bedridden patients, the lesions may be confined to the back.
- A primary lesion is usually a 2- to 5-mm keratotic papule, although rarely there are papulovesicles. An atypical presentation includes large lesions that are often more pruritic and more erythematous (Fig. 7.20).
- The color varies from skin-colored to reddish-brown to reddish.
- Typically, there are numerous lesions.
- Symptoms are typically pruritic, usually minimal to modest in severity.

Diagnosis

- The clinical presentation is usually diagnostic, although some cases can be difficult to differentiate from low-grade folliculitis or even miliaria (heat rash).

- The diagnosis can be established by doing a small shave biopsy. The histologic findings can be seen in other disorders (e.g., Darier disease, Hailey-Hailey disease); however, when combined with the clinical presentation, a definitive diagnosis can be made.

Treatment

- Intense sweat-inducing activities (e.g., prolonged hot tub or sauna use, prolonged exercise) should be avoided.
- No treatment is an option because individual attacks disappear after the cessation of repeated sweat-inducing activities in some but not all patients.
- Topical antipruritic pramoxine-containing agents are useful for symptomatic relief.
- Weak (e.g., 1% hydrocortisone) to moderate strength (e.g., 0.1% triamcinolone) cream applied once or twice daily is helpful in reducing inflammation and pruritus but does alter the course.
- Trichloroacetic acid peeling has been used rarely, with some success.
- Psoralen and ultraviolet A (PUVA) or narrow-band UVB light is helpful in severe symptomatic cases.
- Triple antibiotic ointment (neomycin-polymyxin B-bacitracin) applied qd to affected areas for 1 month produces almost complete clearing in some patients.

Prognosis

Most therapies do not work well and provide only symptomatic relief. Despite the name transient acantholytic dermatosis, some cases are chronic and may persist for years due to repeated thermal stimulation.

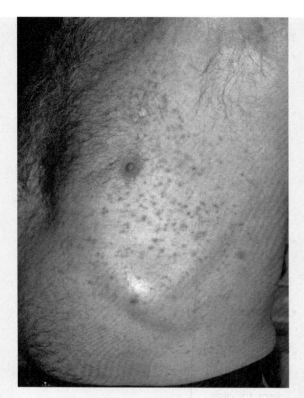

Fig. 7.18. Patient with Grover disease. There are numerous brownish-red, hyperkeratotic, uniform lesions on the trunk. (From the Fitzsimons Army Medical Center Collection, Aurora, CO.)

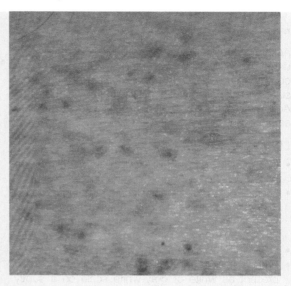

Fig. 7.19. Close-up of typical lesions in a patient with Grover disease demonstrating brownish-yellow to reddish-brown keratotic papules that are virtually identical to the primary lesions of Darier disease (From the Fitzsimons Army Medical Center Collection, Aurora, CO.)

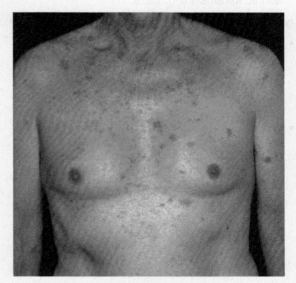

Fig. 7.20. Patient with atypical presentation of Grover disease demonstrating larger, more erythematous lesions. This presentation is usually associated with significant pruritus.

Pathogenesis

Actinic keratoses are precancerous lesions of the epidermis produced by UV light. They are much more common in fair-skinned individuals and immunosuppressed patients, especially transplant patients. Actinic keratoses have the potential to evolve into squamous cell carcinoma (SCC).

Clinical Features

- It is usually seen in fair-skinned individuals with a background of significant sun damage.
- Lesions are predominantly located on sun-exposed skin surfaces, with the head, neck, proximal forearms, and backs of the hands being the most severely affected.
- Lesions can be solitary but are usually multiple.
- Primary lesions are of variable size and usually present as white or gray-white scale on a subtly indurated papule (Figs. 7.21 and 7.22).
- The background color adjacent to the scale varies from being skin-colored to violaceous to red.
- Clinical variants include **atrophic actinic keratosis, pigmented actinic keratosis,** and **hypertrophic actinic keratosis** (Fig. 7.23).

Diagnosis

- An irregularly scaly papule of variable size on the sun-exposed skin of a patient with dermatoheliosis is an actinic keratosis until proven otherwise. In some patients, it may be difficult to differentiate from seborrheic keratosis, xerosis in the elderly, and SCC.
- Lesions that demonstrate significant induration that are suspicious for early SCC in situ or SCC should be biopsied. In most cases, a deep shave biopsy is adequate; however, a 3- or 4-mm punch biopsy is preferred for problematic lesions.

Treatment

- Cryotherapy with liquid nitrogen is the most commonly used therapy by clinicians, and a greater than 90% cure rate with a single treatment can be expected if done correctly.
- Topical 5-fluorouracil is available as multiple products, including Efudex (2% and 5% solutions, 5% cream), Fluoroplex (1% solution, 1% cream), and Carac (0.5% micronized cream). It should be applied qd to bid for 2 to 6 weeks. In general, the face requires 2 to 4 weeks of treatment (Fig. 7.24); the forearms and backs of the hands require 4 to 6 weeks of treatment. About 70% to 80% of lesions will resolve with this treatment regimen.
- Topical diclofenac can be applied bid for 3 months. The cure rate is about 50% if the entire 3-month course is completed. Although this is less than that seen with topical 5-fluorouracil, this treatment is tolerated by patients better than 5-fluorouracil.
- Topical retinoids (e.g., tretinoin) used for months to years on a daily basis produce about a 50% reduction in the number of actinic keratoses.
- Δ amino levulinic acid photodynamic therapy is inconvenient; it requires two office visits and specialized equipment that is usually limited to dermatologists.
- Topical imiquimod is applied twice or three times weekly for 16 weeks. It is as good (if not better) than topical 5-fluorouracil but is an expensive therapeutic modality.

Clinical Course

The exact risk of progression to SCC is controversial. Based on several studies, the calculated risk of an individual actinic keratosis developing into SCC is between 0.025% and 20%. It is reasonable to tell patients that the risk of development of untreated actinic keratoses into SCC is approximately 5%.

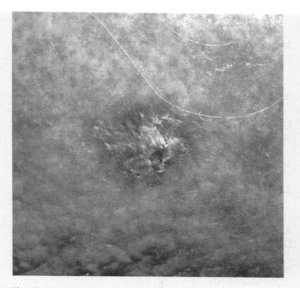

Fig. 7.21. Patient with actinic keratosis, with white scale and background erythema. Note the severely sun-damaged skin with yellowish discoloration, which represents solar elastosis.

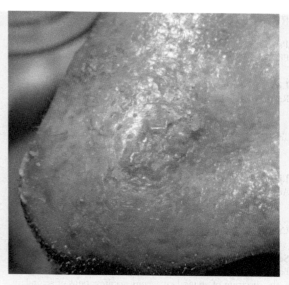

Fig. 7.22. Multiple papules with yellowish scale on the nose in sun-damaged skin. The patient has background erythema due to rosacea. (From the Fitzsimons Army Medical Center Collection, Aurora, CO.)

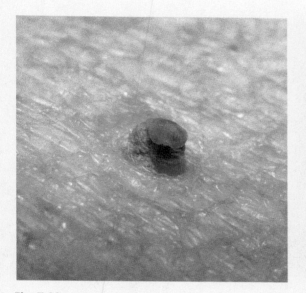

Fig. 7.23. Patient with hypertrophic actinic keratosis with a small cutaneous horn on sun-damaged skin. These lesions are more likely to be biopsied to rule out squamous cell carcinoma.

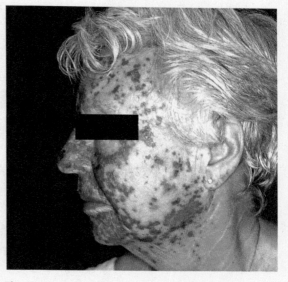

Fig. 7.24. Patient with numerous actinic keratoses after 4 weeks of topical 5-fluorouracil demonstrating the necrosis of actinic keratoses. This is an excellent but uncomfortable treatment.

References

Psoriasis

Pfingstier LS, Maroon M, Mowad C. Guttate psoriasis outcomes. *Cutis.* 2016;97:140-144.

Lichen Nitidus

Rallis E, Verros C, Moussatou V, et al. Generalized purpuric lichen nitidus. Report of a case and review of the literature. *Dermatol Online J.* 2007;13:5.

Tay EY, Ho MS, Chandran NS, et al. Lichen nitidus presenting with nail changes—case report and review of the literature. *Pediatr Dermatol.* 2015;32:386-388.

Lichen Planus

Atzmoney L, Reiter O, Hodak E, et al. Treatments for cutaneous lichen planus: a systematic review and meta-analysis. *Am J Clin Dermatol.* 2016;17:11-22.

Usatine RP, Tinitigan M. Diagnosis and treatment of lichen planus. *Am Fam Physician.* 2011;84:53-60.

Secondary Syphilis

Balagula Y, Mattei PL, Wisco OJ, et al. The great imitator revisited: the spectrum of atypical cutaneous manifestations of secondary syphilis. *Int J Dermatol.* 2014;53:1434-1441.

Molluscum Contagiosum

Bard S, Shiman MI, Bellman B, Connelly EA. Treatment of facial molluscum contagiosum with trichloroacetic acid. *Pediatr Dermatol.* 2009;4:425-426.

Brown M, Paulson C, Henry SL. Treatment of anogenital molluscum contagiosum. *Am Fam Physician.* 2009;80:864.

Grover Disease

Hanson M, Hsu S. Pruritic papules on the chest and back. Grover's disease. *Am Fam Physician.* 2006;74:641-642.

Julliard KN, Milburn PB. Antibiotic ointment in the treatment of Grover disease. *Cutis.* 2007;80:72-74.

Scheinfeld N, Mones J. Seasonal variation of transient acantholytic dyskeratosis (Grover's disease). *J Am Acad Dermatol.* 2006;55:262-268.

Actinic Keratosis

Lebwohl M. Actinic keratosis: epidemiology and progression to squamous cell carcinoma. *Br J Dermatol.* 2003;149:31S-33S.

Rossi R, Mori M, Lotti T. Actinic keratosis. *Int J Dermatol.* 2007;46:895-904.

Spencer JM, Hazan C, Hsiung SH, Robins P. Therapeutic decision making in the therapy of actinic keratosis. *J Drugs Dermatol.* 2005;4:296-301.

Chapter 8
Plaques With Scale

Scaly plaques includes an unrelated admixture of neoplastic and inflammatory disorders characterized by larger, usually sharply defined palpable lesions, with variable scale.

IMPORTANT HISTORY QUESTIONS

How long has the lesion(s) been present?

Although all the lesions can be chronic, mycosis fungoides and psoriasis are often present for years.

Have you had a similar lesion(s) in the past?

A "yes" answer favors a disorder with a genetic basis, such as psoriasis, whereas pityriasis rubra pilaris is usually a onetime occurrence.

Do any of your immediate relatives have psoriasis?

A "yes" answer indicates a predisposition for the development of psoriasis. Rarely, pityriasis rubra pilaris can also be familial.

How are you treating your skin condition?

Many patients use home-based, over-the-counter (OTC), or prescription remedies that can alter the appearance of the condition.

Has the skin condition ever been biopsied?

This could be helpful in regard to any of the conditions in this chapter; however, it is especially important in mycosis fungoides. If this is a clinical consideration, have all previous biopsies reviewed by a pathologist or dermatopathologist with expertise in this area because the diagnosis is often missed.

Are you taking any medications?

Some medications may precipitate or aggravate some of the disorders discussed in this chapter. For example, psoriasis can be worsened by beta blockers, lithium, and terbinafine. Pityriasis rubra pilaris is also notoriously resistant to treatment with topical and systemic corticosteroids. We have seen more than one example in which this was the first clue to a diagnosis of evolving pityriasis rubra pilaris.

Have you had any recent illnesses or infections?

This is a very important question because psoriasis and reactive arthritis are genetic disorders that are often triggered by an infection. In particular, you would be interested in streptococcal infections for psoriasis and either an enteric infection or sexually acquired disease for reactive arthritis.

IMPORTANT PHYSICAL FINDINGS

What is the distribution of the lesions?

Some of the cutaneous disorders demonstrate a characteristic location. For example, psoriasis frequently affects areas that are susceptible to trauma, such as the elbows and knees, whereas mycosis fungoides often begins in the girdle area.

Is the Koebner phenomenon present?

Of the disorders with large plaques and scale, only psoriasis demonstrates lesions at the sites of minor trauma.

Is the oral mucosa involved?

Although reactive arthritis frequently has oral involvement, psoriasis only rarely involves the oral cavity, whereas pityriasis rubra pilaris and mycosis fungoides almost never present with oral lesions.

Are the nails normal or abnormal?

The nails are frequently involved in psoriasis and reactive arthritis, whereas those with mycosis fungoides and pityriasis rubra pilaris usually have normal nails.

Is there any historical or clinical evidence of arthritis?

This is an extremely important question, not only from a diagnostic standpoint but also from a therapeutic standpoint, because joint involvement is the finding that usually dictates therapy for psoriasis and reactive arthritis.

Plaque Psoriasis ICD10 code L40.0

Drugs Implicated in Triggering or Aggravating Psoriasis

- Beta blockers (most common)
- Infliximab—paradoxic effect
- Lithium
- Terbinafine

Pathogenesis

Psoriasis is a common hereditary disease with a chronic course that primarily affects the skin, with variable involvement of joints and oral mucosa. It has been estimated that up to 7 million Americans have psoriasis. Psoriasis is a genetic disorder that usually arises in adolescents and adults after a trigger, such as a streptococcal infection, recent life crisis, skin injury, drugs, and alcohol and tobacco use.

Clinical Features

- Psoriasis may affect any area of the body; however, there is a distinct predilection to involve areas of trauma, such as the elbows, knees, and intergluteal fold.
- The primary lesion in a developed disease is an erythematous papule or plaque, with white adherent scale (Figs. 8.1–8.3). Scale is often absent in inverse psoriasis (Fig. 8.4), where the skin is moist.
- The Koebner phenomenon occurs in about 5% of patients.
- Nail involvement is common but not always present; it usually consists of variable numbers of distinct nail pits. Less common nail manifestations include yellowish-brown areas of discoloration below the nail (so-called oil spots) and full-thickness nail dystrophy (see Chapter 25).
- Patients may also demonstrate pustular lesions and may actually report a history of transforming back and forth between classic papulosquamous lesions and pustular lesions.

Diagnosis

- The clinical presentation of a papulosquamous eruption, with a distinct edge and silvery scale, in a characteristic distribution is usually diagnostic. Psoriasis is usually not pruritic in 80% of cases.
- The presence of the Koebner phenomenon is strongly supportive of the diagnosis.
- The presence of significant nail pitting or oil spots in the nail bed is strongly suggestive of psoriasis.
- In regard to family history, first-degree relatives with psoriasis can be identified in about one-third of patients.
- Rare cases may require a 3- or 4-mm punch biopsy of a well-developed lesion (more likely diagnostic).

Treatment

The selection of therapy depends on the patient's age and general health, cost, local availability of specialized treatment facilities, type of psoriasis (e.g., pustular vs. plaque), distribution of psoriatic lesions, extent of involvement, experience of the health care provider, and motivation of the patient.

- Topical options include corticosteroids of varying strength, depending on the location, severity of disease, and response to therapy. Approximately 80% of patients treated with topical corticosteroids will demonstrate significant clearance.
- Other commonly used topical options include calcipotriol, coal tar products, salicylic acid, tazarotene, and tacrolimus. Patients who do not respond to topical therapy should be evaluated by a dermatologist for alternative therapy.
- Ionizing radiation therapies include natural sunlight (cheapest option), ultraviolet B (UVB) phototherapy (to include narrow-band UVB), Goeckerman regimen (UVB + coal tar), PUVA phototherapy (methoxsalen + UVA), and 308-nm excimer laser.
- Systemic therapy options include methotrexate, mycophenolate, acitretin, cyclosporine, alefacept, infliximab, adalimumab, secukinumab, and etanercept.
- In patients with guttate psoriasis, or patients with a sudden flare of psoriasis, consider empiric oral antibiotics to eliminate infectious triggers.
- Discontinue any drugs implicated in triggering or aggravating psoriasis.

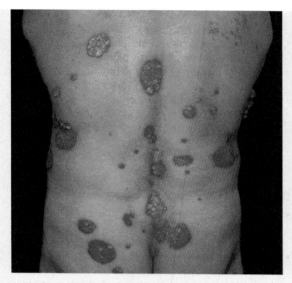

Fig. 8.1. Patient with numerous well-demarcated plaques of variable size, with focal marked scaling on the back. (From the Fitzsimons Army Medical Center Collection, Aurora, CO.)

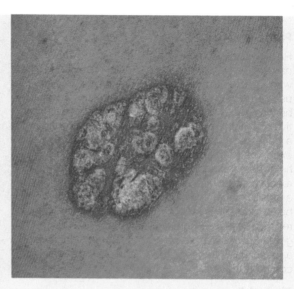

Fig. 8.2. Close-up view of a characteristic lesion of a patient with psoriasis, with sharply demarcated borders and marked white scale. (From the Fitzsimons Army Medical Center Collection, Aurora, CO.)

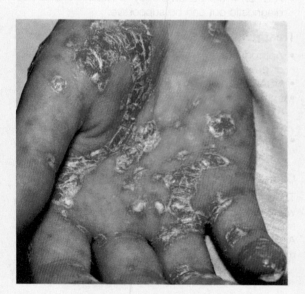

Fig. 8.3. Psoriasis of the palms and soles may show sharply demarcated plaques, as seen here, or may have a diffuse pattern resembling that of hand dermatitis. (From the William Weston Collection, Aurora, CO.)

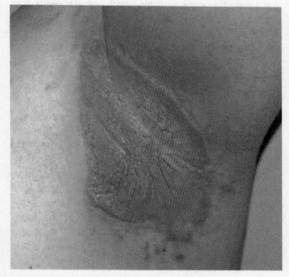

Fig. 8.4. Patient with inverse psoriasis of the axillae. Psoriasis in moister intertriginous areas often lacks scale; however, in contrast to dermatitis, the lesions are usually sharply demarcated, as demonstrated here.

Reactive Arthritis (Reiter Disease) ICD10 code M02

Pathogenesis

Reiter disease, now called *reactive arthritis*, was named after a German army lieutenant, Hans Reiter, who reported this disease in 1916. In recent years, the use of his name has become controversial because he was convicted of being a Nazi war criminal. Reactive arthritis, like psoriasis, is seen in individuals with a genetic predisposition to develop the disease after exposure to the proper trigger. Epidemiologic studies have demonstrated that there is a 10% incidence of reactive arthritis among relatives of the proband, with a positive human leukocyte antigen B27 (HLA-B27) being present in about 70% of white patients with reactive arthritis. Enteric pathogens, including *Shigella, Salmonella, Yersinia,* and *Campylobacter* spp. and sexually transmitted *Chlamydia,* are the most common triggers.

Clinical Features

- There is often a history of enteric infection or *Chlamydia* infection 1 to 4 weeks before the onset of symptoms.
- The classic triad of Reiter disease is nongonococcal urethritis, conjunctivitis, and arthritis, with the classic triad being present at the time of presentation in only 40% of cases. The mucocutaneous findings are often critical in establishing the diagnosis. These are as follows:
  - Nail changes—often associated with keratodermia blennorrhagica. These consist of pitting, subungual hyperkeratosis, and onycholysis, which are clinically indistinguishable from the nail changes seen in psoriasis. Erythema and pustulation may occur in the paronychial tissues (Fig. 8.5).
  - Keratodermia blennorrhagica—skin lesions that begin as pinpoint erythematous papules that progress to pustules, hyperkeratotic papules, and plaques . Texts on this subject invariably only show pictures on the bottom of the feet, but these lesions frequently occur on the scalp, elbows, knees, buttocks, and genitalia. This occurs in approximately 30% to 50% of patients.
  - Circinate balanitis (balanitis circinata)—occurs on the glans penis as shallow, annular (circinate) erosions, ulcerations, or scaly plaques (Fig. 8.7). This occurs independently of the urethritis and is seen in up to 50% of patients. Women may experience an analogous circinate vulvitis.
  - Stomatitis is present in 40% of patients and presents as nonspecific painless erythema, erosions, or ulcerations on the palate, tongue (may resemble geographic tongue), gums, buccal mucosa, or lips.

Diagnosis

- Clinical presentation—the diagnosis is difficult because there is no single test. It requires both correlation and the exclusion of other possibilities.
- Useful laboratory tests include a blood test to detect the genetic factor HLA-B27. A positive test does not establish a diagnosis of reactive arthritis but is supportive. Negative results for an antinuclear antibody (ANA) and rheumatoid factor are helpful in excluding other clinical possibilities.
- A 3- or 4-mm punch biopsy of lesional skin is not diagnostic but can be supportive.

Treatment

- Appropriate antibiotic treatment for the suspected or proven bacterial trigger
- NSAIDs as initial therapy of arthritis
- Immunosuppressive agents (e.g., methotrexate) or biologic agents such as tumor necrosis factor-α (TNF-α) inhibitors for severe or recalcitrant cases
- Topical therapy of choice for the cutaneous manifestations—usually topical corticosteroids

Clinical Course

The initial episode typically lasts from 2 to 6 months, with 10% of patients experiencing chronic reactive arthritis lasting more than 12 months (Fig. 8.8). Approximately 50% of patients will experience two or more additional episodes.

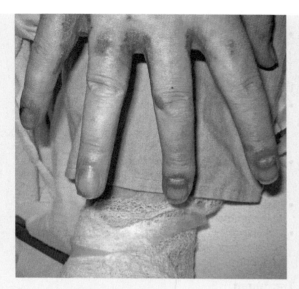

Fig. 8.5. Patient with acute reactive arthritis, with proximal acute paronychia and onycholysis. A lesion on the foot of this patient is shown in the adjacent photograph (Fig. 8.6).

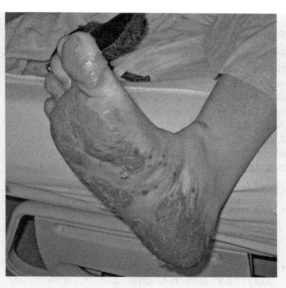

Fig. 8.6. Patient with keratodermia blennorrhagica demonstrating an admixture of erythematous papules and red plaques with scale. Note that there is also a lesion on the leg.

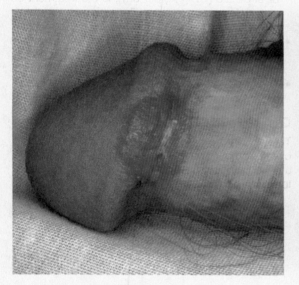

Fig. 8.7. Patient with balanitis circinate presenting as a small scaly plaque on the penis. (From the Fitzsimons Army Medical Center Collection, Aurora, CO.)

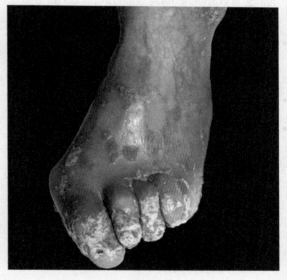

Fig. 8.8. This 25-year-old man with chronic reactive arthritis had persistent scaly plaques and nail changes. The trigger in this case was a *Shigella* infection acquired in Turkey.

Pityriasis Rubra Pilaris ICD10 code L44.0

Pathogenesis

Pityriasis rubra pilaris (PRP) is an uncommon chronic skin disorder that may be acquired (most common) or familial (rare). The pathogenesis is not understood, but occasional reports of low serum levels of retinol-binding protein and resemblance to vitamin A deficiency have suggested an anomaly of vitamin A metabolism. This is important given the frequent response to retinoids. Familial pityriasis rubra pilaris has also been associated with *CARD14* mutations.

Clinical Features

- The much more common acquired form usually presents in middle-aged or older adults; the rare familial variant (autosomal dominant) is more likely to present in children.
- The primary lesions are typically erythematous and scaly (often salmon-colored) and characteristically develop in a cephalad to caudad fashion (Fig. 8.9), with islands of sparing (Figs. 8.10 and 8.11).
- Early in the course, this is usually confused with severe seborrheic dermatitis. Characteristic follicular papules, often on the dorsal aspects of the hands and fingers, have been described as feeling like a "nutmeg grater"; these are distinct and are not seen in seborrheic dermatitis.
- Hyperkeratotic palms (Fig. 8.12) and soles typically develop as the disease progresses and have been described as sandal-like. These are important clinical findings.
- Most patients experience variable pruritus; however, it is usually not as severe as that seen in dermatitis.
- Rarely, patients may eventuate into an exfoliative dermatitis. Patients with human immunodeficiency virus infection are more likely to develop severe pityriasis rubra pilaris.

- Paraneoplastic pityriasis rubra pilaris has also been very rarely reported; a specific associated malignancy has not been identified.

Diagnosis

- The diagnosis is often established by the clinical presentation of relentless, sharply demarcated areas of erythema, with a cephalad to caudad progression that becomes increasingly scaly.
- In some cases, the later manifestations of islands of sparing and hyperkeratotic lesions of the palms and soles are needed to confirm the diagnosis.
- The failure to respond to systemic corticosteroids is also common and is supportive of the diagnosis.
- Skin biopsies are often done. Although they are not usually diagnostic, in some cases they are strongly supportive.

Treatment

- Topical treatment with emollients improves the patient's symptoms and provides comfort without changing the course of the disease.
- An oral retinoid, isotretinoin (1.0–1.5 mg/kg per day) or etretinate (1 mg/kg per day), is the treatment of choice for most patients. The response rate at 4 months is about 75%.
- Oral methotrexate (10–25 mg/kg per week) is the second-line therapy. In our experience, the response rate is lower than with oral retinoids.
- There have been rare isolated case reports of response to biologic agents, such as infliximab.

Clinical Course

The acquired adult form carries a good prognosis because most patients spontaneously involute over a period of months, but the prognosis for the familial form is poor.

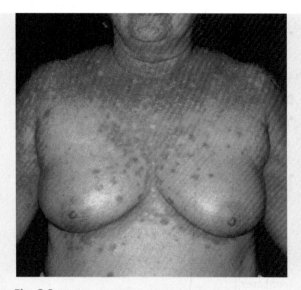

Fig. 8.9. Patient with erythematous macules coalescing into plaques, with variable scale. Note the cephalad to caudad progression. (From the Fitzsimons Army Medical Center Collection, Aurora, CO.)

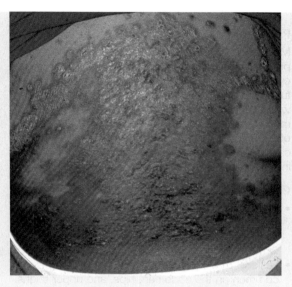

Fig. 8.10. Pityriasis rubra pilaris in a patient with darker skin. The scale is more prominent and darker in color. Note the development of islands of sparing. (From the Fitzsimons Army Medical Center Collection, Aurora, CO.)

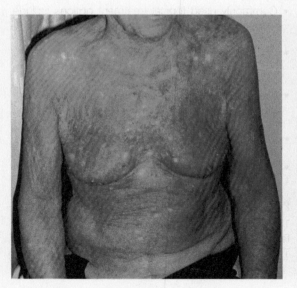

Fig. 8.11. Patient with resolving pityriasis rubra pilaris, with scattered islands of sparing. Note that the upper part of the body demonstrates evidence of resolution in a cephalad to caudad pattern. (From the Fitzsimons Army Medical Center Collection, Aurora, CO.)

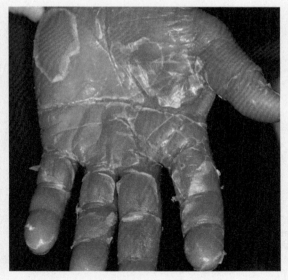

Fig. 8.12. Marked erythema and scale on the palms of an elderly man with pityriasis rubra pilaris.

Mycosis Fungoides ICD10 code C84.0

Pathogenesis

Mycosis fungoides (MF) is a cutaneous T cell lymphoma caused by atypical epidermotropic lymphocytes (Fig. 8.13) that demonstrate the phenotypic and functional qualities of helper T cells. Clinical confusion with chronic eczematous dermatitis and papulosquamous diseases such as psoriasis and pityriasis rubra pilaris frequently occurs. Approximately 2000 new cases of mycosis fungoides are diagnosed each year in the United States.

Clinical Features

- This may occur at any age, including childhood, with the average age of onset being from 45 to 55 years. Males are more commonly affected than females.
- Lesions may occur anywhere but are especially common on the abdomen, hips, and upper thighs.
- The primary lesions in early disease are typically sharply demarcated areas of erythema with variable scale, with variable pruritus that is usually mild (Figs. 8.14 and 8.15).

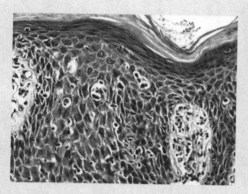

Fig. 8.13. Early mycosis fungoides (MF) demonstrating atypical lymphocytes in the epidermis. It is difficult to distinguish MF from eczematous dermatitis (H&E, 400×).

- As the lesions progress, they typically thicken into plaques and eventually tumors, which can even ulcerate (Fig. 8.16). Patches, plaques, and tumors may be present in the same patient.

Diagnosis

- The diagnosis of MF should be considered or suspected in any patient who demonstrates chronic scaly plaques that are refractory to treatment with emollients and corticosteroids.
- The diagnosis of MF is based on a biopsy. Early MF may be very difficult to diagnose; it is often missed (usually signed out as a nonspecific dermatitis) and frequently requires more than one biopsy. Because the histologic diagnosis is difficult, it is best to send biopsies of suspected cases to a dermatopathologist with expertise in this area.

Treatment

The treatment options in MF are complicated and numerous. In most cases, patients with MF should be referred to a dermatologist or, better yet, to a tertiary referral center with expertise in the management of MF.

- Commonly used topical treatment options include nitrogen mustard, carmustine (BCNU), imiquimod, and corticosteroids.
- Ionizing radiation therapy options include PUVA, RePUVA (retinoids plus PUVA), and electron beam and local radiation.
- Oral treatment options include isotretinoin, bexarotene, interferon-α, and systemic chemotherapy (usually for late-stage disease).
- Photophoresis (for Sézary syndrome or late-stage disease) may be offered.
- Biologic agents that are used include romidepsin and vorinostat.

Prognosis

The treatment of mycosis fungoides is not totally satisfactory, and in most cases a cure cannot be attained. The 5-year survival rate is from 85% to 90%.

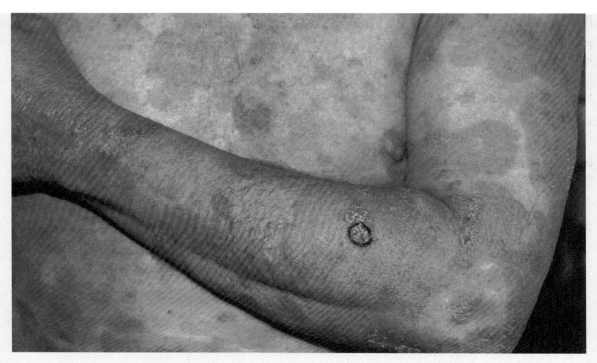

Fig. 8.14. Patient with scaly patches and plaques of mycosis fungoides characterized by variable-sized scales and induration. The ink marking is the site of a planned punch biopsy.

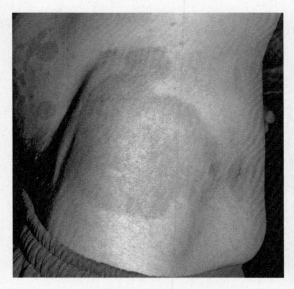

Fig. 8.15. Patient with large plaques with subtle scale that had been present for 8 years. The pelvic girdle is a common location for early lesions. (From the Fitzsimons Army Medical Center Collection, Aurora, CO.)

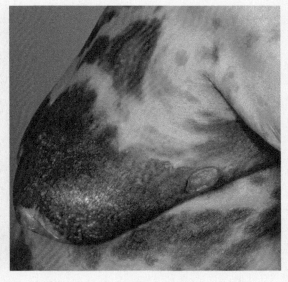

Fig. 8.16. Patient with pigmented mycosis fungoides with patches, plaques, and even two tumors, which are ulcerated.

References

Psoriasis

Mallbris L, Larsson P, Bergqvist E, et al. Psoriasis phenotype at disease onset: clinical characterization of 400 adult cases. *J Invest Dermatol*. 2005;124:499-504.

Nestle FO, Kaplan DH, Barker J. Psoriasis. *N Engl J Med*. 2009;361:496-509.

Severs GA, Lawlor TH, Purcell SM, et al. Cutaneous adverse reaction to infliximab: report of psoriasis developing in 3 patients. *Cutis*. 2007;80:231-237.

Reactive Arthritis (Reiter Disease)

Ajene AN, Fischer Walker CL, Black RE. Enteric pathogens and reactive arthritis: a systematic review of *Campylobacter, Salmonella* and *Shigella*-associated reactive arthritis. *J Health Popul Nutr*. 2013;31:299-307.

Tuuminen T, Lounamo K, Leirsalo-Repo M. A review of serological tests to assist diagnosis of reactive arthritis. *Front Immunol*. 2013;4:418.

Pityriasis Rubra Pilaris

Leger M, Newlove T, Robinson M, et al. Pityriasis rubra pilaris. *Dermatol Online J*. 2012;18:14.

Mercer JM, Pushpanthan C, Anandakrishnan C, Landells ID. Familial pityriasis rubra pilaris: case report and review. *J Cutan Med Surg*. 2013;17:226-232.

Mycosis Fungoides

Sidiropoulos KG, Martinez-Escala ME, Yelamos O, et al. Primary cutaneous T-cell lymphoma: a review. *J Clin Pathol*. 2015;68:1003-1010.

Vollmer RT. A review of survival in mycosis fungoides. *Am J Clin Pathol*. 2014;141:706-711.

Chapter 9
Scaly Disorders

Key Term
Two feet–one hand syndrome

Scaly disorders are a heterogeneous presentation of skin diseases that primarily manifest with scale. This group includes inherited disorders (e.g., ichthyosis vulgaris), acquired disorders (e.g., xerosis), and infections (e.g., tinea pedis).

IMPORTANT HISTORY QUESTIONS

How long has the lesion(s) been present?

This is an important question to distinguish between a genodermatosis, such as ichthyosis vulgaris, from an acquired disorder, such as xerosis.

Have you had a similar lesion(s) in the past?

Some disorders, such as tinea pedis, tend to be one-time events, whereas tinea versicolor and xerosis are often characterized by episodic disease.

Do any of your immediate relatives have a similar disorder?

A "yes" answer indicates a possible genodermatosis; however, the answer has to be weighed against the possibility that the disorder is acquired as an infection from an immediate family member. For example, it is not uncommon for multiple family members to have tinea versicolor or tinea pedis.

How are you treating your skin condition?

Many patients use home-based, over-the-counter (OTC), or prescription remedies that can alter the appearance of the condition. Some home remedies may actually make the condition worse.

Has the skin condition ever been biopsied?

This of course could be helpful in regard to any of the conditions in this chapter; however, not all of the disorders have specific histologic findings. If there is a history of previous biopsies, consider having the biopsy reviewed by a dermatopathologist or a pathologist with expertise in this area because subtle clues to the diagnosis may be missed in scaly disorders.

Are you taking any medications?

This is an important question because some disorders, such as palmoplantar keratodermas, xerosis, and ichthyoses, may be produced by medications.

IMPORTANT PHYSICAL FINDINGS

What is the distribution of the lesions?

Some of the cutaneous disorders demonstrate a characteristic location. For example, ichthyosis vulgaris involves the extensor surfaces of the extremities and spares the intertriginous areas. Tinea pedis and palmoplantar keratodermas are most commonly restricted to palmoplantar areas. Tinea versicolor tends to affect the trunk and usually but not always spares the face.

Are the nails normal or abnormal?

Nail findings may suggest a diagnosis. For example, in tinea pedis there is often accompanying fungal nail disease, whereas in palmoplantar keratodermas, the nails are often unaffected.

What is the color of the scale?

The majority of the scaly disorders demonstrate white scale; however, there are important exceptions, notably tinea versicolor, which has a fine brownish scale, and ichthyosis vulgaris, which has a yellowish-brown scale. Thickened keratin on the palms and soles may have a yellow-brown hue, which may be a clue to an inherited palmoplantar keratoderma.

What are the size and shape of the scale?

Not all scale has the same appearance. For example, tinea versicolor has a fine branlike scale, whereas ichthyosis vulgaris often has a larger rhomboidal scale. Xerosis demonstrates small white scale, which may crack.

Pathogenesis

Tinea versicolor is a common superficial fungal infection produced by the yeast *Malassezia furfur* and other species in this genus. This yeast is a normal part of the cutaneous microflora; however, under certain conditions, it will convert to the mixed hyphal and yeast form, which produces clinical disease. *Malassezia* spp. require lipids for growth and are not dermatophytes. Tinea versicolor is more common in warm humid climates, where it may affect up to 50% of adults.

Clinical Features

- It typically affects adolescents and young adults.
- Tinea versicolor is usually asymptomatic, although occasional patients may complain of a burning sensation or mild pruritus.
- Primary lesions are tan or fawn-colored macules that may coalesce into large patches (Figs. 9.1 and 9.2).
- Close inspection reveals a fine branlike scale that covers the entire macule or patch.
- The affected areas usually display a truncal distribution, although extension to acral areas may occur.
- Hypopigmented macules (Fig. 9.3), due to the production of biochemical products by the yeast that interfere with melanin synthesis and packaging, is a less common presentation. This decrease in pigmentation is more noticeable when the patient has darker skin or is well tanned.

Diagnosis

- A clinical presentation of a predominantly truncal eruption with fine scale that is fawn-colored or hypopigmented is usually diagnostic.
- A potassium hydroxide (KOH) examination can be done by scraping or using clear tape. The finding of an admixture of yeast and short hyphae (so-called spaghetti and meatballs) is diagnostic (Figs. 2.8 and 9.4).

- Rare or atypical cases may require a shave or punch biopsy. The yeast and short hyphae can be seen in the stratum corneum on routine H&E stain; however, special stains make it easier for the pathologist or dermatopathologist to identify the organisms.
- Culture can be done on scrapings but is not recommended because most laboratories have little or no experience preparing special lipid-augmented (usually olive oil) media.

Treatment

- Limited tinea versicolor is best and most easily treated with any of the topical imidazole antifungal creams, including bifonazole, clotrimazole, econazole, ketoconazole, oxiconazole, and tioconazole. There are no differences in efficacy among these agents; price and availability are the driving factors behind the choice. These are typically applied twice per day for 2 to 4 weeks.
- Larger areas of tinea versicolor are better treated with liquid preparations, such as flutrimazole shampoo and ketoconazole shampoo; these are typically applied for 5 minutes before rinsing. Treatment typically lasts 2 to 4 weeks. Topical 2.5% selenium sulfide can also be used in a similar fashion; however, it can be a significant irritant and is not preferred.
- Itraconazole, 200 mg/day for 7 days, or a single dose of 400 mg, has been used effectively and has an expected cure rate of over 80%. Another oral alternative is fluconazole, which is generally used in a dose of 300 mg once weekly for 2 weeks.

Clinical Course

In humid climates, in patients prone to tinea versicolor, the recurrence rate is almost 50% at 6 months after therapy. In one double-blind, placebo-controlled study, itraconazole prophylaxis, using a regimen of 200 mg taken orally each month for 6 months, reduced the relapse rate to 12%.

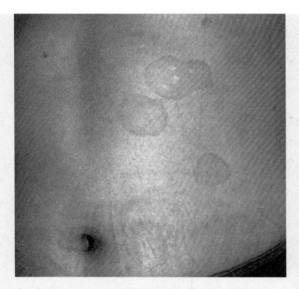

Fig. 9.1. Patient with sharply defined, asymptomatic, fawn-colored patches on the trunk. Note involvement of the navel, an area that is frequently affected.

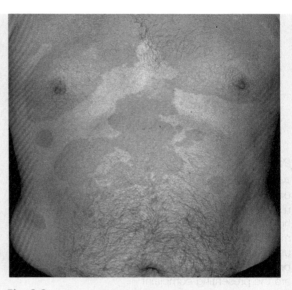

Fig. 9.2. Patient with large confluent plaques of tinea versicolor presenting on the trunk. Once again, note involvement of the naval area.

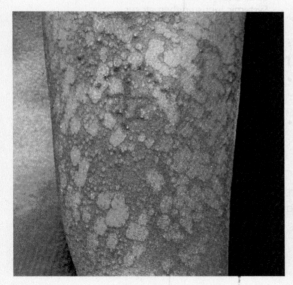

Fig. 9.3. Patient with hypopigmented tinea versicolor presenting as sharply hypopigmented plaques with fine scale on a patient with a darker skin type. (From the Fitzsimons Army Medical Center Collection, Aurora, CO.)

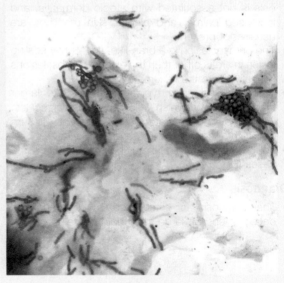

Fig. 9.4. Tape preparation of a sample stained with methylene blue demonstrating diagnostic short hyphae and clusters of yeast (400×).

Drug-Induced Ichthyosis
- Acitretin
- Cholesterol-lowering drugs (e.g., pravastatin)
- Clofazimine
- Hydroxyurea
- Kava
- Lithium
- Nicotinic acid

Pathogenesis

Acquired ichthyosis is associated with a number of underlying conditions, including malignancies (particularly Hodgkin lymphoma), sarcoidosis, graft-versus-host disease, lupus erythematosus, and some medications (see box). This disorder of keratinization usually parallels the course of the underlying disease process. In some cases, the ichthyosiform changes are the presenting complaint.

Clinical Features

- As the name implies, acquired ichthyosis is not present at birth; most cases occur in adults, including the elderly.
- In contrast to ichthyosis vulgaris, acquired ichthyosis is not associated with atopic dermatitis, and increased palmar and plantar skin markings are usually not present.
- The primary lesion is a bran-like, fine, lightly scaling lesion in areas other than the extensor limbs; lesions typically spare the flexures and face.
- The legs and arms typically demonstrate larger brownish or brownish-yellow rhomboidal scales, which may demonstrate a subtle tendency to turn out at the edges (Figs. 9.5 and 9.6).
- Follicular hyperkeratosis may be prominent in some cases (Fig. 9.7).

Diagnosis

- The diagnosis is established by the acquired development of large rhomboidal scales of the extremities and absence of a family history of a similar disorder.
- Once a diagnosis of acquired ichthyosis is suspected, the patient needs a complete review of systems, review of medications, and complete physical examination to identify a systemic cause.
- In most patients in whom an immediate cause is not identified, a chest x-ray is recommended to screen for sarcoidosis or malignancy.
- In some cases, a 3- or 4-mm punch biopsy can be helpful in establishing the diagnosis. For example, the sarcoidal granulomas can sometimes be identified in the underlying dermis in sarcoidal ichthyosis. Another example is the patient shown in Fig. 9.9, whose biopsy identified foreign material in macrophages consistent with a degradation product of clofazimine.

Systematic Causes of Ichthyosis
- Dermatomyositis
- Graft-versus-host disease
- HIV infection
- Leprosy
- Malignancy
- Sarcoidosis
- Systemic lupus erythematosus
- Thyroid disease

Treatment

- The disorder is cured by removing the offending drug or treating the primary disease that is producing the altered keratinization.
- Immediate improvement can be obtained by using emollients, especially those that contain ammonium or sodium lactate.

Clinical Course

The condition typically gradually resolves over a period of several weeks following withdrawal of the drug.

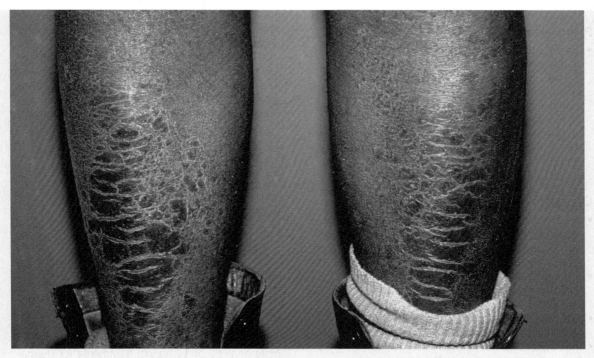

Fig. 9.5. Acquired ichthyosis vulgaris. This patient had sarcoidosis and large, brownish, rhomboidal scale on the anterior legs, indistinguishable from the genetic form of ichthyosis vulgaris. In some cases, a biopsy taken from this area will demonstrate underlying sarcoidal granulomas. (From the Walter Reed Army Medical Center Collection, Washington, DC.)

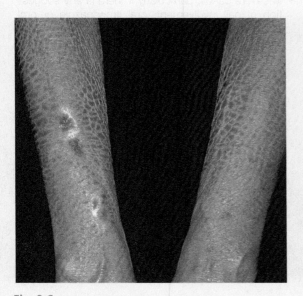

Fig. 9.6. Patient with large brownish rhomboidal scales on the arms secondary to clofazimine. (From the Fitzsimons Army Medical Center Collection, Aurora, CO.)

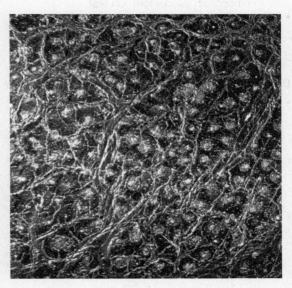

Fig. 9.7. Close-up of lesions of a patient with acquired ichthyosis vulgaris secondary to HIV infection. Note the presence of follicular hyperkeratosis, a feature that is variably present. (From the Fitzsimons Army Medical Center Collection, Aurora, CO.)

Pathogenesis

- The term *athlete's foot,* tinea pedis, is applied to dermatophyte infections of the feet. In the United States, it is the most common superficial fungal infection. Tinea manuum refers to dermatophyte infections of the hand; it is frequently associated with tinea pedis. The most common causative organisms are *Trichophyton rubrum,* followed by *Trichophyton mentagrophytes* and *Epidermophyton floccosum.* Most infections are acquired from other people with a fungal infection.

Clinical Features

- Hyperkeratotic variants of tinea pedis are characterized by diffuse white and yellowish scale that is usually confined to the bottom of the feet (so-called moccasin-like forms).
- Hyperkeratotic moccasin-like forms are often asymptomatic; many patients believe they simply have dry feet.
- It may affect one foot (Fig. 9.8) but usually affects both feet (Fig. 9.9).
- Interdigital variants of tinea pedis appear confined to the interdigital spaces. The hyperkeratosis may demonstrate distinct rings of scale or aggregates of scale (Fig. 9.10).
- Hyperkeratotic variants of tinea manuum present as diffuse scaling of the palms, similar in appearance to the moccasin sandal form on feet.
- Most cases of tinea manuum are unilateral and are associated with bilateral infection of the feet, producing what is known as the *two feet–one hand syndrome* (Fig. 9.11).

Diagnosis

- In some cases, the presence of a unilateral scaly hand or foot, interdigital scaly space, or two feet–one hand syndrome is strongly suggestive of a dermatophyte infection.
- The presence of a thickened nail or nails is a physical finding supportive of a dermatophyte infection.
- The diagnosis is ultimately dependent on identifying a fungus by KOH (Figs. 2.3 to 2.7) or fungal culture.
- Rare cases may require a biopsy and fungal stains.

Clotrimazole-Betamethasone Dipropionate?

In a large study of 176 patients with tinea pedis, the mycologic cure rate after 4 weeks of therapy was 73% for topical naftifine and only 45% for topical clotrimazole-betamethasone dipropionate. The naftifine-treated group also had a lower relapse rate.

Treatment

- Treatment depends upon severity, extent of disease, and cost factors. Options include topical imidazole creams (e.g., clotrimazole, miconazole, econazole, ketoconazole, luliconazole, sertaconazole, sulconazole), topical allylamines (e.g., butenafine, naftifine, terbinafine), or topical ciclopirox olamine. In a meta-analysis of 14 topical treatments for dermatophytes, there was no significant difference in the cure rate among the antifungals, although there was a decreased recurrence rate when allylamines were used.
- In severe cases, particularly if there is any suggestion of nail involvement, oral itraconazole or oral terbinafine is the treatment of choice. There is some evidence that oral terbinafine is more effective.

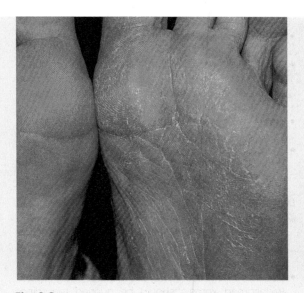

Fig. 9.8. Patient with tinea pedis presenting as a unilateral yellow and white scale. Unilateral presentations are strongly suggestive of a fungal infection.

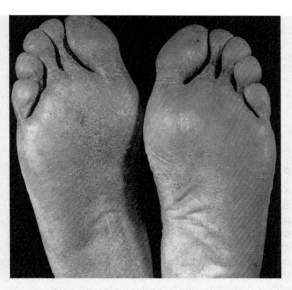

Fig. 9.9. Tinea pedis presenting as bilateral, diffuse, hyperkeratotic white and yellowish scale (moccasin sandal feet). This variant can be difficult to differentiate from dry feet.

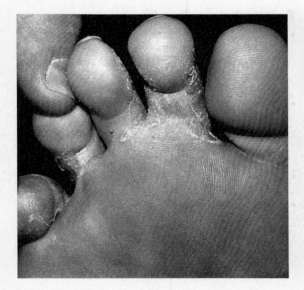

Fig. 9.10. Interdigital hyperkeratotic tinea pedis. As seen here, this pattern almost always affects the space around the fourth toe and is most likely to spare the interdigital space next to the big toe.

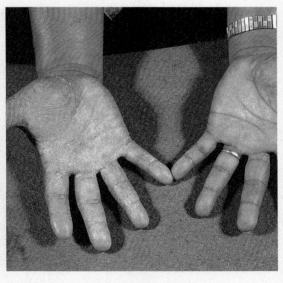

Fig. 9.11. Tinea manuum presenting as unilateral hyperkeratosis. This presentation, when combined with involvement of both feet (two feet–one hand syndrome), is clinically diagnostic.

Drug-Induced Xerosis
- Acitretin
- Anti–tumor necrosis factor inhibitors (e.g., infliximab)
- Cimetidine
- Epidermal growth factor inhibitors (e.g., cetuximab)
- Hydroxyurea
- Isotretinoin

Pathogenesis

Xerosis, which is more commonly known as dry skin, is arguably the most common skin condition in some parts of the world, especially in the elderly. As individuals age, the epidermis becomes thinner, has lower levels of its most important humectant, hyaluronic acid, and loses intercellular lipids. The condition is most often seen and is most severe in individuals with a hereditary predisposition who are exposed to dry climates or topical irritants, such as harsh soaps. Xerosis is most common during the winter months in cold, dry climates when homes are being heated. Less commonly, xerosis may be induced by some drugs (see box).

Systemic Causes of Xerosis
- Diabetes mellitus
- HIV infection
- Hypothyroidism
- Malignancy
- Renal failure
- Sjögren syndrome

Clinical Features

- The primary lesion is a fine white scale, with varying degrees of severity, producing a skin surface that is dry to the touch (Fig. 9.12).
- Pruritus is variably present and is the complaint that is most likely to present in the urgent care setting.

- In severe cases, the dry flakes will develop focal redness.
- A subset of patients may even develop erythema or fissuring in severe cases. The term *erythema craquelé* is sometimes used for these cases (Fig. 9.13).
- Some cases may demonstrate variable follicular hyperkeratosis, which can be prominent (Fig. 9.14).
- Xerosis is often most severe on the hands and feet, where there can be marked hyperkeratosis (Fig. 9.15).

Diagnosis

- Xerosis is such a common clinical disorder that the diagnosis is usually but not always evident to the patient and health care provider, and the diagnosis can be made on clinical grounds.
- Patients who present with acute onset of significant widespread xerosis should be queried regarding their medications and symptoms or physical findings that could support a systemic cause.
- Rare cases may require biopsies; however, the histologic findings are not specific and, at best, are only supportive of the diagnosis.

Treatment

- Treatment with an emollient is the cornerstone of initial therapy, and many emollients are helpful. However, the best immediate results are obtained by using emollients containing a strong humectant, such as urea.
- The best long-term strategy for treatment of chronic xerosis is to use emollients that contain sodium lactate or ammonium lactate. These emollients often have a slightly unpleasant odor and may burn if there are fissures.
- Switch the patient to a synthetic soap, such as Dove.
- Xerotic dry heels may also be treated with manual débridement, such as a pumice stone.

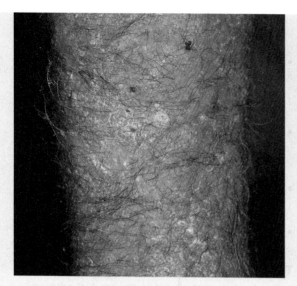

Fig. 9.12. Severe xerosis on the arm of an elderly man. Several of the thicker lesions are actinic keratoses, and it was clinically difficult to differentiate between the two processes.

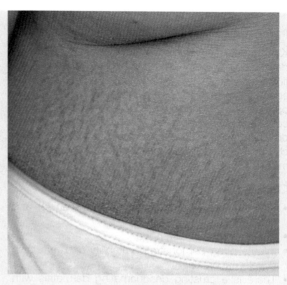

Fig. 9.13. Patient with erythema craquelé. There is moderately severe xerosis on the lateral trunk, with fine fissures and variable erythema.

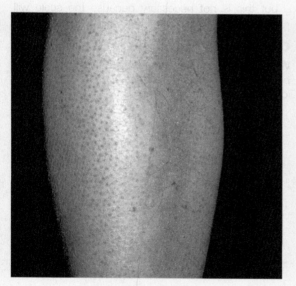

Fig. 9.14. This man presented for the acute development of xerosis, with prominent follicular hyperkeratosis. A clinical history and laboratory evaluation identified profound hypothyroidism as the cause.

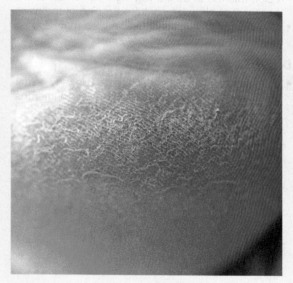

Fig. 9.15. Patient with mildly xerotic heels, one of the most common cutaneous afflictions. Prominence at the lateral edge of the heel is a physical finding that is a clue to the diagnosis. Severe cases frequently demonstrate cracking and fissuring.

Pathogenesis

Kwashiorkor is a nutritional deficiency caused by a deficiency of dietary protein. This results in impaired fluid recovery in the lymphatic system and causes edema. It is primarily seen in those in underdeveloped countries during times of famine. In developed countries, it can be seen in chronic malabsorption disorders (e.g., cystic fibrosis), with fad diets, or with children's medical diets that exclude milk (e.g., a rice milk diet to treat atopic dermatitis).

Clinical Features

- Pitting edema is most prominent in the ankles and feet.
- The abdomen is distended.
- Infants often demonstrate irritability and may also develop anorexia.
- There is a crusting desquamating dermatitis with what appears to be attached scale that flakes. This is referred to as the flaky paint sign or enamel paint sign; it is very distinctive (Figs. 9.16 and 9.17).
- Patients who have alternating periods of improved protein nutrition may develop bands of different hair color, referred to as the flag sign (Fig. 9.18), or the patient may also demonstrate thinning of the hair.
- Other signs of nutritional deficiencies may also be present (e.g., marasmus, pellagra).

Diagnosis

- Kwashiorkor should be suspected in any infant on a diet that excludes milk. There are numerous examples in developed countries of nontraditional fad diets that have produced protein deficiency in infants.
- Retained fluid with pitting edema is the defining sign of kwashiorkor and should be looked for in infants on nontraditional diets. Remember that the infant may appear to have a normal growth curve because the retained fluid may mask true growth failure.
- A skin examination will usually demonstrate a characteristic scaly disorder of keratinization manifesting as flaky paint that peels, leaving what may appear to be normal skin.
- In addition to thinning of the hair, a subset of patients may demonstrate alternating bands of hair color, which is very distinctive.
- A serum total protein will usually demonstrate depressed values.

Treatment

- The treatment of choice is the gradual reintroduction of milk products or other proteins to the diet. However, introduction of large amounts of protein into the diet may overwhelm the capacity of the liver to process the protein and may even result in death.
- The scaly dermatitis can be treated with emollients, but this is not necessary because the scale will resolve with an improved diet.

Clinical Course

With a proper diet, the infant will fully recover, without permanent sequelae. In one study, untreated kwashiorkor had a mortality rate of 19%.

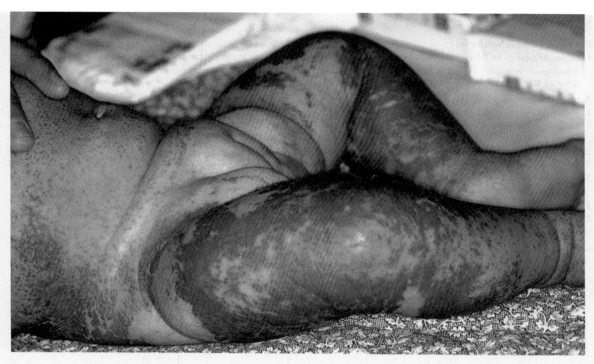

Fig. 9.16. A 5-month-old female infant on a milk-free diet presenting with edema of the lower extremities, hepatomegaly, and characteristic sharply demarcated scale that peels. The infant had maintained a normal weight for her age. (From the William Weston Collection, Aurora, CO.)

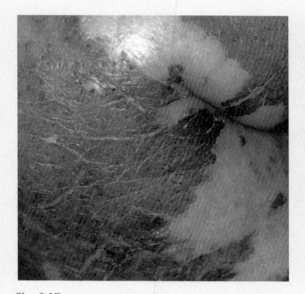

Fig. 9.17. Close-up demonstrating the classic enamel paint sign. (From the William Weston Collection, Aurora, CO.)

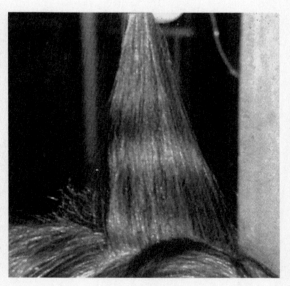

Fig. 9.18. Alternating bands of hair color (flag sign) in a patient with kwashiorkor. (From the William Weston Collection, Aurora, CO.)

References

Pityriasis (Tinea) Versicolor
1. Gupta AK, Lyons DC. Pityriasis versicolor: an update on pharmacological treatment options. *Expert Opin Pharmacother.* 2014;15:1707-1713.

Acquired Ichthyosis Vulgaris
1. Kelley BP, George DE, LeLeux TM, Hsu S. Ichthyosiform sarcoidosis: a case report and review of the literature. *Dermatol Online J.* 2010;16:5.
2. Sparsa A, Boulinguez S, Le Brun V, et al. Acquired ichthyosis with pravastatin. *J Eur Acad Dermatol Venereol.* 2007;21:509-550.
3. Word AP, Cayce R, Panya AG. Beware of underlying malignancy: acquired ichthyosis. *Am J Med.* 2014;127:202-204.

Tinea Pedis
1. Fivenson DP. Clotrimazole/betamethasone diproprionate: a review of costs and complications in the treatment of common cutaneous fungal infections. *Pediatr Dermatol.* 2002;19:78-81.

2. Rotta I, Ziegelman PK, Otuki MF, et al. Efficacy of topical antifungals in the treatment of dermatophytosis: a mixed-treatment comparison meta-analysis involving 14 treatments. *JAMA Dermatol.* 2013;149:341-349.

Xerosis (Asteatosis)
1. Paul C, Maumus-Robert S, Mazereeuw-Hautier J, et al. Prevalence and risk factors for xerosis in the elderly. *Dermatology.* 2011;223:260-265.

Kwashiorkor
1. Buño IJ, Morelli JG, Weston WL. The enamel paint sign in the dermatologic diagnosis of early-onset kwashiorkor. *Arch Dermatol.* 1998;134:107-108.
2. Liu T, Howard RM, Mancini AJ, et al. Kwashiorkor in the United States. Fad diets, perceived and true milk allergy, and nutritional ignorance. *Arch Dermatol.* 2001;137:630-636.

Chapter 10
Dermatitis (Eczematoid Reactions)

Key Terms

Seborrheic Dermatitis
  Cradle cap

Dandruff
Sebopsoriasis
Seborrhea petaloides

*D*ermatitis, a term interchangeable with the term *eczema*, represents the most common cause of skin-related visits to health care providers in the United States. Histologically, dermatitis is characterized by variable epidermal edema (spongiosis), with inflammatory cells infiltrating the epidermis and dermis. Clinically, dermatitis presents with variable erythema and edema; it can appear to weep or even vesiculate. In many cases, a specific diagnosis cannot be made without clinical data, so the following questions are important to ask of all persons with possible dermatitis.

IMPORTANT HISTORY QUESTIONS

How long has the dermatitis (rash) been present?

Attempt to ascertain if the condition is acute or chronic. Atopic dermatitis, nummular dermatitis, and seborrheic dermatitis are often chronic conditions, albeit with waxing and waning moments. Allergic contact dermatitis, id reactions (autoeczematous eruptions), and eczematous drug eruptions are more likely to be acute in nature.

Have you had a similar rash in the past?

An affirmative answer favors repeated exposures to an allergen in allergic contact dermatitis, an exacerbation of a chronic dermatitis (e.g., atopic dermatitis), or repeated exposure to a drug in a drug-induced eczematous process.

Where did the rash start?

Ascertaining the point of initial involvement may provide an important clue in allergic contact dermatitis (ACD) or irritant contact dermatitis (ICD). Be suspicious of a low-grade allergic contact dermatitis when the condition begins on the thin skin of the eyelids.

Do any of your immediate relatives have eczema, asthma, or hay fever?

When multiple persons in a family have these conditions, an atopic diathesis is suggested. It is important to remember that many laypersons refer to atopic dermatitis as childhood eczema.

Do you have allergies or sensitivity to things that come into contact with your skin?

An affirmative response should prompt additional questioning about a specific allergen and allergic contact dermatitis, or it may again suggest an atopic diathesis; persons with atopy often describe their skin as being sensitive.

What sort of work do you do?

Occupational exposure to an irritant or allergen is an important question. For example, a 2001 study of 1200 health care workers identified an irritant or allergic hand dermatitis in more than one-third of participants.

Have you started any new medications in the past month?

Although eczematous drug eruptions represent just 1% to 4% of drug eruptions, the condition with discontinuation of the offending drug.

How are you treating the rash?

Many patients use home remedies, over-the-counter medications, or borrowed or inappropriate prescription medications that can worsen (or improve) dermatitis.

What else do you put on your skin, and what type of soap do you use?

Many patients use lye-based soaps that are irritants or heavily fragranced soaps that can cause an allergic dermatitis. Dermatitis will improve if synthetic soaps are used instead of harsh, lye-based soaps.

IMPORTANT PHYSICAL FINDINGS

What is the distribution of the dermatitis?

Some types of dermatitis have characteristic patterns of involvement (e.g., flexural involvement in atopic dermatitis, involvement of the scalp, eyebrow, eyelid, and nasolabial folds in seborrheic dermatitis).

Is there a distinct pattern to the dermatitis?

Allergic contact dermatitis is initally sharply circumscribed and assumes linear configurations that begins after contact with the allergen. A sharply circumscribed edge, with central clearing, forming an annulus, should raise concern for a dermatophyte infection rather than a dermatitis.

Pathogenesis

Allergic contact dermatitis (ACD) is a delayed type hypersensitivity process (type IV reaction) that occurs when a low-molecular-weight antigen (hapten) is processed by antigen-presenting cells of the skin. These antigen-presenting cells then travel to the lymph nodes and promote expansion of clonal effector T-cells. The T-cells traverse back to the skin to produce inflammation. The memory T-cells serve to facilitate a quicker immune response upon rechallenge. This process of initial sensitization requires 5 to 21 days to foment, but, upon rechallenge, the elicitation of a second response can occur in 24 to 72 hours.

Clinical Features

- ACD occurs about 5 to 21 days after exposure if the patient is not already sensitized to the antigen or 1 to 3 days after re-exposure if the patient is already sensitized.
- Acute ACD is intensely pruritic and causes erythema and variable edema. Allergic dermatitis is the most likely of all forms of dermatitis to present with blisters (see Chapter 11).
- ACD often demonstrates peculiar configurations, reflecting the points of contact; hence, it may produce linear (Figs. 10.1 and 10.2) or round dermatitis (Figs. 10.3 and 10.4).
- In severe ACD the dermatitis can spread past the point of contact (Fig. 10.5).
- ACD often presents on the thin skin of the eyelids (Fig. 10.6), neck (Fig. 10.7), and web spaces between the fingers.

Diagnosis

- Elicitation of a detailed exposure history is critical in ACD. The exposure period of interest is usually about 1 to 3 days but can be as long as 3 weeks with an initial episode.
- A skin biopsy is not diagnostic but may exclude other diseases that can mimic ACD.
- Patients with exposure to multiple potential allergens, such as a woman with facial dermatitis who

uses facial soaps, creams, and other cosmetics, may require all topical preparations be discontinued. One single agent is then added back each week to identify the agent that produced the ACD.
- Some cases may require patch testing by a dermatologist to identify the offending agent or ingredients.

Treatment

"Rule of 78" for Poison Ivy
For ACD caused by poison ivy, it is often useful to prescribe 78 5-mg tablets of prednisone. Then ask the patient to take 12 tablets the first day, 11 the second day, 10 the third day, and so on, until all the tablets have been taken.

- Mild cases of ACD may respond simply to withdrawal but can also be treated with a mild steroid (e.g., 1% hydrocortisone) or moderate steroid (e.g., 0.1% triamcinolone), applied bid.
- Ointments are a useful choice for ACD because these agents do not contain preservatives that could be involved in the process. Hydrocortisone, 1% ointment, is useful for eyelid dermatitis.
- Severe cases of ACD, especially those on thicker skin, may require potent topical corticosteroids applied bid (e.g., fluocinonide, clobetasol).
- Oral antihistamines (e.g., cetirizine, hydroxyzine) are used for relief of pruritus and provide sedation at night.
- Severe or generalized cases may require oral prednisone (40–100 mg PO qd) for 5 to 7 days. Some haptens, such as those in poison ivy, bind irreversibly to the skin, and new lesions may occur for up to 3 weeks. Prednisone may need to be continued for up to 3 weeks in these cases (see "Rule of 78" inset).
- Skin barrier creams (e.g., Stokogard, Hollister Moisture Barrier, Hydropel, Ivy Shield) are partially effective in preventing ACD to poison ivy.

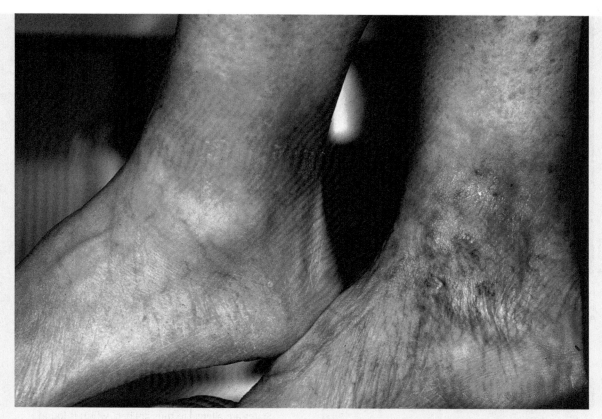

Fig. 10.1. Patient with allergic contact dermatitis to elastin in socks. (From the Fitzsimons Army Medical Center Collection, Aurora, CO.)

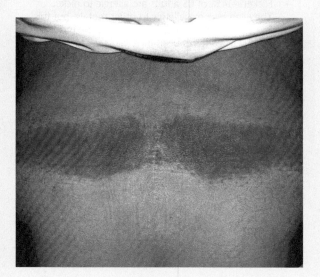

Fig. 10.2. Patient with allergic contact dermatitis to elastin in waistband of underwear. (From the Fitzsimons Army Medical Center Collection, Aurora, CO.)

Contact Dermatitis to Elastic
As demonstrated by the two patients shown in Figs. 10.1 and 10.2, ACD to elastic in clothing can occur. In some cases, it is due to compounds called rubber accelerators that are used during production of the elastic. In other cases, it is due to chemical changes from bleach. In patients with this type of reaction, switching to new clothing and not using bleach avoids the problem.

Allergic Contact Dermatitis (cont.)

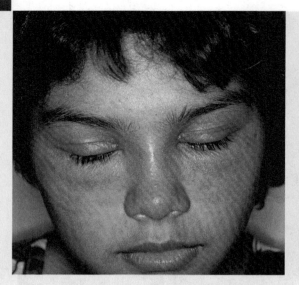

Fig. 10.3. Patient with eyelid dermatitis demonstrating a line of demarcation to the erythema. (From the Fitzsimons Army Medical Center Collection, Aurora, CO.)

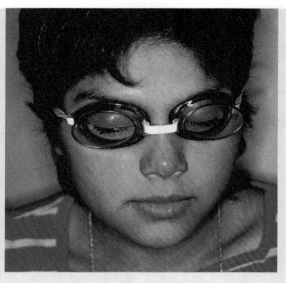

Fig. 10.4. Area of eyelid dermatitis corresponds to goggles worn during swimming. This patient was allergic to one of the rubber accelerators. (From the Fitzsimons Army Medical Center Collection, Aurora, CO.)

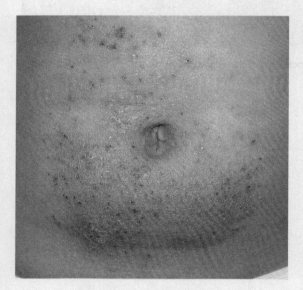

Fig. 10.5. Patient with allergic contact dermatitis due to the nickel found in the metal snap of the jeans. More than 14% of all adults are allergic to nickel. Note that the dermatitis has spread past the point of contact.

Common Causes of Allergic Contact Dermatitis
- Plant allergens—57% of all adults in the United States are allergic to rhus antigen, which is found in poison ivy, poison oak, and poison sumac. It is also found in a variety of related plants (e.g., mango, cashew nut trees)
- Nickel—14% of US adults are allergic to nickel. They can become allergic to other metals, but this is uncommon. It is worth noting that the incidence of ACD to gold has been increasing.
- Formaldehyde and formaldehyde releasers (quaternium-15)
- Neomycin—9% of US adults
- Rubber (thiuram, carba mix)
- Fragrances—8% of US adults

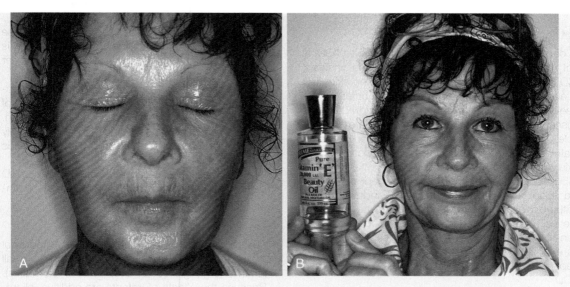

Fig. 10.6. A, Patient with acute onset of markedly pruritic dermatitis. B, The culprit turned out be topical vitamin E. Despite consumer perception, so-called natural products may produce allergic reactions. (From the Fitzsimons Army Medical Center Collection, Aurora, CO.)

Eyelid Dermatitis

Figs. 10.3 and 10.4 demonstrate an important physical finding—namely, involvement of the eyelids. Because the eyelid skin is so thin, it is frequently involved in ACD. It is not uncommon for low-grade ACD to be confined to the eyelids. In a large study of 203 patients with eyelid dermatitis, ACD was the cause in 74% of cases. The remaining patients usually had atopic dermatitis, seborrheic dermatitis, psoriasis, dry eyes, dermatomyositis, and irritant contact dermatitis.

Guin JD: Eyelid dermatitis: experience in 203 patients, *J Am Acad Dermatol* 47:755-765, 2002.

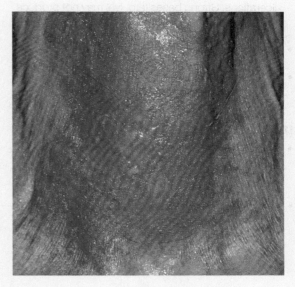

Fig. 10.7. Patient with oozing dermatitis of the thin skin of the anterior neck due to topical neomycin, one of the most common causes of allergic contact dermatitis. (From the Joanna Burch Collection, Aurora, CO.)

Pathogenesis

In contrast to ACD, irritant contact dermatitis (ICD) is not mediated by an immunologic cascade. Instead, ICD is produced by direct toxic injury to the skin. ICD is affected by the nature of the toxic substance, the degree and duration of exposure, and individual skin susceptibility. Some skin sites may be more susceptible, elderly skin is more susceptible, and repeated water exposure damages the barrier function of the skin, making it more susceptible to irritants. Most ICD is caused by soap (e.g., bath soap, dishwashing soap), cleaning products (e.g., window cleaner, bathtub cleaner), alcohols in medications and cosmetics, and glues, cements, and deodorants. ICD can also be caused by minor physical trauma such as exposure to fiberglass, sand, cement, and rough paper. ICD is four- to five-fold more common than ACD.

Clinical Features

- Strong irritants, such as strong acids, produce an immediate burning or stinging with exposure, followed by erythema, edema, and even blisters or ulcerations. Strong bases (e.g. lye) may not produce the same sensory changes but can be just as damaging to the skin.
- Mild irritants, such as soaps, may produce dermatitis through cumulative insult over days or weeks.
- In contrast to ACD, irritant dermatitis is limited to exposed skin, and new lesions do not continue to develop after exposure is terminated.

Diagnosis

- Acute ICD may be self-evident because the patient may observe an immediate and direct relationship to an exposure (Fig. 10.8). Acute ICD follows points of contact with the skin (Figs. 10.9 and 10.10).
- Low-grade and chronic ICD can be difficult to distinguish from other causes of dermatitis; the diagnosis may be established only with a careful exposure history and physical examination (Fig. 10.11).

- In general, biopsy of ICD is not helpful because only nonspecific features of spongiotic dermatitis are observed, but it may be useful in excluding other forms of dermatitis.
- Patch testing may be used to exclude ACD. Provocative use testing can be used, with application of the suspected irritant to a specific area of skin, only if the suspected substance is not excessively harmful. Do not use such testing with strong acids or strong bases.
- In many cases, the diagnosis of low-grade ICD depends on observed improvement with discontinuation of the suspected irritant.

Treatment

- The cornerstone of treatment for ICD is withdrawal of the offending agent, with protection from all irritants (e.g., gloves for irritant hand dermatitis). Because the effects of irritants are additive, all irritants should be avoided.
- The most common irritants are bath soaps, so instruction on proper bathing is important. Dove Sensitive Skin Body Wash, Olay Sensitive Body Wash, Aveeno Daily Moisturizing Body Wash, and Cetaphil skin-cleansing products are excellent choices when ICD is suspected.
- Severe irritant dermatitis (e.g., cantharone blister) is essentially a second-degree burn, and topical treatments are not helpful.
- Moisturizers should be recommended in cases of chronic irritant dermatitis, particularly those with ammonium lactate or sodium lactate, because these agents make the skin less susceptible to irritants. It may take 4 to 6 weeks of continued use to realize the effects of lactate-containing moisturizers.
- Mild to moderate potency topical corticosteroids may be of some benefit in chronic ICD.
- Patients should be cautioned that once the skin is irritated, normal barrier function may not return for 4 weeks and, during this time, the skin is more susceptible to all irritants.

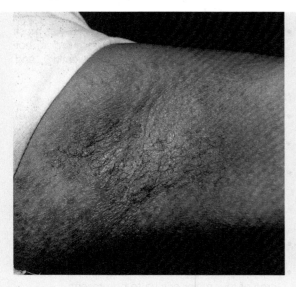

Fig. 10.8. Patient with acute, severe, irritant dermatitis of the axillae due to a topical epilating agent. (From the Fitzsimons Army Medical Center Collection, Aurora, CO.)

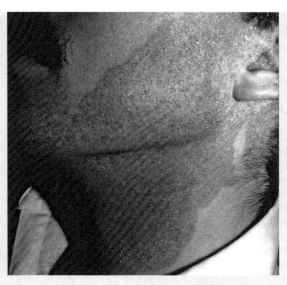

Fig. 10.9. Patient with acute severe irritant dermatitis of the face due to topical epilating agent. (From the Fitzsimons Army Medical Center Collection, Aurora, CO.)

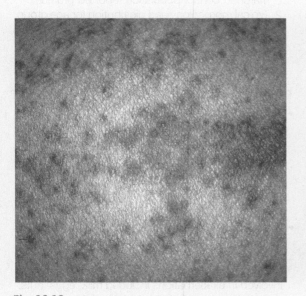

Fig. 10.10. Patient with papular irritant dermatitis caused by exposure to fiberglass that followed a weekend of insulating an attic. (From the Fitzsimons Army Medical Center Collection, Aurora, CO.)

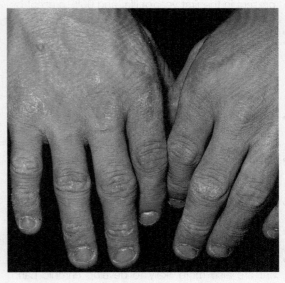

Fig. 10.11. Chronic, low-grade irritant dermatitis due to repeated exposure to soaps in a patient who worked as a car washer. (From the Fitzsimons Army Medical Center Collection, Aurora, CO.)

Pathogenesis

The precise incidence of atopy is unknown, but current evidence suggests that 9% to 20% of all individuals in the United States have an atopic diathesis. Atopy is inherited, and 70% of persons with atopic dermatitis (AD) have a family history of asthma, allergic rhinitis, and/or AD. Evidence suggests that an atopic diathesis is determined by the varied expression of 20 or more genes and is also affected by various environmental stimuli. The immunologic aberrations of atopy are poorly understood, but patients with AD manifest an increased release of histamine from mast cells and basophils, blood and tissue eosinophilia, and exaggerated immunoglobulin E (IgE) response mechanisms. Persons with atopy can be exquisitely sensitive to pruritic stimuli and have depressed cell-mediated immunity. Recent studies have linked some cases of AD to mutations in filaggrin, a protein important in the barrier function of the stratum corneum of the epidermis.

Clinical Features

- Most cases of AD present in childhood—60% present in the first year of life, and 90% present by the age of 5 years.
- During the infantile phase (2 months–2 years), patients demonstrate marked pruritus, excoriations, and diffuse dermatitis that usually involves the head, portions of the trunk, and diaper area (Figs. 10.12–10.14). Half of these patients will clear by the age of 3 years.
- During the childhood phase (3–11 years), lichenified plaques are common on the wrists, ankles, buttocks, and antecubital and popliteal fossae.
- During the adolescent phase (12–20 years), lichenified plaques are common on the face, neck, upper arms, back, and flexures (Figs. 10.15 and 10.16).
- AD persists in adulthood in only 10% of patients, but, when this occurs, the disease presents in much the same way as in the adolescent phase (Figs. 10.17–10.19).
- Adult patients with AD may experience only xerosis but are also more likely to develop chronic hand dermatitis.
- Other physical findings common in patients with AD include xerosis (see Chapter 9), keratosis pilaris, ichthyosis vulgaris, Dennie-Morgan lines (linear transverse folds below the lower eyelids), pityriasis alba (see Chapter 27), and transverse nasal creases (the so-called allergic salute).
- Patients with AD are more likely to harbor *Staphylococcus aureus* (~64% in one study) and are also susceptible to viral superinfection of inflamed skin (e.g., herpes simplex virus [HSV]—eczema herpeticum, vaccinia—eczema vaccinatum, or coxsackievirus A16—eczema coxsackium).

- In a large study of over 2500 children, AD was most often exacerbated by sweating from exercise, hot weather (possibly also because of sweating), and fabrics (especially wool).

Diagnosis

- A careful personal and family history and review of past skin disease are important.
- Unexplained pruritic dermatitis occurring in a child should prompt consideration of AD.
- AD cannot be diagnosed with any single laboratory test, but often patients with AD have an elevated serum IgE level and, possibly, peripheral eosinophilia. A raised total or allergen-specific IgE level was found in 74% of 1097 children with AD.
- A skin biopsy is usually nondiagnostic but may exclude other diseases that can mimic AD.
- A proposed diagnostic scheme for AD requires three of four major criteria to be present:
  1. Pruritus—some authorities believe that this is the principal problem (the itch that rashes). In one study, 52% of patients with AD reported pruritus, even without skin lesions, whereas only 6% of a matched control population reported pruritus.
  2. Typical morphology and distribution for age group (e.g., flexural areas)
  3. Chronic or chronically relapsing dermatitis
  4. Personal or family history of atopy (e.g., allergic rhinitis, asthma, AD)

Treatment

- Removal of cutaneous irritants (soaps, wool) improves AD. Dove Sensitive Skin Body Wash, Olay Sensitive Body Wash, Aveeno Daily Moisturizing Body Wash, and Cetaphil skin-cleansing products are excellent choices for persons with AD. Fragrance-free laundry detergents and fabric softeners can be helpful but generally are not as important as gentle skin bathing choices.
- Food elimination diets are controversial. One study of 160 patients with AD has reported that 28% of individuals experienced exacerbations of AD when challenged with certain foods. The foods most often involved in exacerbations included milk, eggs, nuts, soy, wheat, and seafood. Note that food elimination diets need to proceed with extreme caution because there have been reports of such diets producing malnutrition in children (see discussion of kwashiorkor in Chapter 9). Consultation with a dietician is an option.
- Generous and liberal lubrication is critical. Ammonium lactate– or sodium lactate–containing moisturizers (e.g., AmLactin, Lac-Hydrin) are effective, if tolerated, but these agents may produce a burning sensation. Eucerine Smoothing Repair and Eucerin Intensive Repair, which also contain urea, are lotions that contain sodium lactate in weaker

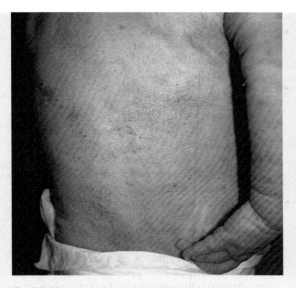

Fig. 10.12. Infant with atopic dermatitis demonstrating eczematoid dermatitis. Note the active excoriation and white dermatographism. (From the Fitzsimons Army Medical Center Collection, Aurora, CO.)

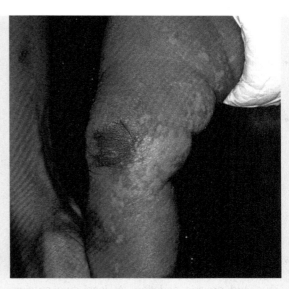

Fig. 10.13. Infant with chronic atopic dermatitis. Note the presence of hyperpigmented and hypopigmented areas. (From the Fitzsimons Army Medical Center Collection, Aurora, CO.)

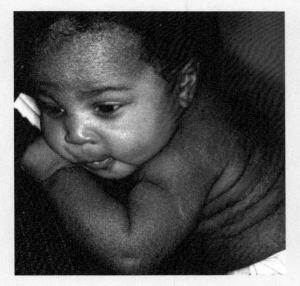

Fig. 10.14. Infant with atopic dermatitis demonstrating extensive scale, a common finding in atopic dermatitis. (From the Fitzsimons Army Medical Center Collection, Aurora, CO.)

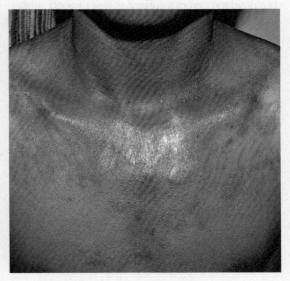

Fig. 10.15. Adolescent with atopic dermatitis of the flexural area of the neck. Some of the lesions demonstrate round configurations and resemble nummular dermatitis.

concentrations, and they are less likely to produce a burning sensation.

- Acutely inflamed or oozing skin may benefit from the application of open wet compresses. Some dermatologists use tap water, and others prefer a modified Burow solution (e.g., Domeboro).
- Topical corticosteroids are a mainstay of therapy for AD. The strength of the corticosteroid must to be tailored to the anatomic site involved and severity of disease. Mild disease may respond to 1% hydrocortisone cream, but more significant disease may require more potent topical corticosteroids, such as triamcinolone, fluocinonide, or even clobetasol for a short period. Severe AD may require corticosteroids under occlusion in conjunction with wet-dry wraps and/or with hospitalization.
- Oral antihistamines (e.g., cetirizine, hydroxyzine, diphenhydramine) are often used to decrease pruritus and provide sedation. At least two studies have demonstrated hydroxyzine to be effective in reducing pruritus in AD. One study has demonstrated that 0.7 mg/kg tid of hydroxyzine was as effective as 1.4 mg/kg tid in reducing the pruritus in children, with lesser sedation. Children or infants with severe AD not only keep themselves awake but drain the parent's energy as well through familial sleep deprivation.

- Rare patients may require short-term oral corticosteroids for severe outbreaks. This should be avoided, if possible, due to the young ages of typical patients with AD and chronicity of the disease.
- Secondary infections, usually due to *S. aureus*, should be treated with appropriate oral antibiotics (e.g., cephalexin, dicloxacillin). In a study of 306 children with AD, 64% of patients were colonized with *S. aureus*. Clinical and experimental studies have supported the concept that topical steroids plus antistaphylococcal antibiotic therapy is more effective than topical steroids alone.
- Bleach baths may be effective in controlling staphylococcal infections and may even be antipruritic. However, the bleach bath must be dilute—½ cup of unscented household bleach in a full tub of water, approximately 1 tsp/gallon). Soaks should last 5 to 10 minutes. Explain to parents that the desired concentration is the same as that of pool water, and too much bleach can cause an irritant dermatitis.
- Topical tacrolimus and topical pimecrolimus can be used as alternatives for many patients, but both carry a black box warning with regard to use in patients younger than 2 years.

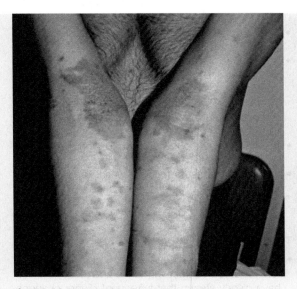

Fig. 10.16. Classic atopic dermatitis in an adolescent involving both antecubital fossae. (From the Fitzsimons Army Medical Center Collection, Aurora, CO.)

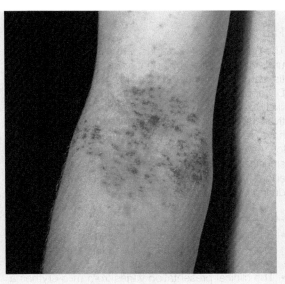

Fig. 10.17. Man with flexural atopic dermatitis demonstrating excoriations and yellow crust due to secondary staphylococcal infection. (From the Fitzsimons Army Medical Center Collection, Aurora, CO.)

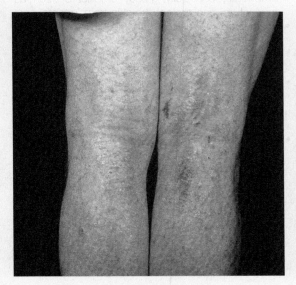

Fig. 10.18. Flexural atopic dermatitis in an adult demonstrating secondary linear excoriation. (From the Fitzsimons Army Medical Center Collection, Aurora, CO.)

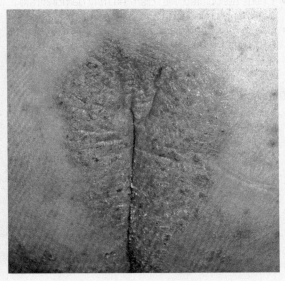

Fig. 10.19. Patient with atopic dermatitis of the sacral area demonstrating thick skin, with increased skin markings indicating secondary lichenification. (From the Fitzsimons Army Medical Center Collection, Aurora, CO.)

Diaper Dermatitis

Pathogenesis

The pathogenesis of diaper dermatitis (DD) is not fully understood, but it is thought to be an irritant dermatitis, caused by urine and feces in contact with the skin. DD appears to be more common in patients with AD, likely because of an impaired epidermal barrier. Multivariate analyses of children in the United Kingdom have revealed the presence of oral candidiasis, a low frequency of diaper changes, and diarrhea to be significant associations. Older texts have noted that about 20% of all infants will develop DD at some time during their first 2 years of life.

Clinical Features

- By definition, DD occurs in infants and young children who wear diapers, but adult cases can be observed in those who are infirm.
- The clinical presentation varies from mild erythema due to chafing to eczematous reactions with variable scale and even shallow erosions (Figs. 10.20–10.23).
- Mild cases often affect the inguinal skin but may spare the deep fold itself, where urine and feces do not actually touch skin.
- Cases associated with diarrhea may demonstrate a perianal prominence.
- Secondary candidiasis is present in some cases and may be associated with flexural accentuation and characteristic satellite pustules, common in candidiasis.

Diagnosis

Differential Diagnosis

- Allergic contact dermatitis (Fig. 10.24)
- Atopic dermatitis
- Candidiasis
- Diaper dermatitis (irritant)
- Langerhans cell histiocytosis
- Seborrheic dermatitis
- Psoriasis

- In most cases, the diagnosis of DD is clear to the parents and health care provider.
- In cases with severe erythema (a beefy red appearance), satellite pustules should suggest secondary candidiasis, and the oral cavity should be examined for thrush. Candidiasis can also be established through performance of a potassium hydroxide (KOH) prep or fungal culture.
- In cases of acute onset occurring in the diaper area, ACD must be excluded.
- In persistent cases, the differential diagnosis also includes psoriasis and Langerhans cell histiocytosis. A shave or punch biopsy may necessary to include or exclude these diagnostic possibilities.

Treatment

- The cornerstone of treatment is reducing prolonged and repeated contact with urine and feces. Studies have clearly shown that infrequent diaper changes and diarrhea are associated with DD. More frequent diaper changes represent an important treatment strategy. Some pediatric dermatologists recommend restricted fluid intake before bed to reduce wet contact during the sleeping hours.
- Emollients, especially greasy emollients such as petrolatum, can protect the skin from irritants.
- Associated candidiasis should be treated with topical nystatin or imidazole. Sulconazole is a particularly strong choice because it has also been shown to have antiinflammatory properties.
- Topical corticosteroids are not widely recommended because this is an occluded site, but, if such a strategy is needed, topical 1% hydrocortisone cream or ointment can be used.
- Some compounding pharmacies offer triple paste or butt paste, which is zinc oxide, hydrocortisone 1% cream, and nystatin cream in a 1 : 1 : 1 ratio.

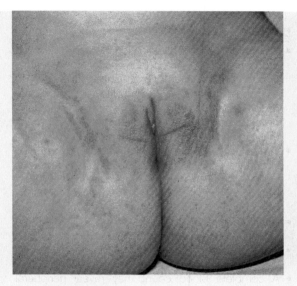

Fig. 10.20. Infant with mild diaper dermatitis with accentuation in the inguinal fold, which is common in mild cases. (From the William Weston Collection, Aurora, CO.)

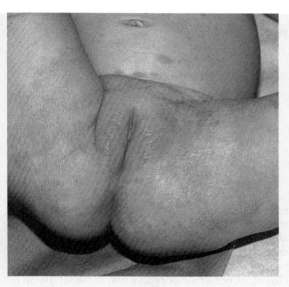

Fig. 10.21. Infant with severe diffuse diaper dermatitis. (From the William Weston Collection, Aurora, CO.)

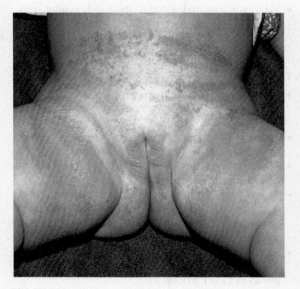

Fig. 10.22. Infant with severe diffuse diaper dermatitis. The small red papules in the waistband area most likely represent miliaria rubra or, less likely, candidiasis. (From the William Weston Collection, Aurora, CO.)

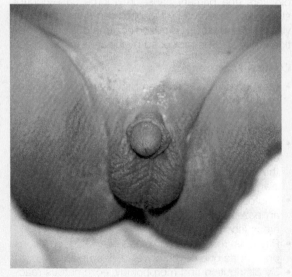

Fig. 10.23. Infant with allergic contact dermatitis to Bag Balm mimicking diaper dermatitis. (From the William Weston Collection, Aurora, CO.)

Pathogenesis

Common Drugs
- Calcium channel blockers
- Carbamazepine
- Gold
- Griseofulvin
- Phenytoin
- Piroxicam
- Sulfonamides
- Thiazide diuretics
- Vitamin K

Eczematous (spongiotic) drug eruptions are drug eruptions that resemble dermatitis (eczema). Eczematous drug eruptions account for just 1% to 4% of all drug eruptions but are an important cause to consider because the condition resolves with discontinuance. Like most eczematous processes, eczematous drug eruptions are mediated by a T cell–derived allergic response. A subset of eczematous drug eruptions also requires light exposure to produce a reaction (photoallergic drug eruptions). Notorious causes of photoallergic drug eruptions include calcium channel blockers (the primary cause in a large case-control study), hydrochlorothiazide, piroxicam, and griseofulvin (see Chapter 19). Localized eczematous drug eruptions may also be produced by injected medications.

Clinical Features
- Most eczematous drug eruptions are composed of papules and plaques, of varied size, that may erode or vesiculate. Individual lesions can be indistinguishable from those of ACD (Figs.10.24 and 10.25).
- Eczematous reactions confined to injection sites e.g., (heparin, interferon) develop 2 to 7 days after the injection. They consist of pruritic erythematous plaques that may vesiculate (Fig. 10.26).
- Photoallergic drug-induced dermatitis manifests as an eczematous process confined to sun-exposed areas (see Chapter 19).
- Pityriasis rosea–like or plaquelike drug eruptions present as one or more well-defined plaques.
- By distribution and morphology, eczematous reactions can mimic other forms of dermatitis, such as AD (Fig. 10.27) or nummular dermatitis.

Diagnosis
- The relationship of medication use to the onset of dermatitis is an important observation because eczematous drug eruptions usually develop 1 to 14 days after starting a drug. However, there are exceptions to this rule, and some patients can develop eczematous drug eruptions from drugs that they have used for many years.
- The absence of another identifiable cause is also important because, if the patient has a known history of AD, nummular dermatitis, or any other well-documented cause of dermatitis, this may affect the likelihood of an eczematous drug eruption.
- Pruritic dermatitis at the site of an injection is often a localized eczematous drug eruption.
- A skin biopsy is not typically diagnostic but can be useful in ruling out other causes of dermatitis.
- A complete blood count may reveal peripheral eosinophilia. Although this may be supportive evidence of a drug-induced hypersensitivity process, one must recognize that a drug-induced process may be present with peripheral eosinophilia and that other causes of peripheral eosinophilia exist.
- In many cases, resolution of the reaction after withdrawal of the suspected medication, possibly with recurrence on rechallenge, provides the most definitive evidence of a drug-induced process.

Treatment
- Withdraw the offending drug, recognizing that it can take 1 to 3 weeks for complete resolution of the reaction.
- Midpotent to ultrapotent topical steroids may be prescribed for a short duration until resolution.
- Antihistamines (e.g., cetirizine, hydroxyzine) may be used for severe pruritus.
- Topical anesthetic or soothing creams may be used, such as hydrocortisone acetate– and pramoxine (Pramosone, Epifoam, Novacort)–based creams, foams, or lotions.
- Sunscreens with broad protection (including ultraviolet A [UVA]) are necessary for patients with photo-induced processes.

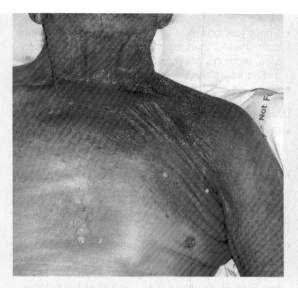

Fig. 10.24. Intense eczematoid dermatitis due to lisinopril. The patient also demonstrated a peripheral eosinophilia.

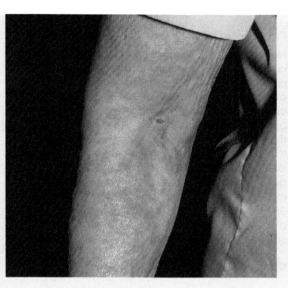

Fig. 10.25. Patient with eczematoid drug eruption due hydroxychloroquine. (From the Fitzsimons Army Medical Center Collection, Aurora, CO.)

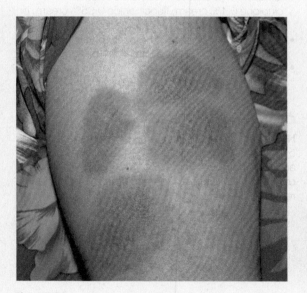

Fig. 10.26. Patient with eczematoid drug eruption due to four vitamin K injections.

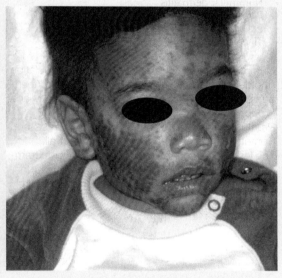

Fig. 10.27. Eczematoid drug eruption due to trimethoprim-sulfamethoxazole in a young child that mimics facial infantile atopic dermatitis. (From the Fitzsimons Army Medical Center Collection, Aurora, CO.)

Nummular Dermatitis ICD10 code L30.0

Pathogenesis

Nummular dermatitis is derived from the Latin word *nummulus*, which means "coinlike." The condition produces round, coin-shaped, areas of dermatitis, often on the lower extremities. The condition is more common in areas of low humidity and in winter, suggesting that excessive drying of the skin is involved in the pathologic process. Also, individual lesions tend to recur at sites of prior involvement, suggesting some localized susceptibility. As in AD, soaps, wool, frequent bathing, and other irritants may worsen nummular dermatitis. Staphylococcal species colonize 95% of skin lesions but may or may not be involved directly in causation. In contrast to atopic dermatitis, serum IgE levels are usually normal.

Clinical Features

Differential Diagnosis of Coin-Shaped Plaques of Dermatitis
- Atopic dermatitis
- Eczematoid drug eruptions
- Mycosis fungoides
- Nummular dermatitis
- Parapsoriasis
- Pityriasis rosea
- Tinea corporis

- Nummular dermatitis affects a biphasic population of older men (>50 years) and young women (teenagers and young adults), but it can affect any age group.
- Pruritus is usually present and can be severe. Sometimes, patients report no pruritus at all.
- The lesions are usually located on the lower extremities (Fig. 10.28) but may also involve the upper extremities and trunk. The head and neck are rarely involved.

- Primary lesions exist as round to oval erythematous coin-shaped plaques studded with pinpoint vesicles, erosions, and crusts (Figs. 10.29 and 10.30). Individual lesions vary from 1 to 10 cm in size.
- Chronic lesions may develop lichenification.

Evaluation

- The diagnosis of nummular dermatitis is based on history, distribution, and characteristic appearance of the lesions.
- Skin biopsy may be useful in excluding other diseases with a similar presentation, such as mycosis fungoides and dermatophyte (tinea) infections.

Treatment

- Most cases of nummular dermatitis can be improved with generous emollient use and avoidance of irritants. Recommended soaps include Dove Sensitive Skin Body Wash, Olay Sensitive Body Wash, Aveeno Daily Moisturizing Body Wash, and Cetaphil skin-cleansing products.
- Many cases require the addition of midpotent to ultrapotent topical corticosteroids, such as triamcinolone 0.1% cream, fluocinonide 0.05% cream, or even clobetasol 0.05% cream in recalcitrant cases.
- Many dermatologists add empiric antistaphylococcal antibiotics, such as dicloxacillin or cephalexin.
- Severe cases may require short-duration oral corticosteroids or phototherapy with narrow-band (NB) UVB light.

Clinical Course

Nummular dermatitis may resolve spontaneously but often persists or waxes and wanes with the seasons and with ambient humidity. In one 2-year study, only 22% of patients demonstrated spontaneous remission.

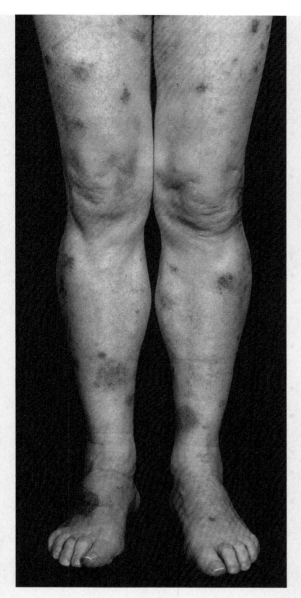

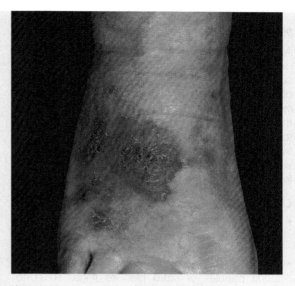

Fig. 10.29. Close-up of a patient with nummular dermatitis demonstrating erythema, scale, and crust. This lesion was secondarily infected with *Staphylococcus aureus.* (From the Fitzsimons Army Medical Center Collection, Aurora, CO.)

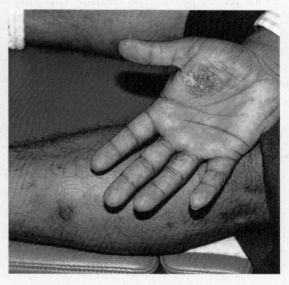

Fig. 10.28. Patient with classic nummular dermatitis of the lower extremities demonstrating numerous round pruritic eczematoid lesions. (From the Fitzsimons Army Medical Center Collection, Aurora, CO.)

Fig. 10.30. Patient with nummular dermatitis of the leg and palm. (From the Fitzsimons Army Medical Center Collection, Aurora, CO.)

Pathogenesis

An id reaction is a secondary immunologic host response that follows a primary eczematous process, such as stasis dermatitis or an infection (tinea). The other term for an id reaction is *autoeczematous response*. For example, as the primary event, a patient may have ACD, infected stasis ulcer, or intense dermatophyte infection, and then the immunologic system triggers an id reaction (autoeczematous response), which leads to inflamed and affected skin well away from the primary process.

Clinical Features

- By definition, the patient must have an identifiable primary skin problem, usually a dermatophyte infection, stasis ulceration, or other form of dermatitis.
- The id reaction consists of erythematous eczematous papules or small plaques (Figs. 10.31 to 10.34).
- Id reactions are often but not always intensely pruritic.
- Less often, id reactions may be bullous or scaly.
- In general, id reactions tend to be more severe near to the primary process and decrease in intensity with distance from the primary process, but there are exceptions. For example, patients with tinea pedis may have id reactions that consist of scaling of the palms, well away from the feet.

Diagnosis

- An id reaction is a challenging diagnosis in dermatology because it may only be definitively established by treating the primary process and producing a remission in the secondary id process.
- A high index of suspicion for an id reaction is necessary in the following situations:
  - A patient with a known primary dermatitis (especially chronic ulcers and superficial fungal infections) with dermatitic lesions that spread the site of involvement of the primary disease
  - A patient with a dermatitis or ulcer that appears secondarily infected and who has a sudden onset of dermatitic lesions of the palms and/or soles
  - Dermatitic lesions that appear to develop from drainage of serum or pus from a primary lesion
- Cultures often grow *S. aureus,* and this may be involved as a superantigen that incites the id reaction.
- A skin biopsy may be helpful in excluding other causes, but the histologic findings are not diagnostic of only an id reaction and cannot be distinguished from those of ACD, AD, nummular dermatitis, and spongiotic drug eruptions.

Treatment

- Management focuses on treatment of the primary skin disorder (e.g., infected ulcer, dermatophyte infection).
- The treatment of pruritus includes topical menthol-camphor or lidocaine-menthol preparations.
- Antihistamines at night (e.g., hydroxyzine, diphenhydramine) are beneficial for sedation and relief of pruritus.
- Treatment with topical steroids requires moderate or potent agents (e.g., triamcinolone, fluocinonide).
- Severe cases may require a 3- to 7-day burst of oral prednisone (40 mg PO qd × 3-7 days).

Clinical Course

- Most acute id reactions last only 2 to 3 weeks as long as the primary process is treated.
- Id reactions may be chronic when the stimulus continues (e.g. continued infection of a leg ulcer).

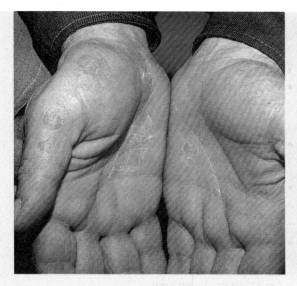

Fig. 10.31. Patient with KOH-negative, low-grade eczematoid reaction on the palms due to tinea pedis. The id reaction resolved with treatment of the feet. (From the Fitzsimons Army Medical Center Collection, Aurora, CO.)

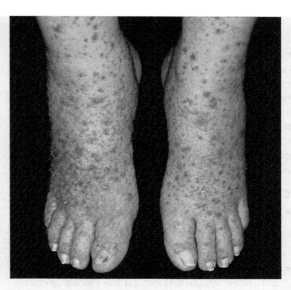

Fig. 10.32. Patient with severe id reaction of the lower extremities due to onychomycosis (note the right great toenail) and tinea pedis. (From the Fitzsimons Army Medical Center Collection, Aurora, CO.)

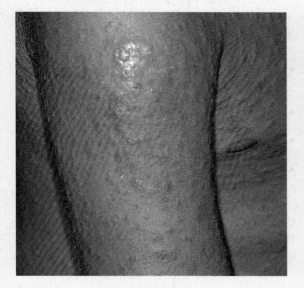

Fig. 10.33. Patient with severe id reaction to a topically applied henna tattoo. The outline of the tattoo is vaguely visible in the center of the arm. (From the Joanna Burch Collection, Aurora, CO.)

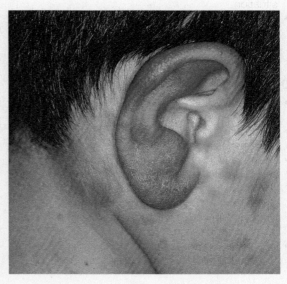

Fig. 10.34. Severe id reaction of the ear and face of a young child due to a kerion of the scalp. (From the William Weston Collection, Aurora, CO.)

Dyshidrosis (Pompholyx) ICD10 code L30.1

INTERNAL ETIOLOGY

Pathogenesis

Dyshidrosis is hand-foot dermatitis of uncertain pathogenesis. A study of 104 patients has f ound that 50% of patients with dyshidrosis have a personal or family history of atopy compared with only 11.5% of patients in a control group with this same personal or family history. Although many patients cannot identify aggravating factors, some patients implicate hyperhidrosis, changing seasons, exposure to harsh chemicals, or even stress.

Clinical Features

- Dyshidrosis is most common in middle-aged women (20–50 years) but also affects men and women of all ages. The condition is uncommon in adolescents or children.
- Often, the condition begins as erythematous skin with eczematous features on the plantar surfaces of the hands (Fig. 10.35) and feet.
- In some patients, clear fluid-filled, tapioca-like vesicles may appear on the lateral digits (Fig. 10.36).
- Less often, the vesicular lesions may be larger and more bullous on the palmoplantar surface; some may refer to the condition as *pompholyx* in this situation.
- Some patients may demonstrate only erythema, without vesiculation, whereas others may demonstrate hyperkeratosis that resembles psoriasis (Fig. 10.37).

Diagnosis

- The diagnosis is established chiefly by history and physical examination.
- The family and personal history should include specific queries regarding atopy.
- Because ACD may mimic dyshidrotic hand dermatitis, a careful exposure history and patch testing should be considered. Patch testing usually needs to be done by a dermatologist but should be considered, especially for those patients with persistent or recurrent disease.
- In unusual cases, a punch biopsy may be useful to exclude other conditions, such as bullous pemphigoid, which can present as blisters on the hands and feet or bullous tinea infections.

Treatment

- Poor barrier function is common in dyshidrosis, particularly given the association with atopy. Excessive wet work, handwashing, and exposure to irritants should be minimized.
- Patients should clean their hands only with gentle cleansers; harsh lye-based soaps should be avoided.
- Hands should be protected from excessive water exposure using vinyl or neoprene or powder-free latex gloves placed over a white cotton glove (the latter for moisture absorption).
- Hand moisturizers with dimethicone (e.g., Thera-Seal Hand Protection, Gloves in a Bottle) may be useful in providing further barrier protection (so-called barrier creams).
- For mild disease, triamcinolone ointment, fluocinolone ointment, or betamethasone diproprionate ointment may be effective. In severe cases, clobetasol ointment or halobetasol ointment may be necessary. Using occlusion with white cotton gloves (with or without vinyl gloves on top) or white cotton socks can increase the penetration of steroids. Tell patients to soak their hands in tap water briefly, apply steroids, cover with gloves or socks, and repeat for 2 to 5 nights.
- Consider 7 to 10 days of treatment with antistaphylococcal antibiotics if the lesions are crusting or oozing.
- Topical bexarotene, 1% gel, applied once or twice daily, is a useful but expensive therapy.
- Severe cases may require short bursts of oral corticosteroids (40–60 mg PO qd for 2–5 days).
- Recalcitrant cases may require topical psoralen and UVA (PUVA) therapy or methotrexate. Refer the patient to a dermatologist.

Clinical Course

The disease tends to be chronic in nature (years) but may disappear spontaneously.

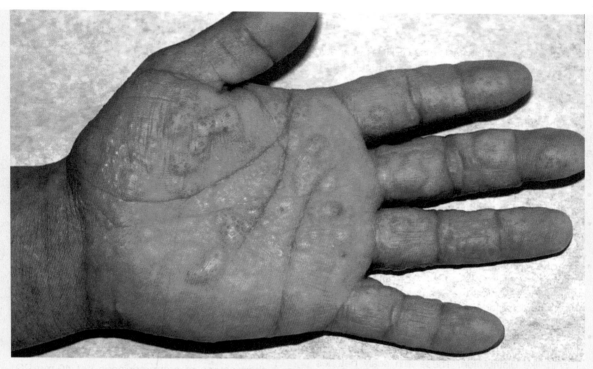

Fig. 10.35. Patient with severe, acute vesicular dyshidrotic hand dermatitis. (From the Fitzsimons Army Medical Center Collection, Aurora, CO.)

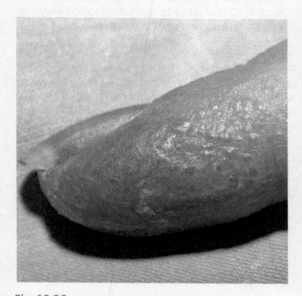

Fig. 10.36. Close-up of dyshidrotic hand dermatitis demonstrating typical small vesicles on the lateral aspects of the fingers. (From the Fitzsimons Army Medical Center Collection, Aurora, CO.)

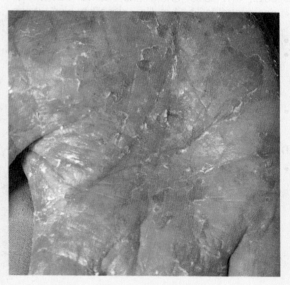

Fig. 10.37. Patient with dyshidrotic hand dermatitis, with erythema and marked scale. (From the Fitzsimons Army Medical Center Collection, Aurora, CO.)

Pathogenesis

The pathogenesis of pityriasis rosea (PR) is not known with certitude, but it has been proposed that the condition is related to viral, bacterial, fungal, or *Mycoplasma* infection, insect bites, or autoimmune disease. The disease has many hallmarks of a viral infection. Recently, some researchers have implicated human herpesvirus 6 and 7 as the cause of PR, but not all authorities agree.

Clinical Features

- Most patients with PR are between 10 and 35 years of age. Women are affected more often than men.
- About 25% of patients with PR report a prodrome of headache, fever, malaise, arthralgias, and gastrointestinal symptoms.
- PR often presents first with a so-called herald patch, present in 12% to 94% of patients, which consists of a solitary erythematous plaque, 2 to 10 cm in diameter (Fig. 10.38). In 5% of cases, the herald patches are multiple.
- About 7 to 14 days after the herald patch (range, 3 hours–84 days), daughter lesions occur in a truncal, T shirt–like distribution. These thin scaly patches and plaques occur along skin tension lines, producing a Christmas tree–like pattern (Fig. 10.39).
- Individual lesions demonstrate an erythematous color, thin scale, and slightly darker center that demonstrates a branlike desquamation when stretched or scratched.
- About one-third of patients complain of pruritus.
- Clinical variants include cases with an inverse pattern (10% to 15%), unilateral pattern, bullous lesions, lichenoid lesions, hemorrhagic lesions, and erythema multiforme–like lesions.
- Oral lesions may be present in 9% of patients (Fig. 10.40).

Diagnosis

- The clinical differential includes dermatophyte infection, nummular dermatitis, PR-like drug eruptions, and secondary syphilis.

- Because PR is self-limited, the diagnosis is often made on a clinical basis, with reassessment in 6 to 12 weeks if the process has not completely resolved.
- Patients with oral lesions or lymphadenopathy should have a screening test (rapid plasma reagin [RPR] test, venereal disease research laboratory [VDRL] test) for syphilis because secondary syphilis may resemble PR.
- A skin biopsy of PR (punch biopsy is preferred) is not typically diagnostic but may suggest the diagnosis and will help exclude other diseases.

Treatment

- Patients do not usually require therapy because the disease is self-limited and is usually asymptomatic.
- Pruritic patients may be treated with topical corticosteroids and antihistamines for symptomatic relief.
- Severe cases can be treated with UVB therapy, typically using five consecutive erythemogenic (mild sunburn-inducing) doses. At least one study has demonstrated that this shortens the duration of disease.
- A short course of oral prednisone (20–40 mg PO qd, for 3 to 7 days) is used for some severe cases.
- A 2000 study of 90 persons showed oral erythromycin (250 mg PO qid × 14 days) resulted in clearance in 73% of patients, compared to no clearance in a placebo-dosed control group.

Clinical Course

PR typically lasts for about 6 weeks, but, in some patients, the condition may last up to 12 weeks. Nearly all cases of PR resolve within 3 months; if the condition does not resolve, the diagnosis of PR should be reconsidered.

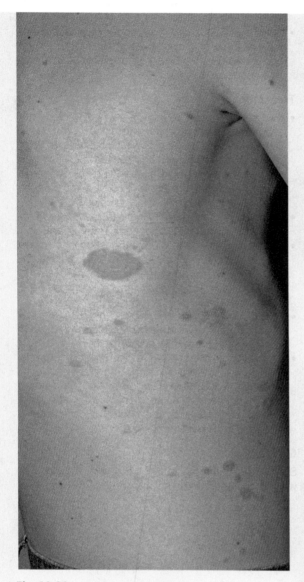

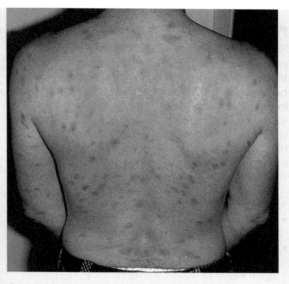

Fig. 10.39. Patient with explosive onset of the secondary lesions of pityriasis rosea demonstrating a vague Christmas tree pattern. (From the Fitzsimons Army Medical Center Collection, Aurora, CO.)

Fig. 10.38. Patient with classic pityriasis rosea demonstrating a typical herald patch near the axilla associated with a shower of secondary round to oval lesions. The herald patch will typically be the first lesion to resolve. (From the Fitzsimons Army Medical Center Collection, Aurora, CO.)

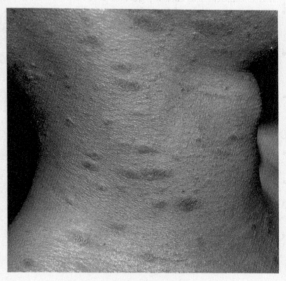

Fig. 10.40. Closer view of pityriasis rosea demonstrating orientation of oval lesions along skin lines. The leading edge also demonstrates a trailing scale. (From the Fitzsimons Army Medical Center Collection, Aurora, CO.)

Seborrheic Dermatitis ICD10 code L21.9

Pathogenesis

Seborrheic dermatitis (SD) is a ubiquitous condition, possibly irritant in nature, that is related to an unidentified antigen or product of commensal lipophilic yeast belonging to the *Malassezia genus*. This yeast exists in the sebum-rich areas of the skin, which accounts for the characteristic distribution of the condition. The yeast's need for sebum also explains the occurrence of SD in infants, when they have high maternal hormones, and the disappearance of the disease during childhood, with a later re-emergence after puberty.

Clinical Features

- SD usually affects the scalp, eyebrows, eyelids, nasolabial folds, ears, and genital folds (Fig. 10.41).
- Cradle cap is the lay term applied to infantile SD. SD in the genital area of infants may also mimic diaper dermatitis.
- Adolescents and adults usually manifest slightly lesser scalp involvement than infants (Figs. 10.42–10.44). Dandruff is the lay term applied to mild SD of the scalp. Less often, areas of involvement include the axillae, genitalia, and midchest.
- Close inspection of the plaques of SD reveals erythema with variable scale, which may be white to yellowish and slightly greasy.
- Clinical variants include annular lesions (seborrhea petaloides) and markedly scaly lesions (sebopsoriasis, which resembles psoriasis).
- Symptoms of SD vary from none at all to moderately pruritic.

Diagnosis

- The diagnosis of SD is established chiefly by history and physical examination.
- The distribution is important because involvement of classic sites is a supportive clinical clue, even when other unusual findings are present.
- Skin biopsy is usually reserved for atypical presentations. In most cases, the histologic findings are consistent with SD but are not diagnostic of only that condition.

Treatment

- Mild scalp disease (dandruff) can be treated with shampoos, including zinc pyrithione–based (e.g., Head & Shoulders), ketoconazole, tar, salicylic acid, ciclopirox olamine, and 5% tea tree oil shampoos (40% response rate). Patients who fail shampoo therapy can be treated with once-daily topical fluocinolone solution or fluocinonide solution.
- Eyelid SD or cradle cap in infants is best treated with gentle cleansing using Johnson's Baby Shampoo.
- Glabrous skin (non–hair-bearing skin) should be treated with a mild topical corticosteroid cream, such as 1% hydrocortisone acetate or desonide 0.05% cream. Rare cases require hydrocortisone valerate.
- Topical antifungals may also be used; all topical imidazoles are basically equally effective (e.g., clotrimazole, ketoconazole, sulconazole).
- In severe or extensive disease, oral itraconazole (200 mg PO qd for 3–7 days) may be used, with the dosage and duration tailored to fit the disease and response. Often, additional doses are used (200 mg PO) on the first day(s) of each month (≈two-thirds of patients will respond).

Clinical Course

SD can be managed but not cured; a waxing and waning course can be anticipated.

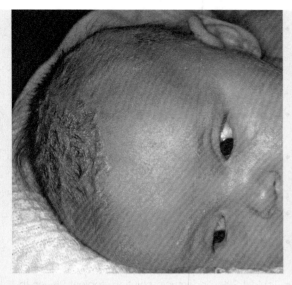

Fig. 10.41. Infantile seborrheic dermatitis (cradle cap) with characteristic involvement of the scalp, eyebrows, eyelids, and ear. (From the Fitzsimons Army Medical Center Collection, Aurora, CO.)

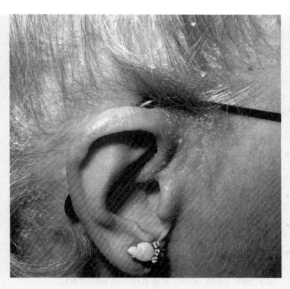

Fig. 10.42. Patient with classic seborrheic dermatitis with involvement of the scalp (dandruff) and ears. (From the Fitzsimons Army Medical Center Collection, Aurora, CO.)

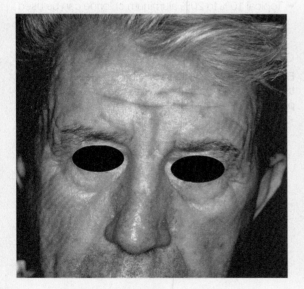

Fig. 10.43. Patient with classic seborrheic dermatitis with involvement of the scalp, facial wrinkles, and a melolabial fold. (From the Fitzsimons Army Medical Center Collection, Aurora, CO.)

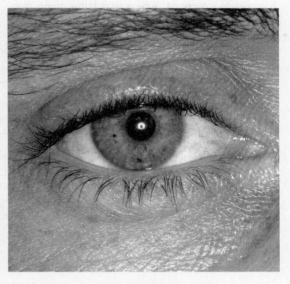

Fig. 10.44. Patient with characteristic involvement of seborrheic dermatitis on the eyelid margin. (From the Fitzsimons Army Medical Center Collection, Aurora, CO.)

Erythrasma ICD10 code L08.1

Introduction

Erythrasma can mimic a low-grade dermatitis, but it is actually a minor superficial bacterial infection. It is more common in humid climates and is caused by infection with *Corynebacterium minutissimum,* a short, gram-positive diphtheroid.

Clinical Features

- Erythrasma presents as sharply demarcated patches of red or red-brown skin covered by a fine white scale (Fig. 10.45).
- In patients with darker skin, there is lesser erythema or minimal to modest hyperkeratosis (Fig. 10.46).
- Erythrasma can be asymptomatic or may be associated with some pruritus.
- The condition is usually confined to the anogenital area, with the inner upper thighs being often affected. Less often, the axilla is affected.

Diagnosis

- Subtle erythema, particularly with red-brown tints and subtle scale, involving the anogenital region or axilla, should suggest the diagnosis. Erythrasma often lacks a distinctive annular edge, whereas dermatophyte infections, which affect the same skin areas, usually have sharp annular shapes.
- The diagnosis is confirmed by demonstrating a coral red fluorescence with Wood light (Fig. 10.47). The often spectacular fluorescence that is observed is due to a porphyrin produced by the bacteria. The skin may not fluoresce if the patient has bathed recently, since the porphyrin is water-soluble, and if this is suspected, the patient should be retested before bathing.

- A skin biopsy is not usually employed but, if performed, the bacteria can be identified in large numbers in the stratum corneum. Note that it is important to list the suspicion of erythrasma on the accession sheet so that the pathologist will know to look for these organisms.
- A scraping of scale, with KOH examination, may be used to exclude dermatophytosis, candidiasis, and tinea pityriasis versicolor.
- Cultures are not usually carried out. The organism is notoriously difficult to culture.

Treatment

- Erythromycin (250 mg PO qid × 5 days) is the most common treatment used.
- Clarithromycin (1 g PO) as a single dose has also been reported to be successful; it costs about the same as a 5-day course of erythromycin.
- Topical 2% clindamycin solution, topical 2% erythromycin solution, or 4% topical erythromycin gel, applied bid for 5 to 7 days, is equally effective. These regimens can be used by patients who do not want to take oral antibiotics or when there are medication interactions.
- Topical 10% to 20% aluminum chloride can be used bid for 5 to 7 days in patients who do not want to use antibiotics.

Clinical Course

Erythrasma is easily cured with topical or systemic therapy. Some patients may reacquire the infection, particularly in humid climates.

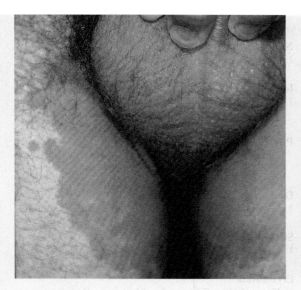

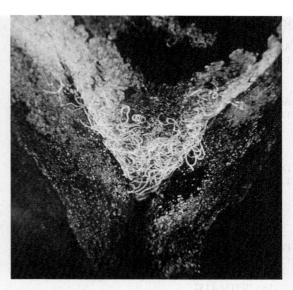

Fig. 10.45. Patient with erythrasma demonstrating characteristic reddish-brown scaly dermatitis. (From the Fitzsimons Army Medical Center Collection, Aurora, CO.)

Fig. 10.47. Striking coral red fluorescence with Wood light examination in a patient with erythrasma. (From the Fitzsimons Army Medical Center Collection, Aurora, CO.)

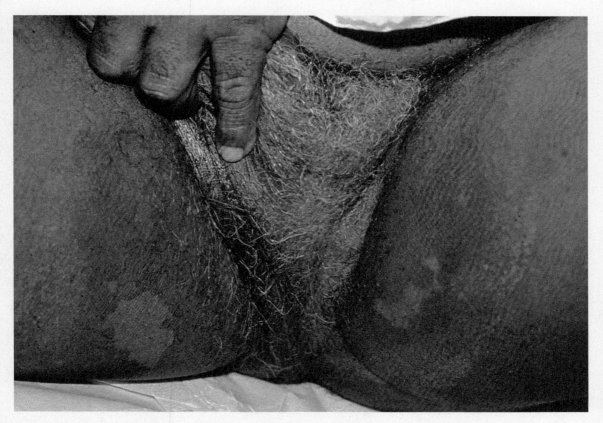

Fig. 10.46. Patient with scaly erythrasma with a subtle brownish-red background. (From the Fitzsimons Army Medical Center Collection, Aurora, CO.)

References

Allergic Contact Dermatitis

1. Gehrig KA, Warshaw EM. Allergic contact dermatitis to topical antibiotics: epidemiology, responsible allergens, and management. *J Am Acad Dermatol*. 2008;58:1-21.

Atopic Dermatitis

1. Eichenfield GF, Tom WL, Berger TG, et al. Guidelines of care for the management of atopic dermatitis. Section 2. Management and treatment of atopic dermatitis with topical therapies. *J Am Acad Dermatol*. 2014;71:116-132.

Diaper Dermatitis

1. Adam R. Skin care of the diaper area. *Pediatr Dermatol*. 2008;25:427-433.
2. Stamatas GN, Tierney NK. Diaper dermatitis: etiology, manifestations, prevention, and management. *Pediatr Dermatol*. 2014;31:1-7.

Eczematoid Drug Eruptions

1. Guillet G, Delaire P, Plantin P, Guillet MH. Eczema as a complication of heparin therapy. *J Am Acad Dermatol*. 1989;20:1130-1132.
2. Joly P, Benoit-Corven C, Baricault S, et al. Chronic eczematous eruptions of the elderly are associated with chronic exposure to calcium channel blockers: results from a case-control study. *J Invest Dermatol*. 2007;127:2766-2771.

Nummular Dermatitis

1. Poudel RR, Belbase B, Kafle NK. Nummular eczema. *J Community Hosp Intern Med Perspect*. 2015;5:27909.

Id Reactions

1. Ilkit M, Durdu M, Karakas M. Cutaneous id reactions: a comprehensive review of clinical manifestations, epidemiology, etiology, and management. *Crit Rev Microbiol*. 2012;38:191-202.

Pityriasis Rosea

1. Drago F, Broccolo G, Rebora A. Pityriasis rosea: an update with critical appraisal of its possible herpesviral etiology. *J Am Acad Dermatol*. 2009;61:303-318.

Dyshidrotic Hand Dermatitis

1. Bikowski JB. Hand eczema: diagnosis and management. *Cutis*. 2008;82(suppl 4):9-15.

Seborrheic Dermatitis

1. Elewski BE. Safe and effective treatment of seborrheic dermatitis. *Cutis*. 2009;83:333-338.

Erythrasma

1. Wharton JR, Wilson PL, Kincannon JM. Erythrasma treated with a single dose of clarithromycin. *Arch Dermatol*. 1998;134:671-672.

Chapter 11
Blisters and Vesicles

Key Terms

Herpes Zoster
  Herpes zoster ophthalmicus
  Ramsey-Hunt syndrome

Herpes Simplex
  Disseminated infection
  Eczema herpeticum
  Herpes gladiatorum

Herpetic whitlow
Hutchinson sign
Neonatal herpes simplex virus
  infections

Blisters and vesicles represent a common category of cutaneous disease. Blisters are an important physical finding because only a limited number of diseases present in this fashion. Usually, in bullous conditions, the clinical presentation, biopsy results, and results of direct immunofluorescent studies will allow for a singular diagnosis. A biopsy from a fresh blister is of greater use in the diagnosis because blisters can occur by different mechanisms (e.g., spongiosis, acantholysis). Blisters may be broadly divided into fragile and and tense blisters.

Fragile Blisters
- Bullous impetigo
- Hailey-Hailey disease
- Pemphigus (all variants)
- Staphylococcal scalded skin syndrome

Tense Blisters
- Allergic contact dermatitis (severe)
- Bullous pemphigoid
- Bullous drug eruption
- Bullous eruption of diabetes
- Bullous fixed drug eruption
- Cicatricial pemphigoid
- Dermatitis herpetiformis
- Dyshidrotic hand dermatitis
- Epidermolysis bullosa acquisita
- Epidermolysis bullosa (genetic)
- Erythema multiforme
- Hand, foot, and mouth disease
- Herpes simplex virus infection
- Herpes gestationis
- Linear immunoglobulin A (IgA) bullous dermatosis
- Porphyria cutanea tarda
- Second-degree sunburn
- Smallpox
- Toxic epidermal necrolysis
- Vaccinia infection
- Varicella-zoster virus infection

IMPORTANT HISTORY QUESTIONS

How long have the blisters been present?

Some conditions, such as allergic contact dermatitis due to poison ivy, may cause acute blistering, whereas other processes, such as bullous pemphigoid, may be chronic in nature.

Have you had blisters before, and do the blisters occur at the same site(s)?

Repetitive blistering could indicate an ongoing exposure, such as poison ivy, ongoing drug use or drug exposure (e.g., fixed drug eruption, repeat Stevens-Johnson syndrome), recurrent bullous erythema multiforme, or recurrent herpes simplex infection.

Are the blisters symptomatic?

Some vesiculobullous disorders are asymptomatic (bullous diabeticorum), whereas others are painful (e.g., toxic epidermal necrolysis) and others are pruritic (e.g., dermatitis herpetiformis).

Are you taking any medications?

Medications may produce blistering disorders, such as bullous drug eruptions, drug-induced linear IgA bullous dermatosis, drug-induced pemphigus, toxic epidermal necrolysis, bullous fixed drug reactions, and Stevens-Johnson syndrome or toxic epidermal necrolysis. Also, some other vesiculobullous diseases may be aggravated by medications.

IMPORTANT PHYSICAL FINDINGS

How old is the patient?

Some blistering disorders occur chiefly in neonates (incontinentia pigmenti), whereas other disorders are more likely to occur in children (e.g., chickenpox), in young adults (e.g., erythema multiforme), in middle-aged adults (e.g., porphyria cutanea tarda), or in geriatric patients (e.g., bullous pemphigoid).

Is the patient a woman of childbearing years, is she pregnant, or has she just delivered a baby?

Gravid or recently gravid status is important in establishing a diagnosis of herpes gestationis.

What is the distribution of the blisters?

Some blisters have characteristic distributions or configurations. For example, sharp lines or irregular shapes often suggest an exogenous origin, such as contact dermatitis or toxic injuries to the skin.

Is the oral mucosa (or other mucosal surfaces) involved?

Mucosal surfaces are often involved in herpes simplex infections and in erythema multiforme (Stevens-Johnson syndrome), toxic epidermal necrolysis, and pemphigus vulgaris or paraneoplastic pemphigus.

Pathogenesis

Impetigo caused by staphylococcal infection is usually associated with group II (phage group 71) *Staphylococcus aureus*. The blister is caused by a toxin, elaborated by the bacterium that lyses an adhesion molecule (desmoglein 1) necessary for keratinocyte adhesion. The split occurs in the superficial aspects of the skin. Infections are more common in the summer months and in humid climates.

Clinical Features

- Bullous staphylococcal impetigo is more common in neonates, small children (Fig. 11.1), and HIV-infected individuals.
- The primary lesions are small vesicles that progress rapidly to flaccid, pus-filled, and fragile bullae.
- The purulence inside the blister space may layer out, with a turbid yellow color (Figs. 11.2 and 11.3).
- The surrounding skin demonstrates minimal or mild erythema.
- Blisters collapse easily, yielding a varnished appearance to the skin where the blister was located.
- Some variations demonstrate only yellow-colored exudative erosions, without active blisters.

Diagnosis

- The clinical presentation of flaccid, pus-filled bullae, with yellow crusting, is often diagnostic.
- Gram-positive cocci in flaccid blisters, as demonstrated with a Gram stain, supports the diagnosis but does not allow for accurate differentiation between streptococcal and staphylococcal causes.
- The diagnostic test of choice is a surface culture, with antibacterial sensitivity testing.
- The diagnosis may be made by biopsy, but this is not usually required.

Treatment

- Topical mupirocin or retapamulin ointment (applied bid for 5 days) is a suitable treatment for limited disease.
- More generalized cases of bullous impetigo are treated empirically with a β-lactam antibiotic, such as oral dicloxacillin (250 mg PO qid for 7–10 days) or cephalexin (250–500 mg PO tid to qid for 7–10 days), because most community-acquired bullous impetigo is not methicillin resistant; this may vary in different areas. This is in contrast to staphylococcal folliculitis, furunculosis, and dermal abscesses.
- Any antibiotic regimen prescribed empirically can be altered once antibiotic susceptibility studies have concluded, based upon the results of culture.
- Oral erythromycin or azithromycin may be used for penicillin-allergic patients, although erythromycin-resistant staphylococci are prevalent (19%–50% of strains) in some regions of the country.
- Methicillin-resistant strains (MRSA) can be treated with ciprofloxacin, trimethoprim, doxycycline (in older children or adults), or topical mupirocin. The management of recurrent impetigo, often due to colonization of *S. aureus*, is a complex issue beyond the scope of this text.

Clinical Course

Most cases do not require follow-up but if the patient continues to get new lesions, beyond 3 days after starting the antibiotic, the veracity of the diagnosis should be reassessed. Correlation with culture or bacterial susceptibility studies should be made. Some patients may become chronic carriers of impetigo-producing *S. aureus* strains.

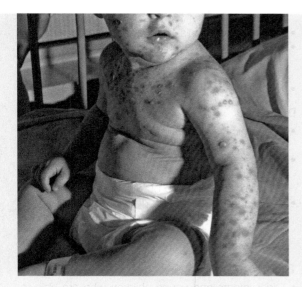

Fig. 11.1. Bullous impetigo in an infant. (From the Fitzsimons Army Medical Center Collection, Aurora, CO.)

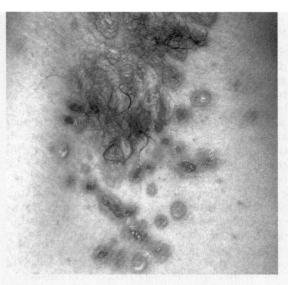

Fig. 11.2. Patient whose axilla demonstrated numerous flaccid blisters in various stages of development. (From the Fitzsimons Army Medical Center Collection, Aurora, CO.)

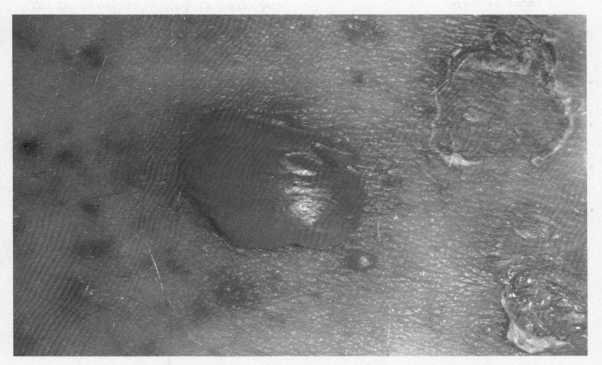

Fig. 11.3. Patient with a flaccid blister demonstrating layering of pus at the base, a finding sometimes seen in bullous impetigo. Note that the superficial blister on the right has broken. (From the Fitzsimons Army Medical Center Collection, Aurora, CO.)

Pathogenesis

Staphylococcal scalded skin syndrome (Ritter disease; SSSS) is caused by infection with group II (often phage group 71) *S. aureus*. Blisters are caused by exfoliative toxins elaborated by the bacteria that lyse an attachment molecule (desmoglein 1) located between keratinocytes. The result is a superficial split in the epidermis in the area of the granular layer. It is thought that infants and young children are more susceptible because immature kidney function does not clear the toxins. This is the same reason why an increased incidence of SSSS is observed in adults with renal disease. Increased susceptibility in immuno-compromised adults is poorly understood but may be due to impaired neutralization of the toxin.

Nikolsky Sign

The Nikolsky sign refers to the production or extension of a blister by lateral or rotating pressure on the epidermis with a finger or a pencil. It is usually associated with the following diseases:

- Pemphigus vulgaris
- Staphylococcal scalded skin syndrome
- Toxic epidermal necrolysis

Clinical Features

- The condition occurs most often in neonates and young children (<5 years).
- The primary site of infection is often unapparent but a prodrome of fever, malaise, lethargy, and irritability is often observed.
- In children and neonates, the disease often begins in the perioral region (Fig. 11.4) and on the neck, axillae, and groin (Fig. 11.5).
- Early lesions are tender and erythematous and manifest variable edema, with superficial bullae and skin fissuring.
- Blisters are fragile, and sloughing leaves shallow bullae, with a moist erythematous surface (Fig. 11.6).

- The Nikolsky sign is often present (see box).
- Adults who experience SSSS frequently have impaired renal function or are immunocompromised and may also develop a staphylococcal cellulitis.
- Mucosal sites are rarely involved.

Diagnosis

- The clinical presentation is usually diagnostic in neonates, infants, and children.
- Because the process is caused by a systemic toxin, Gram staining and cultures of blister cavity fluid are negative, in contrast to bullous impetigo.
- The diagnosis may be suggested on biopsy, with a cleavage plane immediately below the granular layer, but a biopsy is not usually required. The histologic findings of pemphigus foliaceus overlap.

Treatment

- Older infants and young children who are able to eat and drink, and who are with limited cutaneous disease, can be treated with oral antibiotics sufficient to cover *S. aureus* and with local skin care.
- Neonates and children with more severe disease may require admission for intravenous antistaphylococcal antibiotics such as nafcillin, oxacillin, vancomycin, or linezolid.
- Bland emollients (white petrolatum) may be used to decrease pain and promote re-epithelialization.
- NSAIDs and other drugs that impair renal function should be avoided.

Clinical Course

Desquamation occurs over 3 to 5 days, and lesions heal without permanent sequelae in 1 to 2 weeks. The mortality rate in neonates and children has been reported to be 3%, but this figure may be high due to reporting bias at tertiary institutions.

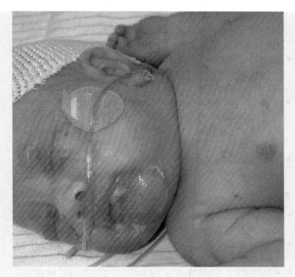

Fig. 11.4. Patient with periorificial erythema and superficial blister formation, a very common location.

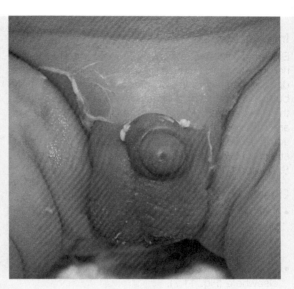

Fig. 11.5. Patient with erythema and superficial blister formation in the genital area, another common location.

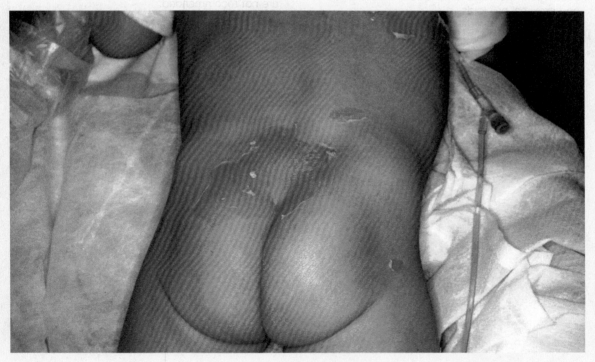

Fig. 11.6. Patient with diffuse erythema and extensive desquamation in the buttocks area. (From the Fitzsimons Army Medical Center Collection, Aurora, CO.)

Blistering Distal Dactylitis ICD10 code L08.9

Introduction

Blistering distal dactylitis is an uncommon bacterial infection that causes superficial blisters on the distal fingers of young children. In reality, it is simply bullous impetigo of acral skin; however, because of the thick stratum corneum on the hands, the blisters are tense. It is a distinctive disorder that presents in acute fashion. It is caused most often by β-hemolytic strains of *Streptococcus pyogenes* and less often by *S. aureus*.

Clinical Features

- Characteristically, the condition affects children and, less often, adolescents. Adults are rarely affected, with most adult cases occurring in those who are immunocompromised.
- Occasionally, classic impetigo may also be present elsewhere (Fig. 11.7).
- The disorder yields rapidly evolving tense and painful bullae on the anterior fat pads of the distal fingertips (Figs. 11.8 and 11.9). Older lesions may become crusted.
- Less often, the bullae extend to involve the lateral and proximal nail folds.

Diagnosis

- The clinical presentation is suggestive of blistering distal dactylitis, but the differential diagnosis includes traumatic blisters, thermal and chemical burns, and herpetic whitlow (herpes simplex infection of the finger).
- The blisters of distal dactylitis are typically unilocular, whereas the blisters of herpetic whitlow are usually multilocular; this is an important diagnostic clue.
- In an urgent care or office setting, the blisters can be aspirated, with Gram staining performed on the fluid and with abundant gram-positive cocci apparent.
- The aspirate can be cultured with antibiotic sensitivities used to guide management.

Treatment

- Tense blisters may be drained, but there is no evidence that this speeds recovery.
- Dicloxacillin at a dose of 3.125 to 6.25 mg/kg may be used for children weighing less than 40 kg.
- Alternative treatments include cephalexin, erythromycin, or another oral antibiotic that covers streptococcal and staphylococcal infection.
- Because of the thickness of the blister roof and frequent presence of β-hemolytic strains of *S. pyogenes*, topical antibiotics, at least as solo therapy, are not recommended.

Clinical Course

The patient should start to demonstrate improvement within 72 hours. If this does not occur, the diagnosis and treatment need to be reassessed.

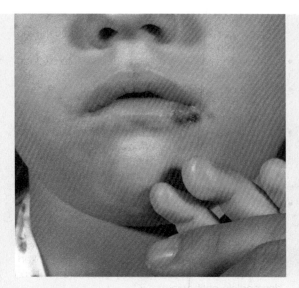

Fig. 11.7. Patient with both streptococcal impetigo and blistering distal dactylitis. (From the Fitzsimons Army Medical Center Collection, Aurora, CO.)

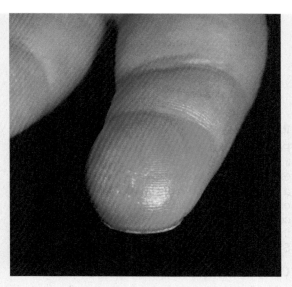

Fig. 11.8. Close-up of older lesion of blistering distal dactylitis demonstrating early crusting. (From the Fitzsimons Army Medical Center Collection, Aurora, CO.)

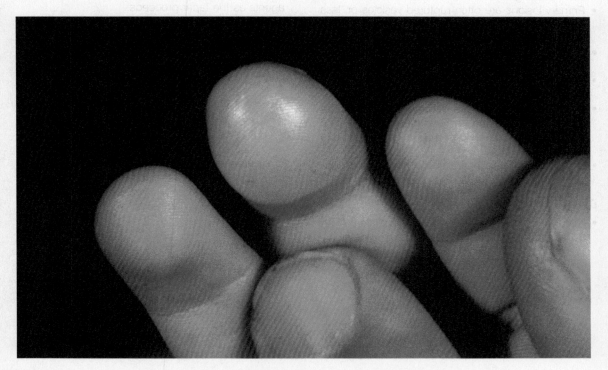

Fig. 11.9. Close-up of classic tense blister of blistering distal dactylitis on the digital pad. (From the Fitzsimons Army Medical Center Collection, Aurora, CO.)

Causes of Drug-Induced Pemphigus Foliaceus

- Captopril (common)
- D-Penicillamine (common)
- Enalapril (rare)
- Sulfasalazine (rare)

Pathogenesis

Pemphigus foliaceus (PF) is an uncommon auto-immune bullous condition caused by immunoglobulin G (IgG) autoantibodies directed against desmoglein 1, a molecule involved in the normal cohesion of keratin-ocytes. In this condition, the split occurs below the cornified layer or in the superficial granular layer. This is the same location as the split in bullous impetigo and SSSS. PF can also be induced by some medications.

Clinical Features

- Middle-aged and older adults are usually affected, but, on occasion, children may be affected.
- There is a predilection for the head and trunk, but in some cases it may involve the entire body surface area, causing erythroderma.
- Primary lesions are often ruptured vesicles or, less often, intact bullae that arise on normal or erythe-matous skin (Figs. 11.10 and 11.11).
- In some cases, the blister may become cloudy or even appear pustular.
- The Nikolsky sign is present in many cases (see p. 166).
- Scaling and crusting are common, and, in some cases, the condition may resemble dermatitis (Fig. 11.12). Verrucous lesions may even resemble a seborrheic keratosis.
- Drug-induced PF appears clinically identical to idio-pathic cases (Fig. 11.13).

Diagnosis

- Recurrent, superficial, often ruptured blisters, with a background of scaling and crusting, are highly suggestive of the diagnosis. There should be no oral involvement.
- It is useful to culture the blister contents to exclude bullous impetigo.
- A shave or punch biopsy, performed at the edge of the lesion, is necessary to establish an acantholytic blistering disorder; this is a cardinal feature of PF.
- DIF of perilesional skin is the diagnostic method of choice. This can be performed using a shave (pre-ferred) or punch biopsy. The tissue must be placed in immunofluorescence transport media, normal saline (for periods of <24–48 hours), or snap frozen.
- If a direct immunofluorescent medium is not readily available, blood can be drawn in a red-top tube (serum separator tube) and sent to an immuno-fluorescence laboratory for indirect immunofluores-cence or to a reference laboratory for enzyme-linked immunosorbent assay (ELISA) measurement of desmoglein antibodies.

Treatment

- First-line therapy is oral prednisone (0.5–1.0 mg/kg per day) with a slow taper, using steroid-sparing agents as the taper proceeds.
- Other medications and/or steroid-sparing agents include methotrexate, azathioprine, dapsone, cyclo-phosphamide, and rituximab.
- Any drug known to induce PF should be discontin-ued or substituted with an unrelated agent.

Clinical Course

The disease is often chronic and may last for years. Children are more likely to demonstrate a short course of disease. In contrast to pemphigus vulgaris, PF has a more benign course, and fatal outcomes are uncommon. Patients with drug-induced PF typically demonstrate resolution over weeks to months, after withdrawal of the inciting medication.

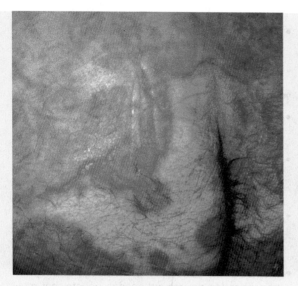

Fig. 11.10. Large erythematous plaques of pemphigus foliaceus, with an edge of flaccid blisters. (From the Fitzsimons Army Medical Center Collection, Aurora, CO.)

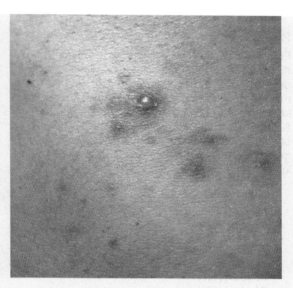

Fig. 11.11. Close-up of a more subtle example of pemphigus foliaceus presenting as red papules, with flaccid vesicles. (From the Fitzsimons Army Medical Center Collection, Aurora, CO.)

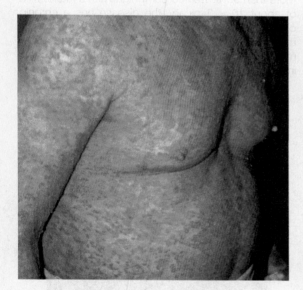

Fig. 11.12. Severe generalized pemphigus foliaceus that, at first glance, has the appearance of dermatitis rather than a blistering disorder. (From the Fitzsimons Army Medical Center Collection, Aurora, CO.)

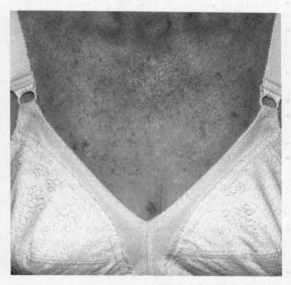

Fig. 11.13. Subtle case of pemphigus foliaceus induced by D-penicillamine. (From the Fitzsimons Army Medical Center Collection, Aurora, CO.)

Pathogenesis

Pemphigus vulgaris is a serious autoimmune bullous disorder caused by autoantibodies directed against desmoglein 1 and desmoglein 3 (Fig. 11.14). These molecules are involved in the normal cohesion of keratinocytes, and hence, the condition leads to large flaccid bullae that are easily ruptured. The mouth is often involved. Rarely, pemphigus vulgaris is triggered by drugs (see box) or foods such as garlic and leeks.

Drug-Induced Pemphigus
- Captopril (common)
- ᴅ-Penicillamine (common)
- Amoxicillin (rare)
- Ampicillin (rare)
- Cephalosporins (rare)
- Penicillin (rare)
- Rifampin (rare)

Clinical Features

- The condition typically affects older adults (40–60 years old).
- Persons of Jewish or Hispanic heritage are more often affected.
- The condition may be localized (often on the head or trunk), or it may eventuate as a generalized eruption (Fig. 11.15).
- Vesicles and bullae (up to several centimeters) arise on normal or erythematous skin (Fig. 11.16).
- The Nikolsky sign may be present.
- Blisters rupture in 1 to 3 days, with a painful, raw, erythematous base.
- Scaling and crusting of older lesions are common.
- Oral involvement is present in more than 90% of patients (Fig. 11.17) during the course of the illness, and often it is the initial site of the presentation.

Diagnosis

- A vesiculobullous disorder with marked mucosal involvement suggests the diagnosis, especially if the Nikolsky sign is present.
- A shave or punch biopsy from the edge of the lesion should always be done.
- DIF using perilesional skin may be performed on a shave biopsy (preferred) or punch biopsy and submitted in immunofluorescent transport media, in saline (for up to 24–48 hours), or snap frozen.

- If a direct immunofluorescent medium is not available, blood can be drawn in a red-top (serum separator) tube and sent for indirect immunofluorescence examination or ELISA testing.

Treatment

- First-line therapy is oral prednisone (0.5–1.0 mg/kg per day) with a slow taper, using steroid-sparing agents as the taper proceeds.
- Pulse corticosteroids (250–1000 mg/day of methylprednisolone sodium succinate) for 1 to 5 days may be used for severe disease or for patients with a poor response to oral prednisone.
- Intravenous immunoglobulin (IVIG), 400 mg/kg per day for 5 days, with the addition of cyclophosphamide (100–150 mg/day) in severe cases, results in clearing in 80% of patients within 2 weeks.
- Methotrexate, azathioprine, rituximab, and cyclophosphamide are steroid-sparing agents that may be used in select cases.

Clinical Course

Untreated, pemphigus vulgaris has a fatality rate of more than 90%. Treated pemphigus has a fatality rate of about 10%. Typically, the disease has a chronic course, lasting years, but spontaneous remissions may occur. Maintenance of hydration and proper nutrition are challenges in those with marked mucosal involvement.

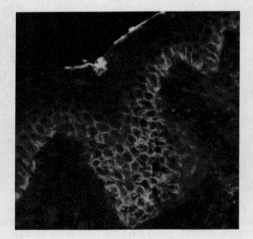

Fig. 11.14. Netlike deposition of IgG autoantibodies in the epidermis in a patient with pemphigus vulgaris.

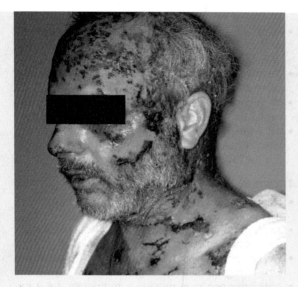

Fig. 11.15. Generalized pemphigus vulgaris demonstrating a classic admixture of crusts, erosions, and superficial blisters. (From the Fitzsimons Army Medical Center Collection, Aurora, CO.)

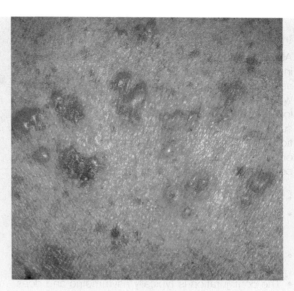

Fig. 11.16. Flaccid vesicles and bullae of pemphigus vulgaris on the trunk, with crusting of an older lesion.

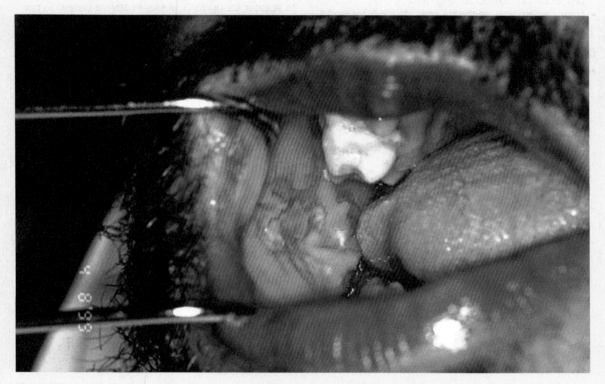

Fig. 11.17. Typical oral pemphigus vulgaris demonstrating erosions. Blisters are not typically seen in oral lesions. (From the Fitzsimons Army Medical Center Collection, Aurora, CO.)

Introduction

Allergic contact dermatitis (ACD) is discussed in depth in Chapter 10. Although most cases of ACD present as an eczematous process, severe ACD may present with marked blistering, particularly if contact is prolonged or if the host response is intense. One should suspect a bullous ACD when blisters are in a distribution (linear) that suggests an exogenous process and/or when pruritus is extreme. Some allergens, such as poison ivy, are well recognized to produce blisters.

Clinical Features

- This presents with erythema and blisters 24 to 72 hours after contact in sensitized patients (Fig. 11.18).
- The distribution initially follows points of contact but may involve adjacent areas later in the course.
- The configuration is typically asymmetric and does not follow normal anatomic lines. Sharp unnatural lines are often present (Fig. 11.19) due to contact with the exogenous agent.
- Bullous ACD is nearly always intensely pruritic.
- In bullous ACD, overlying tense blisters may be unilocular or multilocular (Fig. 11.20).
- New blisters and erythema may develop for up to 3 weeks, even without additional exposure.

Diagnosis

- Bullous ACD should be suspected in any blistering condition with an asymmetric and exogenous distribution pattern, particularly when linear arrangements are present.

- A careful history of potential recent exposures to allergens, such as poison ivy or topical medications, is important in establishing the diagnosis.
- A shave or punch biopsy may be useful to rule out other bullous conditions.
- In rare cases, a perilesional skin biopsy may be useful to exclude autoimmune bullous disorders.
- In patients for whom an allergen cannot be otherwise identified, patch testing may be used to establish the diagnosis and cause.

Treatment

- Remove or discontinue suspected and/or potential allergens.
- Apply potent or ultrapotent topical steroids (e.g., fluocinonide, clobetasol) bid until resolution.
- Generalized cases may require oral prednisone (20–40 mg qd for 7–21 days).
- Antihistamines may provide symptomatic relief for pruritus but do not shorten the disease course.

Clinical Course

Even though the patient may have only had a single exposure to an allergen, new lesions may continue to appear for up to 3 weeks in severe cases. In particular, the allergen in poison ivy (uroshiol) binds irreversibly to the skin and will require treatment for up to 21 days. So-called dose packs of steroids, used for about 5 days, should be avoided because the patient will frequently rebound and flare after the dose pack is completed.

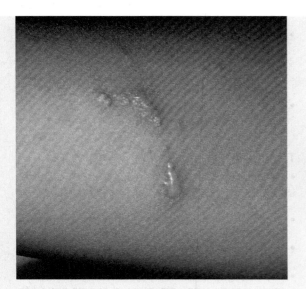

Fig. 11.18. Classic linear distribution of blisters seen in poison ivy contact dermatitis. (From the Fitzsimons Army Medical Center Collection, Aurora, CO.)

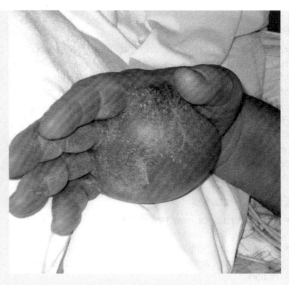

Fig. 11.19. Unilateral, severe, bullous allergic contact dermatitis caused by benzocaine (Lanacane). The patient was mistakenly diagnosed as having toxic epidermal necrolysis and was transferred from the emergency room to the burn unit.

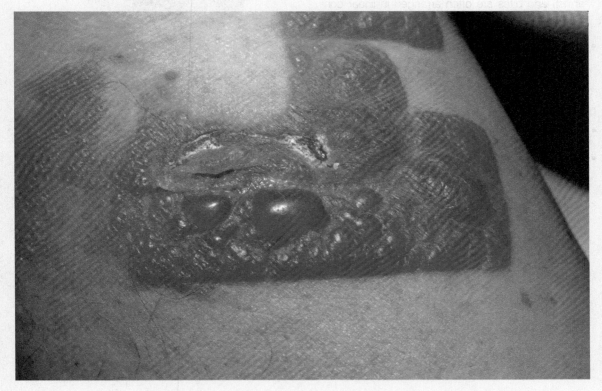

Fig. 11.20. Bullous allergic contact dermatitis due to contact with adhesive tape. Note the multilocular nature of the blisters, a finding seen in many types of intraepidermal blisters. (From the Fitzsimons Army Medical Center Collection, Aurora, CO.)

Bullous Insect and Arthropod Reactions ICD10 code T14.1

Pathogenesis

Insects and arthropods can produce hypersensitivity reactions in the skin. Saliva from the bite of the organism (e.g., bedbugs, ticks) or feces (e.g., scybala of scabies) may serve as an allergen. When allergen exposure is limited, the host response is usually minor. However, when the antigen exposure is more substantial, or the host response is exaggerated, a vesiculobullous reaction can ensue. Common causes of bullous arthropod reactions include bedbugs (Cimex lectularius), fleas (Fig. 11.21), and chiggers.

Clinical Features

- Patients may or may not recall the insect or arthropod bite.
- Lesions are often located on exposed areas of the body and range from urticarial papules to bullae.
- Lesions may be solitary or multiple, and lesions can be grouped, especially in bedbug bites.
- The blister may be unilocular or multilocular on an erythematous base (Figs. 11.22 and 11.23).
- Bedbug bites occur most often on parts of the body exposed during sleep (face, neck, hands, and arms), and bites are often arranged in linear configurations (so-called breakfast, lunch, and dinner arrangement).
- Bullous insect and arthropod bite reactions are nearly always intensely pruritic, except for blistering reactions caused by cutaneous exposure to members of the blister beetle family.

Diagnosis

- In some cases, the patient may bring in the offending insect or arthropod (see Fig. 11.21).
- Bedbugs are a particular problem of travelers, and a travel history should be elicited.

- According to a major national extermination company, the top 10 cities for bedbugs includes Detroit, Philadelphia, Cleveland, Los Angeles, Dayton, Chicago, Columbus, Cincinnati, Dallas–Fort Worth, and San Francisco.
- A shave or punch biopsy is not usually indicated but, in problematic cases, the findings in a biopsy can be supportive of the diagnosis.

Treatment

- Sedating antihistamines (e.g., diphenhydramine) may be used at night for symptomatic relief and to promote sleep.
- Potent or ultrapotent forms may be used in a directed manner for a limited duration.
- Oral antibiotics may be appropriate if a secondary bacterial infection is suspected.
- Depending on the clinical situation, other treatments might include repellants, removal of pets or wildlife (e.g., an abandoned bird's nest near a bedroom window), and/or professional extermination.

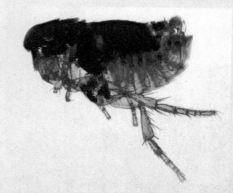

Fig. 11.21. Dog flea recovered from the carpet of a patient's home. Dog fleas and cat fleas are nearly identical in appearance.

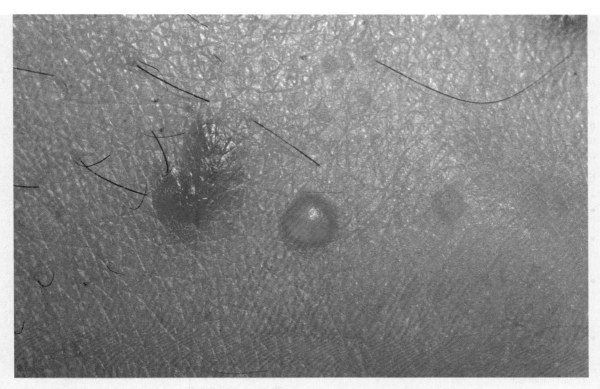

Fig. 11.22. Two arthropod reactions received at the same time. One is a crusted papule that never blistered, whereas the second demonstrates a pruritic, tense, unilocular blister.

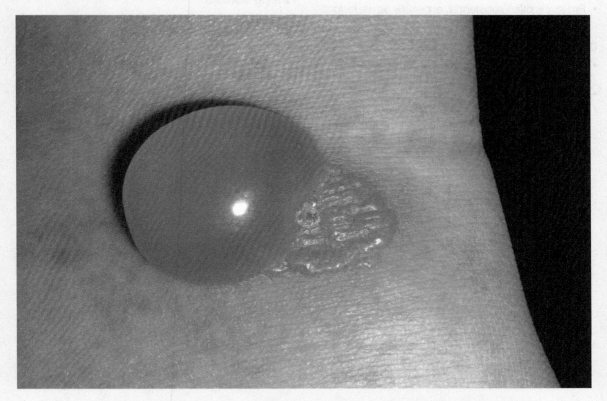

Fig. 11.23. Arthropod reaction demonstrating a central punctum that represents the bite site. This bite is instructive in that it shows that both unilocular *(left side)* and multilocular *(right side)* blisters can occur in an arthropod reaction. (From the Fitzsimons Army Medical Center Collection, Aurora, CO.)

Chickenpox ICD10 code B01.9

Pathogenesis

Chickenpox, or varicella, is a primary infection with the varicella-zoster virus (VZV). Prior to the introduction of a live attenuated vaccine in 1995, there were about 4 million new cases/year, with approximately 100 deaths annually. Since mass vaccinations began, there has been a continued progressive decline in reported cases. VZV is acquired mostly in an aerorespiratory fashion.

Clinical Features

- The incubation period is 14 to 17 days.
- A prodrome of mild upper respiratory tract infection—malaise, low-grade fever—may be present.
- Primary lesions are 1- to 4-mm vesicles arising on an erythematous base (so-called dewdrops on a rose petal; Figs. 11.24 and 11.25).
- Typically, primary varicella yields crops of lesions in different phases of evolution, with some lesions being vesicular and others crusted over. The rash persists for about 2 to 7 days.
- VZV is distributed chiefly on the trunk and proximal extremities, although any site may be affected, including the oral mucosa, ocular mucosa, and nasal mucosa.
- The number of lesions is highly variable and may vary from a few or a dozen to several hundred.
- Pruritus is often substantial, especially as the lesions evolve into later stages.

Diagnosis

- The clinical presentation (dewdrops on a rose petal, with a centripetal predominance) is suggestive.
- A biopsy is diagnostic of herpes family infections, but a routine (H&E) examination cannot distinguish between VZV and herpes simplex virus (HSV) infection.

- Some laboratories have immunohistochemical stains for VZV and HSV and can make a specific diagnosis from biopsy specimens within 24 hours.
- A Tzanck preparation demonstrates acantholytic keratinocytes and multinucleated keratinocytes with cytopathic effect (see Figs. 2.17 to 2.22); this is also indicative of herpes family infections, but, again, HSV and VZV cannot be distinguished without additional studies or clinical correlation.
- Although viral culture used to be performed, all major reference laboratories have now abandoned tissue culture in favor of polymerase chain reaction (PCR)-based molecular techniques that are faster and more reliable.

Treatment

- Observation is reasonable for a young healthy patient because primary VZV is usually self-limited.
- Antiviral drugs, such as acyclovir (children, 20 mg/kg daily for 5 days; adults, 800 mg five times daily for 7 days), valacyclovir, and famciclovir, decrease the number of lesions and promote rapid healing when initiated in the first 24 hours of the rash.
- Varicella-zoster immune globulin (VZIG) is effective in treating serious infections in immunocompromised children and adults.

Clinical Course

Crusted lesions heal within 2 weeks, generally without scarring. Isolated lesions may produce small, round, depressed scars that are often most notable on the face. Complications include varicella-zoster pneumonia (more common in adults), varicella gangrenosa (gangrenous changes secondary to infection with bacteria), and Reye syndrome (particularly with coadministration of salicylates).

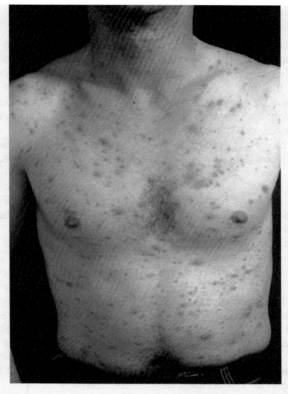

Fig. 11.24. Early chickenpox in a young adult demonstrating lesions in the same stage of development. (From the Fitzsimons Army Medical Center Collection, Aurora, CO.)

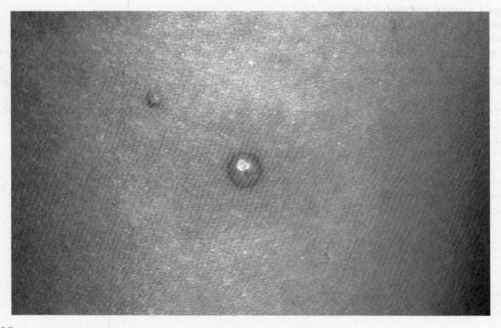

Fig. 11.25. Developed chickenpox demonstrating small vesicles on an erythematous base (so-called dewdrops on a rose petal).

Herpes Zoster ICD10 code B02.0-B02.9

Pathogenesis

Herpes zoster (shingles) is caused by the reactivation of VZV that resides in the dorsal root ganglia after a primary varicella infection (chickenpox) subsides. As the patient's immunity to the virus wanes, often because of age, but also because of another stressor, trauma, or immune suppression, the virus can again successfully replicate. It extends down the nerves associated with the dorsal root ganglia, leading to a classic dermatomal eruption of shingles.

Clinical Features

- Herpes zoster may occur at any age, but most cases occur in geriatric patients.
- Initial symptoms include discomfort or pain, in a dermatomal distribution, that begins 1 to 10 days before the rash is visible. Other changes, such hyperesthesia to touch or contact with clothing, may be noted.
- Early lesions consist of erythematous papules and erythema in a dermatomal distribution.
  - A thoracic dermatome is most often affected, followed by the trigeminal, cervical, and lumbar dermatomes (Fig. 11.26).
  - **Ramsey-Hunt syndrome** is caused by involvement of the geniculate ganglion. It consists of blisters on the pinna, auditory canal, and anterior two-thirds of the tongue, with associated Bell palsy, tinnitus, deafness, vertigo, impaired taste, and, rarely, viral meningitis.
  - **Herpes zoster ophthalmicus** (Fig. 11.27) is caused by involvement of the first division of the trigeminal nerve. It presents as conjunctivitis, scleritis, episcleritis, keratitis, optic neuritis, and other ophthalmic symptoms. An early clinical clue is the **Hutchinson sign,** lesions on the tip or one side of the nose.
- Developed lesions include grouped vesicles (1–4 mm in size) on an erythematous base and located in a dermatomal distribution. Large bullae are rare. Older lesions may appear be pustular (Fig. 11.28).
- Vesicles crust over in 2 to 5 days, but immunocompromised patients may develop ulcers or hemorrhage.

Diagnosis

- The clinical presentation of painful grouped vesicles on an erythematous base, in a dermatomal distribution, is essentially diagnostic of zoster. Mild cases may resemble recurrent HSV infection.
- A biopsy can be diagnostic, if combined with immunohistochemical staining, but is not usually necessary,
- PCR-based studies, which have replaced culture at all reference laboratories, are also of diagnostic use.
- A Tzanck preparation demonstrates acantholytic keratinocytes, multinucleated keratinocytes, and cytopathic effects (see Figs. 2.17–2.22), but, again, HSV and VZV cannot be distinguished in a simple Tzanck preparation.

Treatment

- No treatment is reasonable if the blisters are older than 72 hours, and the patient is not at risk for postherpetic neuralgia. Nonspecific measures include pain medications and cool compresses.
- Antiviral agents are useful when started in the first 72 hours; these include acyclovir (800 mg PO five times daily for 7–10 days), valacyclovir (1000 mg PO tid for 7 days), and famciclovir (500 mg PO tid for 7 days).
- Oral prednisone (40–60 mg PO qd, tapered over 2–3 weeks), in combination with an antiviral agent, has been used to prevent postherpetic neuralgia in patients older than 50 years, but the benefit is controversial.

Clinical Course

Patients with a recent eruption of herpes zoster are not at immediate risk for another episode. Most persons have only one episode of shingles in a lifetime. Up to 40% of patients older than 60 years will develop postherpetic neuralgia (dermatomal pain lasting >12 weeks after the rash has subsided).

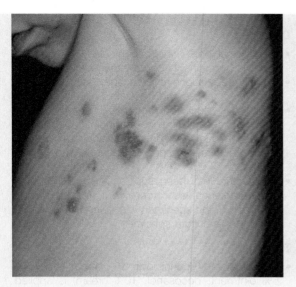

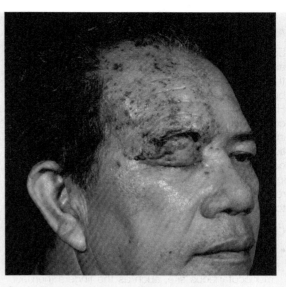

Fig. 11.26. Early herpes zoster in a thoracic dermatome in a pediatric patient. (From the Fitzsimons Army Medical Center Collection, Aurora, CO.)

Fig. 11.27. Resolving herpes zoster ophthalmicus demonstrating scaling and crusting. (From the Fitzsimons Army Medical Center Collection, Aurora, CO.)

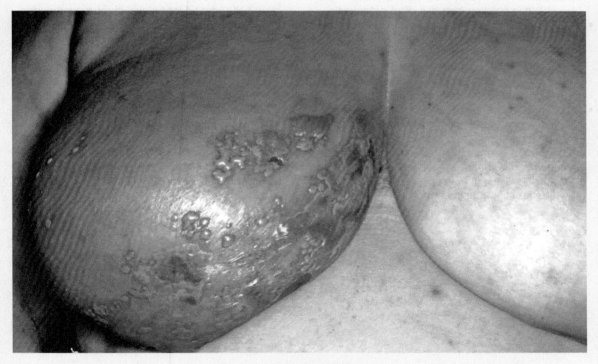

Fig. 11.28. Developed case of herpes zoster in a thoracic dermatome demonstrating an admixture of vesicles, pustules, and erosions. (From the Fitzsimons Army Medical Center Collection, Aurora, CO.)

Pathogenesis

Epidemiologic studies have shown that about 80% of adults have antibodies to HSV-1, which affects chiefly the oral mucosa, and 25% of young adults have antibodies to HSV-2, which affects chiefly the genitalia. HSV infection occurs by direct inoculation via physical contact with an infected person. The virus replicates in keratinocytes and neurons at the site of inoculation and eventually makes its way to the dorsal root ganglia, where it enters quiescence. Various stimuli, including fever, sunburn, and stress, can stimulate replication, with extension down the sensory nerves to the skin, yielding recurrent lesions.

Clinical Features

- Certain strains of HSV affect the oral mucosa (HSV-1) or genital mucosa (HSV-2) more often. Actually, any mucocutaneous site, such as the fingers (herpetic whitlow), may be affected by either strain.
- Primary HSV infections are more severe and may include a prodrome of fever, localized edema, and lymphadenopathy (Fig. 11.29). Primary herpetic infections of the mouth may yield significant oral ulcerations in children (herpetic gingivostomatitis).
- Recurrent herpes outbreaks may yield a prodrome of burning, tingling, or itching (usually 12–24 hours before blisters). Later, small grouped vesicles form on an erythematous base and last for days to weeks. The recurrences occur at the same anatomic site as the primary eruption (Fig. 11.30).
- Other variants include neonatal herpes simplex virus infection (generalized infection that occurs during birth), herpes gladiatorum (occurs in wrestlers and other contact combatants), disseminated infection (in immunocompromised persons; Fig. 11.31), and eczema herpeticum (HSV superinfection that develops in preexisting atopic dermatitis; Fig. 11.32).

Diagnosis

- The clinical presentation, particularly in recurrent herpetic infections, is typically diagnostic.
- Tzanck preparations reveal acantholytic multinucleated keratinocytes and cytopathic effects.
- A biopsy is usually only required in atypical cases, but the histologic findings are indicative only of a herpes family infection. Immunohistochemical staining can confirm the specific diagnosis in about 24 hours.
- Viral culture has been supplanted by PCR at all major reference laboratories, but, from a clinical perspective, the specimen is obtained in the same manner as a culture specimen.

Treatment

- Topical therapy (penciclovir, 1% cream; acyclovir, 5% ointment; docosanol, 10% cream) is applied multiple times per day. In general, topical treatment is often less effective than oral medication.
- Oral therapies include the following:
  - Acyclovir (primary HSV, 400 mg tid or 200 mg five times/day for 10 days; recurrent HSV, 400–800 mg tid for 5 days; chronic suppression, 400 mg PO bid; pregnant HSV patients in their third trimester, 400 mg tid until delivery; disseminated HSV, 5–10 mg/kg IV for 7 days)
  - Famciclovir (primary HSV, 250 mg tid for 10 days; recurrent HSV, 500 mg tid for 5 days, 125 mg bid for 5 days, or 1 g PO bid for 1 day; chronic suppression, 250 mg bid)
  - Valacyclovir (primary HSV, 1 g bid for 10 days; recurrent HSV, 500 mg bid for 3 days; chronic suppression, 250–1000 mg qd).
- Foscarnet and cidofovir are reserved for acyclovir-resistant HSV infections.

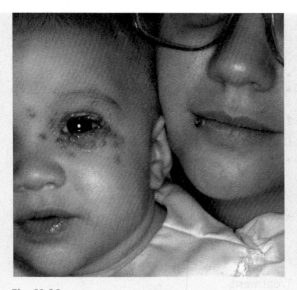

Fig. 11.29. Recurrent herpes labialis in a mother associated with primary facial herpes simplex infection in her daughter. This case demonstrates that primary infection is typically more severe than recurrent infection. (From the Fitzsimons Army Medical Center Collection, Aurora, CO.)

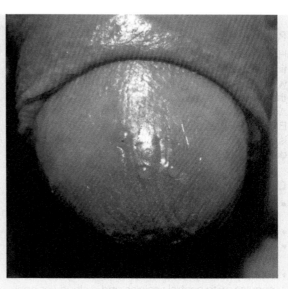

Fig. 11.30. Recurrent herpes progenitalis demonstrating small grouped uniform blisters on an erythematous base. (From the Fitzsimons Army Medical Center Collection, Aurora, CO.)

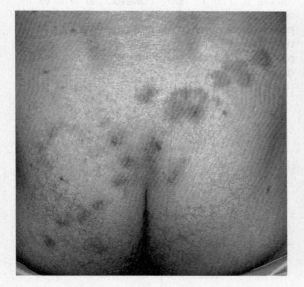

Fig. 11.31. Patient with underlying lymphoma and localized progressive sacral herpes simplex infection. (From the Fitzsimons Army Medical Center Collection, Aurora, CO.)

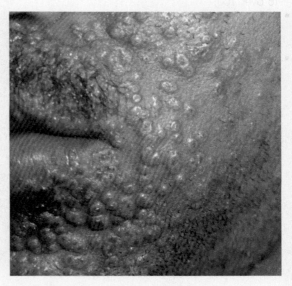

Fig. 11.32. Eczema herpeticum in a patient with underlying atopic dermatitis and generalized small uniform blisters. (From the Fitzsimons Army Medical Center Collection, Aurora, CO.)

Pathogenesis

Hand, foot, and mouth disease (HFMD) is an infection caused chiefly by coxsackievirus group A viruses, with the most common cause being A16. Less often, the disease may be caused by coxsackievirus groups A4, A5, A6, A7, A9, and A10, coxsackievirus groups B1, B2, B3, and B5, or enterovirus 71. Transmission is fecal-oral. HFMD tends to occur in miniepidemics during the summer months.

Clinical Features

- Typically, young children are affected, but the virus may also affect adolescents and adults on occasion.
- The incubation period is brief (3–6 days).
- A brief prodrome of low-grade fever, malaise, anorexia, and abdominal pain may be present.
- Primary lesions are round to oval erythematous papules, with central vesicles and a cloudy or opalescent appearance.
- Lesions arise most often on the hands (Fig. 11.33) and feet (11.34). At other anatomic sites, the primary lesions may simply be red macules, with variable scale or crust.
- The number of lesions varies widely, from only a few to over 100.
- Although the hands and feet are most often involved, other common sites include the anogenital area (Fig. 11.35), buttocks, and flexural areas.
- An enanthem may affect the buccal mucosa, tongue, soft palate, or gingiva and is seen in about 90% of patients as round to oval erosions on an erythematous base, which can be painful (Fig. 11.36).
- One or more nails can be shed (onychomadesis).
- Lymphadenopathy is present in about 20% of cases.
- Lesions resolve without scarring.

Diagnosis

- The clinical presentation of a young child (usually <4 years old) with low-grade fever and lesions on the hands, feet, and oral mucosa is usually sufficient for a presumptive diagnosis.
- Problematic or severe cases may be diagnosed with viral cultures of the oral pharynx or the fluid aspirated from vesicles. Material from these same sites can also be tested by PCR-based modalities.

Treatment

- The disease is self-limited and only symptomatic, and supportive treatments are used. There is no specific antiviral therapy.

Clinical Course

The lesions of the skin and mucous membranes resolve in 3 to 10 days; however, the virus excretion in stool may persist for up to 2 weeks and can provide a source of infection to others. Cases caused by enterovirus 71 are more likely to cause neurologic problems, including encephalitis, and/or cardiopulmonary involvement.

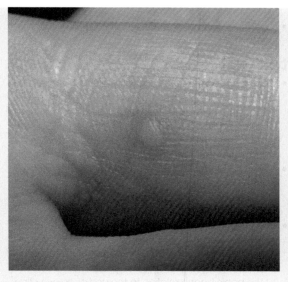

Fig. 11.33. Characteristic oval opalescent blister of hand, foot, and mouth disease on an erythematous base of a finger in a young child. (From the Fitzsimons Army Medical Center Collection, Aurora, CO.)

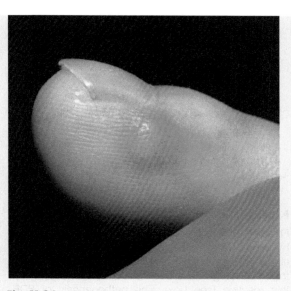

Fig. 11.34. Oval opalescent blister of hand, foot, and mouth disease on an erythematous base on the toe. (From the Fitzsimons Army Medical Center Collection, Aurora, CO.)

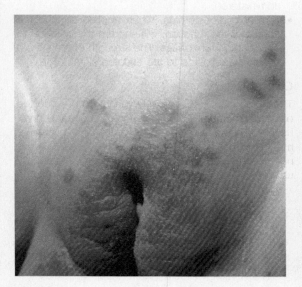

Fig. 11.35. Rare oval blisters of hand, foot, and mouth disease with crusted macules on the genital area of a young girl. Lesions that are not located on the hands and feet are frequently not vesiculated.

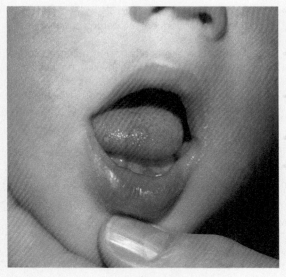

Fig. 11.36. Two typical erosions of hand, foot, and mouth disease on an erythematous base on the tongue of a child. (From the William Weston Collection, Aurora, CO.)

Common Causes of Fixed Drug Eruption
- Acetaminophen
- Antimalarials
- Barbiturates
- Fluoroquinolones
- Nonsteroidal antiinflammatory drug (NSAIDs)
- Penicillins
- Phenolphthalein
- Tetracyclines (class effect)
- Trimethoprim-sulfamethoxazole

Pathogenesis

Fixed drug eruptions (FDEs) are reactions produced by drugs—and rarely by foods—that are localized (fixed) to one or more mucocutaneous sites. More than 100 drugs have been documented to produce this reaction (see box). The pathogenesis of FDE remains unknown, but studies have suggested that T and B cells are stimulated by the causative drug, and skin damage is due to antibody-dependent cell cytotoxicity.

Clinical Features

- An initial episode occurs 1 to 2 weeks after drug exposure, but subsequent exposures can trigger an effect within hours.
- Usually, only one site is affected in a first episode, but subsequent episodes can involve the initial site and one or more additional sites.
- The primary lesion is an erythematous macule that rapidly becomes an erythematous plaque (Fig. 11.37).
- The erythema may subside or the lesion may become bullous or ulcerated (Fig. 11.38 and 11.39).
- The lesion resolves with residual hyperpigmentation.

- The face and male genitalia are the sites affected most often.

Diagnosis

- The diagnosis is usually established on clinical grounds, with the presentation of one or more discrete bullous lesions, following ingestion of a drug. The diagnosis is further established if a history reveals that this same site has been involved in other reactions precipitated by the same drug.
- Rare cases may require a drug challenge or a 3- or 4-mm punch biopsy. The histologic findings are not usually specific for only FDE but can strongly suggest the diagnosis.
- Because FDE is common on the male genitalia, and doxycycline is a drug used for a variety of sexually transmitted diseases but can cause FDE, it is often important to establish precisely when an ulceration of the penis began relative to the use of doxycycline.

Treatment

- The implicated drug needs to be discontinued immediately because the lesions will typically progress to ulceration if the drug continues to be administered.
- Topical corticosteroids, when applied early in the course of the reaction, will shorten the duration of the inflammatory phase. The strength of the steroid should be adjusted to the affected skin.

Clinical Course

The duration of FDE is highly variable, but once the offending medication is discontinued, the reaction will usually subside over 1 to 2 weeks. Residual hyperpigmentation may persist for months. If the medication is not discontinued, the lesions may become chronically ulcerated.

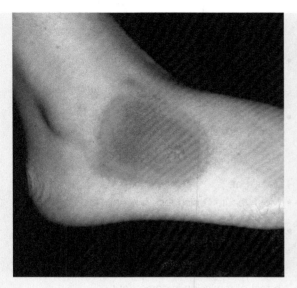

Fig. 11.37. Fixed drug eruption produced by trimethoprim-sulfamethoxazole demonstrating an erythematous plaque with early vesiculation.

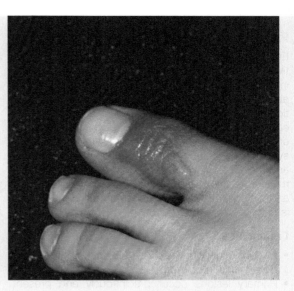

Fig. 11.38. Bullous fixed drug eruption on the big toe produced by ibuprofen. (From the William Weston Collection, Aurora, CO.)

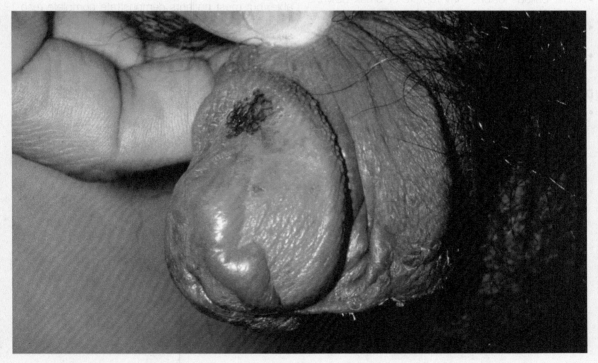

Fig. 11.39. Bullous fixed eruption on the head of the penis due to tetracycline. Note the focal area of hyperpigmentation, which could indicate pigmentary incontinence from one or more previous episodes.

Bullous Erythema Multiforme ICD10 code L51

Pathogenesis

Erythema multiforme (minor) is an inflammatory reactive condition induced by numerous agents and insults. Recurrent herpes simplex infections cause about 70% of cases. Other causes include medications, other infections (viral, bacterial, and fungal), and collagen vascular diseases. The relationship between erythema multiforme (minor) and Stevens-Johnson syndrome (erythema multiform major) is controversial, and there is clinical overlap. Most cases of erythema multiforme minor are not bullous; the more annular and/or targetoid form of erythema multiforme (minor) is discussed in Chapter 16.

Clinical Features

- Lesions usually develop 7 to 10 days after the causative infection or drug.
- Primary lesions occur precipitously and present as erythematous papules or small plaques, which often (but not always) have a targetoid appearance.
- Some cases demonstrate a central blister, and bullous lesions with classic targetoid lesions may coexist (Figs. 11.40 and 11.41).
- Older bullous lesions may rupture or break down, yielding erosions and shallow ulcers (Fig. 11.42).
- Sites often affected include acral areas, the oral mucosa, and genital areas.
- Lesions may occur in sites of trauma (Koebner or isomorphic phenomena; Fig. 11.43).

Diagnosis

- The presentation of bullous lesions, admixed with targetoid lesions, occurring in a chiefly acral distribution, is usually sufficient for establishing the diagnosis.
- A history of previous episodes (recurrent erythema multiforme) and/or a history of HSV infection (HSV-1 or HSV-2) is important historical information that supports the diagnosis.
- Occasional cases may require a shave or punch biopsy (preferred) to establish the diagnosis better. The histologic findings, although not specific, can strongly support the diagnosis.

Treatment

- Most acute episodes do not require therapy because the condition is self-limited.
- Cases associated with recurrent HSV infection may be treated with suppressive acyclovir, valacyclovir, or famciclovir. A typical suppressive dose of acyclovir is 400 mg PO bid for up to 6 months, and then a test of remission is carried out.
- The use of oral corticosteroids for bullous erythema multiforme is controversial.

Clinical Course

Disease activity in erythema multiforme (minor) is variable, but most patients demonstrate complete resolution of lesions in 1 to 3 weeks. Patients with darker skin may demonstrate residual hyperpigmentation that lasts for months.

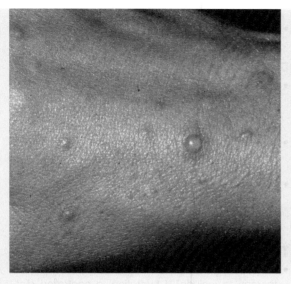

Fig. 11.40. Small classic targetoid lesions of erythema multiforme, with some demonstrating small central blisters.

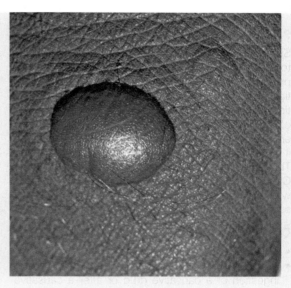

Fig. 11.41. Bullous erythema multiforme with an unusually large blister. Note the adjacent, nonblistered, red papular lesion.

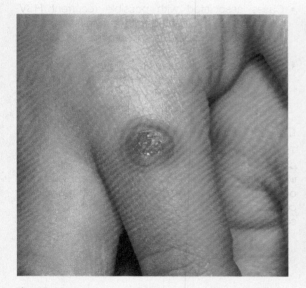

Fig. 11.42. Bullous herpes simplex–induced erythema multiforme, with collapsed blister.

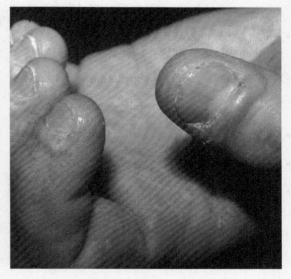

Fig. 11.43. Bullous erythema multiforme demonstrating the Koebner phenomenon due to work-related trauma around the nails.

Pathogenesis

Stevens-Johnson syndrome (SJS), sometimes referred to as erythema multiforme major, is a hypersensitivity process usually caused by drugs, including antiepileptics, antibiotics, and NSAIDs, and sometimes by infections (e.g., HSV, *Mycoplasma*). The precise nosology of SJS is controversial, with some authorities considering it a disorder sui generis and others considering it on a spectrum with toxic epidermal necrolysis (TEN). This latter viewpoint has prevailed in recent years. Classic SJS is defined as a vesiculobullous disorder with targetoid lesions that affects at least two mucosal surfaces.

Clinical Features

- SJS may affect persons of any age.
- Clinical lesions develop about 1 to 3 weeks after ingestion of a causative drug or after a causative infection, although sometimes SJS may occur within a few days if it is a recurrent episode.
- Patients often demonstrate a prodrome of fever, malaise, and myalgias.
- Cutaneous lesions resemble targetoid lesions of erythema multiforme minor (Fig. 11.44) and may become bullous (Fig. 11.45).
- Lesions may involve the following:
  - <10% of body surface area—considered classic SJS
  - 10% to 30% of body surface area—considered SJS-TEN overlap
  - >30% body surface area—often considered simply as TEN
- Lesions are often painful and/or may produce a burning sensation.
- Older bullous lesions may rupture or collapse, with the epidermis shed, yielding superficial ulcers.
- The ocular mucosa, lips, oral mucosa (see Fig. 11.44), anogenital mucosa (Fig. 11.46), and lung mucosa (e.g., pneumonitis, bronchitis) may be involved.

- Lesions may occur in sites of trauma (Koebner or isomorphic phenomena).

Diagnosis

- The classic presentation of admixed bullous lesions, atypical bullous targetoid lesions, and involvement of at least two mucosal surfaces is sufficient for establishing the diagnosis.
- A history of new medications within the past 3 weeks, or an infection, especially with *Mycoplasma,* supports the diagnosis.
- Biopsies should be performed for standard H&E examination and for DIF studies to exclude autoimmune bullous conditions that can mimic SJS (e.g., paraneoplastic pemphigus).

Treatment

- All patients should be hospitalized for supportive therapy to include IV hydration, a controlled diet, thermoregulation, pain control, and mouth rinses and emollients.
- Potentially causative drugs must be discontinued as soon as possible.
- Cases associated with possible recurrent HSV infection may be treated with antivirals; cases of suspected *Mycoplasma* pneumonia should be treated with antibiotics.
- Use of oral corticosteroids in bullous erythema multiforme is controversial, but most evidence suggests that high-dose, short-duration steroid regimens may be used early in the disease course.

Clinical Course

The degree of severity in SJS is variable, but most patients demonstrate complete resolution of lesions in 2 to 3 weeks. Some morbidity may occur when the ocular mucosa is involved, and liberal ophthalmologic consultation should be used. The mortality rate in severe cases approaches 5%.

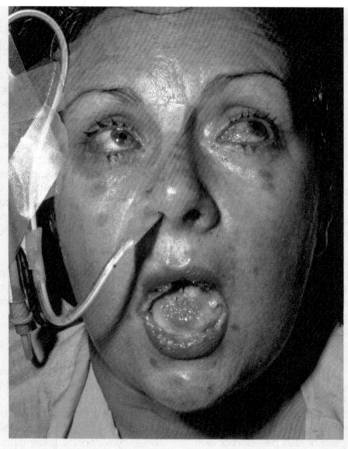

Fig. 11.44. *Mycoplasma*-induced Stevens-Johnson syndrome, with involvement of the ocular mucosa, lips, oral mucosa, and skin. All patients with ocular involvement should have an ophthalmologic consultation.

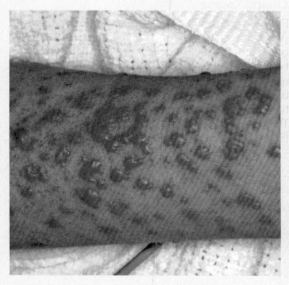

Fig. 11.45. Uniform vesicles and bullae of Stevens-Johnson syndrome on the arm. The extremities are the cutaneous site that is most likely to be affected.

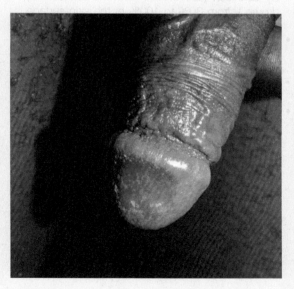

Fig. 11.46. Erosions on the male genitalia in a case of Stevens-Johnson syndrome precipitated by herpes labialis.

❶ Toxic Epidermal Necrolysis ICD10 code L51.2

Common Causes of Toxic Epidermal Necrolysis

- Drugs
  - Allopurinol
  - Barbiturates
  - Hydantoin
  - NSAIDs
  - Penicillins
  - Sulfonamides
- Immunizations
- Infections
  - Herpes simplex
  - *Mycoplasma*
  - Systemic fungal infections

Pathogenesis

TEN is a life-threatening, severe hypersensitivity reaction to a drug (most common), infection or, rarely, an immunization and represents a dermatologic emergency. Many authorities consider it to be a severe variant of Stevens-Johnson syndrome (see previous section). For some drugs, there is evidence of a genetic predisposition to develop TEN.

Clinical Features

- TEN may affect any age group.
- Lesions develop about 1 to 3 weeks after a causative drug (or infection), but some drug-induced cases may develop quickly.
- Patients typically complain of skin pain and/or skin burning and may develop erythema of the skin, which rapidly becomes confluent, resembling a sunburn (Fig. 11.47).
- By definition (see earlier, "Stevens-Johnson Syndrome"), from 30% to 100% of the skin surface is involved.
- Fully developed lesions consist of sheets of necrotic epidermis that shear easily, leaving an erythematous raw base (Figs. 11.48 and 11.49).
- The Nikolsky sign may be present, where the skin will denude with lateral pressure.
- The ocular mucosa, lips, oral mucosa, anogenital mucosa, and sinopulmonary epithelium may be involved.

Diagnosis

- The classic presentation of painful erythema, resembling severe sunburn, that easily denudes and occurs after ingestion of a new medication, is strongly suggestive of the diagnosis.
- A positive Nikolsky sign is also strongly supportive of the diagnosis (see page 166).
- All cases should be biopsied for H&E and direct immunofluorescence because this clinical pattern maybe mimicked by other severe bullous disorders, such as pemphigus, paraneoplastic pemphigus, and drug-induced, linear, IgA bullous dermatosis.
- All patients should have a complete blood count (CBC) and comprehensive metabolic panels (to include kidney and liver function).

Treatment

- All patients should be hospitalized, preferably in a burn unit, for supportive therapy. This should include proper hydration, a controlled diet, thermoregulation, mouth rinses, eye care, analgesics, and emollients.
- Immediately withdraw any potentially causative drugs.
- As the skin denudes, replacement with some form of appropriate dressing should be considered.
- Prophylactic antibiotics are not used, but the threshold for culture and starting antibiotics is low.
- Second-line and controversial therapies include IVIG, cyclosporine, plasmapheresis, and systemic corticosteroids.
- There should be liberal ophthalmology consultation for patients with any possible ocular involvement.

Clinical Course

Poor prognostic factors include age older than 40 years, associated malignancy, more than 10% of the body surface detached, tachycardia more than 120 beats/min, and elevated serum urea (>10 nmol/L), elevated serum glucose (>14 nmol/L), and low serum bicarbonate (<20 nmol/L) levels. The mortality rate has approached 40% in some studies (Fig. 11.49). There is a validated prognostic scale for clinical use (SCORETEN) that may be used.

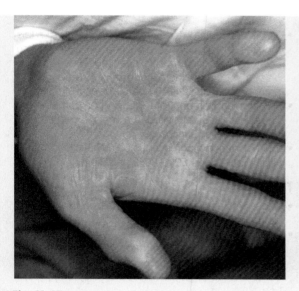

Fig. 11.47. Hydantoin-induced early toxic epidermal necrolysis manifesting as painful erythema. Note the early blister formation on the small finger.

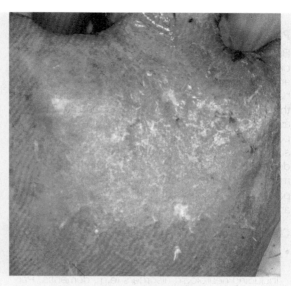

Fig. 11.48. Developed toxic epidermal necrolysis demonstrating sheets of partially detached epidermis and a raw denuded base.

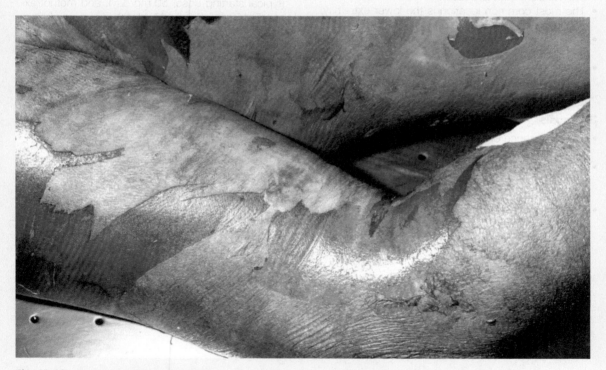

Fig. 11.49. Fatal case of captopril-induced toxic epidermal necrolysis demonstrating sheets on partially detached epidermis associated with a glistening denuded base. (From the Fitzsimons Army Medical Center Collection, Aurora, CO.)

Pathogenesis

Bullous pemphigoid (BP) is an autoimmune bullous disease that usually occurs in elderly patients, although any age group may be affected. The incidence of BP has tripled in the past 10 years as the population of the United States has aged. BP is mediated by IgG autoantibodies (BPAg1 and BPAg2) directed against portions of the hemidesmosome, a structure necessary for normal attachment of the epidermis to the dermis. This deposition results in an inflammatory milieu that causes chemotaxis of inflammatory cells, particularly eosinophils. It is unknown why these autoantibodies develop.

Clinical Features

- Typically BP affects elderly patients, and it is more common in patients with multiple comorbidities, including neurologic disorders (e.g., dementia, Parkinson disease).
- Urticarial plaques, or tense blisters, are common (Figs. 11.50 and 11.51). Either or both forms of disease may be present in the same patient.
- The Nikolsky sign is absent.
- The most common location is the lower extremity, although any skin surface may be affected.
- Older lesions demonstrate a raw, denuded base (Fig. 11.52).
- Oral lesions are uncommon, although some studies have reported that 20% of patients have mucosal lesions.

Diagnosis

- The occurrence of fixed urticarial lesions and tense bullae is suggestive, especially in an elderly patient.
- Some bullous drug eruptions mimic BP, clinically and histologically, and a careful drug history must be taken.
- A biopsy (shave, punch, or small excision) of an early urticarial lesion, or a new blister, is useful to establish the diagnosis.

- DIF is also useful to establish the diagnosis; this requires a biopsy from perilesional skin (≈0.5–1 cm away from a blister). This specimen needs to be placed in immunofluorescent transport medium, in normal saline (for 24–48 hours), or snap frozen.
- DIF studies demonstrate IgG and/or complement component C3 deposited in a linear fashion at the dermoepidermal junction.
- Indirect immunofluorescent studies have lesser sensitivity (positive in 50%–80% of patients).

Treatment

- Those with a mild case and/or localized disease may be managed with potent topical corticosteroids.
- Moderate to severe cases are managed first with oral prednisone (≥0.5 mg/kg per day), with the understanding that many elderly patients have comorbidities (e.g., diabetes) that may complicate use.
- After controlling the disease with oral corticosteroids, steroid-sparing agents are generally used. These may include doxycycline (100 mg PO bid) with nicotinamide (500 mg PO qid), dapsone (typical starting dose, 50 mg/day), and methotrexate (5–15 mg as a weekly dose).
- Treatments used less often include azathioprine, cyclophosphamide, mycophenolate, methotrexate, chlorambucil, plasmapheresis, IV gamma globulin, and rituximab.

Clinical Course

BP is often considered to be an autoimmune disease with a low mortality rate, but the degree of discomfort (especially pruritus) experienced by elderly patients is substantial. Moreover, elderly persons with extensive disease demonstrate increased mortality rates (as high as 31% in 6 months). Current literature has indicated that half of patients will go into clinical remission within 2.5 to 6 years although, for some patients, the disease may continue for 10 years or longer.

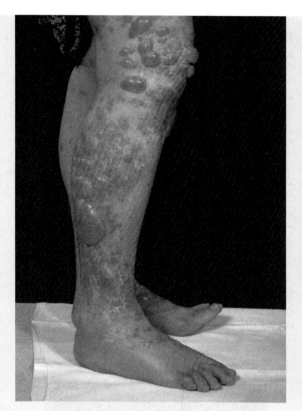

Fig. 11.50. Typical tense blisters of bullous pemphigoid on an erythematous base. (From the Fitzsimons Army Medical Center Collection, Aurora, CO.)

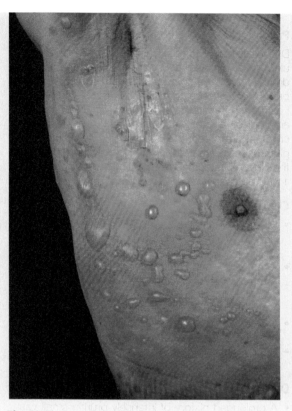

Fig. 11.51. Tense blisters of bullous pemphigoid in combination with urticarial lesions. (From the Fitzsimons Army Medical Center Collection, Aurora, CO.)

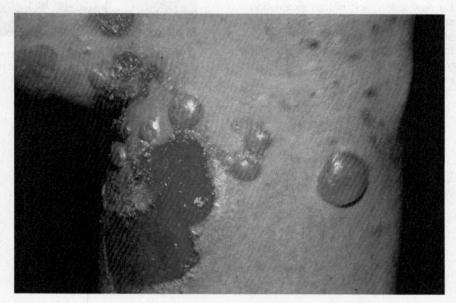

Fig. 11.52. Tense blisters of bullous pemphigoid with a typical eroded base when the blisters break. (From the Fitzsimons Army Medical Center Collection, Aurora, CO.)

Pathogenesis

Dermatitis herpetiformis (DH) is a subepidermal vesiculobullous disease caused by IgA autoantibodies directed against a component of the basement membrane zone, tissue transglutaminase 3 (Fig. 11.53). Less often, antireticular antibodies, antiendomysial antibodies, and/or antigliadin antibodies (especially children) are present. DH is strongly associated with gluten-sensitive enteropathy. The prevalence of DH in the United States has been estimated to be between 1 and 39 cases per 100,000 persons.

Clinical Features

- Males and females are equally affected and, most often, the disease begins in the fifth decade of life. Actually, any age group may be affected.
- Primary lesions are small (1–5 mm), intensely pruritic blisters on an erythematous base (Figs. 11.54–11.56) that are often grouped (herpetiform). Large bullae are uncommon.
- Often, the appearance is complicated by excoriations because of the intense pruritus.
- Characteristic sites of involvement include the elbows, knees, buttocks, and occipital scalp.

Diagnosis

- A prolonged history of intensely pruritic small vesicles, in characteristic areas, suggests the diagnosis. The occurrence of lesions on the scalp, buttocks, elbows, and knees is a pattern not seen in most other bullous disorders.
- A biopsy of a new lesion, and not an excoriation, may suggest strongly the diagnosis.
- The diagnosis may be further substantiated by DIF studies performed on perilesional skin. DH is characterized by the deposition of granular IgA in the papillary dermis (Fig. 11.53).

Treatment

- The treatment of choice for DH is dapsone (25–150 mg/day), with improvement occurring rapidly after initiating the drug.
- Alternative treatments include sulfapyridine (2–4 g PO daily) or colchicine (up to 0.6 mg PO tid) in patients who cannot tolerate dapsone.
- A gluten-free diet may be used, but adherence can be problematic, and it may take 3 to 12 months to demonstrate significant improvement.
- It is also important to realize that iodides and NSAIDs, especially indomethacin, may exacerbate DH.
- Because of the strong association with gluten-sensitive enteropathy (celiac disease), patients should be referred to a gastroenterologist for further testing.

Clinical Course

DH is a chronic lifelong disease that frequently wanes in intensity as patients age.

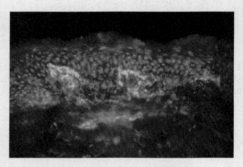

Fig. 11.53. Direct immunofluorescence demonstrating deposition of granular IgA along the basement membrane zone in a patient with dermatitis herpetiformis.

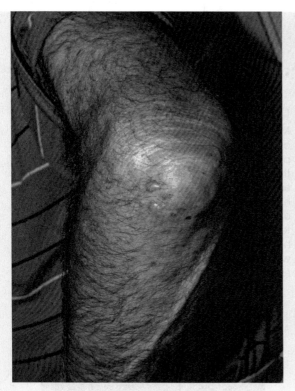

Fig. 11.54. Dermatitis herpetiformis, with blisters and excoriations. (From the Fitzsimons Army Medical Center Collection, Aurora, CO.)

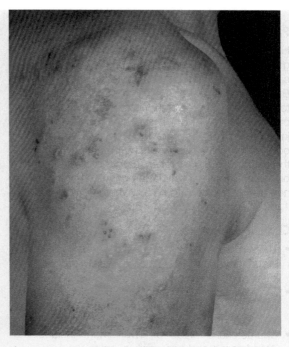

Fig. 11.55. Dermatitis herpetiformis presenting primarily with excoriations. (From the Fitzsimons Army Medical Center Collection, Aurora, CO.)

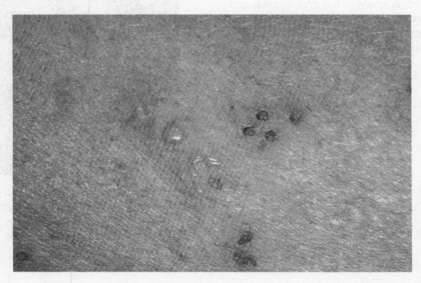

Fig. 11.56. Close-up of dermatitis herpetiformis demonstrating admixture of small unilocular vesicles and excoriations. (From the Fitzsimons Army Medical Center Collection, Aurora, CO.)

Herpes Gestationis ICD10 Code O26.4

Pathogenesis

Herpes gestationis (gestational pemphigoid, pemphigoid gestationis) is an autoimmune bullous condition caused by IgG antibodies directed primarily against BPAg2 (occasionally BPAg1), a structure necessary for adherence of the epidermis to the basement membrane zone (Fig. 11.57). It is, in essence, BP occurring in gravid or recently gravid women. The condition occurs nearly exclusively during pregnancy or shortly thereafter and is less often associated with trophoblastic malignancy or molar pregnancy. The incidence has been calculated to be anywhere from 1 : 3000 to 1 : 60,000 pregnancies.

Clinical Features

- The condition affects pregnant women or recently pregnant women. The disease usually occurs in the latter portion of pregnancy or following delivery.
- Lesions can be fixed, red, urticarial plaques, tense blisters, or a combination of these two primary lesions (Figs. 11.58–11.60).
- Characteristic areas of involvement include the intertriginous and periumbilical areas.
- The symptoms are typically pruritic.

Diagnosis

- The clinical presentation of a pregnant or recently pregnant woman who presents with a sudden onset of fixed red plaques, with or without blisters, is highly suggestive of the diagnosis.
- Characteristic involvement of the intertriginous and periumbilical areas also supports the diagnosis.
- A punch biopsy of lesional skin should be done for routine histologic examination. The findings are diagnostic not only of herpes gestationis but also can strongly support and exclude other clinical possibilities.
- A biopsy of perilesional skin should be performed for DIF studies. Linear deposition of C3, with or without IgG, at the dermoepidermal junction is diagnostic in this context.

Treatment

- Treatment of choice is oral prednisone, with a usual initial dose being 40 to 60 mg. Because the disease is generally self-limited and resolves over a period of days, weeks, or months after delivery, the therapy usually does not have to be sustained.
- Rare patients may demonstrate disease for years afterward, and steroid-sparing agents are used.

Clinical Course

Most cases resolve in the postpartum period, usually over days, weeks, or months. Occasional cases may persist for years or be perpetuated by use of oral contraceptives. Although early studies have suggested an adverse effect on the fetus, more recent studies have concluded that there is usually no adverse effect on the fetus. Herpes gestationis may be transmitted to the neonate, but this is very rare. Neonates with herpes gestationis experience spontaneous resolution within weeks after birth as the maternal antibodies are lost.

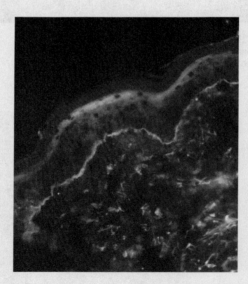

Fig. 11.57. Linear IgG directed against the basement membrane zone in a patient with herpes gestationis.

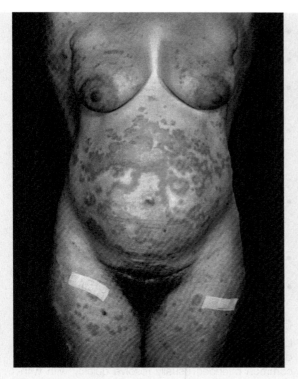

Fig. 11.58. Arcuate urticarial lesions in herpes gestationis. Note involvement of the umbilicus. (From the Fitzsimons Army Medical Center Collection, Aurora, CO.)

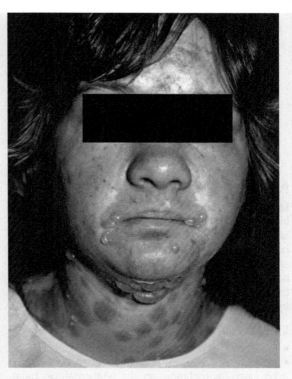

Fig. 11.59. Postpartum herpes gestationis demonstrating urticarial lesions and tense blisters. (From the Fitzsimons Army Medical Center Collection, Aurora, CO.)

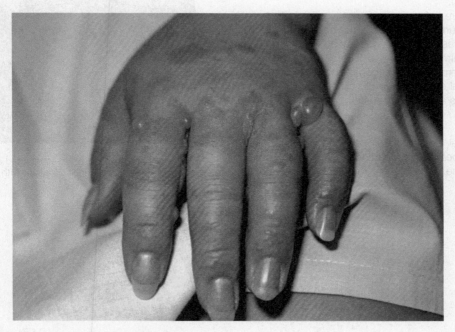

Fig. 11.60. Tense blisters and urticarial lesions in herpes gestationis. Interdigital blisters are common in this disorder. (From the Fitzsimons Army Medical Center Collection, Aurora, CO.)

Drug-Induced Linear IgA Bullous Dermatosis
- Ampicillin-sulbactam (rare)
- Benazepril (rare)
- Carbamazepine (rare)
- Ceftriaxone-metronidazole (rare)
- Gemcitabine (rare)
- Naproxen (rare)
- Piroxicam (rare)
- Sulfadimethoxine (rare)
- Vancomycin (common)

Pathogenesis

Linear IgA bullous dermatosis (LABD) is a rare auto-immune bullous condition in which IgA autoantibodies are directed against a structural component of the basement membrane zone between the epidermis and dermis (Fig. 11.61). Most cases are idiopathic, but a significant number of cases are drug-induced (see box). When it occurs in children, it has also been termed *chronic bullous disease of childhood*.

Clinical Features

- LABD may affect children and adults.
- Both minute vesicles and large tense bullae may be seen, sometimes on an erythematous base (Fig. 11.62).
- Blisters may be arranged in groups or annular configurations, sometimes likened to a string of pearls (Fig. 11.63), or with sausage or beanlike shapes (Fig. 11.64).
- Lesions are often symmetrically distributed on extensor surfaces, especially the back and neck.
- In severe cases, the blisters may be large and generalized, mimicking those of TEN.
- Oral involvement is rather common and usually consists of oral erosions and ulcerations.
- The blisters are usually pruritic.

Diagnosis

- The clinical presentation, particularly in a child, can be persuasive, particularly because other autoimmune disorders are relatively uncommon in children.

- Annular configurations of blisters, arranged as a string of pearls, strongly suggest the diagnosis.
- In adults, vancomycin use should prompt consideration of drug-induced LABD.
- A shave or punch biopsy is often useful in suggesting the diagnosis, but other autoimmune blistering diseases share similar histologic features.
- The diagnosis is established definitively via a punch or shave biopsy of perilesional skin for DIF studies to demonstrate a linear band of IgA autoantibodies.

Treatment

- Oral prednisone is used initially for quick control, usually at a dose of 0.5 to 1.0 mg/kg per day, with tapering as the condition improves or as steroid-sparing agents are added.
- Dapsone (25–100 mg PO qd) is the steroid-sparing drug used most often.
- Sulfapyridine and colchicine are other steroid-sparing agents that are used less often.

Clinical Course

LABD may last for months or years, especially in children. Drug-induced forms of LABD (vancomycin is a common offender) usually resolve quickly with withdrawal of the offending drug.

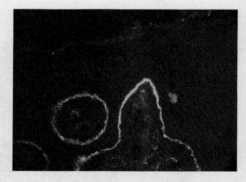

Fig. 11.61. Linear IgA autoantibodies directed against the basement membrane zone in a patient with linear IgA bullous dermatosis.

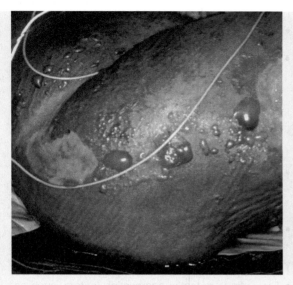

Fig. 11.62. Small to large tense blisters associated with erosions in a patient with vancomycin-induced, linear IgA bullous dermatosis. (From the Fitzsimons Army Medical Center Collection, Aurora, CO.)

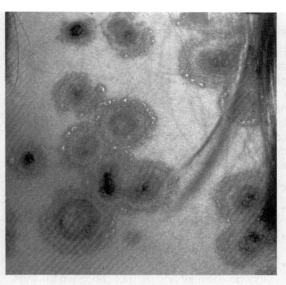

Fig. 11.63. Chronic bullous disease of childhood demonstrating characteristic blisters, with a string of pearls arrangement.

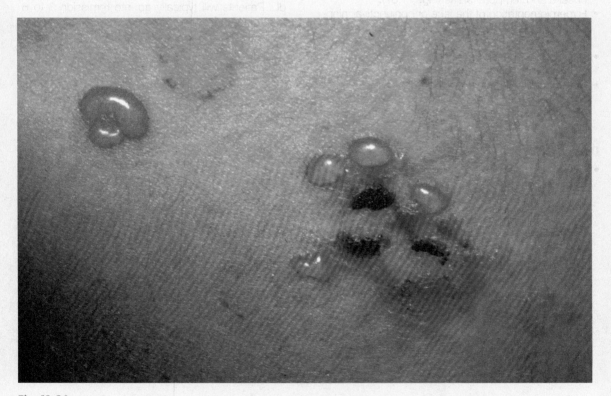

Fig. 11.64. Close-up of a child with chronic bullous disease of childhood with tense blisters, some of which demonstrate a bean or sausage shape. (From the Fitzsimons Army Medical Center Collection, Aurora, CO.)

Porphyria Cutanea Tarda ICD10 code E80.1

Pathogenesis

Porphyrias represent a group of inherited, or rarely acquired, disorders of porphyrin metabolism, which produce blisters in the skin. Porphyria cutanea tarda (PCT) is the most common of these disorders, with an estimated incidence of about 1:25,000 in the United States. It is due to an inherited deficiency of uroporphyrinogen decarboxylase. Precipitating and/or aggravating factors include hepatitis C infection, alcohol abuse, estrogens, and general iron overload.

Clinical Features

- PCT may occur at any age, but it usually affects middle-aged individuals of both genders.
- Primary lesions include thick-walled blisters, often on the back of the hands (photoexposed skin).
- The blisters often lack erythema or inflammation, although hemorrhage is not uncommon (Figs. 11.65 and 11.66).
- Patients often report that minor trauma produces blisters or erosions (see Figs. 11.65 and 11.66) on the back of the hands and fingers.
- Hypertrichosis may be noticeable on the upper cheeks and temporal areas (Fig. 11.67).
- Hyperpigmentation of the face or conjunctival injection (so-called traveling salesman eyes) may be noted.
- Patients can develop scarring and milia formation at the sites of previous blisters.
- Rare patients demonstrate induration of the scalp, arms, or upper trunk indistinguishable from that of morphea or even progressive systemic sclerosis (scleroderma).

Diagnosis

- PCT should always be included in the differential diagnosis of tense blisters on the hands.

- A skin biopsy, although not diagnostic only of PCT, often strongly suggests the diagnosis.
- If high levels of porphyrins are present in the urine, a freshly voided sampled will demonstrate coral red fluorescence when examined with a Wood lamp (Fig. 11.68). If more moderate levels of porphyrins are present, the urine will demonstrate coral red fluorescence only in the meniscus (Fig. 2.1). Sometimes, examination of the urine will not demonstrate any remarkable findings, even when PCT is present.
- The diagnosis is best established by measuring a 24-hour urine collection for total porphyrins. Values of 300 µg (or >800 µg if active lesions are present) will be observed.
- Serum iron levels, a CBC, and liver function tests (LFTs) should be done on all patients.

Treatment

- Discontinue potential aggravating factors, such as estrogen or alcohol.
- Phlebotomy is a safe and effective method for depleting hepatic iron and results in improvement. Typically, 1 unit of blood (500 mL) is removed each week until the hemoglobin level reaches 11 g/dL. Patients will typically go into remission 3 to 6 months after beginning therapy.
- Hydroxychloroquine may be used cautiously— 250 mg PO once or twice weekly. Note that daily doses may lead to liver failure in this patient population.

Clinical Course

Because this is a genetic disorder, it cannot be cured but, in general, the withdrawal of exacerbating agents, phlebotomy, and/or low-dose hydroxychloroquine will place most patients in complete remission.

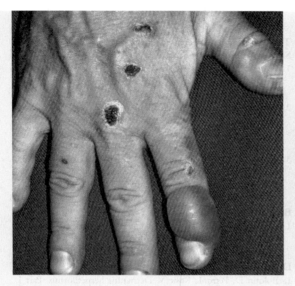

Fig. 11.65. Large bulla of the finger of a patient with porphyria cutanea tarda associated with numerous erosions and crusts. (From the Fitzsimons Army Medical Center Collection, Aurora, CO.)

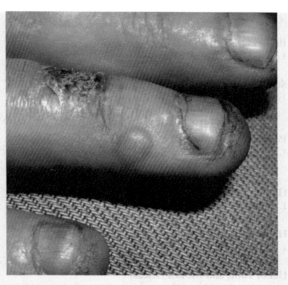

Fig. 11.66. Close-up of a tense blister and finger in a patient with porphyria cutanea tarda. (From the Fitzsimons Army Medical Center Collection, Aurora, CO.)

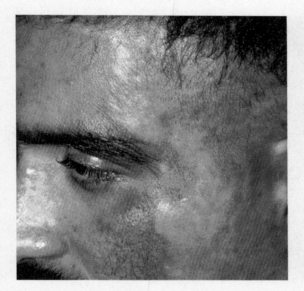

Fig. 11.67. Hypertrichosis and hyperpigmentation in a patient with chronic porphyria cutanea tarda. (From the Fitzsimons Army Medical Center Collection, Aurora, CO.)

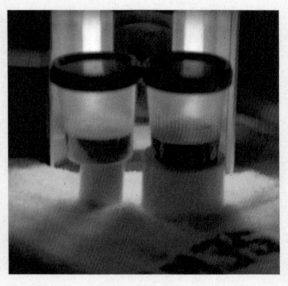

Fig. 11.68. Wood light examination of normal urine *(left)* and urine with coral red fluorescence from a patient with porphyria cutanea tarda *(right)*.

References

Bullous Impetigo

1. Brown J, Shriner D, Schwartz RA, Janniger CK. Impetigo: an update. *Int J Dermatol.* 2001;42:251-255.

Staphylococcal Scalded Skin Syndrome

1. Braunstein I, Wanat KA, Abuabara K, et al. Antibiotic sensitivity and resistance patterns in pediatric staphylococcal scalded skin syndrome. *Pediatr Dermatol.* 2014;31:305.

Pemphigus

1. Allen KJ, Wolverton SE. The efficacy and safety of rituximab in refractory pemphigus: a review of case reports. *J Drugs Dermatol.* 2007;6:883-889.

Herpes Zoster

1. Cohen JI. Clinical practice: herpes zoster. *N Engl J Med.* 2013;369:255-263.

Herpes Simplex Infections

1. Emmert DH. Treatment of common cutaneous herpes simplex virus infections. *Am Fam Physician.* 2000;61:1697-1706.

Hand, Foot, and Mouth Disease

1. Stewart CL, Chu EY, Introcaso CE, et al. Coxsackievirus A6-induced hand-foot-mouth disease. *JAMA Dermatol.* 2013;149:1419-1421.

Toxic Epidermal Necrolysis and Stevens-Johnson Syndrome

1. Fromowitz JS, Ramos-Caro FA, Flowers FP. Practical guidelines for the management of toxic epidermal necrolysis and Stevens-Johnson syndrome. *Int J Dermatol.* 2007;46:1092-1094.
2. Schwart RA, McDonough PH, Lee BW. Toxic epidermal necrolysis. Part I. Introduction, history, classification, clinical features, systemic manifestations, etiology, and immunopathogenesis. *J Am Acad Dermatol.* 2013;69:173-184.
3. Schwartz RA, McDonough PH, Lee BW. Toxic epidermal necrolysis. Part II. Prognosis, sequelae, diagnosis, differential diagnosis, prevention, and treatment. *J Am Acad Dermatol.* 2013;69:187-202.

Bullous Pemphigoid

1. Brick KE, Weaver CH, Savica R, et al. A population-based study of the association between bullous pemphigoid and neurologic disorders. *J Am Acad Dermatol.* 2014;71:1191-1197.

Dermatitis Herpetiformis

1. Bolotin D, Petronic-Rosic V. Dermatitis herpetiformis. Part I. Epidemiology, pathogenesis, and clinical presentation. *J Am Acad Dermatol.* 2011;64:1017-1024.

Porphyria Cutanea Tarda

1. Balwani M, Desnick RJ. The porphyrias: advances in diagnosis and treatment. *Blood.* 2012;120:4496-4504.

Chapter 12
Pustular Eruptions, Nonfollicular

Key Terms

Acrodermatitis continua of
   Hallopeau

Impetigo herpetiformis
Pustulosis of the palms and soles

Pustules are defined as papular lesions filled with an exudate of acute inflammatory cells. In most cases, the acute inflammatory cells are neutrophils; however, less often the cells are eosinophils or an admixture of the two cell types. This chapter excludes pustular lesions that are follicular based (acute folliculitis), which is discussed in Chapter 23. Not all pustular eruptions are discussed in this chapter (see box).

> ### Pustular Eruptions
> - Acute generalized exanthematous pustulosis
> - Acropustulosis of infancy
> - Candidiasis
> - Intraepidermal immunoglobulin A (IgA) pemphigus
> - Pustular psoriasis
> - Reactive arthritis (Reiter disease)
> - Pustular arthropod reactions
> - Subcorneal pustular dermatosis
> - Transient neonatal pustular melanosis

IMPORTANT HISTORY QUESTIONS

How long have the pustules been present?

Some pustular reactions develop acutely, such as pustular drug eruptions or pustular arthropod reactions, whereas pustular psoriasis and reactive arthritis may be chronic or recurring.

Do you have a known personal or family history of psoriasis?

Pustular psoriasis can be tricky to diagnose when it initially presents. The presence of a personal or family history of psoriasis would strongly suggest the possibility of pustular psoriasis.

Do you have a past or current history of arthritis or painful joints?

This question is obviously looking for potential joint disease due to psoriasis or reactive arthritis.

Have you started any new medications?

This is a very important questions because pustular drug eruptions are always high in the differential diagnosis. One should be suspicious of any antibiotic, especially if it belongs to the penicillin class. This question is also important even for patients with known psoriasis because a number of drugs (e.g., oral or intramuscular corticosteroids, terbinafine) will precipitate a pustular reaction in an otherwise classic plaque type of psoriasis.

Had you spent any time outdoors before you developed the rash?

This question is directed at finding any potential source of pustular arthropod reactions.

Does anyone else in the family have a rash?

This question is directed at finding a potential common arthropod exposure, such as flea bites.

How are you treating this rash?

Many patients use home-based, over-the-counter (OTC), or prescription remedies that may alter a reaction. One of the most common is a topical corticosteroid, which may actually produce follicular pustules and confuse the clinical picture.

IMPORTANT PHYSICAL FINDINGS

How old is the patient?

Some pustular disorders occur in young children (e.g., acropustulosis of infancy), others are primarily in young adults (e.g., vaccinia infection), and others occur in any age group.

What are the distribution and arrangement of the pustules?

Some pustular disorders have a distinct distribution (e.g., acropustulosis of infancy, acrodermatitis continua). Some pustular disorders present as solitary lesions, whereas others may demonstrates annular or circinate arrangements (e.g., some cases of pustular psoriasis, intraepidermal IgA pemphigus).

Are the pustules based on hair follicles or non-follicular skin?

If the pustules are based on hair follicles, refer to Chapter 23.

Drug-Induced Pustular Drug Eruptions

Analgesics
- Acetaminophen

Antimalarial Agents
- Hydroxychloroquine (Plaquenil)
- Quinidine

Antipsychotic Agents
- Olanzapine

Antibiotics
- Amoxicillin
- Ampicillin
- Cefazolin
- Cephradine
- Cephalexin
- Clindamycin
- Cotrimazole
- Metronidazole
- Penicillin
- Norfloxacin
- Vancomycin

Antiseizure Agents
- Carbamazepine
- Phenytoin

Calicum Channel Blockers
- Nifedipine

Miscellaneous
- Chromium picolinate
- Mercury
- Radiocontrast dye

Pathogenesis

Acute generalized exanthematous pustulosis (AGEP) is a reproducible pustular drug hypersensitivity produced by many drugs; the most common offenders are antibiotics (cephalosporins, cotrimoxazole are most frequently implicated), anticonvulsants, and hydroxychloroquine. This distinct drug eruption has been reproduced with topical patch testing; however, the exact immunologic basis for this reaction is not understood.

Clinical Features

- The patient has a history of a new medication within the past 1 to 5 days.

- There is an acute (often dramatic) onset of macular (typically confluent) erythema that can affect any site, although it usually affects large areas of the trunk and proximal extremities.
- Erythema studded with varying numbers of 1- to 2-mm pustules (Figs. 12.1–12.3) is found. Pustules may be present on some regions of the body and absent on others.
- Less commonly, patients may demonstrate erythematous indurated papules or small plaques that may resemble erythema multiforme.
- Patients may complain of burning, itching, or both.
- A low-grade fever is common.

Diagnosis

- The history of a new drug (especially antibiotics), combined with toxic erythema and pustules, is very strongly suspicious of AGEP.
- Complete blood count (CBC). Leukocytosis is commonly present.
- Typically, a 3- or 4-mm punch biopsy will demonstrate a subcorneal or, less commonly, a follicular-based pustule containing numerous neutrophils, with variable numbers of eosinophils. The biopsy results, although not specific, can be strongly supportive of the diagnosis.

Treatment

- Withdraw the suspected offending drug(s).
- No treatment is necessary in most cases because this is a self-limited disease.
- Sedating antihistamines such as diphenhydramine can be used for patient comfort at night.
- Medium-potency corticosteroids (e.g., triamcinolone, fluocinonide) in a cream or ointment base can be used for for pruritus.
- Severe cases may require a short burst of oral prednisone (typically, 40 mg for 3 or 4 days).
- Patients need to be labeled as allergic to the implicated drug because these reactions will occur with subsequent challenge.

Clinical Course

The erythema typically fades over several days, followed by desquamation similar to that seen in sunburn.

Fig. 12.1. Numerous small pustules on a background of erythema caused by amoxicillin.

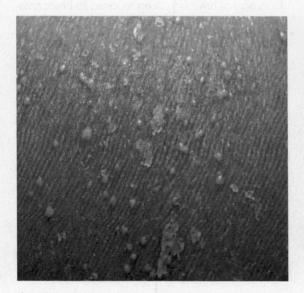

Fig. 12.2. Acute generalized exanthematous pustulosis due to ceftriaxone. This lesion demonstrates uniform pustules, background erythema, and early desquamation.

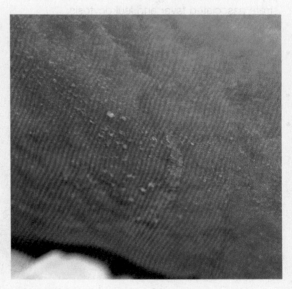

Fig. 12.3. Close-up of a pustular drug eruption due to hydroxychloroquine that demonstrates erythema studded with small pustules. This eruption is several days old, and there is already early desquamation of the top layer of skin.

Pustular Psoriasis ICD 10 codes L40.1, L40.2, and L40.3

Pathogenesis

The pathogenesis of pustular psoriasis is the same as for classic papulosquamous psoriasis in that it is a genetic disorder with a trigger, such as an infection. Patients may demonstrate features of both the papulosquamous and pustular types or move back and forth between the two phenotypic presentations. In some cases, pustular psoriasis may be precipitated by oral corticosteroids. The reason for this is not understood.

Implicated Drugs in Pustular Psoriasis
- Aceclofenac
- Antitumor necrosis factor therapy (e.g., adalimumab, etanercept, infliximab)
- Clopidogrel
- Fexofenadine
- Systemic corticosteroids
- Terbinafine

Clinical Features
- Patients may have a past, present, or family history of plaque-type or pustular psoriasis.
- Patients may demonstrate a localized (e.g., confined to palms and soles) or generalized distribution.
- The primary lesion is diffuse erythema studded with pustules that are not infrequently distributed around the edges in an annular fashion (Fig. 12.4).
- Pustular psoriasis confined to the fingers is frequently associated with marked nail dystrophy and underlying arthritis.
- A patient experiencing acute flares may demonstrate associated fever and leukocytosis.
- Patients are more likely to have associated active psoriatic arthritis.
- Patients with pustular psoriasis are more likely to develop geographic tongue, scrotal tongue, and iritis.
- Rare cases may be life-threatening, with associated shock and/or renal failure.
- **Impetigo herpetiformis** is now considered to be acute pustular psoriasis associated with pregnancy.

- **Pustulosis of the palms and soles** (pustulosis palmaris et plantaris) is a variant that was formerly known as pustular bacterid (of Andrews) in older texts (Fig. 12.5).
- **Acrodermatitis continua of Hallopeau** is a rare variant of pustular psoriasis. It consists of pustules on one or more distal fingers or, less commonly, on the toes (Fig. 12.6). This variant is often associated with nail dystrophy and distal psoriatic arthritis.

Diagnosis
- The diagnosis should be suspected in a patient with a personal or family history of psoriasis who has an acute or chronic pustular eruption.
- Peripheral leukocytosis is commonly present.
- A 3- or 4-mm punch biopsy of a pustular area will demonstrate a subcorneal pustule containing neutrophils. Although not specific, the histologic findings are often supportive.
- X-ray studies are indicated in the acrodermatitis continua of Hallopeau variant to exclude underlying psoriatic arthritis.

Treatment
- Withdraw oral corticosteroids or offending drugs, if possible.
- The recommended treatment is an oral retinoid, with etretinate being the treatment of choice. It can be combined with light therapy (narrow-band ultraviolet B [UVB], UVB, or psoralen and ultraviolet A [PUVA]).
- Treat with a biologic agent, such as adalimumab, etanercept, or infliximab. Paradoxically, some biologic agents have also been reported to precipitate pustular psoriasis.
- Oral cyclosporine, dapsone, and methotrexate have also been anecdotally reported to be useful.
- A medium-potency corticosteroid (e.g., triamcinolone, fluocinonide) in a cream or ointment base is helpful, although most cases only demonstrate partial improvement.

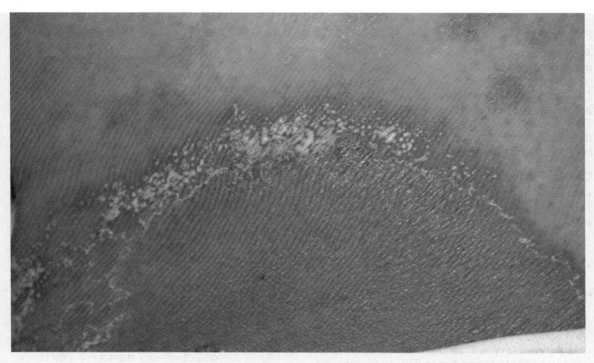

Fig. 12.4. Patient with generalized pustular psoriasis presenting as markedly erythematous plaques, with numerous small pustules arranged around the periphery of the lesions.

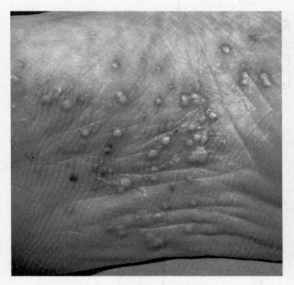

Fig. 12.5. Patient with pustular psoriasis of the palms and soles. This is a close-up of the instep of the foot. (From the Fitzsimons Army Medical Center Collection, Aurora, CO.)

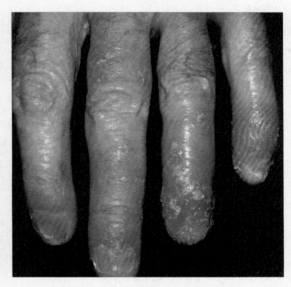

Fig. 12.6. Hand of a patient with acrodermatitis continua demonstrating marked erythema, pustules, crust, and destruction of the nail.

Pathogenesis

Acropustulosis of infancy, also known as **infantile acropustulosis,** is, as the name implies, a pustular disorder that tends to affect the acral areas of infants. The pathogenesis is not understood, although there is a higher than expected incidence of atopic dermatitis. There also appears to be a higher than expected incidence in warmer climates, suggesting the possibility of an exaggerated arthropod reaction.

Clinical Features

- Typically, this first develops in infants between the ages of 2 and 6 months.
- This disorder may affect infants of any ethnic group but is more common in children with a darker skin color.
- Lesions classically recur in crops every 2 to 6 weeks.
- The primary lesion appears as markedly pruritic. 1- to 2-mm pustules on an erythematous base (Fig. 12.7). In some cases, the primary lesions may have the appearance of cloudy vesicles.
- As the name implies, the distribution is primarily to the feet (Fig. 12.8) and hands (Fig. 12.9), although lesions may extend more proximally. In rare cases, lesions may affect the head and neck area or trunk.
- Lesions typically resolve spontaneously over 1 to 3 weeks.

Diagnosis

- The clinical presentation of crops of small pruritic pustules on an erythematous base in an infant, particularly an infant with darker skin, is essentially diagnostic, although the differential diagnosis still includes scabies or another arthropod reaction.

- Important features include the absence of pruritic lesions in other members of the family. If other members of the family are affected, an arthropod reaction, especially scabies, needs to be excluded.
- In difficult cases, the lesions can be scraped for a mineral preparation to exclude scabies. The contents of the blister can also have Wright staining performed because the presence of numerous neutrophils favors acropustulosis of infancy, and the presence of numerous eosinophils would favor an arthropod reaction.
- A biopsy can be done in problematic cases and can be strongly supportive of the diagnosis; however, in most cases, it is not needed.

Treatment

- Topical corticosteroids are the mainstay of therapy. This disorder usually requires potent to superpotent topical corticosteroids.
- In severely pruritic patients, oral antihistamines can be added.
- In very severe cases, oral dapsone, 1 to 2 mg/kg per day, can be added. However, given the side effects associated with oral dapsone in infants, the risk-benefit ratio needs to be carefully considered.
- The patient's parent(s) need to understand that none of these therapies alters the course of the disease.

Clinical Course

This is usually a chronic disorder, with children continuing to get new crops of lesions up to the age of 3 years, although the succeeding attacks tend to diminish in intensity.

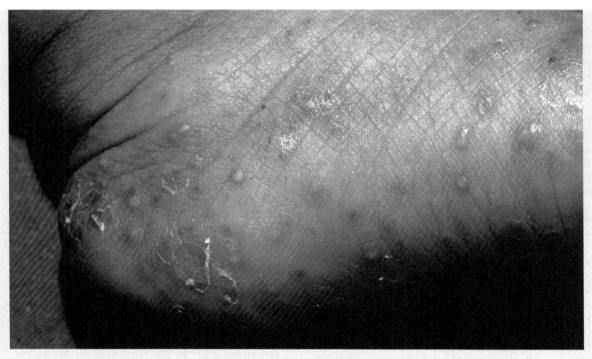

Fig. 12.7. Numerous small pustules and cloudy vesicles on the foot of a child. The lesions are in various stages of development, with some lesions demonstrating resolution and scale. (From the William Weston Collection, Aurora, CO.)

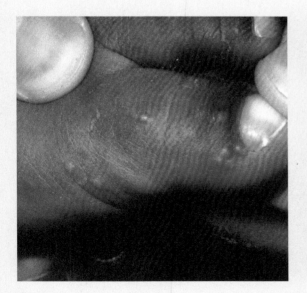

Fig. 12.8. Close-up of typical small pustules and cloudy vesicles on the toe of a young child.

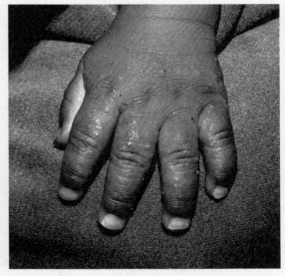

Fig. 12.9. Numerous pustules and cloudy vesicles on the hand of a young child. (From the Fitzsimons Army Medical Center Collection, Aurora, CO.)

Pathogenesis

Pustular arthropod reactions are usually the result of fire ant envenomation, flea bites, and, less commonly, other arthropod reactions. The imported fire ant, *Solenopsis invicta*, is the most commonly implicated species, although at least two other species can also produce pustular reactions. Fire ants have an expanding but limited range that primarily includes the southeastern United States and southwestern United States (Fig. 12.10). Fire ants use their jaws to clamp onto the skin and then pivot, with the stinging apparatus located at the end of the abdomen.

Clinical Features

- Fire ant stings produce an immediate burning sensation, which may last for several minutes.
- The initial reaction is erythema, with a variable wheal-and-flare reaction.
- Lesions are often clustered or circular and can be numerous.
- Over a period of hours to days, the erythema is frequently surmounted by solitary vesiculopustules or pustules (Fig. 12.11).
- Rare patients with fire ant stings experience anaphylaxis.

- Flea bites usually present as one or more pruritic pustules on the lower extremity.
- Scabies may rarely be pustular in children (Fig. 12.12).

Diagnosis

- Fire ant stings are usually diagnostic, because most patients can report a history of fire ant stings.
- In some cases, the lesions may occur in young children who have been outdoors, and the history is not diagnostic. In these cases, the characteristic clustering of the lesions in an endemic area is considered to be supportive of the diagnosis.
- Biopsies are not helpful.

Treatment

- No treatment is an option because the disease is self-limited.
- Ice compresses may provide immediate relief.
- Topical corticosteroids (potent or ultrapotent) can reduce erythema and decrease pruritus.
- Eradication of colonies is often difficult, but a variety of pesticides are useful. A dermatologist with expertise in this area has recommended Amdro fire ant bait as being the most effective.

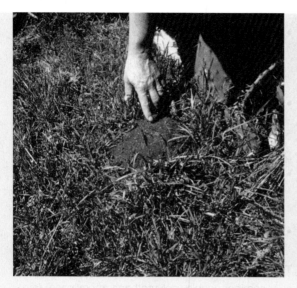

Fig. 12.10. Typical fire ant mound in Georgia. Note that fire ants do not clear the surrounding vegetation like some ant species.

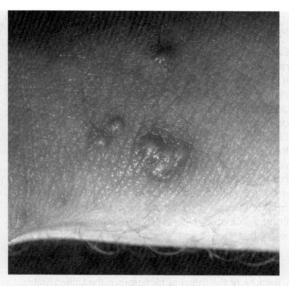

Fig. 12.11. Patient with grouped pustules on an erythematous base that are the result of fire ant stings.

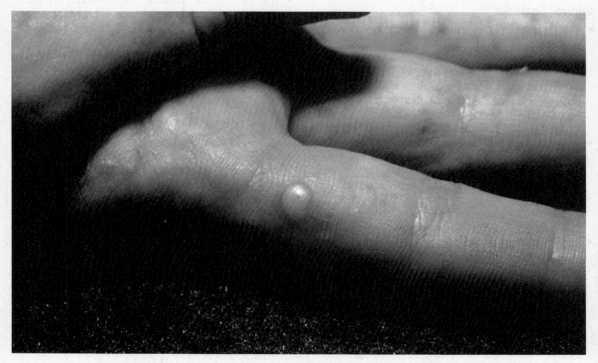

Fig. 12.12. Hand of a patient with pustular scabies. Note the linear burrow leading into the pustule. Pustular scabies does occur but is an uncommon clinical presentation.

Pathogenesis

Cutaneous vaccinia infections are the result of vaccination, which uses a live virus derived from vaccinia, a pox-type virus that is closely related to the smallpox virus. Although routine vaccination has been abandoned, it is still practiced in the military and, to a lesser degree, in civilian and public health care workers. In 2003, about 500,000 individuals were vaccinated in the United States. In more recent years, the use of vaccination has been more selective; however, the number of individuals being vaccinated has not been reported. Although most cases occur because of vaccination, in some cases the virus can be transmitted from vaccinated individuals by direct close contact with other individuals (e.g., between spouses).

Did You Know?

Because of the threat of bioterrorism the United States, the federal government maintains a large enough stockpile of vaccinia to vaccinate everyone in the United States!

Clinical Features

- The vaccination site itself will eventuate into one or more pustules at the site of the introduction of the vaccine (Fig. 12.13). The site usually becomes erythematous within the first 4 days and then rapidly develops a cloudy vesicle, which becomes pustular. Because the vaccination is done with a two-pronged needle that breaks the skin several times, one or more pustules maybe present.
- An autoinoculation vaccination reaction is a second pattern that is perhaps the most common cutaneous complication. It is caused by the patient's touching the vaccination site and spreading it to other sites of her or his body (Figs. 12.14 and 12.15). This reaction pattern usually occurs around thin skin, such as the eye, nose, and genitalia.
- Localized vaccinia infection can spread to others by direct contact. This usually involves a spouse, child, or sexual partner.

- Progressive vaccinia (vaccinia necrosum), as the name implies, consists of progressive localized extension of the vaccinia that does not heal spontaneously. This is most common in immunocompromised individuals.
- Eczema vaccinatum usually occurs in patients with active or quiescent atopic dermatitis. It occurs in about 1 in every 26,000 primary vaccinations.

Diagnosis

- In most cases, the history of a recent smallpox vaccination, associated with one of the patterns described, is sufficient to establish a presumptive diagnosis.
- Rare cases may require a biopsy that, although not diagnostic, will be supportive of the diagnosis.

Treatment

- A semipermeable polyurethane membrane (e.g., Opsite) placed on top of a small gauze pad blocks shedding of the virus at the vaccination site and may reduce autoinoculation and spread to close contacts.
- The Centers for Disease Control and Prevention (CDC) has recommended 0.6 mL/kg of intramuscular vaccinia immune globulin (VIG), divided into multiple doses over several days for severe cases.
- Cidofovir demonstrates in vitro activity against variola and vaccinia and, in theory, could be useful, although there have been no clinical studies to support its routine use.

Clinical Course

Mild autoinoculation infections and localized vaccinia infections are self-limited and will heal without therapy. Patients who are immunocompromised or have eczema vaccinatum have about a 1% to 6% risk of a fatal outcome. All patients presenting with one of these two patterns should be hospitalized for treatment and observation.

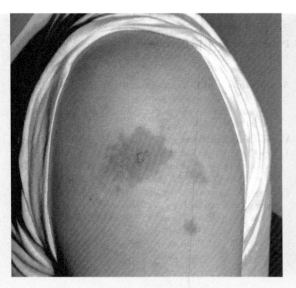

Fig. 12.13. Patient with exuberant erythematous vaccination reaction surrounding several small pustules. Remember that this is an active infection.

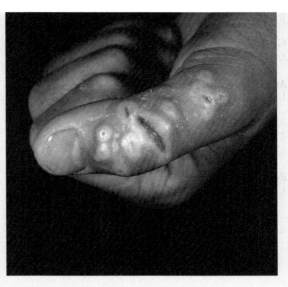

Fig. 12.14. Autoinoculation of vaccinia from a vaccination site to the thumb. (From the Fitzsimons Army Medical Center Collection, Aurora, CO.)

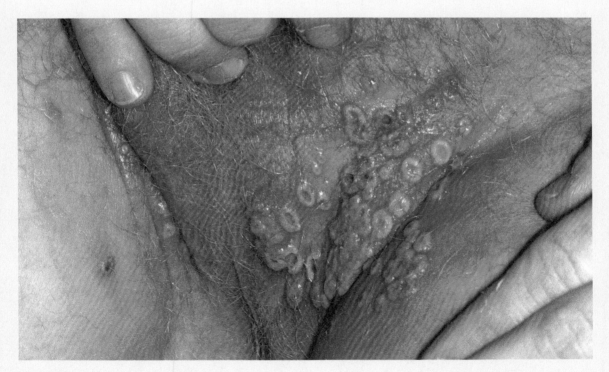

Fig. 12.15. Extensive autoinoculation of vaccinia virus into the groin area of a young soldier presenting as numerous small annular pustules. (From the Fitzsimons Army Medical Center Collection, Aurora, CO.)

References

General

1. Menqesha YM, Bennett ML. Pustular skin disorders: diagnosis and management. *Am J Clin Dermatol.* 2002;3:389-400.

Acute Generalized Exanthematous Pustulosis

1. Hammerbeck AA, Daniels NH, Callen JP. Ioversol-induced acute generalized exanthematous pustulosis. A case report. *Arch Dermatol.* 2009;145:683-687.
2. Momin SB, Del Rosso JQ, Michaels B, Mobini N. Acute generalized exanthematous pustulosis: an enigmatic drug-induced reaction. *Cutis.* 2009;83:291-298.

Pustular Psoriasis

1. Lewis TG, Tuchinda C, Lim HW, Wong HK. Life-threatening pustular and erythrodermic psoriasis responding to infliximab. *J Drugs Dermatol.* 2006;5:546-548.
2. Sheu JS, Divito SJ, Enamamdram M, Merola JF. Dapsone therapy for pustular psoriasis: case series and review of the literature. *Dermatology.* 2016;232:97-101.

Pustular Arthropod Reactions

1. Burroughs R, Elston DM. What's eating you? Fire ants. *Cutis.* 2005;75:85-89.

Acropustulosis of Infancy (Infantile Acropustulosis)

1. Kimura M, Higuchi T, Yoshida M. Infantile acropustulosis treated successfully with topical maxacalcitol. *Acta Derm Venereol.* 2011;91:363-364.

Vaccination Reactions

1. Beachkofsky TM, Carrizales SC, Bidinger JJ, et al. Adverse events following smallpox vaccination with ACAM200 in a military population. *Arch Dermatol.* 2010;146:656-661.
2. Lewis FS, Norton SA, Bradshaw RD, et al. Analysis of cases reported as generalized vaccinia during the US military smallpox vaccination program, December 2002 to December 2004. *J Am Acad Dermatol.* 2006;55:23-31.
3. Spuls PI, Bos JD, Rudikoff D. Smallpox: what the dermatologist should know. *Skinmed.* 2004;3:197-208.

Key Terms

Community-Acquired Methicillin-
  Resistant *Staphylococcus aureus*
  Carbuncle
  Furuncle

Dissecting Cellulitis of the Scalp
  Hoffman disease
  Perifolliculitis capitis abscedens et
    suffodiens

Select Abscesses
- Carbuncle
- Dissecting cellulitis of the scalp
- Furuncle
- Hidradenitis suppurativa
- Kerion
- Mycobacterial furunculosis
- Ruptured epidermoid cyst
- Tungiasis

An abscess results from a neutrophilic host response to something perceived by the immune system to be foreign. As such, abscesses may result from endogenous material, such as keratin from a ruptured follicle or cyst, exogenous foreign material (e.g., injected drugs, suture material), or infectious organisms (e.g., bacteria, fungus, protozoa).

IMPORTANT HISTORY QUESTIONS

How long has the abscess(es) been present?

An abscess may result from an acute event (e.g., ruptured epidermoid cyst), whereas other abscesses may be recurrent (e.g., recurrent furunculosis), or even chronic in nature (e.g., hidradenitis suppurativa).

Do you have any underlying medical conditions?

Immunocompromised patients (e.g., those with HIV infection) are more likely to develop abscesses due to infections. Other conditions, such as end-stage renal disease, and visitation to dialysis centers are associated with methicillin-resistant *Staphylococcus aureus* (MRSA).

Have you recently traveled outside of the country?

This question is a hunt for so-called zebras that might be causing the abscesses (e.g., tropical parasites—myiasis, tungiasis) but also a quick survey for risk factors associated with more germane processes. For example, simply being a traveler, or even being in contact with travelers, is a risk factor for MRSA.

Are you currently taking antibiotics?

In a patient taking an antibiotic, when the condition has not responded or is progressive, there should be prompt consideration of culture and susceptibility studies, a switch in antibiotics, or even reassessment about whether the process was truly infectious in the first place.

Does anyone else in the family have similar lesions?

An affirmative response could indicate an infectious cause—multiple family members with methicillin-sensitive *S. aureus* (MSSA) or MRSA—or could suggest a common exposure among family members (e.g., myiasis, tungiasis).

IMPORTANT PHYSICAL FINDINGS

Is the abscess solitary or multiple?

This is an important physical finding because some conditions are more likely to yield singular abscesses (e.g., ruptured epidermoid cyst), whereas other conditions are more likely to yield multiple abscesses (e.g., hidradenitis suppurativa, recurrent furunculosis).

What is the distribution of the abscesses?

Some abscesses have characteristic distributions. For example, hidradenitis suppurativa occurs in the axillary and groin folds, and dissecting cellulitis occurs on the scalp. Moreover, some infectious processes occur in characteristic locations. Gram-negative bacterial abscesses are more likely to occur in the anogenital region, whereas organisms introduced from the environment (e.g., tungiasis, deep fungal infections) are more likely to occur at acral sites because traumatic inoculation is usually the source of the infection.

Does the abscess demonstrate significant associated erythema or edema?

The presence of erythema, particularly with edema, could indicate an inflammatory host response to the inciting agent but also raises concern for secondary cellulitis, which may affect treatment.

Is the patient febrile?

The presence of fever may implicate an infection. Furthermore, a significant or marked fever could alter management, necessitate use of empiric antibiotics, or even require admitting the patient to the hospital.

Community-Acquired Methicillin-Resistant *Staphylococcus aureus*

Community-acquired MRSA (CA-MRSA) may present with abscesses, abscesses with cellulitis, or as cellulitis alone. Management of CA-MRSA infections is not standardized, but a reasonable approach is as follows.

Healthy Patient With Abscess, With or Without Cellulitis
- Carry out incision and drainage.
- Culture for organism and sensitivity.
- Institute empiric antibiotic therapy (e.g., cephalexin, cefdinir, dicloxacillin, amoxicillin-clavulanate).
- Change to appropriate drug based on culture and sensitivity results.

Unhealthy Patient, High Index of Suspicion for CA-MRSA, and Abscess With or Without Cellulitis, or High-Endemicity Area
- Carry out incision and drainage.
- Culture for organism and sensitivity.
- Institute empiric antibiotic therapy with trimethoprim-sulfamethoxazole ± rifampin, minocycline-doxycycline ± rifampin, or clindamycin ± rifampin.
- Change to appropriate drug based on culture and sensitivity results.

Severe Infection With High Index of Suspicion for CA-MRSA
- Carry out incision and drainage.
- Culture for organism and sensitivity.
- Treat initially with intravenous vancomycin.
- Change to appropriate drug based on culture and sensitivity results.

Pathogenesis

Furuncles (boils) represent a follicle-situated infection caused by lipase-producing strains of *S. aureus* that break down lipids derived from the sebaceous glands.

Strains of CA-MRSA are increasingly prevalent, and CA-MRSA is more likely to present as a furuncle with surrounding cellulitis. Less often, furunculosis is caused by other bacteria, such as streptococci and gram-negative organisms.

Clinical Features
- Furunculosis may occur at any age.
- Lesions may be solitary or multiple.
- Furunculosis may occur on any hair-bearing surface.
- The primary lesion is a painful, follicle-based nodule (Fig. 13.1) that becomes a red fluctuant abscess (Fig. 13.2) that drains purulent material spontaneously or with incision and drainage (Fig. 13.3).
- Some cases demonstrate surrounding erythema and induration indicative of associated cellulitis (Fig. 13.4).
- A **carbuncle** is simply a larger lesion that is caused by the confluence of adjacent infected follicles.

Diagnosis
- A presumptive diagnosis is made based on clinical findings, as supported by results of a Gram stain.
- The diagnosis is more fully established based on the results of culture and sensitivity studies of purulent debris and/or the anterior nasal vestibule.

Treatment
- Incision and drainage of singular abscesses is most often adequate therapy, even for CA-MRSA strains.
- Initial antibiotic therapy is based on the clinical situation (see box) but often includes cephalexin, dicloxacillin, and/or amoxicillin-clavulanate.

Clinical Course

Most cases of furunculosis are self-limited and will resolve, perhaps with some scarring or dyspigmentation. About 10% to 20% of patients will develop recurrent furunculosis.

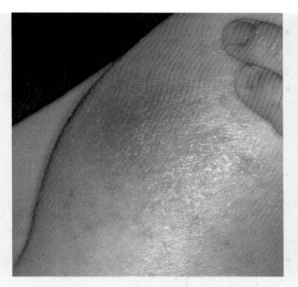

Fig. 13.1. Patient with an early furuncle presenting as a tender erythematous nodule that is not yet fluctuant. (From the William Weston Collection, Aurora, CO.)

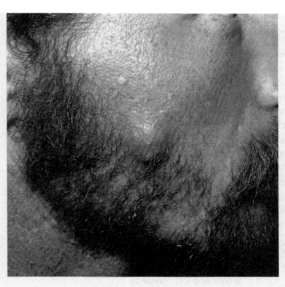

Fig. 13.2. Patient with a developed fluctuant furuncle that has started to point as a pustule on the central hair follicle.

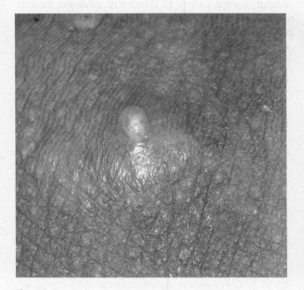

Fig. 13.3. Patient with an older furuncle that has spontaneously ruptured, demonstrating yellowish pus.

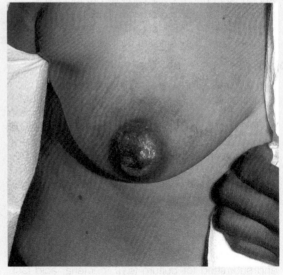

Fig. 13.4. Patient with a large furuncle of the nipple, with marked erythema, raising the possibility of CA-MRSA or cellulitis. (From the Fitzsimons Army Medical Center Collection, Aurora, CO.)

Pathogenesis

Atypical mycobacteria (AMB), including *Mycobacterium marinum*, *Mycobacterium fortuitum*, and *Mycobacterium chelonae* (Fig. 13.5) can produce boil-like lesions in the skin. These AMB are ubiquitous in nature and are often found in soil, water, and decaying organic matter. AMB can be acquired through accidental breaks in the skin, surgical procedures, and even via pedicures or water baths. Although AMB infections may present initially as one or more follicle-based lesions, the condition may progress to a sporotrichoid pattern (see Chapter 18). Many AMB species common to dermatology are so-called rapid-growing species.

Clinical Features

- AMB infections often involve acral skin but can occur anywhere on the skin.
- Early lesions present as one or more red, indurated, usually tender nodules.
- Lesions enlarge and become suppurative, often with the discharge of yellow-white pus (Figs. 13.6 to 13.8).
- Secondary changes are variable but include scale, purulent crusting, and/or ulceration.
- Some patients develop lymphocutaneous (sporotrichoid) spread or satellite abscesses (Fig. 13.9).

Diagnosis

- The clinical features of AMB infections are not singularly diagnostic. It is not uncommon for AMB infections to be managed first as staphylococcal furuncles or foreign body granulomas. It is a failed response to initial management that often triggers consideration—and correct diagnosis—of AMB infection.
- The history of a woman with one or more abscesses of the lower extremity, unresponsive to standard management, and with a history of pedicures at salons, should trigger suspicion of AMB furunculosis.
- The diagnosis is further established by a punch (at least 4 mm) or incisional biopsy that is bisected and submitted for culture (e.g., bacteria, acid-fast bacillus [AFB], fungus) and histologic examination.

- Organisms can be visualized using special AFB stains, but speciation is not possible without culture.

Treatment

- Treatment of cutaneous mycobacterial infections is not standardized. If mycobacterial organisms were detected only by special stains, oral minocycline (100 mg PO bid) is a reasonable empiric therapy while awaiting the results of culture and sensitivity testing that will further refine therapy.
- Once sensitivity is known, drugs often used in addition to minocycline include rifampin, clarithromycin, azithromycin, ciprofloxacin, and cotrimoxazole. Treatment is often continued for 2 to 4 months, and occasional unresponsive cases may require multidrug therapy.
- Physiotherapy (the purposeful warming of an area above 37°C [98.6°F]) may be used as an adjunctive intervention for some species (e.g., *M. marinum*) that are particularly temperature-sensitive.

Clinical Course

Most cases of AMB infection resolve spontaneously without therapy over 2 to 6 months, whereas treated cases respond more quickly. Rare cases, particularly in those who are immunocompromised, may result in dissemination.

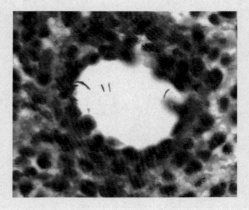

Fig. 13.5. Ziehl-Neelsen stain demonstrating *M. chelonae* from the patient depicted in Fig. 13.7 (1000×).

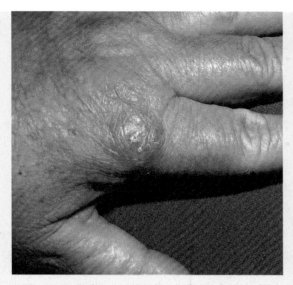

Fig. 13.6. *Mycobacterium marinum.* This abscess over the knuckle was initially thought to be a foreign body granuloma and was initially treated with intralesional triamcinolone.

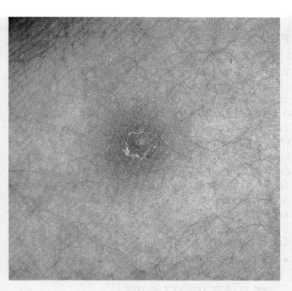

Fig. 13.7. *Mycobacterium chelonae.* This solitary abscess developed at the site of a tick bite. (From the Fitzsimons Army Medical Center Collection, Aurora, CO.)

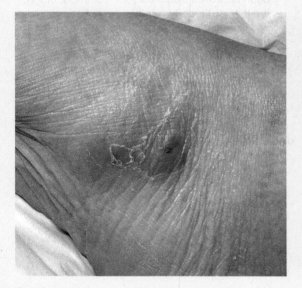

Fig. 13.8. *Mycobacterium chelonae.* There is a large abscess on the medial foot that spontaneously ruptured. (From the Fitzsimons Army Medical Center Collection, Aurora, CO.)

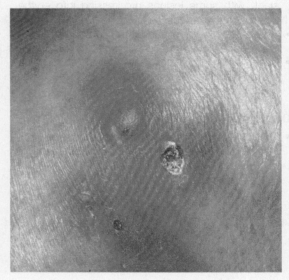

Fig. 13.9. *Mycobacterium chelonae.* This erythematous plaque on the knee was studded with multiple small abscesses and superficial ulcers. (From the Fitzsimons Army Medical Center Collection, Aurora, CO.)

Pathogenesis

Hidradenitis suppurativa (HA) is a chronic disease that involves abscesses and draining sinuses of the axillae and inguinal folds. Careful studies have demonstrated that the first causative step in HA is follicular hyperkeratosis, which occludes the apocrine glands that empty into the hair follicle. This explains why HA appears in other disorders of follicular occlusion, such as severe acne, dissecting cellulitis of the scalp, and pilonidal cyst. Although bacteria are found in some abscesses of HA, and this exaggerates the host response, studies have suggested that these are secondary events.

Clinical Features

- HA typically begins in adolescents or young adults but, due to chronicity of the disease, is frequently seen in older patients as well.
- Women may demonstrate premenstrual flaring.
- The distribution includes apocrine-rich areas such as the axillae (Fig. 13.10), inguinal folds, and inframammary and perianal regions, although isolated lesions may extend away from the apocrine areas.
- Early lesions resemble a folliculitis that may be transient, with some lesions progressing into erythematous tender abscesses (Fig. 13.11).
- Abscesses may point and rupture, gradually resolve, or produce sinus tracts and scarring (Fig. 13.12).
- Patients with HA typically have multiple attacks, ultimately resulting in confluent plaques of abscesses, sinus tracts, and cicatrix.

Diagnosis

- The clinical presentation of a postpubertal individual presenting with recurrent abscesses in apocrine-rich areas, such as the axilla and inguinal folds, is strongly suggestive of the diagnosis.
- If the process is confined to the perianal region, the differential diagnosis should be expanded to include lymphogranuloma venereum, cutaneous amebiasis, and localized extension of Crohn disease.

Treatment

- Early disease (isolated abscesses without sinus tracts or scarring)
  - Intralesional triamcinolone (2.5–5 mg/mL)
  - Topical clindamycin solution bid for 3 months
  - Oral tetracycline or minocycline
  - Consideration of oral isotretinoin because this is the stage at which it is most likely to be effective
  - Women with premenstrual flares—antiandrogen therapy with spironolactone or cyproterone acetate occasionally useful
- Established disease (abscesses, sinus tracts, and scarring)
  - Surgical extirpation or surgical unroofing of areas of sinus tracts and scarring is the treatment of choice.
  - Adalimumab, a TNF-alpha inhibitor, has now been approved specifically for treatment of HA.
  - If either of these two is not an option, consider oral isotretinoin, although the results are generally not as effective in advanced disease.
  - If these are not options, treat with the same modalities as for early disease, realizing that at best there will be only some improvement.

Clinical Course

HA is usually a chronic, unrelenting, progressive disease that typically causes scar tissue to be formed.

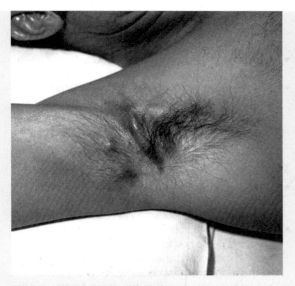

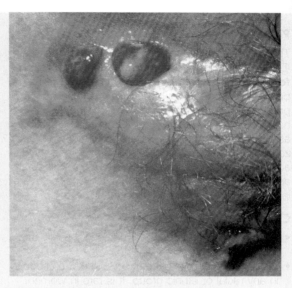

Fig. 13.10. Patient with hidradenitis suppurativa of the axilla presenting as indurated red abscesses with a large sinus tract.

Fig. 13.11. Patient with hidradenitis suppurativa of the groin presenting as a ruptured suppurative abscess that is exuding yellowish pus.

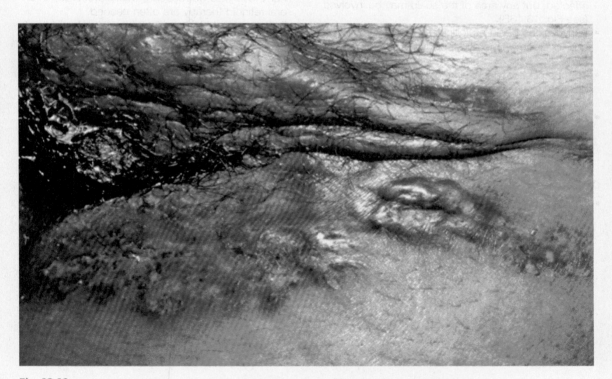

Fig. 13.12. Patient with end-stage hidradenitis suppurativa of the left inguinal fold with abscesses, sinus tracts, and scar formation. (From the Fitzsimons Army Medical Center Collection, Aurora, CO.)

Dissecting Cellulitis of the Scalp ICD10 code L66.3

Pathogenesis

The pathogenesis of dissecting cellulitis of the scalp (DCS), also known as **Hoffman disease** or **perifolliculitis capitis abscedens et suffodiens**, is poorly understood. However, it seems that the initial precipitating event is occlusive hyperkeratosis of the hair follicle. This hypothesis is supported by a strong association with other disorders of follicular keratinization, including hidradenitis suppurativa and severe acne. These diseases are often referred to collectively as the follicular occlusion triad or, if pilonidal cysts are included, the follicular occlusion tetrad.

Clinical Features

- DCS occurs in postpubertal persons, usually adolescents or young men.
- Black men are more often affected, but it can occur in any racial or ethnic group. It is rare in women.
- Other occlusive follicular disorders, such as severe acne (Fig. 13.13A), HA, and pilonidal cyst, may be present in the patient or in family members.
- The vertex and posterior scalp are most often affected, but any area of the scalp may be involved (see Fig. 13.13B).
- Early lesions begin as follicularly situated pustules, but, over time, more deeply situated abscesses form.
- The number of lesions is variable, but, as the disease progresses, sinus tracts form to drain and connect the abscesses (Fig. 13.14).
- Alopecia develops over time. In early lesions, the hairs above the abscesses are easily removed; in later lesions, scarring with permanent hair loss ensues (Fig. 13.15).

Diagnosis

- The clinical presentation of a young man with one or more deep abscesses on his scalp, and with scarring and resultant hair loss, is suspicious for DCS.
- Bacterial and fungal culture (to exclude tinea capitis/kerion) of pus should be carefully considered.
- A 4- to 6-mm punch biopsy or incisional biopsy is useful to confirm the diagnosis. In most cases, the findings will be diagnostic of or consistent with DCS. Special stains may also be used to exclude fungal infection.

Treatment

- Intralesional triamcinolone acetonide (5–10 mg/mL) injection into the abscesses provides rapid diminution of the host response, with reduction of pain.
- Tetracycline antibiotics are useful in reducing the microflora in the hair follicles and directly inhibit neutrophil migration. The senior author (JEF) has had the most anecdotal success with minocycline.
- Oral isotretinoin, dosed in the same fashion as for acne, is effective when used early in the course of the disease but is less effective once extensive scarring and sinus tract formation have occurred. For those who do respond, multiple courses of an oral retinoid therapy are often needed.
- Tumor necrosis factor-α inhibitors have been used, with anecdotal success.
- For patients with severe and/or intractable disease, therapeutic options include surgical drainage of individual abscesses (with only a temporary respite), surgical removal of scar and sinus tracts (requires general surgery in most cases), and radiation therapy at an epilating dose.

Clinical Course

DCS is typically a chronic, unrelenting progressive disease that usually results in scar tissue and permanent alopecia.

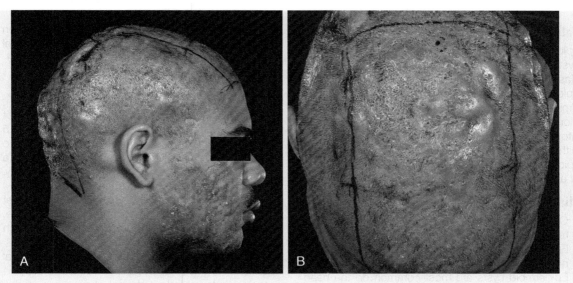

Fig. 13.13 A, Patient with severe dissecting cellulitis of the scalp associated with acne conglobata. B, Close-up demonstrating alopecia, abscesses, and sinus tracts. (From the Fitzsimons Army Medical Center Collection, Aurora, CO.)

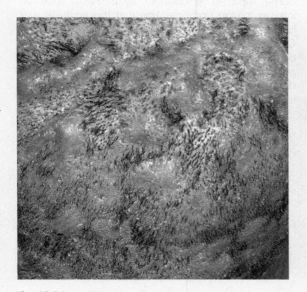

Fig. 13.14. Patient with dissecting cellulitis of the scalp with alopecia, abscesses, scars, and an unusually large sinus tract at the top.

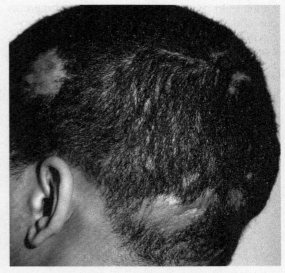

Fig. 13.15. Patient with residual scar and alopecia from dissecting cellulitis treated with oral isotretinoin. (From the Fitzsimons Army Medical Center Collection, Aurora, CO.)

Ruptured Epidermoid Cyst ICD10 code L72.0

Pathogenesis

Epidermoid cysts (also known as epidermal inclusion cysts or sebaceous cysts) are common benign neoplasms that arise from the upper third of the hair follicle. Epidermoid cysts demonstrate a thin epithelial lining, similar to the normal epidermis, which ruptures easily. Moreover, rupture of the cyst, with release of keratin into the dermis, produces a foreign body reaction, with vigorous inflammation. Because of their ubiquity, epidermoid cysts are easily the most common cause of a cutaneous abscess.

Clinical Features

- Often, there is history of a long-standing cyst that rapidly enlarges and becomes painful.
- Epidermoid cysts can occur in areas of previous nodulocystic acne.
- Epidermoid cysts are most common on the head and neck, followed by the trunk.
- The primary lesion is a tender cystic structure, often inflamed or suppurative (Fig. 13.16A), perhaps with surface changes, such as erosion, ulceration, hemorrhage, or discharge of pus.
- An inflamed cyst usually contains an admixture of pus and foul-smelling keratin. Less often, hemorrhage may be present, especially if the patient has manipulated the cyst (see Fig. 13.16B).

Diagnosis

- The clinical presentation of a long-standing cyst that suddenly changes color and/or becomes spontaneously painful is usually sufficient for diagnosis.

- In problematic cases, the most fluctuant portion of the lesion can be incised with a no. 11 scalpel blade; the discharge of white, foul-smelling, keratinous debris establishes the diagnosis.

Treatment

- If the cyst is not suppurative, and hence is not yet ready to be drained, initial therapy may be 2.5 to 5.0 mg of intralesional triamcinolone simply to reduce inflammation. In general, it is safer to use a lower dose of steroids on the face to avoid atrophy. In some cases, this will be adequate therapy.
- Lesions that are clearly suppurative are best managed with incision using a no. 11 scalpel blade, followed by gentle compression to remove as much pus and keratin as possible.
- Although there is a compulsion to treat with oral antibiotics, there has been no evidence to support their use for standard dermal abscesses, smaller than 5 cm, without complex loculations.

Clinical Course

Some ruptured epidermoid cysts have such an intense foreign body reaction that the epithelial wall is destroyed, and no additional therapy is required. Other cysts will persist, in whole or in part, and can be excised after the inflammation has subsided. Surgical removal of cysts that have scarred down is more difficult than the surgical removal of epidermoid cysts that have never been inflamed.

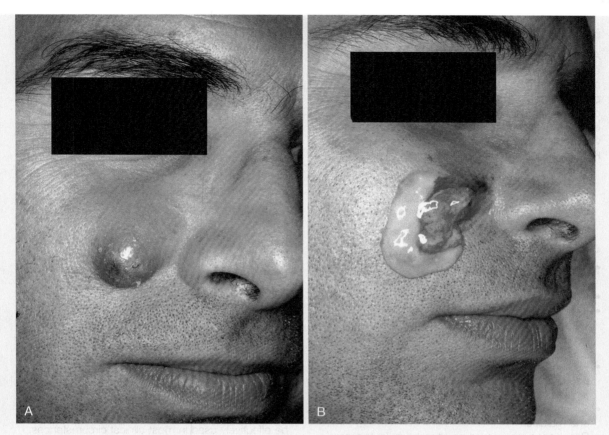

Fig. 13.16 A, B, Typical suppurative ruptured epidermoid cyst of the right cheek of a patient who reported that a small cyst had suddenly enlarged and became painful. The lesion was incised with a no. 11 scalpel blade, revealing contents consisting of an admixture of pus, keratin, and blood. After drainage of the contents, the patient was treated with intralesional triamcinolone, 2.5 mg/mL. The cyst wall was destroyed by the inflammatory host response, and surgical removal was not required. (From the Fitzsimons Army Medical Center Collection, Aurora, CO.)

Pathogenesis

A kerion is a subtype of tinea capitis in which the dermatophyte causes significant inflammation and abscess formation on the scalp. Just like other forms of tinea capitis, most kerions occur in prepubertal children, with peak incidence between 2 and 9 years of age. Most kerions are caused by *Trichophyton* spp., with some cases being caused by *Microsporum* spp. Kerions are often confused with bacterial infections.

Clinical Rule
An abscess and/or pyoderma of the scalp of a prepubertal child is a kerion until proven otherwise!

Clinical Features

- Most kerions affect children between 2 and 9 years of age.
- Kerions can be solitary or multiple.
- Kerions present on the scalp as abscesses with vigorous inflammation and erythema and may be associated with pustular folliculitis, scale, erosions, and/or yellowish scale or crust (Figs. 13.17–13.20).
- Regional lymphadenopathy is often present in the posterior cervical triangle or posterior auricular region.
- Severe cases may be associated with high fevers and malaise.
- Rare cases may cause an id reaction (autoeczematization) of the head and neck area.

Diagnosis

- The clinical presentation of a prepubertal child with one or more deep abscesses on the scalp, with hair loss, is concerning for a kerion. All too frequently, a kerion may be confused with a bacterial abscess and treated with oral antibiotics or, worse, with incision and drainage.

- Broken hairs can be plucked and examined with potassium hydroxide (KOH) for hyphae and spores on or within hair shafts.
- Broken hairs can be plucked and cultured for fungus, or the pus may be cultured for bacteria, but it must be remembered that superinfection with *S. aureus* is not uncommon.
- A 4-mm or larger punch biopsy or incisional biopsy is useful to confirm the diagnosis. In some cases, the histologic findings will be diagnostic (the organisms can be visualized), whereas in other cases, the findings will merely suggest a possible kerion. The biopsy should be bisected, with half sent for fungal culture.

Treatment

- Griseofulvin (microsized, 20–25 mg/kg per day; ultramicrosized, 15 mg/kg per day) for 6 to 8 weeks is the treatment regimen used most often in children; it is widely available as a pediatric suspension.
- Alternatives include terbinafine (3–6 mg/kg per day) for 2 to 4 weeks, itraconazole (3–5 mg/kg per day) for 4 to 6 weeks, or fluconazole (3–6 mg/kg per day) for 6 weeks.
- It has been suggested that terbinafine may be more effective (but more costly) against *Trichophyton* species, while griseofulvin may be more effective against *Microsporum* spp. but at present either may be effectively used in most clinical circumstances.

Clinical Course

In patients with a kerion, about 50% will recover normal hair density on resolution. About 25% will demonstrate focal hair loss that is cosmetically acceptable, and about 25% will demonstrate a cosmetically significant degree of permanent hair loss due to the inflammation.

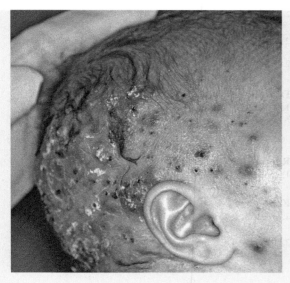

Fig. 13.17. Kerion. This 2-month-old infant had alopecia, pustules, scales, and crusts and multiple small abscesses. (From the Joanna Burch Collection, Aurora, CO.)

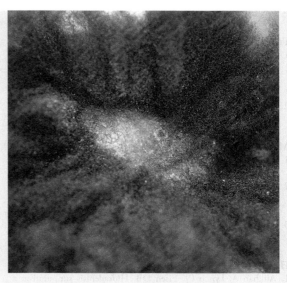

Fig. 13.18. Patient with kerion presenting on the vertex of the scalp as a solitary boggy abscess with alopecia. Also note the associated scale. (From the William Weston Collection, Aurora, CO.)

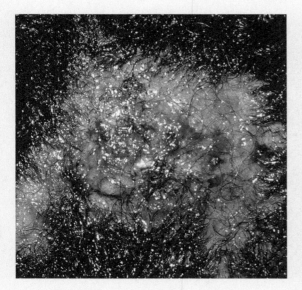

Fig. 13.19. Patient with kerion presenting as a large abscess with alopecia, with marked overlying postulation and crust.

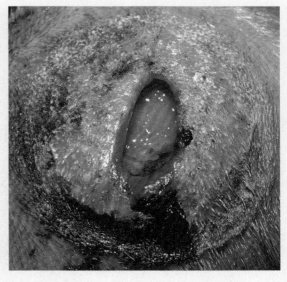

Fig. 13.20. Patient with kerion that was mistakenly thought to be a bacterial abscess and was treated with incision and drainage. (From the William Weston Collection, Aurora, CO.)

References

Furunculosis

1. Cohen PR. Community-acquired methicillin-resistant *Staphylococcus aureus* skin infections: a review of epidemiology, clinical features, management, and prevention. *Int J Dermatol*. 2007;46:1-11.
2. Ibler KA, Kromann CB. Recurrent furunculosis—challenges and management: a review. *Clin Cosmet Invest Dermatol*. 2014;7: 59-64.

Mycobacterial Furunculosis

1. Corboy JE, Sarkar D, Goins WP. Persistent skin furuncle. *Am Fam Physician*. 2013;88:331-332.
2. Dodiuk-Gad R, Dyachenko P, Ziv M, et al. Nontuberculous mycobacterial infections of the skin: a retrospective study of 25 cases. *J Am Acad Dermatol*. 2007;57:413-420.
3. Redbord KP, Shearer DA, Gloster H, et al. Atypical *Mycobacterial* furunculosis occurring after pedicures. *J Am Acad Dermatol*. 2006;54:520-524.

Hidradenitis Suppurativa

1. Alikhan A, Lynch PJ, Eisen DB. Hidradenitis suppurativa: a comprehensive review. *J Am Acad Dermatol*. 2009;60:239-261.

2. Grant A, Gonzalez T, Montgomery MO, et al. Infliximab therapy for patients with moderate to severe hidradenitis suppurativa: a randomized, double-blind, placebo-controlled crossover trial. *J Am Acad Dermatol*. 2010;62:205-217.

Dissecting Cellulitis of the Scalp

1. Mansouri Y, Martin-Clavijo A, Nesome P, Kaur MR. Dissecting cellulitis of the scalp treated with tumour necrosis factor-α inhibitors: experience with two agents. *Br J Dermatol*. 2016;174:916-918.

Ruptured Epidermoid Cyst

1. Zuber TJ. Minimal excision technique for epidermoid (sebaceous) cysts. *Am Fam Physician*. 2002;65:1409-1412.

Kerion

1. Feetham JE, Sargant N. Kerion celsi: a misdiagnosed scalp infection. *Arch Dis Child*. 2016;101:503.
2. LaSenna CE, Miteva M, Tosti A. Pitfalls in the diagnosis of kerion. *J Eur Acad Dermatol*. 2016;30:515-517.

Chapter 14

Necrotic and ulcerative disorders encompass a wide variety of disease, ranging from infections to autoimmune to vascular conditions. There are many diseases that can present with ulcers, but this chapter discusses only those conditions that present principally, or exclusively, as necrotic lesions or ulcerations.

Necrotic and Ulcerative Lesions: Differential Diagnosis
- Anthrax
- Arterial ulcers
- Calciphylaxis
- Factitial ulcers
- Livedoid vasculopathy
- Necrotic arachnidism (spider bite)
- Necrotizing fasciitis
- Pyoderma gangrenosum
- Stasis ulcers

Sexually Transmitted Ulcers
- Chancroid
- Granuloma inguinale
- Herpes progenitalis
- Primary syphilis

IMPORTANT HISTORY QUESTIONS

How long has the condition been present?

Infections, whether localized (e.g., chancroid, necrotizing fasciitis) or systemic (e.g., ecthyma gangrenosum), necrotic arachnidism (spider bites) tend to have an abrupt onset, whereas some disorders, such as vascular disorders (e.g., stasis ulcers), tend to have a gradual onset.

Do you have any underlying systemic disorders?

Always investigate any predisposing condition. For example, inflammatory bowel disease, rheumatoid arthritis, and lymphoproliferative conditions may be associated with pyoderma gangrenosum. Diabetes mellitus may predispose someone to necrotizing fasciitis, whereas renal disease is a predisposition for calciphylaxis. The use of chemotherapy may predispose an individual to ecthyma gangrenosum.

Is there any history of a clotting disorder?

Some ulcerative conditions are associated with clotting disorders (e.g., stasis ulcers), whereas others are associated with livedoid vasculopathy.

When was your last sexual contact, and did you use a barrier device?

This question is usually reserved for someone with genital ulcers, but it is important in that setting.

Have you had exposure to animals?

This is important in rare cases of anthrax, in addition to milker's nodules (cows) and orf (sheep).

IMPORTANT PHYSICAL FINDINGS

What is the distribution of the lesions?

Some ulcerating conditions involve certain areas. For example, sexually transmitted diseases usually affect the genitalia, whereas vascular disorders usually affect the lower extremities. Many infectious causes of ulcers, such as orf or milker's nodules, involve the hands.

How many lesions are present?

Some ulcers are solitary (e.g., syphilis, necrotizing fasciitis, brown recluse spider bite), whereas other ulcers are multiple (e.g., chancroid, pyoderma gangrenosum, ecthyma gangrenosum).

What is the shape of the ulcer?

Some ulcers are round or oval, with a clean base and sharp circumscription (e.g., syphilis chancre), whereas others often demonstrate ragged edges (e.g., chancroid).

How deep does the ulceration extend?

Some ulcers are superficial (e.g., syphilis, herpes progenitalis), whereas others extend into muscle, tendon, or even bone (e.g., pyoderma gangrenosum, calciphylaxis).

What does the base of the ulcer look like?

The base of some ulcers often resembles granulation tissue (e.g., granuloma inguinale), whereas others are usually quite purulent (e.g., chancroid, pyoderma gangrenosum).

Are the peripheral pulses normal and equal in patients with lower extremity ulcers?

Circulatory abnormalities are important to document when considering arterial insufficiency.

Pathogenesis

Necrotizing fasciitis is a life-threatening infection of the skin that involves the deep subcutis and superficial investing fascia. Fournier gangrene represents necrotizing fasciitis of the genitalia and perineum. The current trend is to refer to these conditions, in general, as necrotizing soft tissue infections (NSTIs). Although laypersons may refer to the condition as "flesh-eating Strep," and some cases are due to Streptococcal spp. and/or a single organism, most cases are polymicrobial in nature. Cases of necrotizing fasciitis have been attributed to a number of organisms, including *Streptococcus pyogenes, Staphylococcus aureus, Bacteroides fragilis,* and *Clostridium, Haemophilus, Vibrio,* and *Prevotella* spp. Other rare bacteria and even fungi may be involved in some cases of necrotizing fasciitis.

Clinical Features

- NSTIs occurs in adults and children, with both genders equally affected.
- Patients may be otherwise healthy, but risk factors for NSTIs include diabetes mellitus (≈50% of cases), obesity, alcoholism, intravenous (IV) drug abuse, and recent history of prior surgery.
- Patients with NSTIs may report a history of trauma (or surgery) at that site, or they may have another infection that serves as the source of the bacteria (e.g., odontogenic abscess, remote skin abscesses).
- The primary lesion begins as a painful area that looks much like routine cellulitis (Figs. 14.1 to 14.3). The most common sites are the extremities, followed by the trunk and perineum. The pain is often described as being out of proportion to the clinical findings.
- More developed lesions may manifest with dusky skin hues, hemorrhagic blisters, hemorrhagic necrosis, and ulceration. Crepitus or focal abscess formation may be present with some species.

Diagnosis

- An incision or excision biopsy is preferred that should include a generous amount of subcutaneous fat or soft tissue. A punch biopsy might be useful if done deeply, depending on the clinical circumstances.

- Half of the specimen should be sent for bacterial (aerobic and anaerobic) and fungal cultures.
- The other half of the specimen can be used for a touch prep with Gram staining if there are facilities and knowledge available for this technique. Typically, there are numerous bacteria; this will provide an immediate indication of the infectious organism(s) likely present.
- After doing a touch prep with Gram staining, the rest of the specimen should be submitted for a tradition histopathologic examination and be expedited as much as possible.

- Particularly if there is crepitus, consider soft tissue x-rays to see if a gas-forming organism is present (e.g., *Clostridium*).
- Blood cultures should be performed before initiating antibiotics.
- Minimum laboratory studies should include a complete blood count (CBC), chemistry panel—electrolytes, liver function studies, renal function studies—and urinalysis.

Treatment

- Start IV antibiotics in the emergency room (or in any other setting in which this is possible). Always admit the patient to the hospital because NSTIs are an emergency (flesh-eating bacteria).
- Consult an infectious disease specialist to recommend an empiric antibiotic regimen. If such a consultation is not possible, agents such as ticarcillin-clavulanate, piperacillin-tazobactam, imipenem, or meropenem may be used. IV vancomycin should be added if methicillin-resistant *Staphylococcus aureus* (MRSA) is a concern.
- Immediately call a surgeon because prompt surgical débridement is the treatment of choice. Impress on him or her that this life-threatening situation and time is of the essence.

Clinical Course

In a retrospective study at a major medical center, the mortality rate approached 50% and morbidity was substantial.

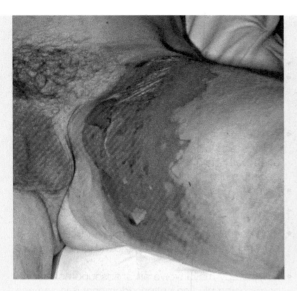

Fig. 14.1. Diabetic patient with *Streptococcus*-induced necrotizing fasciitis, with epidermal necrosis and hemorrhage. (From the Fitzsimons Army Medical Center Collection, Aurora, CO.)

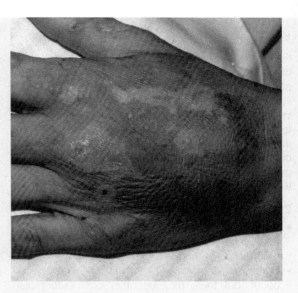

Fig. 14.2. Patient with early necrotizing fasciitis with crepitus due to *Bacteroides* species. (From the Fitzsimons Army Medical Center Collection, Aurora, CO.)

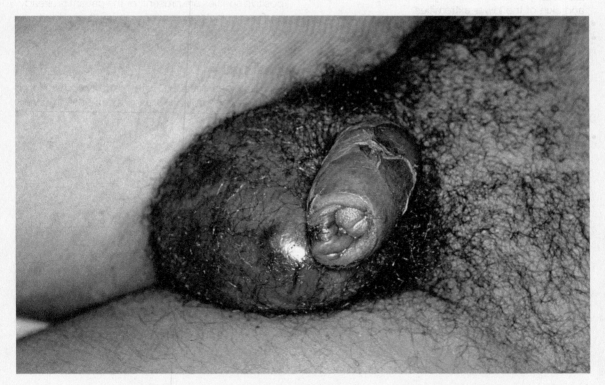

Fig. 14.3. Patient with necrotizing fasciitis of genitalia—Fournier gangrene caused by *Escherichia coli*. (From the Fitzsimons Army Medical Center Collection, Aurora, CO.)

Pathogenesis

Ecthyma gangrenosum (EG) is an infection consisting of sepsis and localized skin necrosis, with the latter at one or more sites. Classic forms of the disease involve neutropenic patients, with the most frequently implicated bacteria being *Pseudomonas aeruginosa,* followed by *Serratia, Escherichia coli, Klebsiella pneumoniae,* and other gram-negative organisms. Some cases of EG are polymicrobial and, in addition to gram-negative bacteria, another gram-positive bacteria may also be involved in the infection.

Pathogenesis

- Patients with EG are usually neutropenic, with the total white blood cell count usually less than 250 cells/mcL.
- Rarely, patients have a normal white blood cell count, but there may be other contributory diseases (e.g., HIV infection, hypogammaglobinemia, lymphoma).
- Signs and symptoms of a systemic infection, including fever, malaise, lassitude, are often present.
- EG usually affects the axillary skin, anogenital skin, and skin of the lower extremities.
- Single or multiple lesions may be present,
- Primary lesions are edematous red macules or patches that rapidly progress to hemorrhagic bullae (Fig. 14.4). Mature lesions demonstrate an eschar (Fig. 14.5) or ulcer (Fig. 14.6), with a rim of erythema.

Diagnosis

- An acute onset of erythematous macules or patches, later with ulceration and hemorrhage, in a patient with neutropenia or another form of immunosuppression, should raise suspicion of EG.
- A CBC to determine neutropenia is always indicated.
- Gram staining of an aspirate or touch prep will demonstrate numerous bacteria (Fig. 14.7) and provide information as to whether this is a gram-positive, gram-negative, or polymicrobial infection.
- A 3- or 4-mm punch biopsy is characteristic, with millions and billions of bacteria typically identified, often with little or no inflammation because the patient is usually neutropenic.
- Culture blood, aspirate, and biopsy material.

Treatment

- Monotherapy is usually with a antipseudomonal antibiotic, such as ceftazidime, imipenem, or cefepime.
- Polytherapy may involve an antipseudomonal aminoglycoside plus an antipseudomonal β-lactamase penicillin (e.g., piperacillin) or ticarcillin-clavulanate potassium.
- If an infected catheter is suspected, there are chemotherapy-induced oral ulcers, known gram-positive species are present, or the patient is already on fluoroquinolone, vancomycin is often added.
- Correction of the neutropenia or another cause of immunosuppression is useful, if possible.

Clinical Course

EG is a serious infection, with mortality rates in the literature of over 30% and as high as 90% in some series.

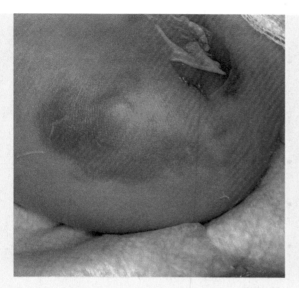

Fig. 14.4. Patient with early ecthyma gangrenosum showing necrosis and hemorrhage. (From the Fitzsimons Army Medical Center Collection, Aurora, CO.)

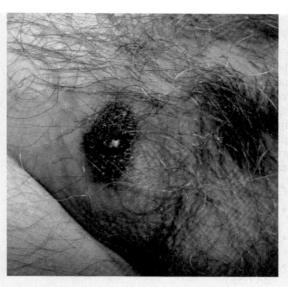

Fig. 14.5. Patient with ecthyma gangrenosum, with black eschar and rim of erythema. (From the Fitzsimons Army Medical Center Collection, Aurora, CO.)

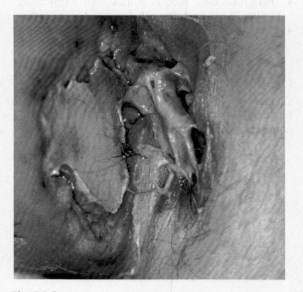

Fig. 14.6. Patient with polymicrobial ulcerated ecthyma gangrenosum. (From the Fitzsimons Army Medical Center Collection, Aurora, CO.)

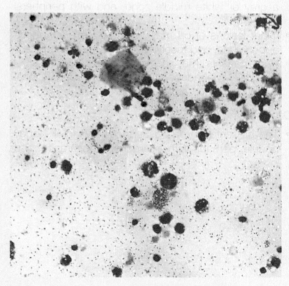

Fig. 14.7. Touch prep from ecthyma gangrenosum showing numerous very short rods of *Serratia marcescens* (Gram stain: 400×).

Orf ICD10 code B08.02

Pathogenesis

Orf is an uncommon viral infection (*Parapoxvirus,* from the family Poxviridae) of the skin that is usually acquired from direct contact with goats or sheep or with fomites in a farm or ranch environment (e.g., fencing, digging in infected soil). Rarely, the infection may also be acquired from deer, musk ox, camel, or pronghorn antelope. A similar but less common viral infection, called milker's nodule, can be acquired from cattle.

Clinical Features

- Orf is acquired through minute breaks in skin and begins 3 to 7 days after inoculation.
- Orf usually occurs on acral skin, but any site may be involved.
- Orf lesions are usually solitary, but multiple lesions can occur.
- Early orf creates round to oval erythematous lesions, with a maculopapular appearance.
- Fully developed orf consists of round to oval boggy nodules, with a targetoid appearance (Figs. 14.8 to 14.10). The center is typically eroded and red, with a gray or white middle zone, and with peripheral erythema.
- Older lesions of orf may demonstrate a verrucous appearance, and resolving lesions may be crusted.
- Rare patients may demonstrate lymphangitis or regional lymphadenopathy, or even constitutional symptoms, such as fever, malaise, and chills.

Diagnosis

- The presentation of a usually solitary, acral, boggy nodule, perhaps with a targetoid appearance, and in a patient with exposure to farm animals or in an agricultural setting, suggests the diagnosis of orf.
- A history of direct contact with sheep, goats, or other more exotic animals or exposure to agricultural settings should be carefully sought because it is thought that the virus may remain dormant for years in soil, wood, or on fomites in an agricultural setting. If there is a history of exposure to cows, then milker's nodule should be suspected.
- A punch or small excision biopsy is usually fairly diagnostic, although it may be difficult to differentiate from a closely related virus (milker's nodule).
- In rare cases, specimens can be submitted for electron microscopy, which is a more specific test. However, this is expensive and rarely done.
- Viral culture, complement fixation tests, and immunofluorescent tests are available in research laboratories but are not typically done in routine clinical settings.

Treatment

- No treatment is required because this is a self-limited viral infection.
- There have been reports of treatment via excision, but this is not recommended.
- Topical idoxuridine or topical cidofovir may accelerate healing, although the reports are anecdotal, and controlled randomized trials have not been done.

Clinical Course

Orf is a benign, self-limited disorder that heals without treatment over 4 to 6 weeks. Rare cases result in permanent scarring.

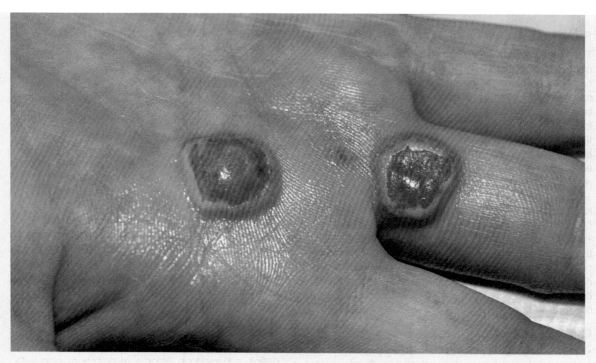

Fig. 14.8. Two superficially ulcerated nodules typical of orf. This was acquired from digging in the backyard of the patient's home in Colorado that had been built on the site of an old sheep ranch. It is important to realize that the virus can remain dormant in the soil and on fomites for decades.

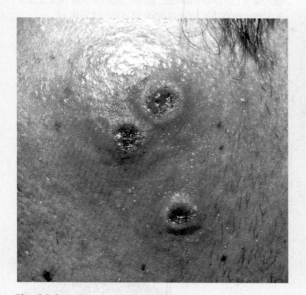

Fig. 14.9. Three ulcerated nodules on the left cheek of a young man from Texas. The source of the infection was never identified. (From the Fitzsimons Army Medical Center Collection, Aurora, CO.)

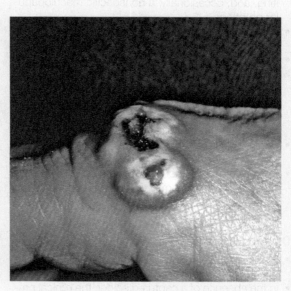

Fig. 14.10. Patient with large linear ulcerated lesion on the dorsum of the hand. The lesion was acquired in Colorado, with no known source. (From the Fitzsimons Army Medical Center Collection, Aurora, CO.)

Pathogenesis

The true prevalence of spider bites is unknown, but about 10,000 spider bites are reported to poison control centers in the United States each year. *Necrotic arachnidism* is the term used for all necrotic spider bites. *Loxoscelism* is a term reserved for reactions to bites of the brown recluse spider and members of that same genus (Fig. 14.11). Brown recluse spiders are normally found outdoors—under rocks, cliffs, and areas that afford protection—but this spider readily adapts to indoor habitats as well. There are 13 species of *Loxosceles*, with 5 causing cutaneous loxoscelism (*Loxosceles reclusa*, *Loxosceles deserta*, *Loxosceles arizonica*, *Loxosceles laeta*, and *Loxosceles rufescens*). The brown recluse is sometimes called the violin spider because of a violin-shaped marking on the dorsum. Brown recluse venom contains at least nine identified protein fractions; the most important to cutaneous reactions is a substance called sphingomyelinase D2.

Clinical Features

- A brown recluse spider bite is usually painless.
- Within 6 to 12 hours, a small papule develops at the bite site, surrounded by edema (Fig. 14.12).
- Constitutional symptoms are variable and include malaise, headache, arthralgias, fever, nausea, vomiting, and, occasionally, a nonspecific maculopapular eruption.
- In about 90% of cases, the response is limited to a local urticaria-like or cellulitis-like reaction.
- In less than 10% of cases, and within 2 to 3 days, the site begins to demonstrate early signs of hemorrhage (Fig. 14.13) and necrosis (Figs. 14.14 and 14.15), with a central gray to violaceous center, surrounded by a white ring, and then by erythema, the so-called red, white, and blue sign.
- Ulcers caused by the brown recluse spider characteristically heal very slowly.
- Rarely reported complications may include a Coombs-positive hemolytic anemia, disseminated intravascular necrosis, seizures, renal failure, and even death.

Diagnosis

- History of a spider bite and identification of the offending spider is the only definitive test.
- In the absence of a captured spider, the clinical presentation remains the principal means of diagnosis.
- Biopsies are not diagnostic but may reveal findings consistent with a spider bite. A biopsy is not typically performed unless there is desire to exclude other ulcerative conditions.

- In severe cases, serial CBC testing because of possible hemolysis and thrombocytopenia and serial urinalysis to rule out hemoglobinuria may be performed.

Treatment

Mild Cases

- RICE therapy—*r*est, *i*ce *c*ompresses for 15 min/hour, and *e*levation
- Aspirin for pain relief and to reduce thrombosis and a tetanus booster shot (if not up to date)

Severe Cases

- Dapsone use is controversial. Animal studies have produced mixed results. In one uncontrolled human study, patients treated with dapsone required less surgery and had better clinical outcomes. Some studies have indicated that to have any efficacy, dapsone must be initiated in the first 36 hours after the bite.
- The use of systemic corticosteroids is advocated by some authorities, but six animal studies and human studies have failed to demonstrate any definitive benefit on lesion size or progression with corticosteroids.
- Surgical excision has been advocated by some, but others think that it is contraindicated and can actually be detrimental. Most authorities advocate surgery only for late-stage, stabilized lesions.
- Brown recluse specific antivenin exists but must be administered within the first 24 hours.

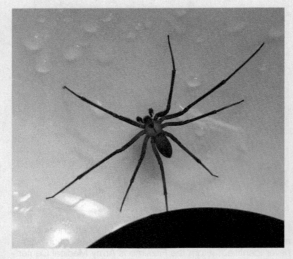

Fig. 14.11. Brown recluse spider in Arkansas demonstrating the characteristic violin marking on the dorsum.

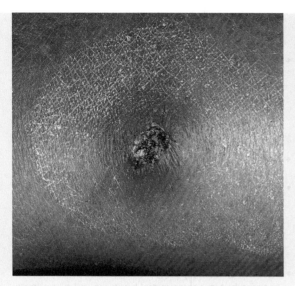

Fig. 14.12. Patient with typical spider bite from an unknown species. Routine spider bite ulcers are often oval because the venom is injected with two fangs.

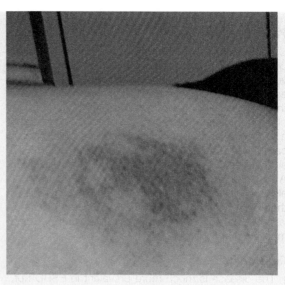

Fig. 14.13. Hemorrhagic brown recluse spider bite on day 2. (Courtesy Dr. Paul Gillum.)

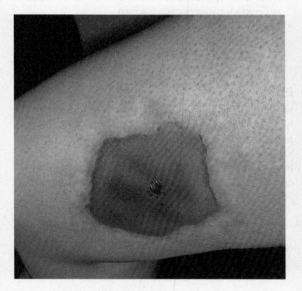

Fig. 14.14. Brown recluse spider bite on day 11. (Courtesy Dr. Paul Gillum.)

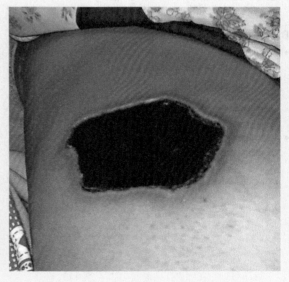

Fig. 14.15. Brown recluse spider bite with black eschar on day 37. (Courtesy Dr. Paul Gillum.)

Pathogenesis

Calciphylaxis is an uncommon and potentially lethal condition caused by occlusive calcification of blood vessels, with resultant tissue necrosis. The pathogenesis is poorly understood, but, in nearly all cases, there are underlying abnormalities in calcium and/or phosphorus metabolism that are often precipitated by a secondary event, such as trauma. Most patients with calciphylaxis have end-stage renal disease (ESRD) and elevated levels of parathyroid hormone (PTH). A high percentage of these same affected patients also receive vitamin D supplementation. However, less than 5% of all persons with ESRD develop calciphylaxis, indicating that the process is likely complex and multifactorial.

Clinical Features

- The disease is much more prevalent in ESRD but, even among persons with ESRD, calciphylaxis is more common in whites and in women (3 : 1).
- Lesions of calciphylaxis may be single or multiple.
- Early lesions present as painful indurated or dusky plaques that manifest a reticulated appearance.
- Later lesions may ulcerate or progress to irregular black eschars (Figs. 14.16 and 14.17).

Diagnosis

- A punch or incision or excision biopsy, to include a generous amount of subcutaneous fat, is necessary. Histologic findings include occlusive calcium deposition in lobular blood vessels, with resultant inflammation (Fig. 14.18). This finding, combined with the clinical situation, is diagnostic.
- Soft tissue x-rays may show calcium in the fat or blood vessels, but this is not diagnostic of only calciphylaxis. For example, elderly persons may have nonocclusive calcification of larger blood vessels,

specifically without the other stigmata of calciphylaxis (Mönckeberg arteriosclerosis).
- When calciphylaxis is suspected, minimum laboratory studies should include determination of blood calcium (abnormal in about 20%), phosphate, and PTH levels. Renal function tests and urinalysis should also be performed.

Treatment

- Calciphylaxis is a medical emergency, and all patients should be admitted to the hospital.
- Sodium thiosulfate, 25 g IV three times per week, may be helpful through the formation of calcium thiosulfate salts that are 250 to 100,000-fold more soluble than other calcium salts, allowing mobilization of the deposits, with subsequent excretion. Treatment must be continued for months.
- Parathyroidectomy has been advocated by some authors but is controversial because not all patients with calciphylaxis manifest elevations of PTH levels. The rationale is that parathyroidectomy reduces hormone levels and normalizes calcium and phosphate homeostasis. It seems reasonable to consider this approach when there is demonstrable secondary hyperparathyroidism.
- Anecdotal evidence supports the use of cinacalcet, 30 mg PO qd. This drug targets the calcium-sensing receptor of the parathyroid gland and lowers PTH levels.

Prognosis

Historically, calciphylaxis has been associated with high mortality. One- and 5-year survival rates may be as poor as 45% and 35%, respectively. Many patients with calciphylaxis die from sepsis. The impact of newer treatments, such as sodium thiosulfate and cinacalcet, on mortality has not yet been fully appreciated.

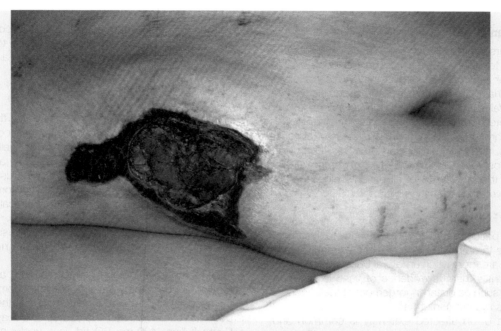

Fig. 14.16. Fatal case of calciphylaxis demonstrating eschar, with central necrosis extending into the fat. (From the Fitzsimons Army Medical Center Collection, Aurora, CO.)

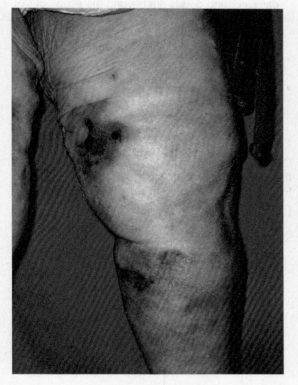

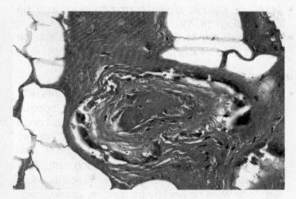

Fig. 14.18. Biopsy of calciphylaxis demonstrating calcium deposition in vessel wall associated with complete obliteration of the vascular lumen. This vascular occlusion accounts for the necrosis seen clinically (H&E;1000×).

Fig. 14.17. Patient with calciphylaxis demonstrating multiple lesions, with dusky appearance of the leg due to anoxia associated with early signs of necrosis. (From the Fitzsimons Army Medical Center Collection, Aurora, CO.)

Pathogenesis

Leg ulcers caused by chronic venous hypertension are due to incompetent valves in the deep venous plexus or incompetent valves in venous perforator vessels that connect the deep and superficial venous plexus. Valve incompetence, in turn, is a complex and multifaceted process, but implicated factors include venous thrombosis, congenital weakness or absence of valves, and injury and aging of valves. Leg ulcers occur most often in the elderly, with some studies showing that about 1% of all patients older than 65 years have at least one leg ulcer.

Clinical Features

- Many patients with leg ulcers have a history of venous thrombosis in the affected extremity.
- Ulcers are more often unilateral but can be bilateral.
- Frequently, there is evidence of venous incompetence, such as distal engorgement of the superficial venous system (Fig. 14.19).
- Edema of an affected extremity is common and, early in the course of disease, may be all that is present.
- Venous ulcers usually present on the medial aspect of the leg, near the malleolus.
- Acute or chronic stasis dermatitis may also be present (Fig. 14.20).
- Scars from previously healed ulcers may also be present (Fig. 14.21).

Diagnosis

- Patch testing should be considered in patients with ulcers that itch or demonstrate significant edema. It has been well recognized that stasis, and hence leg ulcers, predisposes an individual to allergic contact dermatitis. In a study of 235 patients with leg ulcers, 106 underwent patch testing, with 75% demonstrating at least one positive reaction. Most reactions were caused by fragrances, lanolin, colophony, and neomycin.

- Venous ulcers are often ragged, at least in comparison to arterial ulcers, which are more likely to have a punched-out appearance. Arterial ulcers are also more likely to demonstrate an eschar.

Treatment

- Compression hose are a mainstay of therapy because they reduce the chronic venous congestion and hypertension. Hose should be well fitted and with graded compression. Carefully applied elastic bandage (Ace) wraps may also be used.
- Unna boots provide excellent fixed compression and protection and may be used in recalcitrant cases.
- Intermittent pneumatic compression is useful in reducing edema and may also accelerate healing. Many brands are available.
- Mild to moderate topical corticosteroids, applied for 1 to 2 weeks, are useful for the management of the associated dermatitis (and itching), but their use does not otherwise alter the course of disease.
- Pentoxifylline, 400 mg PO tid, is a useful adjunct because it reduces fibrosis, promotes fibrinolysis, and makes erythrocytes more pliable.
- Optimal topical management of ulcers is not standardized, and details are beyond the scope of this chapter. In general, fibrinolytic agents are not useful, and topical antibiotics (e.g., bacitracin, neomycin) should be avoided due to high rates of sensitization in the setting of stasis. Topical petrolatum is a mainstay.
- Split-thickness grafts, pinch grafts, or artificial skin (e.g., Apligraf, Dermagraft) can accelerate healing once a bed of granulation tissue has been achieved.

Clinical Course

Chronic venous hypertension is a chronic condition that requires continuous therapy to prevent ulceration. Patients may be referred to wound centers or wound specialists for longer term care.

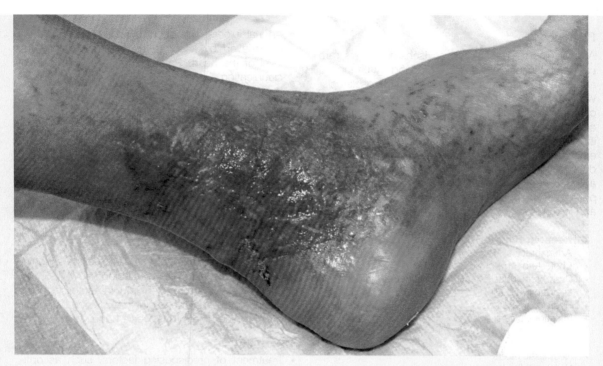

Fig. 14.19. Patient with superficial stasis ulceration and erosion near the medial malleolus area, a common site of venous ulcers. Note the dilated vessels distal to the ulceration. This is a common clinical finding that indicates valvular incompetence and supports the presence of chronic venous hypertension.

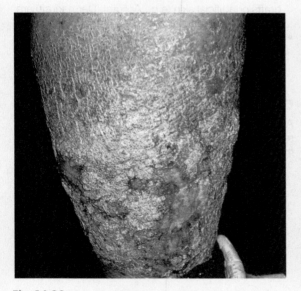

Fig. 14.20. Severe chronic stasis dermatitis, with superficial ulceration and marked hyperkeratosis.

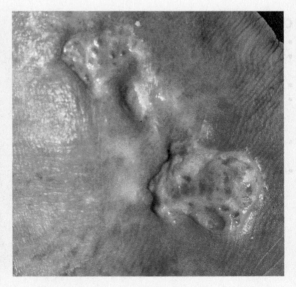

Fig. 14.21. Patient with partially healed venous ulceration, with associated scar from healed ulcers from a previous episode of ulceration.

Pathogenesis

Arterial ulcers, also known as ischemic ulcers, are caused by insufficient delivery of blood by peripheral arteries. Most often this is due to atherosclerosis, which, in turn, causes partial or complete occlusion of one or more peripheral arteries. Although most cases are due to gradual occlusion of the arteries, in some cases the ulcers are caused by cholesterol emboli. These consist of an atheromatous plaque detached from a proximal source, which occludes a distal vessel. Arterial ulcers are more common in patients with diabetes mellitus, in cigarette smokers, and in the elderly.

Differential Diagnosis of Chronic Leg Ulcers
- Arterial ulcers
- Cholesterol emboli
- Dysproteinemias (e.g., cryoglobulinemia, cold agglutinin disease)
- Hydroxyurea ulcers
- Infectious ulcers
- Livedoid vasculopathy
- Necrobiosis lipoidica
- Neoplastic ulcers
- Neuropathic ulcers
- Pyoderma gangrenosum
- Red blood cell disorders (e.g., sickle cell anemia, thalassemia)
- Stasis (venous) ulcers
- Vasculitis (various types)

Clinical Features

- Arterial ulcers may be unilateral or bilateral.
- Arterial ulcers usually affect the distal leg and are more likely to affect the lateral leg than stasis ulcers.
- Distal pulses may be diminished or absent.
- Chronic arterial insufficiency may lead to hair loss and thinned skin in the affected extremity (Fig. 14.22).
- The toes may be purple-red due to vascular insufficiency (see Fig. 14.22).
- Arterial ulcers tend to be have a more punched-out quality and are deeper than stasis ulcers (Figs. 14.23 and 14.24).

- Arterial ulcers are often painful. The pain may be relieved by keeping the extremity below the level of the heart. Patients may also complain of claudication.

Diagnosis

- The clinical presentation of an ulcer in an older patient with known atherosclerotic disease and/or diabetes mellitus should trigger consideration of an arterial ulcer. This concern is augmented when the ulcer appears punched out, when it lies on the lateral leg, or if there are other findings of peripheral artery disease (e.g., loss of hair, shiny skin appearance, purple-red toes).
- Weak or absent distal pulses is a supportive clinical finding.
- Doppler ultrasonographic studies provide a noninvasive means to assess distal blood flow.
- Routine x-rays are rarely helpful in establishing the diagnosis but may be useful in excluding osteomyelitis in deep ulcers that overlie bone.

Treatment

- Treatment of predisposing factors, such as optimizing diabetes management, smoking cessation, and hypertension treatment and/or hyperlipidemia therapy, may slow progression of the disease.
- In contrast to stasis ulcers, compression should be avoided. Wound care is necessary, and skin grafts or artificial skin (e.g., Apligraf, Dermagraft) are helpful once granulation tissue has been achieved.
- The most important immediate treatment is referral to a vascular surgeon for consideration of bypass grafting, angioplasty (with or without stent placement), and atherectomy.

Clinical Course

Arterial ulcers heal poorly unless blood flow is restored. Some patients may lose part(s) of one or more extremities.

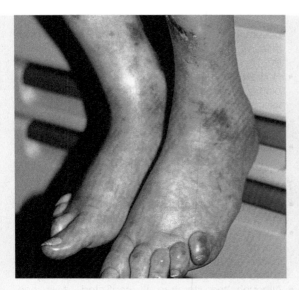

Fig. 14.22. Arterial ulcer of the shin associated with thin, shiny, hairless skin and reddish-purple toes in a patient with diabetes mellitus.

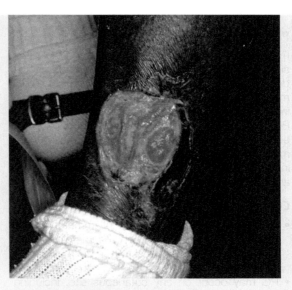

Fig. 14.23. Large, deep, punched-out ulcer in a patient with peripheral artery disease and cholesterol emboli. (From the Fitzsimons Army Medical Center Collection, Aurora, CO.)

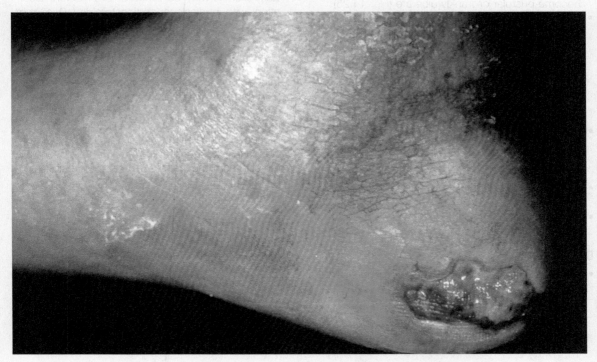

Fig. 14.24. Patient with large, deep sharply defined ulcer on the heel due to peripheral atherosclerotic disease. (From the Fitzsimons Army Medical Center Collection, Aurora, CO.)

Pathogenesis

Pyoderma gangrenosum (PG) is a serious ulcerative skin condition that is often underappreciated, to the detriment of the patient and clinician. Lesions of PG may be easily confused with vascular ulcerations, infections, and spider bites. The pathogenesis of PG is poorly understood. A strong association exists between PG and inflammatory bowel disease, rheumatoid arthritis, and autoimmune hepatitis, suggesting that it is a T cell–mediated autoimmune disorder, although neutrophils represent the effector cells.

Clinical Features

- PG is strongly associated with inflammatory bowel disease (~50% of cases) and rheumatoid arthritis (~10%) of cases. Disease activity in PG may or may not parallel that of the associated condition.
- PG may occur on any cutaneous site, including mucosal surfaces such as the genitalia or conjunctiva. The lower extremities are most often affected.
- Early lesions of PG begin as tender erythematous papules that enlarge to an erythematous nodule but with intact skin. Subsequently, lesions of PG then become pustular or frankly ulcerate (Fig. 14.25).
- Fully evolved PG represents an ulcer that may rapidly and relentlessly enlarge (up to 1–2 cm/day) or may remain stable. Ulcers often demonstrate a marked or even violaceous erythema that extends up to 3 cm away from the ulcer, with a ragged or undermined edge. PG ulcers are of varied depth and may extend into deep underlying structures, including bone and internal organs (Fig. 14.26).
- PG may occur on mucosa (Fig. 14.27) and may develop at sites of trauma (pathergy). Because of this pathergy, the ulcers of PG may expand with surgical débridement, which is contraindicated.
- About one-third of patients with PG have an asymmetric seronegative arthritis.
- Pain is often substantial in PG and may be out of proportion to the physical findings.

Diagnosis

- The clinical presentation, with one or more expanding ulcers and a ragged and undermined border, occurring in a patient with inflammatory bowel disease or rheumatoid arthritis, strongly suggests PG.
- However, PG is a diagnosis of exclusion, and a biopsy for routine histopathologic analysis and tissue culture (for bacterial, fungal, and acid-fast organisms) should be performed from the ulcer's edge.
- Imaging may be useful to exclude osteomyelitis or involvement of deep integument or bone.

Treatment

- Therapy for PG must be individualized, based on the extent of disease and associated conditions.
- Lavage with sterile saline and/or wet compresses may be used to débride necrotic tissue gently. As lesions are brought under control, occlusive hydrocolloid dressing becomes a treatment mainstay.
- Although the literature is conflicted, it is one author's experience (WAH) that collagenase ointment, in some situations, may paradoxically worsen PG, probably because of tissue injury or pathergy mechanisms.
- Early lesions may be aborted, even before ulceration, with intralesional corticosteroids (10–40 mg/mL).
- Once ulcers develop, or if there are extensive lesions, oral prednisone (40–80 mg PO qd) is the initial treatment of choice. Prednisone dosing is tapered based on the clinical response. Reduced pain and lesser erythema are clinical indications of a response. Minocycline may also be added to the regimen.
- Steroid-sparing agents used for PG include cyclosporine (2–4 mg/kg per day), mycophenolate mofetil, tacrolimus, and anti–tumor necrosis factor-α (TNF-α).
- TNF-α agents may be used.

Clinical Course

The clinical course of PG is highly varied. Some patients will have a single episode of PG, whereas other patients will have recurrent episodes that span decades and are often precipitated by minor trauma.

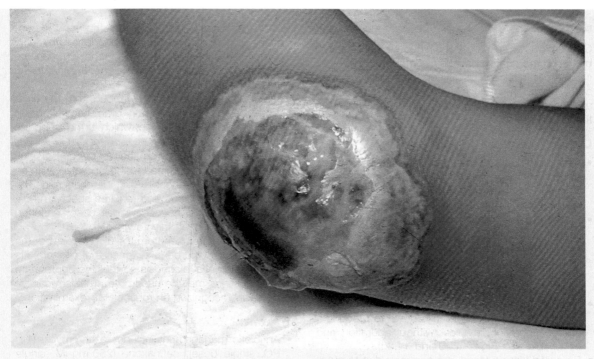

Fig. 14.25. Early pyoderma gangrenosum of the knee, with a rapidly spreading margin, in a young woman. (From the Fitzsimons Army Medical Center Collection, Aurora, CO.)

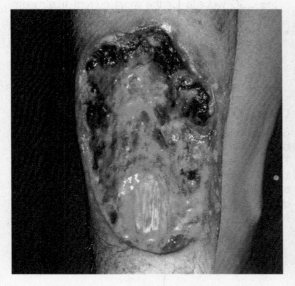

Fig. 14.26. Patient with established lesion of pyoderma gangrenosum, with exposed tendon. (From the Fitzsimons Army Medical Center Collection, Aurora, CO.)

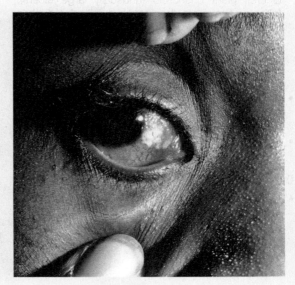

Fig. 14.27. Patient with ocular pyoderma gangrenosum. (From the Fitzsimons Army Medical Center Collection, Aurora, CO.)

Pathogenesis

Chancroid is a sexually transmitted disease caused by the gram-negative bacillus *Haemophilus ducreyi*. It causes painful ulcers, usually on the genitalia, in men and women. The condition is most common in Africa and Asia, but sporadic outbreaks have appeared in the United States.

Clinical Features

- Chancroid has a short incubation period compared to syphilis, ranging from 2 to 5 days in most cases. In some cases, it may take as long as 10 days to develop into visible disease.
- Lesions usually occur on the genitalia, but extra-genital sites may be involved. In men, the prepuce, penile shaft, glans penis, coronal sulcus, and frenulum are most often involved; in women, most lesions occur on the labia majora, fourchette, labia minora, and clitoris.
- The earliest lesion is a painful papule or nodule (Fig. 14.28) that rapidly breaks down to produce a tender, ragged or dirty ulcer, without induration, and of variable size (Figs. 14.29 and 14.30).
- So-called kissing ulcers are common due to auto-inoculation (see Fig. 14.29).
- Variations include dwarf chancroid (small shallow ulcers), giant chancroid (unusually large ulcers), follicular chancroid (begins as a follicular pustule that ulcerates), transient chancroid (superficial ulcer that heals, followed by lymphadenopathy), serpiginous chancroid (often due to multiple ulcers that coalesce), and mixed chancroid (chancroid plus another sexually transmitted disease).
- Regional lymph nodes are usually enlarged and tender and may be fluctuant (Fig. 14.31). Spontaneous rupture of the enlarged node can occur.
- Some patients may have constitutional symptoms, such as low-grade fever and malaise.

Diagnosis

- Recent suspicious sexual contacts, especially occurring in an endemic area, and/or if it occurred with a sex worker, should prompt consideration of chancroid.

- A tender, ragged, dirty ulcer occurring on the genitalia, with tender regional lymphadenopathy, also suggests chancroid, but the condition can be mimicked by a primary herpes simplex virus (HSV) infection.
- Gram staining of material swabbed from the ulcer edge may demonstrate short, gram-negative bacilli arranged as schools of fish, which further supports the diagnosis.
- Culture of a specimen from the ulcer edge is useful, but it should be submitted to the laboratory with an explicit (written) request to exclude chancroid. The organism is fastidious and requires specific media (e.g., enriched gonococcal agar base, enriched Mueller-Hinton agar) for growth.
- Biopsies can be taken from the ulcer edge, but the pathologist should be forewarned that chancroid is in the differential diagnosis so that the appropriate special stains may be used. The organism cannot be easily recognized on routine H&E examination.

Treatment

- Antibiotic management includes azithromycin (1 g PO, single dose), ceftriaxone (250 mg IM, single dose), erythromycin (500 mg PO tid × 7 days), and ciprofloxacin (500 mg PO bid × 3 days). Before instituting therapy, it would be prudent to refer to the CDC website for the most current treatments and dosages.
- All sexual partners encountered in the 10 days preceding symptom onset must be treated, and affected patients cannot engage in sexual activity until the antibiotic therapy is complete and the ulcers have healed.

Clinical Course

Subjective improvement usually occurs within 3 to 7 days of therapy, and the ulcers heal within 2 weeks. The lymphadenopathy may persist for 3 weeks or longer. Scarring, phimosis, balanoposthitis, ruptured buboes with severe pain, fistula formation, and sexual dysfunction due to scarring are rare complications.

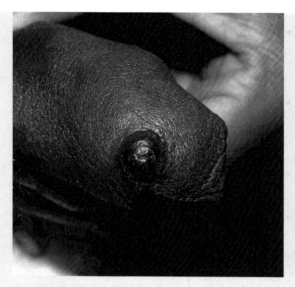

Fig. 14.28. Patient with early chancroid demonstrating painful papulonodular lesion with impending necrosis. (From the Fitzsimons Army Medical Center Collection, Aurora, CO.)

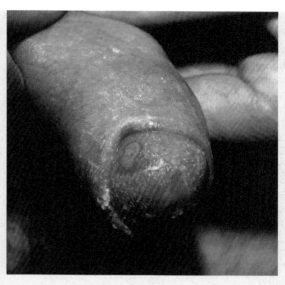

Fig. 14.29. Patient with superficial chancroid ulcers with kissing lesions in an uncircumcised man. (From the Fitzsimons Army Medical Center Collection, Aurora, CO.)

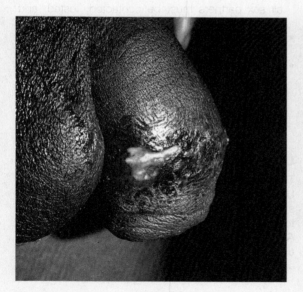

Fig. 14.30. Patient with characteristic large, irregular, and tender nonindurated ulcer of chancroid. (From the Fitzsimons Army Medical Center Collection, Aurora, CO.)

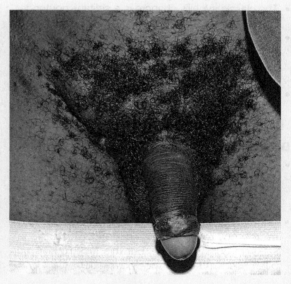

Fig. 14.31. Patient with chancroid ulcer, with associated tender suppurative unilateral lymphadenopathy. (From the Fitzsimons Army Medical Center Collection, Aurora, CO.)

Primary Syphilis

Pathogenesis

Syphilis is an infection caused by the spirochete *Treponema pallidum*. It is transmitted nearly exclusively by sexual contact. Epidemiologic studies have suggested that about one-third of persons who have sexual intercourse with an infected individual will themselves develop infection. About 20,000 cases of primary and secondary syphilis were reported to the Centers for Disease Control and Prevention (CDC) in 2015, but the true incidence is likely much higher. Syphilis is particularly prevalent in the men who have sex with men (MSM) population, but lately the elderly represent the US subpopulation with the greatest observed increases in syphilis incidence.

Clinical Features

- The incubation period is 10 to 90 days (average, 21 days).
- In men, primary syphilis chancres usually involve the prepuce, coronal sulcus, glans, and frenulum of the penis (Fig. 14.32 and 14.33); in women, the labia, urethra, and cervix are preferentially involved. Common extragenital sites include the oral cavity, anus, and fingers (Fig. 14.34).
- The classic syphilis chancre is a solitary, nontender, indurated (rubbery) ulcer, with a clean base.
- Unusual chancres may be painful, multiple (up to 25%), minimally indurated, or purulent (the latter due to secondary infection). Regional lymphadenopathy (firm, nonsuppurated) is often present.
- Sometimes, the mucocutaneous manifestations of secondary syphilis will occur before the primary chancre resolves (Fig. 14.35).

Diagnosis

- A high index of suspicion is necessary to recognize syphilis. In one study, more than 50% of cases of primary syphilis were missed at the initial medical visit.
- Demonstration of the organism by dark-field microscopy remains the gold standard for diagnosis, with 80% sensitivity, but this technique is not often used and is not widely available.

- Smears from the ulcer base can be examined using the direct fluorescent antibody test for *Treponema pallidum* (DFA-TP). Although the sensitivity of this technique approaches 100%, it is also not widely available.
- Serologic testing remains the most widely available technique in an emergency, urgent, or primary care setting. The rapid plasma reagin (RPR) and venereal disease research laboratory (VDRL) tests are used. In general, if the ulcer has been present for only 1 week, only 25% of cases will test positive, but if the ulcer has been present for 4 weeks, almost 100% of cases will test positive.
- Positive results via the RPR and VDRL assays should be confirmed with a *Treponema*-specific test, such as the fluorescent treponemal antibody absorption (FTA-ABS) test and *Treponema pallidum* particle agglutination (TP-PA) test. These latter tests, once positive, usually remain positive for the life of the patient.

Treatment

- Syphilis is a reportable disease. The appropriate public health authorities must be notified, and all sex partners must be contacted, tested, and treated.
- Benzathine penicillin G (2.4 million units IM, single dose) is the treatment of choice for adults.
- For special cases, such as in children and pregnant, HIV-positive, and penicillin-allergic patients, it is strongly recommended that the current treatment recommendations be obtained from the CDC website (http://www.cdc.gov/std/tg2015/syphilis.htm).

Clinical Course

The chancre of syphilis will heal in 2 to 4 weeks. Untreated primary syphilis may progress to secondary syphilis or, rarely, to tertiary syphilis. Nontreponemal testing modalities (RPR, VDRL) titer to disease activity. A four-fold decrease in titer within 6 to 12 months is usually indicative of treatment success.

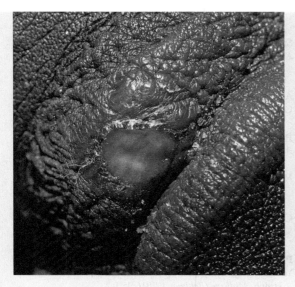

Fig. 14.32. Primary genital syphilis chancre. Note the indurated edge. (From the Fitzsimons Army Medical Center Collection, Aurora, CO.)

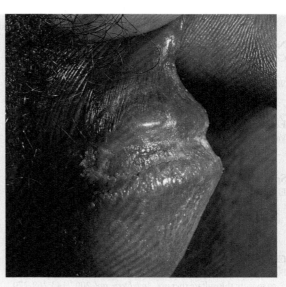

Fig. 14.33. Patient with resolving primary syphilis. Because the primary lesion resolves, some patients fail to seek medical care. (From the Fitzsimons Army Medical Center Collection, Aurora, CO.)

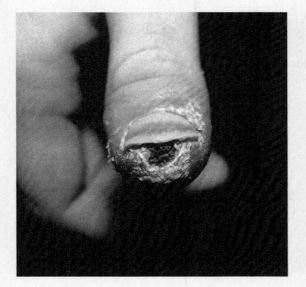

Fig. 14.34. Patient with extragenital primary syphilis chancre. (From the Fitzsimons Army Medical Center Collection, Aurora, CO.)

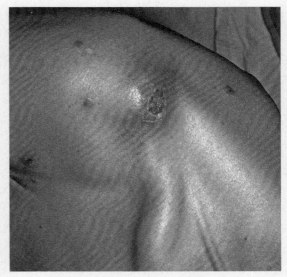

Fig. 14.35. Primary extragenital syphilis with secondary syphilis. The primary lesion occurred when his partner laid his penis on his shoulder while he slept. (From the Fitzsimons Army Medical Center Collection, Aurora, CO.)

References

Necrotizing Fasciitis

Cabrera H, Skoczdopole L, Marini M, et al. Necrotizing gangrene of the genitalia and perineum. *Int J Dermatol.* 2002;41:847-851.

Wang Y-S, Wong C-H, Tay Y-K. Staging of necrotizing fasciitis based on the evolving cutaneous features. *Int J Dermatol.* 2007;46:1036-1041.

Ecthyma Gangrenosum

Vairman M, Lazarovitch T, Heller L, Lotan G. Ecthyma gangrenosum and ecthyma-like lesions: review article. *Eur J Clin Microbiol Infect Dis.* 2015;34:633-639.

Spider Bites

Elston DM, Miller SD, Young RJ III, et al. Comparison of colchicine, dapsone, triamcinolone, and diphenhydramine therapy for the treatment of brown recluse spider envenomation. A double-blind, controlled study in a rabbit model. *Arch Dermatol.* 2005;141:595-597.

Calciphylaxis

Baker BL, Fitzgibbons CA, Buescher LS. Calciphylaxis responding to sodium thiosulfate therapy. *Arch Dermatol.* 2007;143:269-270.

Robinson MR, Augustine JJ, Korman NJ. Cinacalcet for the treatment of calciphylaxis. *Arch Dermatol.* 2007;143:152-154.

Stasis Ulcers

Alavi A, Sibbald G, Phillips TJ, et al. What's new: management of venous leg ulcers. Treating venous leg ulcers. *J Am Acad Dermatol.* 2016;74:643-664.

Arterial Ulcers

Gulati A, Botnaru I, Garcia LA. Critical limb ischemia and its treatments: a review. *J Cardiovasc Surg (Torino).* 2015;56:775-785.

Pyoderma Gangrenosum

Brooklyn T, Dunnill G, Probert C. Diagnosis and treatment of pyoderma gangrenosum. *BMJ.* 2006;333:181-184.

Miller J, Yentzer BA, Clark A, et al. Pyoderma gangrenosum: a review and update on new therapies. *J Am Acad Dermatol.* 2010;62:646-654.

Chancroid

Sehgal VN, Srivastava G. Chancroid: contemporary appraisal. *Int J Dermatol.* 2003;42:182-190.

Primary Syphilis

Yu X, Zheng H. Syphilitic chancre of the lips transmitted by kissing. *Medicine (Baltimore).* 2016;95:1-2.

Chapter 15
Subcutaneous Diseases

Key Terms

Erythema Induratum
  Nodular vasculitis
Lupus Panniculitis
  Lupus erythematosus panniculitis
  Lupus profundus

Subcutaneous Granuloma Annulare
  Deep granuloma annulare
  Pseudorheumatoid nodules

Rheumatoid Nodules
  Rheumatoid nodulosis syndrome

Subcutaneous diseases include those conditions that are classically considered panniculitis (e.g., erythema nodosum, erythema induratum), in addition to diseases that may involve the subcutaneous fat (e.g., rheumatoid nodules, deep granuloma annulare), and even vasculitis, which may affect the vessels of the subcutaneous fat and resemble a panniculitis. It is important to note that later in the course of the disease, some forms of panniculitis may involve the dermis and/or epidermis, resulting in perforation or ulceration.

IMPORTANT HISTORY QUESTIONS

How long have the lesions been present?

Some forms of panniculitis are usually acute and do not last long (e.g., pancreatic panniculitis), whereas others (e.g., lupus panniculitis) tend to be chronic.

Are the lesions painful, and, if so, how painful are they?

Some types of panniculitis are exquisitely painful (e.g., pancreatic panniculitis), whereas others are only tender (e.g., erythema nodosum) and some are typically not painful (e.g., subcutaneous granuloma annulare).

What medications do you take?

This is a very important question, because some forms of panniculitis can be drug induced (e.g., erythema nodosum, pancreatic panniculitis), which may mean that the condition is potentially curable.

Do you have any other medical conditions?

Tuberculosis is of particular interest; this specifically because it is associated with erythema induratum and erythema nodosum. Determine if there is a known history of hepatitis B infection, which is associated with polyarteritis nodosa; pancreatitis, which could indicate pancreatic fat necrosis; and sarcoidosis, which can present as subcutaneous nodules and plaques. The patient should also be asked about any known history of a connective tissue disorder, such as lupus erythematosus.

Have you ever had a positive tuberculosis skin test?

This is a most important evaluation of the patient with possible erythema induratum and, to a lesser extent, erythema nodosum.

How much alcohol do you consume in a week?

This question obviously needs to be used only when pancreatic fat necrosis is a clinical consideration. It needs to be stated with tact.

IMPORTANT PHYSICAL FINDINGS

What is the distribution of the lesions?

Some types of panniculitis are almost always located on the legs (e.g., erythema nodosum, erythema induratum), whereas others are frequently located in other areas. For example, subcutaneous granuloma annulare is not infrequently found on the head in infants and young children.

Are the lesions ulcerated, or is there any evidence of epidermal change?

Some forms of panniculitis are never ulcerated (e.g., erythema nodosum, subcutaneous fat necrosis of the newborn), whereas others, such as erythema induratum and pancreatic fat necrosis, are frequently ulcerated. Rheumatoid nodules can also demonstrate perforation of necrotic collagen.

Is there any physical evidence of active arthritis?

Rheumatoid nodules and pancreatic fat necrosis can both be associated with arthritis. It is not uncommon for erythema nodosum to be associated with arthralgias.

Are there any other types of skin lesions?

This is important, because some diseases, such as subcutaneous granuloma annulare (e.g., annular lesions) or sarcoidosis, may have different types of lesions present on the body, which is diagnostic.

Erythema Nodosum ICD10 code L52

Pathogenesis

The pathogenesis of erythema nodosum is poorly understood. Erythema nodosum, like urticaria, is not a primary disease but rather represents a reaction pattern to a variety of different antigenic insults, with the most common underlying factors being β-hemolytic streptococcal infection, drug therapy (particularly birth control pills), which includes herbal therapy (e.g., Echinacea), sarcoidosis, ulcerative colitis, tuberculosis, viral infections, Crohn disease, deep fungal infections, Behçet syndrome, pregnancy, and underlying malignancy. Patients with β-hemolytic streptococcal infection typically develop erythema nodosum 2 to 3 weeks after the infection, which is usually associated with an elevated antistreptolysin O (ASO) titer.

Drug-Induced Erythema Nodosum

- Azathioprine
- Celecoxib
- Echinacea herbal therapy
- Gold
- Oral contraceptives
- Sulfonamides

Clinical Features

- This is the most common form of panniculitis; it may occur at any age, including children, but the peak incidence is in patients between 20 and 30 years of age.
- It is three to six times more common in women than men.
- Patients may demonstrate a prodrome of fever, malaise, and arthralgias.
- Primary lesions are tender, erythematous subcutaneous nodules of variable size (1–15 cm); they are never sharply demarcated.
- It is predominantly acral, with the classic location being the anterior shins (Fig. 15.1).
- Less common locations include other parts of the leg (Fig. 15.2) and arms (Fig. 15.3).

- There are typically less than 10 lesions; however, more than 50 lesions are seen in rare patients.
- Ulceration does not occur.

Diagnosis

- Clinical presentation is usually characteristic, although the presentation may be mimicked by other forms of panniculitis, such as erythema induratum, or deep vasculitis, such as periarteritis nodosa.
- Routine laboratory tests that should be done include a throat culture to rule out active streptococcal infection and an ASO titer to rule out recent streptococcal infection.
- In select cases, consider testing stool for *Yersinia* infection and/or chest x-ray to rule out sarcoidosis or an underlying deep fungal infection.
- The histologic findings on biopsy—a 5-mm or larger punch biopsy or incisional biopsy that includes fat— is typically needed and is usually diagnostic.

Treatment

- No treatment is needed in mild cases but is always an option, because most cases are self-limited.
- Using nonsteroidal antiinflammatory drugs (NSAIDs) for pain relief and reduction of inflammation is recommended as initial treatment in more severe cases.
- Very painful or severe cases quickly respond to prednisone, 10 to 40 mg per day for 3 to 7 days. This therapy should be used with caution if an underlying infection is suspected.
- Oral potassium iodide (SSKI) is an alternate therapy, starting at two drops tid and increasing up to six drops tid.

Clinical Course

Individual lesions typically last 3 to 6 weeks, although new lesions may continue to develop. Rare patients may develop chronic erythema nodosum that is more likely to be unilateral.

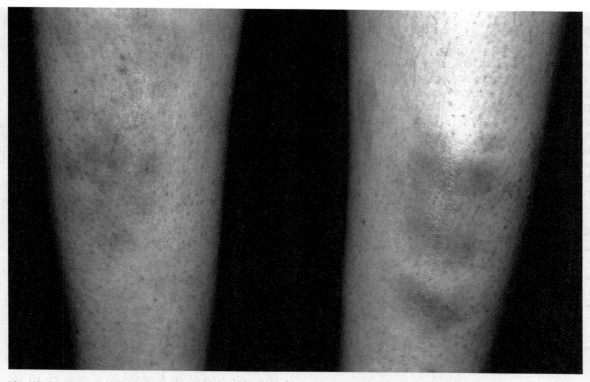

Fig. 15.1. Typical erythema nodosum of the anterior shins in a young woman. Note the discoloration of some of the lesions on the right leg. (From the Fitzsimons Army Medical Center Collection, Aurora, CO.)

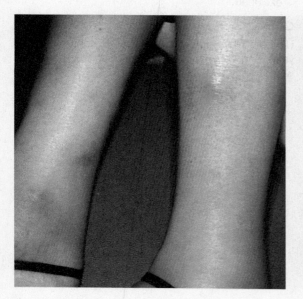

Fig. 15.2. Erythema nodosum on the lateral legs in a patient. (From the Fitzsimons Army Medical Center Collection, Aurora, CO.)

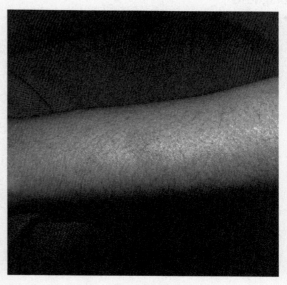

Fig. 15.3. Unusual location for erythema nodosum on the arm of a patient. (From the Fitzsimons Army Medical Center Collection, Aurora, CO.)

Pathogenesis

The term *erythema induratum* (of Bazin) is often used interchangeably with the term nodular vasculitis, although some dermatologists reserve the former for cases that are tuberculosis-associated and the latter term for those that are not. The pathogenesis is not entirely understood, although in cases associated with tuberculosis, polymerase chain reaction (PCR) studies have demonstrated *Mycobacterium tuberculosis* DNA in more than 75% of cases, suggesting that it is a hypersensitivity reaction. Less common associations have included Crohn disease, other infections, and, very rarely, medications (e.g., propylthiouracil).

Clinical Features

- It usually affects young and middle-aged women, although any age or gender can be affected.
- It is more common in clinical populations with a strong exposure to tuberculosis.
- It is usually located on the calves and shins, although the trunk, upper extremities, and even the face can be affected.
- The primary lesion is comprised of one or more painful, erythematous, subcutaneous nodules (Fig. 15.4).
- Ulceration is frequently present in one or more lesions (Figs. 15.5 and 15.6), a finding that is not found in erythema nodosum.

Diagnosis

- In regard to the clinical presentation, be particularly suspicious in a patient with a known history of tuberculosis or exposure to individuals with active tuberculosis. The differential diagnosis includes erythema nodosum, lupus panniculitis, polyarteritis nodosa, and other rare forms of panniculitis.

- The diagnosis is typically established by a 5- to 8-mm punch biopsy or incisional biopsy. It is critical that the biopsy includes adequate subcutaneous fat. The histologic findings may be strongly suggestive or diagnostic. Cases associated with tuberculosis are culture negative and do not demonstrate organisms with special stains; they can only be demonstrated by PCR assay, which is not routinely available.
- Chest x-rays and a purified protein derivative (PPD) skin test are strongly recommended in all cases to exclude evidence of tuberculosis. If tuberculosis is strongly suspected, consider diluting the PPD to 1:10, because patients may demonstrate very exuberant reactions.

Treatment

- The treatment of choice is to identify any underlying cause (e.g., tuberculosis) and treat that disorder or withdraw any potentially offending drug.
- Oral potassium iodide (SSKI) is an alternate therapy, starting at two drops tid and increasing up to six drops tid.
- NSAIDs may be used to reduce pain and inflammation.
- Use oral prednisone, starting at a dose of 10 to 40 mg/day, that is tapered as quickly as possible as the patient responds to therapy. Prednisone is not recommended until active tuberculosis has been excluded.

Clinical Course

Untreated lesions tend to persist for months or even years and, when the lesions resolve, they may heal with atrophy and variable scarring.

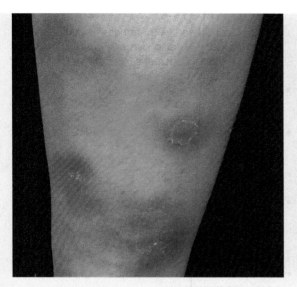

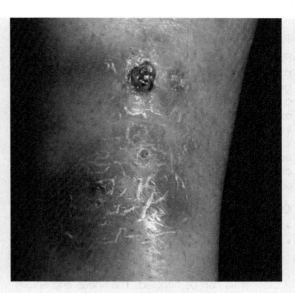

Fig. 15.4. Classic location of erythema induratum on the posterior aspect of the calf of a patient. (From the Fitzsimons Army Medical Center Collection, Aurora, CO.)

Fig. 15.5. Patient with indurated subcutaneous plaques of erythema induratum, with early ulceration. (From the Fitzsimons Army Medical Center Collection, Aurora, CO.)

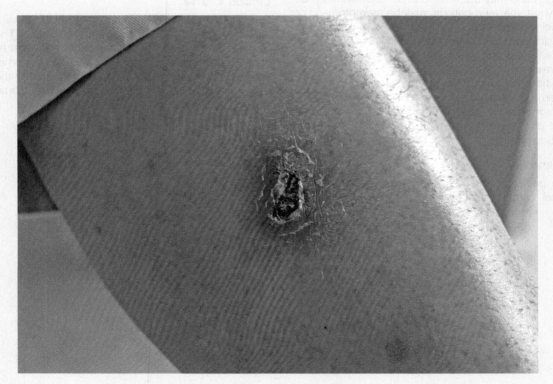

Fig. 15.6. Patient with ulcerated erythema induratum of the thigh that was secondary to undiagnosed tuberculosis.

Pathogenesis

Pancreatic panniculitis is the result of damage to the pancreas that releases enzymes such as lipase and/or amylase, which then digest and damage the subcutaneous fat. This damage to the fat (saponification) results in necrosis and the accumulation of acute inflammatory cells and calcium. Although pancreatitis is the most common cause, other cases have been associated with pancreatic cancer and, rarely, medications. Approximately 2% of all patients with pancreatitis will develop pancreatic panniculitis.

Clinical Features

- It typically affects adult patients.
- There is an acute onset of single or, more commonly, multiple subcutaneous nodules, which are primarily distributed on the lower legs, although other sites can be affected. The knees and ankles are especially common sites of involvement.
- Initially, nodules are typically very erythematous (Figs. 15.7 and 15.8).
- Developed nodules may become fluctuant (Fig. 15.9) and may ultimately drain a yellowish material.
- Symptoms vary; patients may be asymptomatic or feel extreme pain.
- Painful acute arthritis and, less commonly, polyserositis (e.g., pleuritis, pericarditis, synovitis) may be present.
- Lytic bone lesions are variably present due to the same process occurring in the intraosseous fat.
- Abdominal ascites may be present. This can be due to pancreatic disease or panniculitis of the intraabdominal fat.

Diagnosis

- In particular, the clinical presentation may involve the combination of very painful subcutaneous nodules associated with arthritis and abdominal pain. Patients may also demonstrate all the other features of acute pancreatitis (e.g., low-grade fever, tachycardia, hypotension).
- Pancreatic enzyme studies should be carried out. Serum amylase and lipase levels should always be ordered.
- A complete blood count (CBC) should be done; leukocytosis, eosinophilia, and an elevated erythrocyte sedimentation rate (ESR) are frequently present.
- A computed tomography (CT) scan can also be used to support the diagnosis of pancreatitis.
- A 4-mm or larger punch biopsy or incisional biopsy can yield findings that are histologically specific and can be diagnostic, even in the absence of a history.

Treatment

- There is no specific recommended treatment of the pancreatic panniculitis.
- Treatment is aimed at management of the primary pancreatitis (e.g., analgesics, intravenous fluids, no oral alimentation).

Clinical Course

The cutaneous lesions often drain and resolve over a period of weeks, leaving variable atrophy and scar. The patient's clinical outcome is dependent on the course of the pancreatitis or pancreatic adenocarcinoma, both of which can be fatal, as demonstrated by the patient depicted in Fig. 15.7, who had a fatal outcome from his alcoholic-induced acute pancreatitis.

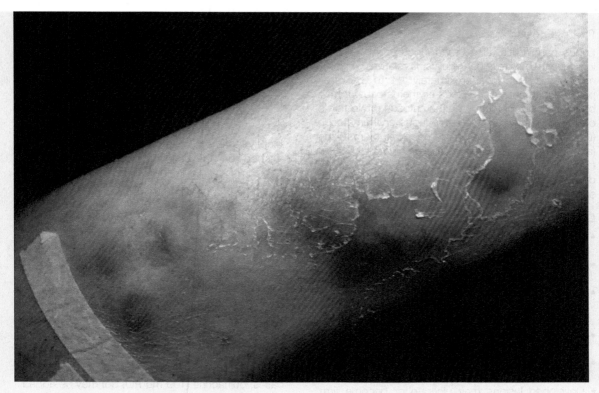

Fig. 15.7. Pancreatic panniculitis in a patient with fatal acute pancreatitis. (From the Fitzsimons Army Medical Center Collection, Aurora, CO.)

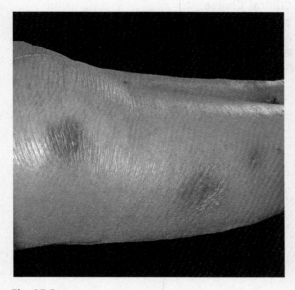

Fig. 15.8. Patient with bilateral tender erythematous nodules of pancreatic fat necrosis.

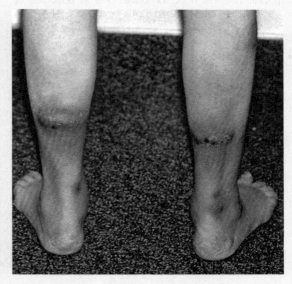

Fig. 15.9. Bilateral suppurative pancreatic fat necrosis that localized to the tops of the patient's boots. (From the Fitzsimons Army Medical Center Collection, Aurora, CO.)

Lupus Panniculitis ICD10 code L92.2

Pathogenesis

Lupus panniculitis, also called lupus profundus and lupus erythematosus panniculitis, is relatively uncommon but is seen in approximately 1% to 3% of all patients with cutaneous lupus erythematosus. It may be seen in discoid lupus erythematosus (≈two-thirds of cases), subacute cutaneous lupus erythematosus (uncommon), and systemic lupus erythematosus (about 5% of cases) and may arise de novo. Like other forms of lupus erythematosus, it is an autoimmune disease; however, the reasons why it localizes to the subcutaneous fat in some patients is not known.

Clinical Features

- The patient is typically adult or elderly, with a median age of 48 years in one study (range, 20–71 years).
- Like most forms of lupus erythematosus, women are more commonly affected than men.
- It tends to affects fatty areas, such as the breasts (Fig. 15.10), periorbital region (Fig. 15.11) upper lateral arms (Fig. 15.12), thighs, and buttocks.
- There is an acute onset of single or, more commonly, multiple subcutaneous nodules.
- The primary lesions are erythematous nodules or subcutaneous plaques, which may be tender.
- Developed lesions may ulcerate or become firm due to fibrosis and sclerosis, which develops in persistent lesions.
- Patients may demonstrate lupus erythematosus panniculitis de novo or develop it in association with discoid or systemic lupus erythematosus.

Diagnosis

- The clinical presentation of subcutaneous nodules in a patient with known discoid or systemic lupus erythematosus should strongly raise the possibility of lupus erythematosus panniculitis.

- Panniculitis with overlying skin changes of discoid lupus erythematosus (e.g., hypopigmentation or hyperpigmentation, follicular hyperkeratosis) is also obviously strongly suggestive.
- Diagnostic treatment of choice is a 5- to 8-mm punch biopsy or incisional biopsy that includes adequate fat. In most cases, the diagnosis can be established by the histologic findings from a single biopsy if enough fat is present. Patients should be warned that the biopsies in lupus erythematosus panniculitis frequently break down and form ulcers that may take weeks to months to heal.
- Direct immunofluorescence of lesional skin is useful in select cases.
- Patients should have routine screening laboratory tests for lupus erythematosus, including screening antinuclear antibody (ANA, and ANA panel if positive) and total complement activity (CH50) tests, CBC, and determinations of levels of blood urea nitrogen (BUN), creatinine, and uric acid (UA).

Treatment

- Hydroxychloroquine (200 mg PO, qd or bid) is the drug most commonly used as a corticosteroid-sparing agent for long-term management. In recalcitrant cases, quinacrine (100 mg PO, qd) may be added.
- Severe or recalcitrant cases may require oral prednisone, typically in the 20- to 40-mg per day dose range, which is titered to the patient's response.

Clinical Course

This form of panniculitis tends to be persistent and chronic and, even with even optimal therapy, the lesions may ulcerate, develop scar, or leave permanent areas of fat atrophy.

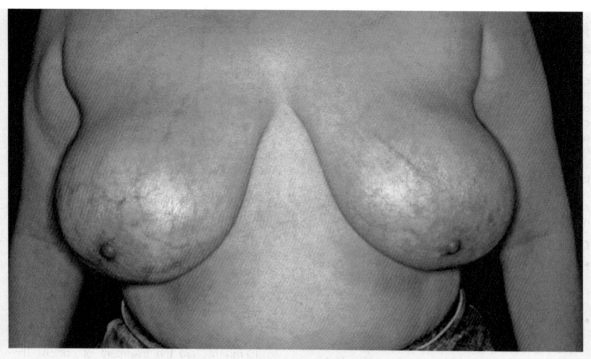

Fig. 15.10. Lupus panniculitis affecting the subcutaneous tissue of the breast in a patient with systemic lupus erythematosus. (From the Fitzsimons Army Medical Center Collection, Aurora, CO.)

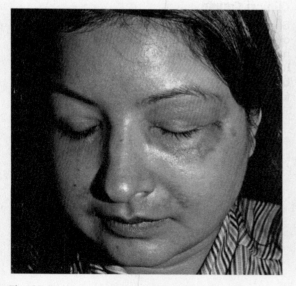

Fig. 15.11. Patient with lupus panniculitis affecting the subcutaneous tissue of the orbit. (From the Fitzsimons Army Medical Center Collection, Aurora, CO.)

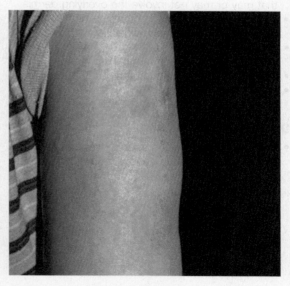

Fig. 15.12. Patient with lupus panniculitis affecting the upper arm, with atrophy and a surface scar. (From the Fitzsimons Army Medical Center Collection, Aurora, CO.)

Pathogenesis

Granuloma annulare is a relatively common granulomatous disease of uncertain pathogenesis in which collagen is destroyed by a granulomatous host response (necrobiotic granuloma). In most cases, the disease is confined to the dermis. However, in some cases, the process affects the collagen of the dermis and subcutaneous tissue or is directed against the collagen only of the subcutaneous tissue. Although it is usually called deep granuloma annulare or subcutaneous granuloma annulare because of the clinical resemblance to rheumatoid nodules, this deeper presentation has also been referred to as pseudorheumatoid nodules.

Clinical Features

- GA typically affects young children, with most cases occurring between the ages of 3 and 6 years. Adults and even infants younger than 1 year can develop this disorder.
- Lesions are usually found on the lower extremities, with a predilection for the anterior pretibial areas, toes (Fig. 15.13), and ankles (Fig. 15.14).
- In infants and young children, the head (Fig. 15.15) is not uncommonly involved and may raise clinical concern for a neoplastic process.
- The primary lesion is a deep subcutaneous nodule that may or may not involve the overlying dermis.
- The lesions may be skin colored or demonstrate a subtle violaceous discoloration.
- The number of lesions is highly variable and can vary from one lesion to multiple lesions.
- The primary lesions are usually asymptomatic.
- In about 25% of patients, there may be more characteristic superficial lesions, which are annular.

Diagnosis

- The clinical presentation of asymptomatic subcutaneous nodules of the lower legs in an infant or young child is suggestive but not specific. This is because other inflammatory disorders, including sarcoidosis, foreign body granulomas, and rheumatoid nodules, in addition to benign tumors (e.g., giant cell tumor of the tendon sheath) and malignant tumors, would be in the clinical differential diagnosis.
- The presence of the typical superficial lesions of granuloma annulare is an important finding that would so strongly support the diagnosis that a biopsy would not be needed.
- The diagnosis can only be established with certitude with a deep 4-, 5-, or 6-mm punch biopsy or incisional biopsy that includes the subcutis. The histologic findings are diagnostic.

Treatment

- No treatment is a viable option because this is an asymptomatic benign condition that will typically resolve on its own.
- For patients for whom there is parental pressure to treat the lesion, or if there is discomfort from the lesions when pressure is put on the lesion by footwear, intralesional corticosteroids, from 2.5 to 10 mg/mL, are the treatment of choice. The response can be monitored; if there is no or minimal response at 4 to 6 weeks, the treatment can be repeated and dose increased, if needed.

Clinical Course

Subcutaneous granuloma annulare is a chronic disorder that usually slowly improves over a period of months or even years. It should be noted that we have seen patients for whom a partial biopsy has been therapeutic, with all the lesions being resolved following the procedure.

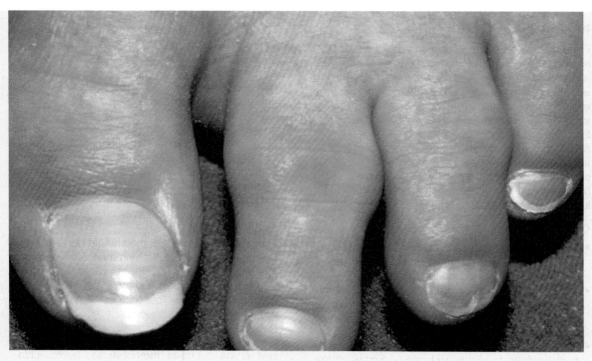

Fig. 15.13. Patient with subcutaneous granuloma annulare presenting as subcutaneous nodules, with focal violaceous discoloration on the second and third toes. (From the Fitzsimons Army Medical Center Collection, Aurora, CO.)

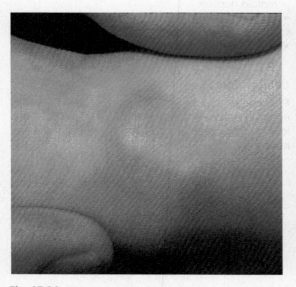

Fig. 15.14. Subcutaneous granuloma of the ankle of a young child. (From the William Weston Collection, Aurora, CO.)

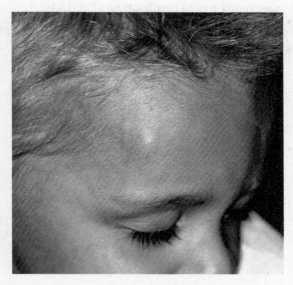

Fig. 15.15. Subcutaneous presentation of granuloma annulare on the forehead of a young child. (From the Joanna Burch Collection, Aurora, CO.)

Rheumatoid Nodules ICD10 code M06.3

Pathogenesis

Rheumatoid nodules represent a granulomatous host response that surrounds necrotic collagen. It may be associated with juvenile and classic adult rheumatoid arthritis. A rare variant, called rheumatoid nodulosis syndrome, consists of the rapid onset of rheumatoid nodules associated with a high-titer rheumatoid factor and no evidence of active arthritis. In about 10% of patients, rheumatoid nodules are present at the time of presentation. Although not discussed in this section, it is important to understand that rheumatoid nodules may affect other structures of the body (e.g., lungs, vocal cords).

Clinical Features

- Rheumatoid nodules are seen in about 10% of cases of juvenile rheumatoid arthritis and in about 25% of cases of adult rheumatoid arthritis.
- The lesions are usually distributed over the elbow, proximal ulnar bony surfaces (Fig. 15.16), interphalangeal joints of the fingers (Fig. 15.17), feet, and sacrum.
- The primary lesions are usually skin colored to slightly erythematous to slightly violaceous dermal and/or subcutaneous nodules, which may be movable or demonstrate attachment to periosteum or tendons.
- The size of the lesions is highly variable and may vary from 1 mm to over 5 cm (see Fig. 15.16).
- Typically, patients are asymptomatic unless they are traumatized.
- The overlying epidermis is typically intact and uninvolved, although some patients may demonstrate perforation of necrotic collagen at two or more sites (Fig. 15.18) or may demonstrate ulceration due to trauma or infection.

Diagnosis

- The clinical presentation of subcutaneous nodules in a patient with known rheumatoid arthritis is usually diagnostic.

- The diagnosis can only be established with certitude with a deep 4-, 5-, or 6-mm punch biopsy or incisional biopsy that includes the subcutis. The histologic findings are usually diagnostic, although rare cases may be difficult to differentiate from subcutaneous granuloma annulare.
- If the patient does not have known rheumatoid arthritis, an initial screening evaluation might include x-rays of joints with evidence of arthritis, rheumatoid factor (RF), CBC (patients may have anemia and/or thrombocytosis), ESR, C-reactive protein, and screening ANA (≈25% of patients with rheumatoid arthritis will have a positive ANA).

Treatment

- The primary treatment of rheumatoid nodules is the management of the underlying rheumatoid arthritis. The lesions usually but not always slowly resolve with treatment of the rheumatoid arthritis.
- Initial therapy usually consists of NSAIDs, with or without low-dose prednisone.
- Patients who do not respond to this therapeutic regimen are usually treated with immunosuppressive drugs such as methotrexate, hydroxychloroquine, minocycline, cyclosporine, and biologic agents. Methotrexate and biologic agents have been paradoxically reported to exacerbate rheumatoid nodules.
- Large lesions that interfere with activity can be excised, although some lesions do recur.
- Large lesions can also be injected with 10 to 40 mg/mL of triamcinolone.

Clinical Course

Rheumatoid nodules are chronic in untreated patients and may continue to enlarge. In treated patients, the lesions slowly resolve with management of the rheumatoid arthritis.

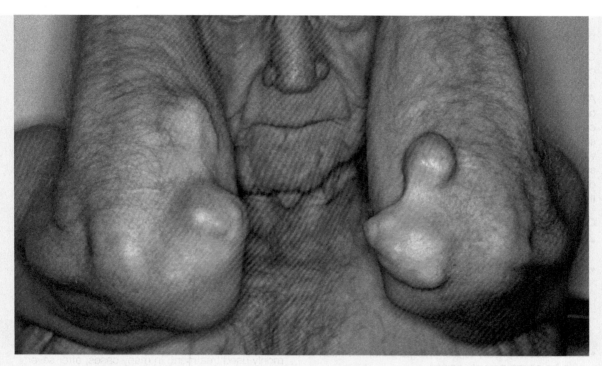

Fig. 15.16. Patient with numerous, unusually large rheumatoid nodules of the elbow and forearm. (From the Fitzsimons Army Medical Center Collection, Aurora, CO.)

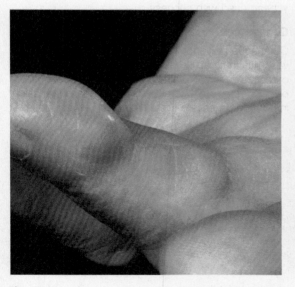

Fig. 15.17. Patient with two smaller, lightly red rheumatoid nodules of the finger. (From the Fitzsimons Army Medical Center Collection, Aurora, CO.)

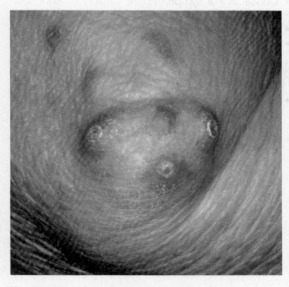

Fig. 15.18. Patient with large rheumatoid nodule, with superficial crusts representing foci of perforation of necrotic collagen. Several smaller nodules are also present.

Cutaneous Polyarteritis Nodosa ICD10 code M30.0

Pathogenesis

Cutaneous polyarteritis (panarteritis) nodosa is a vasculitis that preferentially involves small to medium-sized arteries of the deep dermis or subcutaneous tissue. Although some cases are associated with hepatitis B or C infection or inflammatory bowel disease, most cases do not have an identifiable association. However, some cases also present as subcutaneous nodules, which are indistinguishable from a primary panniculitis such as erythema nodosum. Rare cases have been drug-induced; minocycline and propylthiouracil are the most commonly implicated medications.

Clinical Features

- Cutaneous PAN may affect those of any age, including neonates.
- Bilateral erythematous to reddish-brown nodules that appear to be subcutaneous (Figs. 15.19 and 15.20) are present. Some lesions may show a slight tendency to be linear in configuration. Note that the most superior nodule in Fig. 15.19 demonstrates a linear configuration at its bottom pole.
- It is characteristically tender with palpation and can also be spontaneously painful.
- Lesions may ulcerate, although this is not common.
- Some cases may also be associated with a focal livedo (netlike) pattern of unaffected blood vessels.
- Constitutional symptoms are variably present, but patients frequently report fatigue and myalgia.
- Low-grade fever is frequently present.
- Rarely, patients may have an associated peripheral neuropathy.

Diagnosis

- The clinical presentation of lesions, without any evidence of a linear configuration, is not diagnostic, and the differential diagnosis would usually include erythema nodosum and erythema induratum. If there is any suggestion of a linear lesion, the clinical presentation is strongly supportive of polyarteritis nodosa.
- Diagnosis is confirmed by a 6- to 8-mm punch or an incisional biopsy of lesional skin. The histologic findings are usually diagnostic.
- Direct immunofluorescent studies, in contrast to most forms of vasculitis, yield negative or nonspecific results.
- Laboratory studies could include a CBC with differential (eosinophilia is usually absent in contrast to systemic polyarteritis nodosa), ESR (usually normal or mildly elevated, in contrast to systemic polyarteritis nodosa), antineutrophil cytoplasmic antibody (ANCA) determination, and serologic testing for hepatitis B and C.

Treatment

- Treatment may be supportive with NSAIDs because mild cases often resolve spontaneously.
- Oral prednisone, typically starting at a dose of 40 mg/day with a rapid taper, is the most commonly used treatment. In many cases, after several weeks, the prednisone can be discontinued.
- Alternative treatments, including oral methotrexate (5–15 mg/week), mycophenolate mofetil (1 g PO bid), and azathioprine (50–100 mg/day), have all been used with success.

Clinical Course

Cutaneous polyarteritis nodosa is a relatively benign vasculitis that can usually be successfully brought into complete remission, although occasional cases may be recurrent. Fortunately, only rare cases transition into the more severe systemic polyarteritis nodosa.

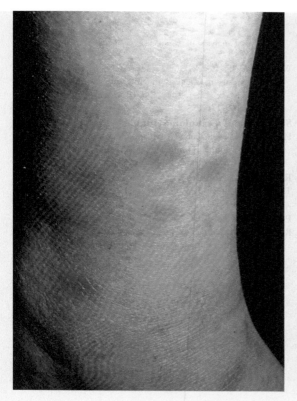

Fig. 15.19. Numerous tender, red, subcutaneous nodules of the lower leg and ankle in a patient with positive hepatitis B serology. (From the Fitzsimons Army Medical Center Collection, Aurora, CO.)

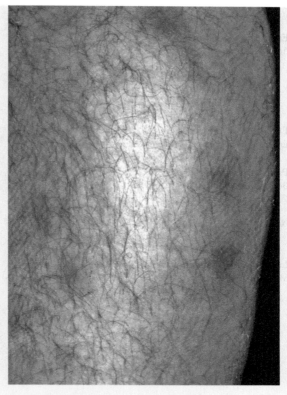

Fig. 15.20. Patient with numerous tender, red, subcutaneous nodules of the lower leg. Note that the most superior lesion has a linear configuration at the bottom pole, a clinical clue suggesting the diagnosis of cutaneous polyarteritis nodosa. (From the Fitzsimons Army Medical Center Collection, Aurora, CO.)

References

Erythema Nodosum

Anan T, Imamura T, Yokoyama S, Fujiwara S. Erythema nodosum and granulomatous lesions preceding acute myelomonocytic leukemia. *J Dermatol.* 2004;31:741-747.

Kakourou T, Drosatou P, Psychou F, et al. Erythema nodosum in children: a prospective study. *J Am Acad Dermatol.* 2001;44:17-21.

Erythema Induratum

Erythema nodosum and erythema induratum (nodular vasculitis): diagnosis and management. *Dermatol Ther.* 2010;23:320-327.

Pancreatic Panniculitis

Bogart MM, Milliken MC, Patterson JW, Padgett JK. Pancreatic panniculitis: associated with actinic cell adenocarcinoma: a case report and review of the literature. *Cutis.* 2007;80:289-294.

Woo SL, Kim MY, Kim SW, et al. Fatal pancreatic panniculitis associated with acute pancreatitis: a case report. *J Korean Med Sci.* 2007;22:914-917.

Lupus Erythematosus Panniculitis

Massone C, Kodama K, Salmhofer W, et al. Lupus erythematosus panniculitis (lupus profundus): clinical, histopathological, and molecular analysis of nine cases. *J Cutan Pathol.* 2005;32:396-404.

Weingartner JS, Zedek DC, Burkhart CN, Morrell DS. Lupus erythematosus panniculitis in children: report of three cases and review of previously reported cases. *Pediatr Dermatol.* 2012;29:169-176.

Subcutaneous Granuloma Annulare

Pimental DR, Michalany N, Milanes MA, et al. Multiple deep granuloma annulare limited to the cephalic segment in childhood. *Pediatr Dermatol.* 2008;25:407-408.

Rheumatoid Nodules

Tilstra JS, Lienesch DW. Rheumatoid nodules. *Dermatol Clin.* 2015;33:361-371.

Polyarteritis Nodosa

Rogalski C, Sticherling M. Panarteritis cutanea benigna—an entity limited to the skin or cutaneous presentation of a systemic necrotizing vasculitis? Report of seven cases and review of the literature. *Int J Dermatol.* 2007;46:817-821.

Chapter 16
Annular and Targetoid Lesions

Key Term
Erythema chronicum migrans

Annular and targetoid lesions are distinct clinical configurations that include many common disorders, such as dermatophyte infections, granuloma annulare, various reactive conditions, and even serious diseases (e.g., Lyme disease, leprosy).

Differential Diagnosis of Annular and Targetoid Lesions

Without Scale
- Actinic granuloma
- Borderline leprosy (can have scale)
- Erythema annulare centrifugum (see below)
- Erythema chronicum migrans
- Erythema multiforme
- Erythema marginatum
- Granuloma annulare
- Necrobiosis lipoidica
- Neonatal lupus erythematosus (can have scale)
- Subacute lupus erythematosus

With Scale
- Erythema annulare centrifugum (see above)
- Pityriasis rosea
- Seborrheic dermatitis (seborrhea petaloides)
- Tinea corporis, tinea cruris, tinea faciei
- Tuberculoid leprosy

IMPORTANT HISTORY QUESTIONS

How long have the lesions been present?

This question is useful in distinguishing among disorders that are typically acute, such as erythema migrans and erythema multiforme, and conditions that tend to be chronic, such as granuloma annulare, tuberculoid leprosy, and necrobiosis lipoidica.

Have you had a similar rash in the past?

Erythema multiforme, for example, tends to occur as repetitive episodes.

What medications do you take?

A medication history is important because erythema multiforme and erythema annulare centrifugum may be drug induced.

Where have you lived?

Leprosy is endemic to much of the world, including, in the United States, Texas and Louisiana.

Where have you been recently?

Travel to an area of the country where Lyme disease is endemic is important (see box).

Have you been camping outdoors or with animals?

Lyme disease is caused by a tick bite, and it is also useful to inquire directly about insect and arthropod bites.

Are you diabetic?

Necrobiosis lipoidica diabeticorum and, to a slightly lesser extent, granuloma annulare are both associated with diabetes.

Lyme Disease in the United States
In 2014, the Centers for Disease Control and Prevention (CDC) reported that 96% of all confirmed cases of Lyme disease were found in these 14 states:

Connecticut	New Jersey
Delaware	New York
Maine	Pennsylvania
Maryland	Rhode Island
Massachusetts	Vermont
Minnesota	Virginia
New Hampshire	Wisconsin

IMPORTANT PHYSICAL FINDINGS

Do the lesions demonstrate scale?

This is an important clinical feature because dermatophyte infections and erythema annulare centrifugum typically demonstrate scale, whereas granuloma annulare, erythema marginatum, and erythema migrans typically lack appreciable scale.

What is the distribution of the lesions?

Distribution is important because some diseases have a characteristic pattern. For example, necrobiosis lipoidica usually affects the pretibial surface, whereas erythema multiforme often involves distal acral skin. Symmetric distribution may also be more characteristic of a systemic reactive condition. Also, some diseases, such as actinic granuloma and neonatal lupus erythematosus, may be photodistributed.

Are there any mucosal lesions?

The presence of mucosal lesions (e.g., ocular, oral, genital) is an important finding in erythema multiforme.

Introduction

When dermatophytes affect glabrous skin, such as the face, groin, and trunk, annular lesions often result—hence, the common name, "ringworm." Dermatophyte infections are usually acquired from other humans but may also be acquired from other animals and from the soil. The three species most often associated with cutaneous infections in humans include *Trichophyton rubrum*, *Trichophyton mentagrophytes*, and *Epidermophyton floccosum*. Outbreaks may be seen among people in close contact, such as wrestling teams (tinea corporis gladiatorum) prisoners or persons who are institutionalized.

Clinical Features

- The primary lesion in dermatophyte infections is an erythematous annular plaque that is nearly always scaly (Figs. 16.1 and 16.2), particularly at the peripheral edge. The amount of scale is variable.
- Rarely, concentric annular lesions may resemble a topographic map.
- In tinea cruris (so-called jock itch), the lesions typically involve the inguinal crease and characteristically spare the scrotum (Fig. 16.3).
- A subset of patients may also demonstrate follicular lesions, especially if a topical corticosteroid has been used by the patient, causing localized immunosuppression.
- In rare cases, the peripheral edge may be pustular, or bullae may form (Fig. 16.4).

Diagnosis

- In many cases, the diagnosis may be strongly suspected on clinical grounds, but it is important to remember that even skilled dermatologists may mistake erythema annulare centrifugum, granuloma annulare, and even tuberculoid leprosy, for a dermatophyte infection.
- A potassium hydroxide (KOH) preparation, taken from the active edge of the lesion and examined by skilled persons, is diagnostic (see Chapter 2).
- A culture of scrapings from the active edge may also be diagnostic.
- The diagnosis may also be made by a skin biopsy, although clearly it is prudent not to perform a biopsy unless necessary. Also, a pathologist may miss the organism without use of special stains, so it is important for clinicians to indicate suspicion of a fungal infection on submission.

Treatment

- First-line treatment of uncomplicated dermatophyte infections of glabrous skin includes topical allylamines, such as terbinafine cream 1%, available over the counter, applied bid to affected areas for 1 week beyond any visible infection. This usually takes 2 to 3 weeks.
- Near-equivalence is seen with topical azoles (e.g., clotrimazole, miconazole) and ciclopirox olamine.
- Systemic therapy should be considered for patients with extensive or follicular involvement. Typically, oral terbinafine (250 mg/day for 7–14 days) or itraconazole (100–200 mg/day for 7–14 days) is used in these cases.
- Tinea infections among athletes may require evaluation of the entire team to prevent or mitigate a larger outbreak. Most cases are acquired by skin-to-skin contact, although rare cases may be acquired from fomites (e.g., wrestling mats). Fomites (e.g., headgear, padding) should be cleaned and not shared.
- Infected teams should be treated with oral medications, if possible, until the outbreak has been controlled.

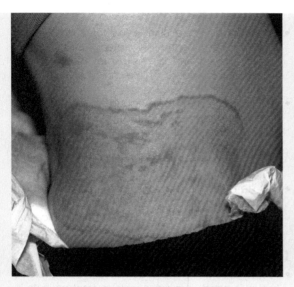

Fig. 16.1. Patient with tinea corporis, with highly inflammatory annular lesions. Note that a very early lesion is not yet annulare. (From the William Weston Collection, Aurora, CO.)

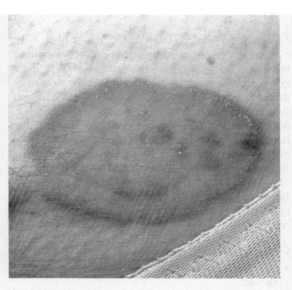

Fig. 16.2. Close-up of a lesion of tinea corporis. Note the trailing scale. The blood is the result of overzealous scraping for a potassium hydroxide (KOH) preparation.

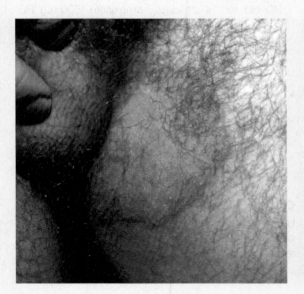

Fig. 16.3. Patient with classic case of tinea cruris, with an annular edge. Note that the scrotum is spared. (From the Fitzsimons Army Medical Center Collection, Aurora, CO.)

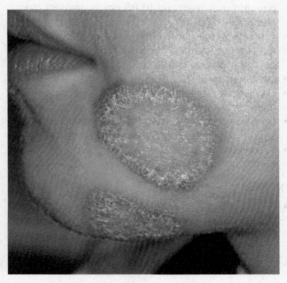

Fig. 16.4. Patient with tinea faciei presenting as annular lesions with marked induration and scale to the point that papulosquamous disease, such as psoriasis, is in the clinical differential diagnosis.

Pathogenesis

Lyme disease is a tickborne systemic infection caused by the spirochete, *Borrelia burgdorferi*. The most common vectors in the United States are the deer tick *(Ixodes scapularis)* and, in the western United States, the black-legged tick *(Ixodes pacificus)*. Although adults and nymphs may transmit the disease, the nymphs are more often the source of infection. Lyme disease has been reported in nearly every state, but a travel history is often involved (see box, above) outside of the East Coast, West Coast, or Great Lakes areas. Because of increased outdoor exposure during the summer months, children are affected more often than adults.

Clinical Features

- In many cases, history of a tick bite cannot be elicited.
- Skin lesions appear between 3 and 30 days after tick attachment, with an average of 9 days.
- The primary lesion is an annular ring of erythema, with variable induration (erythema chronicum migrans), which expands at a rate of 1 to 2 cm/day and may reach up to 60 cm in greatest diameter (Fig. 16.5).
- A small central papule that represents the tick bite may (or may not) be observed, which may give the appearance of a bull's eye (Fig. 16.6).
- Lesions may be pruritic.
- The primary lesion lasts up to 4 weeks and may become hemorrhagic (Fig. 16.7).
- Some patients may get one or more secondary smaller annular lesions (from spirochetemia).
- Associated constitutional findings include fever, lymphadenopathy, headache, and malaise.

Diagnosis

- An erythematous annular lesion after travel to a highly endemic area should raise suspicion of erythema migrans.

- Punch biopsy of a skin lesion for culture (modified Barbour-Stoenner-Kelly medium) is the only diagnostic test and is positive in about 75% of cases within 4 weeks. This technique is not widely available.
- Serologic screening tests include the enzyme-linked immunosorbent assay (ELISA), but immunoglobulin M (IgM) titers become positive after 30 days, and IgG titers become positive between 45 and 60 days; this is not the period in which the rash is observed.
- A 4- to 6-mm punch biopsy can manifest features that are consistent with but not only diagnostic of erythema migrans. In about one-third of cases, special stains may demonstrate the spirochete.

Treatment

- Prophylactic treatment of tick bites is controversial, but, at present, it is reasonable to treat patients in endemic areas with a single dose of doxycycline (200 mg) within 72 hours of a tick bite.
- Adults with suspected or documented erythema migrans are treated with doxycycline (100 mg PO bid for 14–21 days), amoxicillin (500 mg PO tid for 14–21 days), or cefuroxime axetil (500 mg bid for 14–21 days). Doxycycline is also effective against human granulocytic ehrlichiosis, which is a co-infection seen in about 10% of Lyme disease cases.
- Children with suspected or documented erythema migrans may be treated with doxycycline (100 mg PO bid for 14–21 days) if older than 9 years, amoxicillin (30–50 mg/kg per day for 14–21 days), erythromycin (30 mg/kg per day for 14–21 days), or phenoxymethylpenicillin (25–50 mg/kg per day for 14–21 days).

Clinical Course

Untreated erythema chronicum migrans can result in disseminated disease that may involve other organ systems.

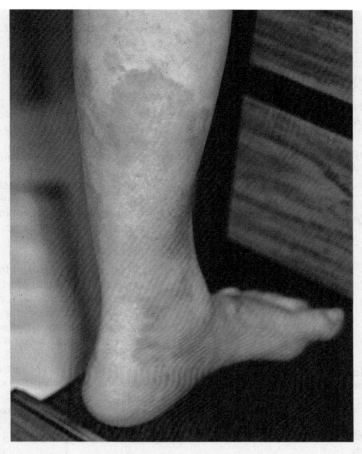

Fig. 16.5. Patient with large, irregular, annular lesion of the lower leg, with a small secondary lesion at the superior pole. (From the William Weston Collection, Aurora, CO.)

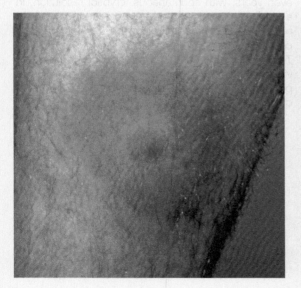

Fig. 16.6. Patient with annular lesion with central bull's eye that represents the site of the tick attachment. (From the Fitzsimons Army Medical Center Collection, Aurora, CO.)

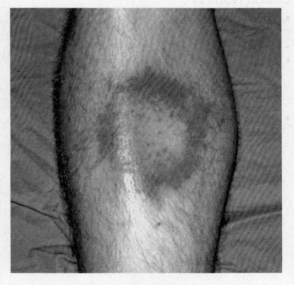

Fig. 16.7. Patient with hemorrhagic annular variant of erythema chronicum migrans. (From the Fitzsimons Army Medical Center Collection, Aurora, CO.)

Erythema Annulare Centrifugum ICD10 code L53.1

Pathogenesis

Erythema annulare centrifugum (EAC), like urticaria or erythema multiforme, is a reactive condition that can result from multiple immunologic stimuli or other systemic perturbations of homeostasis, even conditions such as pregnancy. The precise immunologic mechanism whereby it develops is not well understood.

Known Causes of Erythema Annulare Centrifugum

- Infections
  - Candidiasis
  - Dermatophyte infections
  - Viral infections (molluscum contagiosum, herpes zoster)
- Infestations
  - Ascariasis
  - Phthirus pubis
- Medications
  - Amitriptyline
  - Ampicillin
  - Antimalarials
  - Cimetidine
  - Finasteride
  - Gold
  - Hydrochlorothiazide
  - Nonsteroidal antiinflammatory drugs (NSAIDs)
  - Piroxicam
  - Thiacetazone
- Foods
  - Blue cheese (Penicillium)
- Internal malignancies
- Pregnancy

Clinical Features

- No predilection exists regarding gender, race, or age.
- Multiple lesions are usually present.
- Superficial variants of EAC present as annular or polycyclic lesions, with an erythematous edge and trailing scale, which extend in centrifugal fashion (Figs. 16.8 to 16.10).
- Deeper variants present as annular or polycyclic lesions, with an erythematous edge but without scale and with greater induration, which extend in centrifugal fashion (Fig. 16.11).
- Lesions may be asymptomatic or may produce variable pruritus.

Diagnosis

- In most cases, the clinical history and appearance are distinctive, and a clinical diagnosis may be rendered.
- In some cases, a 3- or 4-mm punch biopsy manifests histology that supports the diagnosis.
- Antinuclear antibody (ANA) testing should be considered as a screening measure because lupus erythematosus and other connective tissue diseases are in the differential diagnosis.

Treatment

- Identification and removal of the antigenic or systemic stimulus represents ideal management.
- Potent topical corticosteroids are usually of minimal benefit but may improve the appearance of the lesions while not affecting the overall clinical course.
- Case reports have documented an anecdotal response to topical calcipotriol.
- Oral antihistamines may relieve pruritus but do not alter the clinical appearance or course of the disease.
- In severe cases, oral hydroxychloroquine (200–400 mg/day) may produce a partial or complete remission over a period of 1 to 3 months.

Clinical Course

Lesions of EAC tend to last weeks to months, or even years, with spontaneous (cryptic) resolution. In a study of 66 cases, the mean duration for spontaneous resolution was found to be 2.8 years. Some cases may recur, even after spontaneous resolution. The most rapid and effective resolution can be provided if the underlying antigenic stimulant or systemic perturbation can be identified and avoided, mitigated, or treated.

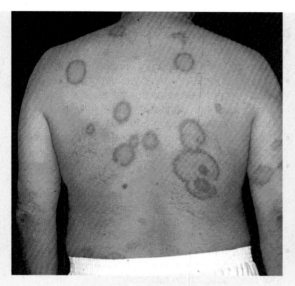

Fig. 16.8. Dramatic example of erythema annulare centrifugum demonstrating lesions within lesions in addition to arciform lesions.

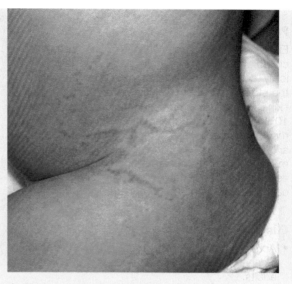

Fig. 16.9. Infant with erythema annulare centrifugum demonstrating incomplete annular lesions. (From the William Weston Collection, Aurora, CO.)

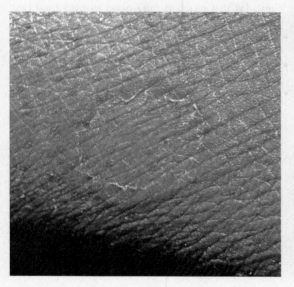

Fig. 16.10. Patient with superficial variant of erythema annulare centrifugum demonstrating the frequently present trailing scale. Note that the erythema is difficult to appreciate in darker skin.

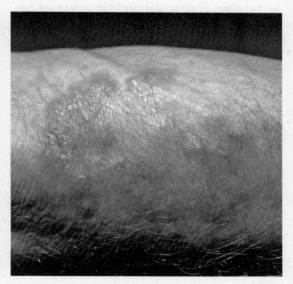

Fig. 16.11. Patient with deep variant of erythema annulare centrifugum, with incomplete annular lesions. Trailing scale is frequently absent in this clinical variant.

Pathogenesis

Erythema marginatum is a cutaneous finding associated with acute rheumatic fever. The lesions typically develop 7 days to months after the onset of the streptococcal pharyngitis or, rarely, streptococcal skin infections. Erythema marginatum occurs in about 10% cases of acute rheumatic fever. Although acute rheumatic fever is less common in the United States and other developed countries, it continues to be a major concern in underdeveloped countries, with an estimated 470,000 new cases occurring worldwide each year, causing 200,000 deaths.

Clinical Features

- Acute rheumatic fever is most common in children older than 3 years and in adolescents and young adults.
- Primary lesions are asymptomatic, erythematous, annular, or polycyclic wheal-like lesions (Figs. 16.12 to 16.14). Some patients may be unaware of the lesions at all.
- The lesions characteristically migrate rapidly (as fast as 2–10 mm in 12 hours), and this movement can be documented with use of permanent ink markers on the skin (see Figs. 16.12 and 16.13).
- Other primary lesions that may be present include erythematous macules (e.g., erythema circinatum), papular lesions (e.g., erythema papulatum), and subcutaneous nodules (e.g., rheumatic fever nodules).
- Lesions are most common on the trunk and proximal extremities and rarely involve the face.

Diagnosis

- Acute rheumatic fever should be excluded in anyone with unexplained migratory annular lesions.
- A recent or active β-hemolytic streptococcal infection or recent history of scarlet fever should raise suspicion of the diagnosis, particularly in children, adolescents, and young adults.
- The throat should be swabbed for testing with a rapid antigen detection test (RADT).
- Other tests that should be performed include throat culture, antistreptolysin O (ASO) titer, anti–deoxyribonuclease B study (these latter two studies may reflect past disease but not necessarily current disease), and electrocardiography, usually with a prolonged PR interval.
- A 3- or 4-mm punch biopsy from the active erythematous edge may reveal supportive histology but is not diagnostic or exclusionary.

Treatment

- Cutaneous lesions do not need to be treated. Rheumatic fever requires treatment that includes antibiotics, aspirin or other NSAIDs, and bed rest. Patients who fail this regimen may need to also take oral prednisone.
- Cardiac and central nervous system (CNS) manifestations must be treated.
- Initial antibiotics may include penicillin G benzathine, penicillin G procaine, and penicillin V and VK.
- Long-term management often includes 5 years or more of prophylactic antibiotics, which may include oral penicillin V or VK, oral erythromycin, or oral sulfadiazine, depending on the circumstances.

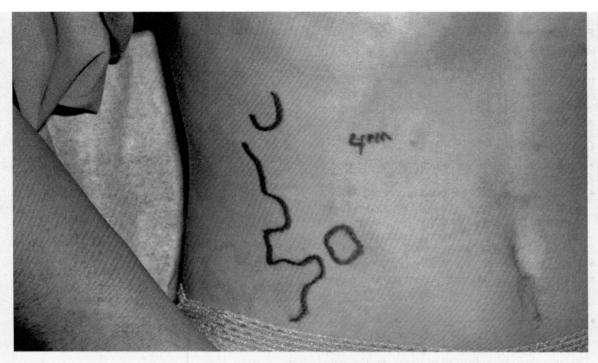

Fig. 16.12. Patient with erythema marginatum presenting as irregular red annular lesions on the trunk. Note that the margins have been marked to evaluate whether the lesions are migratory. The patient also has macular lesions, called erythema circinatum. (From the Fitzsimons Army Medical Center Collection, Aurora, CO.)

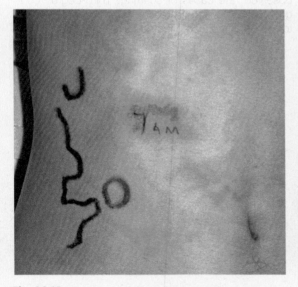

Fig. 16.13. Same patient as depicted in Fig. 16.12 15 hours later demonstrating the significant migration of the annular edges of the lesion.

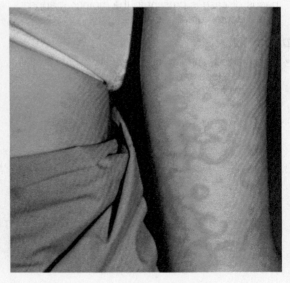

Fig. 16.14. Different patient with dramatic erythematous migratory lesions of erythema marginatum.

Neonatal Lupus Erythematosus

Pathogenesis

Neonatal lupus erythematosus (NLE) is a form of connective tissue disease caused by autoantibodies transmitted from the mother to the fetus. The antinuclear antibody that is invariably present is anti-Ro (anti-SSA) although, less commonly, anti-La (anti-SSB) antibodies may also be present.

Clinical Features

- Lesions may be present at birth or may develop in the first weeks of life.
- Primary lesions affect the head and neck, with the scalp and periocular area being most often involved, leading to a so-called "raccoon eyes" (Fig. 16.15) appearance. Less often, lesions occur on the trunk, extremities, or groin.
- The lesions may be photodistributed.
- Lesions may or may not manifest significant scale (Fig. 16.16) or may even be crusted (Fig. 16.17). Less often, the lesions may be hemorrhagic.
- Internal manifestations include congenital heart block, seen in up to 50% of cases (first-degree, second-degree, or third-degree), hepatobiliary disease, seen in up to 10% of cases, and hematologic manifestations (especially thrombocytopenia), seen in up to 10% of cases.
- The mothers usually appear normal but are positive for ANA–anti-Ro (anti-SSA) autoantibodies. If cutaneous disease is present in the mother, it appears as subacute cutaneous lupus erythematosus.

Diagnosis

- Unexplained annular erythema that preferentially affects the face and scalp of neonates should raise suspicion for the diagnosis.

- Unexplained congenital heart block, which may manifest as cardiomyopathy, hepatobiliary disease, or hematologic disease should mandate a comprehensive evaluation for NLE.
- Serologic testing for ANA–anti-Ro (anti-SSA) autoantibodies establishes the diagnosis.
- Other studies include electrocardiography (most important), liver function tests (LFTs), and complete blood count (CBC).
- A 3- or 4-mm punch biopsy from the active erythematous edge for H&E and direct immunofluorescent studies can be done. The results often support the diagnosis, but this is not usually required.

Treatment

- Skin lesions resolve without treatment, although a low-potency topical corticosteroid, such as hydrocortisone 1% or 2.5% for facial lesions, may be safely employed. Scarring is rare but has been reported by one of the authors (WAH).
- Avoidance of sun exposure is important to prevent the development of new lesions.
- Congenital heart block may require a pacemaker.

Clinical Course

The cutaneous lesions of neonatal lupus typically resolve over a period of weeks to months, with nearly all manifestations gone by 6 months. We have observed rare cases of scarring. Third-degree congenital heart block, if present, is permanent, and up to 20% of infants so affected have a fatal outcome.

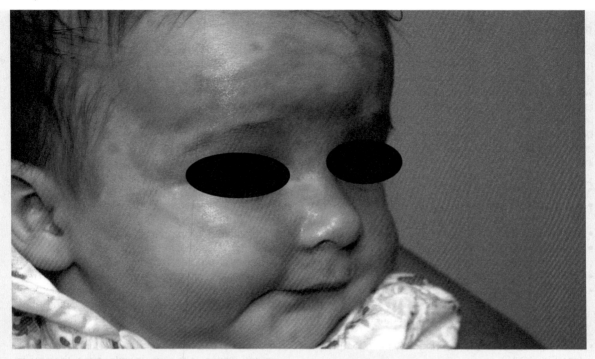

Fig. 16.15. Patient with characteristic raccoon facies of neonatal lupus erythematosus, with a distinct annulare edge without significant scale.

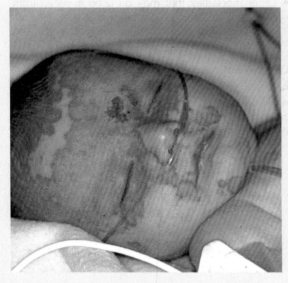

Fig. 16.16. Neonatal lupus erythematosus with scaly annular lesions extending on to the trunk. This patient also had a congenital heart block and hepatitis. (From the William Weston Collection, Aurora, CO.)

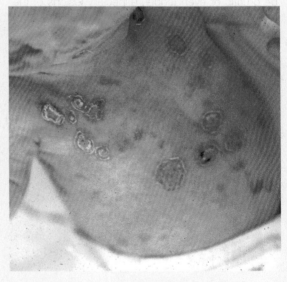

Fig. 16.17. Neonatal lupus erythematosus with scaly, crusted, annular lesions of the trunk in a neonate with cholestatic jaundice and thrombocytopenia. (From the William Weston Collection, Aurora, CO.)

Pathogenesis

Granuloma annulare (GA) is a granulomatous dermatitis of uncertain pathogenesis that leads to alteration or destruction of the collagen of the dermis, with increased mucin accumulation. The condition is usually associated with diabetes. Rarely patients may develop GA at sites of trauma (an octopus bite has done this!) or severe inflammation (herpes zoster). Familial clustering of GA suggests a genetic influence.

Clinical Features

- Most patients with GA are in the first 3 decades of life (age range, 3 months–88 years)
- GA is more common in women (F:M = 2.5 : 1)
- Lesions vary from one annular lesion to hundreds of lesions (disseminated or generalized GA).
- The fingers, hands, and feet are usually affected.
- Primary skin lesions are skin-colored to brownish (Fig. 16.18) to erythematous to violaceous (Fig. 16.19) smooth-topped papules, sometimes with an annular configuration.
- In some lesions, an annular ring may be incomplete (see Fig. 16.19).
- Scarring is not usually observed in the center of the lesion.
- Most patients are asymptomatic but some may be pruritic or even tender, especially lesions of the palms (Fig. 16.20). Palmoplantar lesions are more likely to have red and violaceous hues.
- Clinical variants include disseminated GA (≈5%–10% of cases), subcutaneous GA (see Chapter 15), photodistributed GA (Fig. 16.21), linear GA, and perforating GA, with umbilicated grouped papules with central crust or scale. Photodistributed GA may be difficult to differentiate from actinic granuloma, and some contend it is the same disease.

Diagnosis

- The history and appearance of the lesions are often so distinctive that the diagnosis may be rendered on clinical grounds.
- In occasional cases, a 3- or 4-mm punch biopsy is diagnostic.
- In patients with generalized GA, it is appropriate to consider screening to exclude diabetes mellitus.

Treatment

- No treatment is required because the condition is benign and typically asymptomatic.
- Potent topical corticosteroids are often used but are typically of minimal benefit.
- Corticosteroid-impregnated tape (e.g., Cordran tape) may be useful in select cases.
- Intralesional corticosteroids (e.g., triamcinolone, 1–5 mg/mL) is often a preferred treatment, with resolution expected in about 70% of lesions injected.
- Destructive liquid nitrogen cryotherapy is an option in small and superficial forms of the disease.
- Psoralen and ultraviolet A (PUVA) or narrow-band ultraviolet B (NB-UVB) can be used in severe generalized cases, although maintenance therapy is usually required. UVA penetrates the skin more deeply than UVB, and often PUVA yields a better response than NB-UVB.
- Other modalities that may be used in recalcitrant or extensive disease include hydroxychloroquine, potassium iodide, dapsone, cyclosporine, and chlorambucil.

Clinical Course

Approximately 50% of cases spontaneously clear within 2 years. About 40% of patients who do clear will experience one or more recurrences. Rare cases persist for decades or longer.

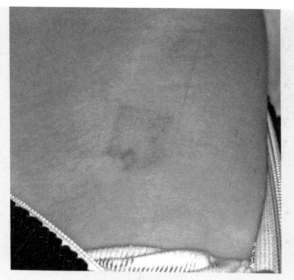

Fig. 16.18. Patient with typical yellow-brown annular lesion without scale or evidence of scarring in the center of the lesion. (From the William Weston Collection, Aurora, CO.)

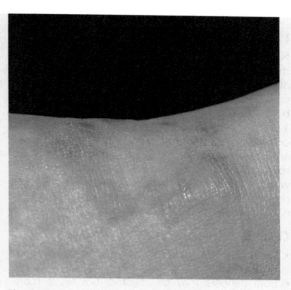

Fig. 16.19. Side view of a larger lesion of granuloma annulare with brownish and violaceous hues.

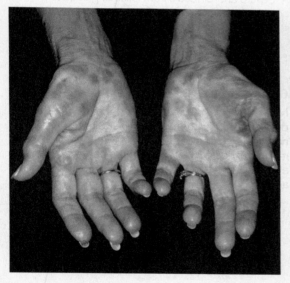

Fig. 16.20. Patient with red to reddish-brown papular lesions, with only several of the lesions being annular. These lesions were painful with pressure.

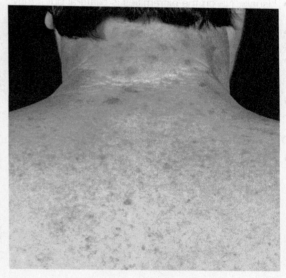

Fig. 16.21. Patient with photosensitive granuloma annulare confined to sun-exposed areas of the back of the neck and V of the chest. This presentation can be difficult to differentiate from actinic granuloma.

Pathogenesis

Necrobiosis lipoidica (NL) is a necrobiotic granulo-matous process, with degeneration of collagen that affects the entire dermis and may extend into the sub-cutis. The pathophysiology of the disease is unknown, but about two-thirds of cases are associated with type 1 or 2 diabetes. Moreover, about 50% of the remaining one-third of patients has an abnormal glucose toler-ance test. Some dermatologists refer to necrobiosis lipoidica as necrobiosis lipoidica diabeticorum (NLD) when evidence of diabetes is present. Although the disease is strongly associated with diabetes, NL is present in less than 1% of diabetics.

Clinical Features

- NL is most common in adults during the second, third, and fourth decades of life.
- Both genders may be affected, but NL is more common in women.
- The anterior pretibial surface is usually affected (Figs. 16.22 and 16.23), but rare cases may involve other areas of the body, including the face (Fig. 16.24) and scalp.
- Usually, NL on the extremities is bilateral but it may vary in degree.
- Early lesions begin as nondiagnostic red papules or plaques.
- Established lesions exist as annular plaques with red, red-brown, brown, or brown-yellow margins and central variable atrophy with telangiectasias.
- Ulceration is seen in about 25% of cases (Fig. 16.25).

Diagnosis

- The diagnosis of early NL may be difficult, but estab-lished lesions, particularly those in typical locations, like the pretibial surface, are clinically distinctive.

- A 4- to 6-mm punch biopsy from the active and erythematous edge, or even the center, is usually diagnostic. However, biopsy is often avoided, if possible, because such sites often heal poorly.
- Patients without a known medical history of diabe-tes should be evaluated for that disorder.

Treatment

- The role of diabetes management in NLD is con-troversial. Although some patients have reported improvement of NLD skin lesions with improved control of blood sugar levels, others have not seen such benefit.
- Cessation of smoking is helpful in some patients with NL (NLD).
- Although treatment of NL (NLD) is often difficult, early lesions can be improved with potent topical corticosteroids (with or without occlusion) and/or intralesional corticosteroids.
- Other treatment options include oral prednisone (with careful monitoring of the blood glucose level), mycophenolate mofetil, cyclosporine, clofazimine, and pentoxifylline.
- Severe and/or recalcitrant lesions, particularly those with ulceration, may be treated carefully with surgi-cal excision to the fascia, followed by split-thickness skin grafts.
- Sometimes phototherapy, particularly UVA-1 ther-apy, may be used by specialty dermatologists.

Clinical Course

NL (NLD) is a chronic disease and, once atrophy has developed, it is permanent. Ulcers in NL (NLD) are notoriously difficult to heal. It is important to have realistic expectations regarding the appearance of the affected skin, even if the disease process can be arrested.

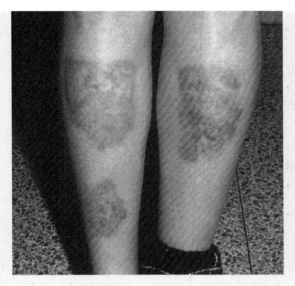

Fig. 16.22. Patient with characteristic pretibial, bilateral, annular plaques, with brown edges and yellowish brown centers. (From the Fitzsimons Army Medical Center Collection, Aurora, CO.)

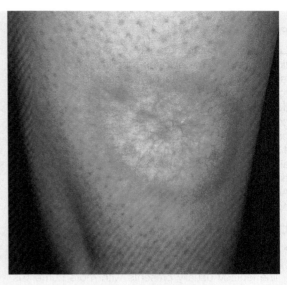

Fig. 16.23. Close-up of annular lesions demonstrating reddish-brown annular edges and centers, with telangiectasia and yellowish hues. (From the Fitzsimons Army Medical Center Collection, Aurora, CO.)

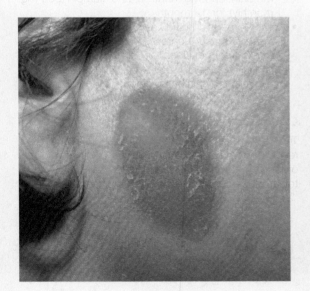

Fig. 16.24. Early lesion of necrobiosis lipoidica diabeticorum on the face of a patient with juvenile diabetes. The lesion is only vaguely annular, with early central atrophy. This patient also had a similar lesion in her scalp.

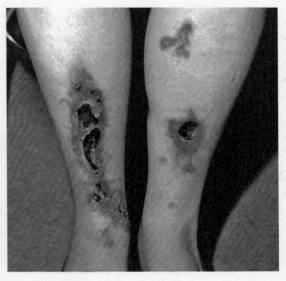

Fig. 16.25. Patient with severe ulcerative necrobiosis lipoidica diabeticorum of the anterior pretibial area. (From the Fitzsimons Army Medical Center Collection, Aurora, CO.)

Pathogenesis

Leprosy is a cutaneous and peripheral nerve infection caused by the acid-fast bacillus *Mycobacterium leprae.* It is believed to be transmitted from person to person primarily via the respiratory route, although the disease may also be contracted by people in contact with the nine-banded armadillo, common in parts of Texas and Louisiana. In 2014, there were 175 new cases reported in the United States, with almost 75% of cases being from Arkansas, California, Florida, Hawaii, Louisiana, New York, and Texas. Annular lesions are usually seen in the tuberculoid and borderline (dimorphic) forms of leprosy.

Clinical Features

- Tuberculoid leprosy is comprised of only one or a few cutaneous lesions at most, whereas borderline leprosy usually presents with more numerous lesions.
- Tuberculoid leprosy usually manifests an asymmetric distribution; borderline leprosy is usually rather symmetric.
- Tuberculoid and borderline leprosy cause a varied number red or red-brown annular lesions (Figs. 16.26 to 16.28). Variable overlying scale may be present.
- The lesion(s) of tuberculoid leprosy tend to be larger than the more numerous lesions of borderline leprosy.
- Lesions of tuberculoid leprosy typically often have central diminished sensation, but borderline leprosy may or may not demonstrate such loss. Perception of temperature is often the first sensation affected.
- Nerve enlargement occurs within or adjacent to skin lesions in both forms of leprosy.

Diagnosis

- Clinical suspicion is important, particularly in patients who are from endemic areas.

- Cutaneous anesthesia may be demonstrated by using a wisp of cotton from a cotton swab; however, it is often sensation of temperature that is first affected.
- Because the lesions of leprosy are not clinically diagnostic, a 3- to 6-mm punch biopsy from the annular edge is often necessary to establish the diagnosis. The organism can be demonstrated with a Fite stain.

Treatment

- New patients with leprosy should be reported to the appropriate local/state health agency.
- The World Health Organization has recommended the following treatments for adults with leprosy:
  - Single-lesion tuberculoid disease—one-time dosing of rifampicin (600 mg), ofloxacin (400 mg), and minocycline (100 mg).
  - Paucibacillary disease (including tuberculoid leprosy with a few lesions)—dapsone (100 mg daily), rifampin (600 mg monthly) for 6 months.
  - Multibacillary disease (including borderline leprosy)—dapsone (100 mg daily), clofazimine (50 mg daily, 300 mg monthly), and rifampin (600 mg monthly) for 12 months.
- Some experts, including those at the National Hansen Disease (Leprosy) Program, in Louisiana, prefer to treat paucibacillary disease for 12 months and multibacillary disease for 24 months. Often, minocycline or clarithromycin may be added to regimens or substituted for other drugs.

Clinical Course

Tuberculoid leprosy often remains stable and may resolve without treatment, whereas borderline forms of leprosy are not stable and, over time, may move toward tuberculoid or lepromatous poles of disease.

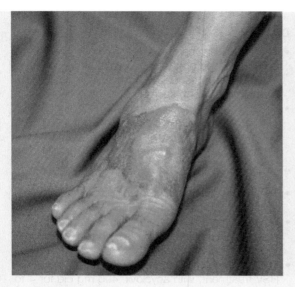

Fig. 16.26. Patient with tuberculoid leprosy demonstrating an annular lesion with scale.

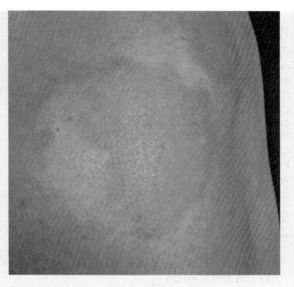

Fig. 16.27. Patient with borderline leprosy demonstrating two red annular lesions of the buttock. (From the Fitzsimons Army Medical Center Collection, Aurora, CO.)

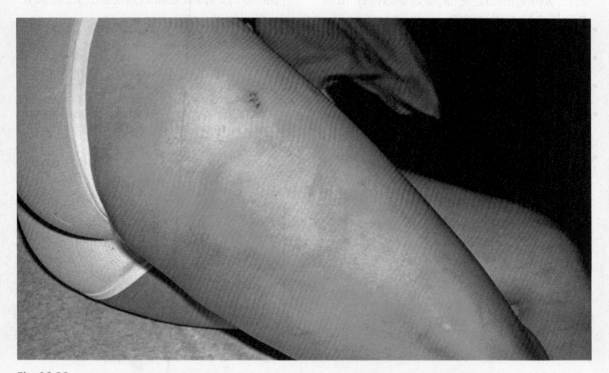

Fig. 16.28. Patient with borderline leprosy. Shown are large red annular lesions of the upper thigh in a patient who emigrated from Thailand. A biopsy site from a smaller nonannular red plaque is also shown. (From the Fitzsimons Army Medical Center Collection, Aurora, CO.)

Erythema Multiforme ICD10 code L51

Pathogenesis

Erythema multiforme (EM) is a mucocutaneous hypersensitivity reaction, with many precipitating causes, including infections (herpes simplex infection being most common), medications, and connective tissue disorders. In some cases, the precipitating event cannot be identified. Classically, EM has been divided into EM minor, which is a milder form of the disease, often associated with herpes simplex virus (HSV) infection, and EM major, which is usually associated with medications and is used synonymously with Stevens-Johnson syndrome (see Chapter 11).

Clinical Features

- EM usually affects distal acral skin, with the dorsal hands being the most often affected sites. The most common mucosal sites involved are the oral mucosa and genitalia.
- The primary lesion is a round macule that quickly develops one or more concentric zones of color change. EM lesions may have two zones of color and appear annular or may develop three zones of color, yielding the classic targetoid lesion (Fig. 16.29 and 16.30).
- Lesion size is variable, and some may be as small as 2 to 3 mm and some larger than 5 cm.
- One or more EM lesions may develop a central blister (see Chapter 11).
- Oral lesions usually present as ulcerations (Fig. 16.31).
- An isomorphic response may be present, with lesions developing at sites of sunburn (Fig. 16.32), trauma, or pressure.
- The lesions may be asymptomatic or may demonstrate mild burning and/or pruritus.

Diagnosis

- The diagnosis can usually be made on clinical grounds based on the appearance and distribution of the lesions, especially if there is an identifiable precipitating event, such as HSV infection.
- A 3- or 4-mm punch biopsy from an early lesion can be done to confirm the diagnosis if the case is unclear. Histologic findings, although not pathognomonic, usually strongly support the diagnosis.

Treatment

- Treat the infection (HSV, *Mycoplasma*) or withdraw suspected drugs.
- Because most cases are self-limited, mild disease may be treated with only supportive therapy or topical corticosteroids.
- For patients with recurrent EM minor, suppressive HSV treatment, with acyclovir, 400 mg bid for 4 to 12 months, is recommended, even if HSV cannot be firmly identified as a cause.
- Alternate therapies used for significant recurrent disease include oral corticosteroids, dapsone, hydroxychloroquine, azathioprine, and cyclosporine.

Clinical Course

Individual outbreaks of EM minor usually last 3 to 6 weeks, with some patients having postinflammatory hyperpigmentation at the sites of involvement. A subset of patients will have recurrent episodes of erythema multiforme, with many of these cases being attributable to recurrent HSV infections, even if subclinical in nature or unrecognized by the patient.

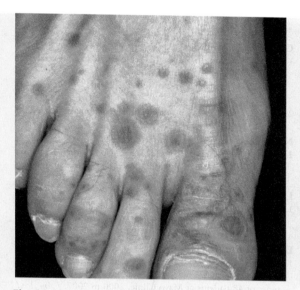

Fig. 16.29. Patient with classic targetoid lesions of erythema marginatum secondary to hydrochlorothiazide. (From the Fitzsimons Army Medical Center Collection, Aurora, CO.)

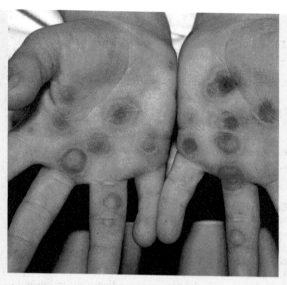

Fig. 16.30. Dramatic example of erythema marginatum of the palms secondary to herpes simplex infection. Some of the lesions are bullous.

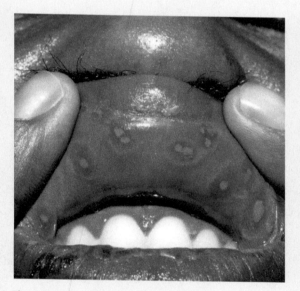

Fig. 16.31. Patient with resolving herpes labialis of the lower lip associated with oral erosive erythema marginatum. (From the Fitzsimons Army Medical Center Collection, Aurora, CO.)

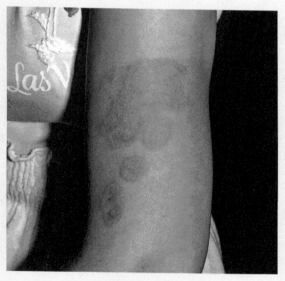

Fig. 16.32. Patient with photosensitive erythema marginatum, with both classic targetoid lesions and unusually large annular lesions demonstrating confluence. (From the Fitzsimons Army Medical Center Collection, Aurora, CO.)

References

Tinea Corporis, Tinea Faciei, and Tinea Cruris

1. Adams BB. Tinea corporis gladiatorum. *J Am Acad Dermatol.* 2002;47:286-290.
2. Patel GA, Widerkehr M, Schwartz RA. Tinea cruris in children. *Cutis.* 2009;84:133-137.

Lyme Disease

1. Montiel NJ, Baumgarten JA, Sinha AA. Lyme disease—Part II: clinical features and treatment. *Cutis.* 2002;69:443-448.

Erythema Annulare Centrifugum

1. Kim KJ, Chang SE, Choi JH, et al. Clinicopathologic analysis of 66 cases of erythema annulare centrifugum. *J Dermatol.* 2002;2:61-67.

Erythema Marginatum

1. Troyer C, Grossman ME, Silvers DN. Erythema marginatum in rheumatic fever: early diagnosis by skin biopsy. *J Am Acad Dermatol.* 1983;8:724-728.

Neonatal Lupus Erythematosus

1. Alkharafi NN, Alsaeid K, AlSumait A, et al. Cutaneous lupus erythematosus in children: experience from a tertiary care pediatric clinic. *Pediatr Dermatol.* 2016;33:200-208.
2. High WA, Costner MI. Persistent scarring, atrophy, and dyspigmentation in a preteen girl with neonatal lupus erythematosus. *J Am Acad Dermatol.* 2003;48:626-628.

Granuloma Annulare

1. Brey NV, Malone J, Callen JP. Acute-onset, painful acral erythema annulare. A report of 4 cases and a discussion of the clinical and histologic spectrum of the disease. *Arch Dermatol.* 2006;142:49-54.
2. Cyr PR. Diagnosis and management of granuloma annulare. *Am Fam Physician.* 2006;74:1729-1734.

Necrobiosis Lipoidica (Diabeticorum)

1. Reid SD, Ladizinski B, Lee K, et al. Update on necrobiosis lipoidica: a review of etiology, diagnosis, and treatment options. *J Am Acad Dermatol.* 2013;69:783-791.

Leprosy

1. Bruce S, Schroeder TL, Ellner K, et al. Armadillo exposure and Hansen's disease: an epidemiologic survey in southern Texas. *J Am Acad Dermatol.* 2000;43:223-238.

Erythema Multiforme

1. Wetter DA, Davis MDP. Recurrent erythema multiforme: clinical characteristics, etiologic associations, and treatment in a series of 48 patients at Mayo Clinic, 2000 to 2007. *J Am Acad Dermatol.* 2010;62:45-53.

Chapter 17
Linear and Serpiginous Lesions

Epidermal Nevus Syndrome
Nevus unius lateralis
Systemized epidermal nevus

Linear and serpiginous presentations of skin disease represent distinctive patterns that are so unique that a diagnosis can often be made without a biopsy or any further testing. In this short chapter, not all linear diseases may be discussed because many rare congenital disorders may present with linear configurations but would be beyond the scope of this practical discourse. It is also important to note that linear and serpiginous patterns should not be confused with sporotrichoid patterns of infection, which appear linear due to lymphatic spread. The sporotrichoid pattern is covered in Chapter 18.

IMPORTANT HISTORY QUESTIONS

Were the lesions present at birth or shortly after birth?

This is an important question because many linear conditions are congenital in nature and were present in the neonatal period (e.g., linear epidermal nevus, incontinentia pigmenti).

Is there a family history of a similar lesion?

In the appropriate clinical circumstances, an affirmative answer would support the diagnosis of incontinentia pigmenti, an X-linked dominant genetic disorder. However, it is important to note that a negative response does not exclude incontinentia pigmenti because spontaneous mutations are common.

How long have the lesions been present?

Some lesions persist for life (e.g., linear epidermal nevus), whereas others have a finite duration (e.g., lichen striatus).

What medications do you take?

This is an important question in patients for whom linear bleomycin-induced erythema or hyperpigmentation is suspected.

Is there a history of recent travel?

This question is designed to include or exclude cutaneous larva migrans. This condition is especially prevalent in the southeast United States and in other subtropical or tropical climates.

IMPORTANT PHYSICAL FINDINGS

What is the distribution of the lesions?

A distribution that follows the lines of Blaschko supports assessment of a linear epidermal nevus or other epithelial hamartoma, whereas cutaneous larva migrans is more common on acral skin.

What color are the lesions?

Linear epidermal nevi are often yellow-brown or brown, flagellate erythema due to bleomycin or cutaneous larva migrans is erythematous, and linear morphea may be white or yellow-white.

Do any lesions demonstrate vesicles or blisters?

Vesiculobullous lesions may be seen in incontinentia pigmenti or cutaneous larva migrans. Although not discussed in this chapter, allergic contact dermatitis may also demonstrate linear vesiculobullous lesions.

Does the lesion demonstrate induration on palpation?

Linear morphea is characterized by marked induration due to thickening of the collagen.

What Are the Lines of Blaschko?

There is no easy answer because the lines of Blaschko do not conform to any known anatomic features. Instead, the lines of Blaschko are somewhat circularly defined as lines that congenital linear abnormalities follow. It has been suggested that the lines are due to cutaneous mosaicism of different clones of cells.

Pathogenesis

Lichen striatus is an uncommon, self-limited dermatosis, of unknown cause; it affects mostly children. Some studies have suggested a more frequent personal or familial atopic diathesis in affected patients.

Clinical Features

- Some studies have reported a slight female preponderance, whereas others studies have reported that both genders are equally affected.
- Most cases occur in preschool children, with a mean age of 3 years, but the condition can also occur in adolescents and young adults as well.
- A unilateral (and rarely bilateral) eruption affects the lower limbs (one-third of cases), followed by the upper limbs, trunk and, rarely, the face (~10%).
- The eruption begins as discrete skin-colored, pink, or red papules (Fig. 17.1), with variable overlying scale. In darker skin types, the condition may appear hyperpigmented (Fig. 17.2) or hypopigmented.
- Less often, the condition may resemble lichen planus or psoriasis.
- Lesion are grouped as continuous or discontinuous lines that generally follow the lines of Blaschko (see box), with some cases manifesting more than one parallel line of involvement (Fig. 17.3).
- Typically, the condition is asymptomatic, but it may be pruritic in about 10% of cases.
- Rare patients may demonstrate extension to a contiguous fingernail or toenail, with onychodystrophy manifesting as thinning, splitting, longitudinal ridging, or onycholysis (Fig. 17.4).

Diagnosis

- The history and clinical appearance are usually diagnostic.
- A skin biopsy is not usually required, but, if the presentation is atypical, a biopsy may be performed. The histologic findings will support the diagnosis, but exclusive pathognomonic findings do not exist.

Treatment

- Reassurance is usually all that is necessary because the condition is self-limited and typically disappears in weeks or months (rarely years), without permanent sequelae.
- Weak to midstrength topical steroids may be used for pruritus.

Clinical Course

The mean duration of disease is 6 to 9 months; however, rare patients may have lesions for up to 3 years. Hypopigmentation may persist for months, even after the lesion resolves. Rare patients may suffer a relapse or even multiple relapses.

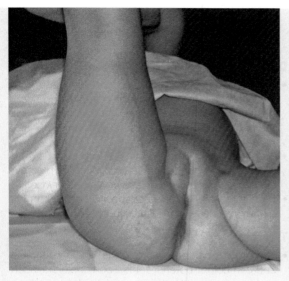

Fig. 17.1. Patient with early lesions of lichen striatus composed of red linear papules. (From the William Weston Collection, Aurora, CO.)

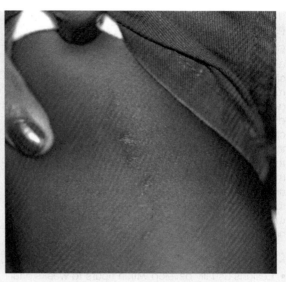

Fig. 17.2. Patient with linear lesions of lichen striatus on the upper thigh demonstrating subtle hyperpigmentation.

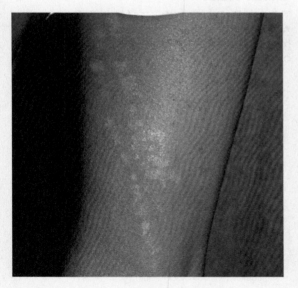

Fig. 17.3. Patient with hypopigmented lichen striatus with two parallel linear lesions following the lines of Blaschko.

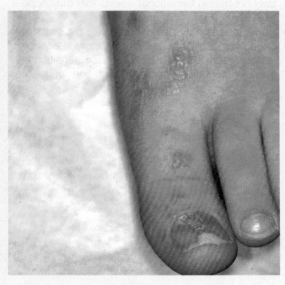

Fig. 17.4. Patient with unusually indurated red linear papules, with associated nail dystrophy. (From the William Weston Collection, Aurora, CO.)

Bleomycin-Induced Flagellate Erythema and Hyperpigmentation

ICD10 code Y43.1

Pathogenesis

Bleomycin is a chemotherapeutic agent that produces a distinct skin eruption with linear erythema that transitions into linear hyperpigmentation. It is most commonly seen at higher cumulative doses, usually in the range of 90 to 285 mg; however, some patients may develop this reaction with the first dose. There is no clear consensus as to how often this adverse reaction transpires, with a reported range in the literature of 6% to 66% of patients who have received the drug. The mechanism whereby the linear lesions are produced is uncertain, but it has been postulated that it is related to scratching because affected patients report pruritus. Attempts to induce lesions with superficial trauma have not always been successful.

Clinical Features

- Lesions usually develop within hours to weeks after taking bleomycin.
- Primary lesions present as linear erythema, with pruritus (Fig. 17.5).
- The lesions transition, usually over days or weeks, into linear hyperpigmented lesions, with some patients having transitional lesions that may appear violaceous (Figs. 17.6 and 17.7).
- Some lesions may demonstrate variable scale.
- Other less distinctive lesions may include erythema over pressure points, which can also transition into hyperpigmentation, hyperpigmentation of palmar and flexural creases, and hyperpigmentation of striae distensae (stretch marks).

Diagnosis

- Early lesions may be difficult to differentiate from dermatographism, but dermatographism usually resolves within hours, whereas the flagellate erythema of bleomycin persists for an extended duration.
- The presence of linear erythema with pruritus and/or hyperpigmentation in a patient receiving bleomycin is a drug eruption, unless proven otherwise.
- Biopsy typically reveals nonspecific findings and is usually not needed to establish the diagnosis.

Treatment

- The pruritus can be managed with an antihistamine and/or medium-potency topical corticosteroid, such as triamcinolone. Sedating antihistamines, such as diphenhydramine, are useful at bedtime.
- No treatment is reasonable if the patient is comfortable and unconcerned.

Clinical Course

This condition represents a self-limited drug reaction. Although the erythema subsides within days, the hyperpigmentation may persist for weeks or months before gradually fading.

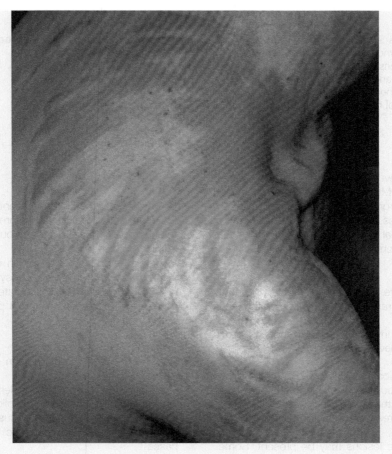

Fig. 17.5. Patient with characteristic flagellate areas of a pruritic erythema produced by bleomycin.

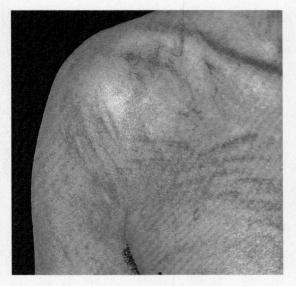

Fig. 17.6. Patient with intermediate lesions induced by bleomycin, with variable erythema, hyperpigmentation, and a focally violaceous hue.

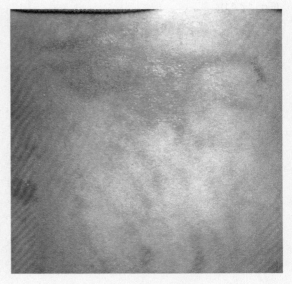

Fig. 17.7. Patient with typical flagellate hyperpigmentation weeks after receiving bleomycin. Note that there is also focal subtle scaling.

Epidermal Nevus Syndrome

Epidermal nevus syndrome consists of an epidermal nevus (usually extensive), with associated skeletal, neurologic, ocular, and cardiac abnormalities. Central nervous system abnormalities are more common when the epidermal nevus involves the head and neck.

Pathogenesis

Linear epidermal nevus (epidermal nevus) is a localized genetic disorder (OMIM 162900) that is characterized as a localized overgrowth of epithelium in a pattern that follows the lines of Blaschko. About one-third of those with epidermal nevi have *FGFR3* mutations that are also found in some seborrheic keratoses.

Clinical Features

- Epidermal nevi are usually present at birth or shortly after birth, but rare cases may present in early adulthood.
- The lesions may involve any part of the skin.
- Once a lesion develops, it may gradually enlarge over years.
- The primary lesion is a yellow-brown to brown aggregate of papules, with variable scale and verrucous features that follow the lines of Blaschko. So-called skip areas are often present (Figs. 17.8 and 17.9).
- Single or multiple lesions may be present. Sometimes, the process involves half of the body (nevus unius lateralis; Fig. 17.10) or nearly the entire body (systemized epidermal nevus).
- Rare cases may involve the oral mucosa (Fig. 17.11).

Linear Malformations of Childhood: Differential Diagnosis

- Goltz syndrome
- Linear adnexal tumors
- Linear Darier disease
- Linear epidermal nevus
- Linear porokeratosis
- Nevus comedonicus
- Nevus sebaceus

Diagnosis

- In most cases, the clinical presentation is diagnostic. Other congenital linear malformations can be in the clinical differential diagnosis but are not covered in this text (see box).
- In problematic cases, the lesion may be biopsied with a 3- to 6-mm punch biopsy. Shave biopsies are not adequate to differentiate epidermal nevi from some of the other clinical possibilities listed in the box.

Treatment

- Because the condition is benign, treatment is not required.
- Surgical excision is a consideration for select lesions. However, the cost, complications, and cosmetic appearance of the scar must be considered.
- Laser ablation is a therapeutic option in some cases.
- Topical therapies that may improve the clinical appearance include ammonium lactate, 12%; calcipotriene ointment or cream, 0.005%; and tazarotene cream, 0.1%.

Clinical Course

Linear epidermal nevi may remain stable or may enlarge gradually, over a period of years or decades.

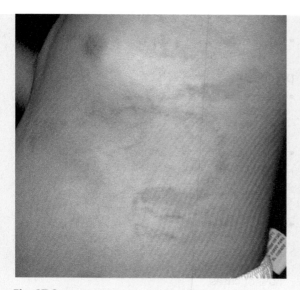

Fig. 17.8. Subtle light brown linear epidermal nevus in a young child that follows the lines of Blaschko.

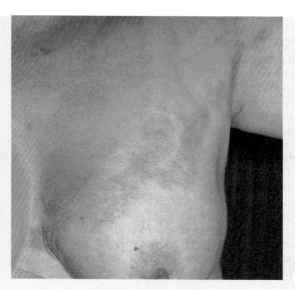

Fig. 17.9. Yellow-brown linear epidermal nevus in a woman. (From the Fitzsimons Army Medical Center Collection, Aurora, CO.)

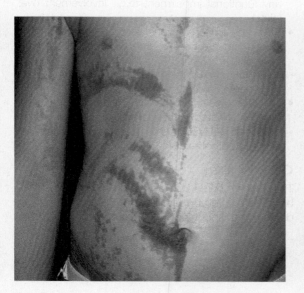

Fig. 17.10. Extensive dark brown papillomatous epidermal nevus involving half of the body in a child. This variant is often termed *nevus unius lateralis.*

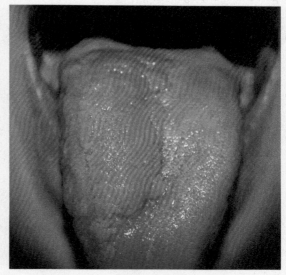

Fig. 17.11. Close-up of a patient with a markedly papillomatous linear epidermal nevus of the tongue.

Pathogenesis

Morphea, also known as localized scleroderma, is a disorder characterized by thickening of the collagen in the dermis and, to a lesser degree, in the subcutaneous tissue and rarely into the fascia. The pathogenesis is not understood; however, there is evidence to support that this is a limited form of an autoimmune connective tissue disease. Some cases in Europe have been associated with infection by *Borrelia* spp. There are several clinical presentations of morphea, including linear presentations that are discussed here. Linear presentations account for about 50% or more of childhood cases and 15% of adult cases. Some cases of linear morphea may demonstrate clinical and histologic features of overlying lichen sclerosus et atrophicus (LS&A); the relationship between these two disorders is not clear.

Clinical Features

- Studies have reported a modest female preponderance in morphea, with most cases occurring in children, adolescents, and young adults, although persons of any age may be affected.
- Lesions are usually linear, solitary, and unilateral, but multiple lesions can occur (Figs. 17.12–17.14).
- Lesions are usually asymptomatic, but some patients may manifest pruritus, or even pain or discomfort, particularly in lesions that cross joint spaces.
- The primary lesion is usually a skin-colored to violaceous area of induration. Many lesions demonstrate a violaceous color at the periphery.
- As lesions evolve, the color may vary from violaceous to hyperpigmented to white or yellow-white. Often, more than one color may be present in the same lesion.
- Established lesions can manifest epidermal atrophy and may be shiny, with fine wrinkling.

- Lesions that cross a joint may impair function and produce contractures (see Fig. 17.14).

Diagnosis

- The diagnosis is usually established on clinical grounds, based on the presence of a linear lesion with marked induration on palpation. White lesions may be difficult to differentiate from LS&A.
- In problematic cases, a 4- to 6-mm punch or incisional biopsy, which includes subcutaneous tissue, will generally be diagnostic, as long as the clinical suspicion of morphea is communicated to the pathologist or dermatopathologist.
- Laboratory tests that may be helpful include a complete blood count (CBC; often a peripheral eosinophilia may be present) and a screening antinuclear antibody (ANA) test, positive in a low titer in about 50% of cases.

Treatment

- The treatment used is dependent on the patient's age, site and extent of involvement, and degree of any functional impairment (e.g., involvement over joints).
- Small or limited lesions without any functional impairment are best treated with topical calcipotriene, 0.005% ointment, bid for 2 to 4 months, with or without occlusion, or tacrolimus, 0.1% bid for 2 to 4 months, with or without occlusion.
- Larger lesions or lesions with functional impairment are best treated with phototherapy (narrow-band ultraviolet B [UVB] or UVA-1), systemic corticosteroids, or methotrexate.

Clinical Course

The clinical course in any individual patient may not be predicted reliably, but about 50% of patients will demonstrate spontaneous remission within 5 years.

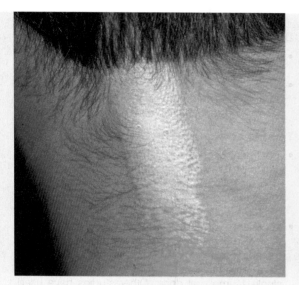

Fig. 17.12. Linear morphea of the back of the neck, with white lichen sclerosus et atrophicus–like hypopigmentation.

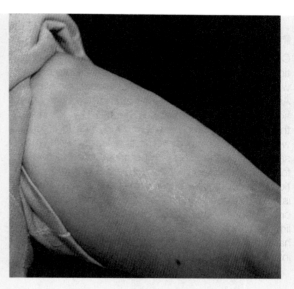

Fig. 17.13. Patient with hyperpigmentation and hypopigmentation in linear morphea of the upper thigh and lower leg. (From the William Weston Collection, Aurora, CO.)

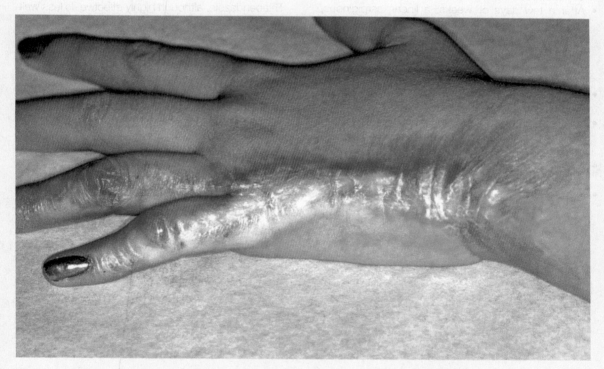

Fig. 17.14. Patient with end-stage linear morphea, with shiny epidermal atrophy that has produced a contracture across the hand. (From the Joanna Burch Collection, Aurora, CO.)

Pathogenesis

Cutaneous larva migrans is a so-called creeping eruption that occurs when human skin comes into contact with soil containing viable larva of animal hookworms. *Ancylostoma braziliense* (the cat and dog hookworm) accounts for 95% of cases. In the United States, the highest incidence is seen in Florida and Georgia, where humans have frequent contact with moist sandy soil. Sandboxes are notorious sites of contact for young children, and beaches are common locations for contact for children and adults. The disease is also an occupational hazard for individuals who crawl under houses (e.g., plumbers). The disease is limited to the skin because the larval worms do not have the proper collagenase enzymes to penetrate into the deeper zones of human skin.

Clinical Features

- Common sites of involvement include the dorsal feet and interdigital spaces between the toes.
- A pruritic papule or dermatitis develops at the site of penetration within one hour.
- After a few days or weeks, a linear, serpiginous, slightly indurated, erythematous tract develops as the larva migrates. Usually, the tract is 2 to 4 mm wide, with some lesions being bullous (Figs. 17.15–17.18). The number of burrows may vary from 1 to a record of 2100 burrows in one patient.
- Rarely, larvae may track down a hair follicle and produce follicular lesions.
- Larvae migrate several millimeters a day. Larvae are 1 to 2 cm ahead of the perceptible end of the lesion.
- Additional manifestations include peripheral eosinophilia and, rarely, Loeffler syndrome.
- In rare cases, a secondary bacterial infection, including streptococcal cellulitis, may develop.

Diagnosis

- The clinical appearance and migratory nature of the burrow (creeping) is distinctive, facilitating diagnosis.
- Biopsy of a burrow demonstrates an eosinophilic infiltrate and a burrow just above the basement membrane zone, but larva are rarely seen on biopsy.

Treatment

- Treatment of choice for limited disease is the application of 10% to 15% liquid thiabendazole suspension or 10% to 15% topical thiabendazole cream (prepared by a compounding pharmacy), applied qid for 1 week (98% success rate in one study).
- In patients with extensive lesions or lesions on the thick skin of the sole, and/or who have failed topical therapy, oral ivermectin is the treatment of choice. Cure rates have varied from 77% to 100% with a single 12-mg oral dose. Other studies have used 200 mg/kg for 3 to 7 days.
- Other oral treatment options include albendazole (400 mg qd in a 1-, 3-, or 5-day regimen) and thiabendazole (50 mg/kg per day in a single dose for 2–4 days), with a 99% cure rate in one study. Thiabendazole, although highly effective, is less well tolerated than ivermectin or albendazole and should be utilized only when the other options are not available.
- Older references have indicated liquid nitrogen cryotherapy as a treatment, to be applied to the advancing edge of the burrow, but because the organism is always present before the visible body reaction, this therapy has a high failure rate, and we do not recommend its use.

Clinical Course

The disease is self-limited, and most larvae die within 2 to 8 weeks—81% of all larvae are dead at 4 weeks. Rare larvae may persist up to 1 year or longer.

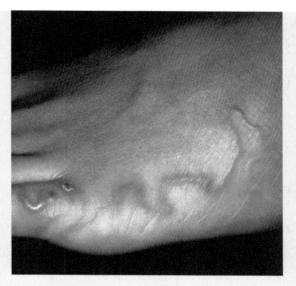

Fig. 17.15. Patient with linear larval burrow on the toe and top of the foot. Note the linear blister at the leading edge. (From the Fitzsimons Army Medical Center Collection, Aurora, CO.)

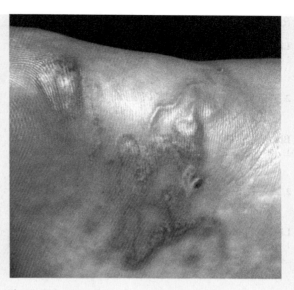

Fig. 17.16. Patient with convoluted linear burrows on the bottom of the foot. (From the Fitzsimons Army Medical Center Collection, Aurora, CO.)

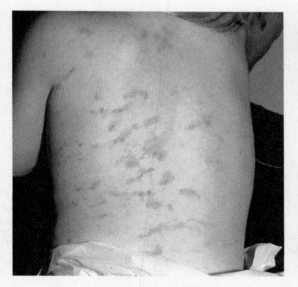

Fig. 17.17. Child with numerous older burrows present for 4 weeks that had been treated as a dermatitis by both the emergency room clinician and her pediatrician. (From the Fitzsimons Army Medical Center Collection, Aurora, CO.)

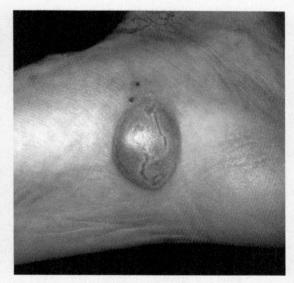

Fig. 17.18. Patient with atypical bullous lesion on the instep of the foot. Careful observation of the lesion demonstrates the serpiginous burrow within the blister.

References

Lichen Striatus

1. Kim M, Jung HY, Eun YS, et al. Nail lichen striatus: report of seven cases and review of the literature. *Int J Dermatol.* 2015;54:1255-1260.
2. Patrizi A, Neri I, Fiorentini C, et al. Lichen striatus: clinical and laboratory features of 115 children. *Pediatr Dermatol.* 2004;21:197-204.

Bleomycin-Induced Erythema and Hyperpigmentation

1. Khmamouchne MR, Debbagh A, Mahfoud T, et al. Flagellate erythema secondary to bleomycin: a new case report and review of the literature. *J Drugs Dermatol.* 2014;13:983-984.
2. Lee HY, Lim KH, Ryo Y, Song SY. Bleomycin-induced flagellate erythema: a case report and review of the literature. *Oncol Lett.* 2014;8:933-935.

Linear Epidermal Nevus

1. Chatproedprai S, Wananukul S, Prasarnnaem T, Noppakun N. Epidermal nevus syndrome. *Int J Dermatol.* 2007;46:858-860.

2. Hafner C, Hartmann A, Vogt T. *FGFR3* mutations in epidermal nevi and seborrheic keratoses: lessons from urothelium and skin. *J Invest Dermatol.* 2007;127:1572-1573.

Linear Morphea

1. Mazori DR, Wright NA, Patel M, et al. Characteristics and treatment of adult-onset linear morphea: a retrospective cohort study of 61 patients in 3 tertiary care centers. *J Am Acad Dermatol.* 2016;74:577-579.
2. Zwischenberger BA, Jacobe HT. A systematic review of morphea treatments and therapeutic algorithm. *J Am Acad Dermatol.* 2011;65:925-941.

Cutaneous Larva Migrans

1. Prickett KA, Ferringer TC. What's eating you? Cutaneous larva migrans. *Cutis.* 2015;95:126-128.
2. Richey TK, Gentry RH, Fitzpatrick JE, et al. Persistent cutaneous larva migrans due to *Ancylostoma* species. *South Med J.* 1996;89:609-611.

Chapter 18
Sporotrichoid Disorders

Sporotrichoid disorders, sometime also termed *nodular lymphangitis,* are defined as nodular abscesses that spread along lymphatics, away from a primary inoculation site. Streaking erythema, along lymphatics, may or may not be present. As the name implies, sporotrichosis is a fungal infection that serves as the prototype for the sporotrichoid presentation pattern.

IMPORTANT HISTORY QUESTIONS

Have you had any recent injuries to your skin?

This is an important question because most sporotrichoid infections of the skin are associated with cutaneous inoculation injury. The classic (overrated) question is "Have you been working in a rose garden?" However, although rose gardening is a potential source of exposure for sporotrichosis, it is not the only way to acquire the infection.

Do you own cats, or have you been exposed to cats?

Cats are the animals most often infected with sporotrichosis, and the scratch of an infected cat can lead to infection. Veterinarians are at particular risk of this infection.

Have you had any fever or chills?

This is an attempt to gauge if there is any evidence of systemic infection.

Do you have any other medical problems?

This question can reveal important clinical information including whether the patient is immunocompromised.

Have you traveled outside of the United States?

Sporotrichosis and atypical mycobacterial infections are ubiquitous in the United States; nocardiosis is common in Mexico. Leishmaniasis requires travel to an endemic area for infection to develop.

Have you had a recent pedicure?

This is an important question if the patient has a suspected infection on the lower extremities, because pedicures represent an important source of mycobacterial infection.

Differential Diagnosis of Sporotrichoid Reactions

Common
- Sporotrichosis
- Atypical mycobacterial infection

Uncommon
- Anthrax
- Nocardiosis
- Leishmaniasis
- Mycetoma
- Staphylococcal abscesses
- Tuberculosis
- Tularemia

IMPORTANT PHYSICAL FINDINGS

What is the distribution of the lesions?

Sporotrichoid infections are unilateral, unless disseminated, and follow a single lymphatic drainage basin. There are only rare exceptions to this rule, with the most common being atypical mycobacterial infections due to pedicures, in which bilateral exposure to contaminated water leads to bilateral infection.

Does there appear to be a lesion that represents a primary point of trauma?

The location of the primary lesion may suggest a potential diagnosis. Lesions on the hand are usually associated with gardening, which favors sporotrichosis. Lesions on the leg, especially in those who get pedicures, suggest a potential atypical mycobacterial infection. Such observations are useful in guiding empiric therapy while awaiting biopsy or culture results.

Are there any lesions outside of the lymphatic drainage basin?

Patients with sporotrichoid skin lesions may suffer dissemination, potentially with life-threatening systemic disease. Dissemination requires aggressive therapy, possibly with hospital admission and consultation with infectious disease specialists.

Pathogenesis

Sporotrichosis is due to a localized infection of the skin by the dimorphic fungus *Sporothrix schenckii*, a ubiquitous saprophytic fungus found in decaying vegetation (e.g., hay, sphagnum peat moss, wood, soil). The organism is found nearly worldwide, in temperate, subtropical, and tropical environs. The fungus is usually introduced into the skin via local injury, such as a thorn prick—hence, the classic question as to whether the patient works in a rose garden. Although many animal species can be infected, cats are notoriously susceptible and may infect humans directly by scratching. Although most sporotrichosis produces a sporotrichoid clinical pattern of infection (~80% of cases), fixed cutaneous infection (10%–15% of cases), disseminated infection, and pulmonary infection can also occur.

Clinical Presentation

- The initial lesion, usually found on extremities, especially the hand, is a tender erythematous papule that usually appears 1 to 3 weeks after the injury.
- The inoculation site often erodes or ulcerates or, more rarely, becomes verrucous or ulcerated.
- Secondary lesions consisting of erythematous nodules or abscesses appear along ascending lymphatics (nodular lymphangitis) en route to regional lymph nodes (Figs. 18.1–18.3).
- The secondary lesions may have no epidermal changes, may ulcerate or, even more rarely, demonstrate verrucous changes.
- Variable lymphadenopathy in the regional lymph nodes is present.

Diagnosis

- A sporotrichoid pattern of infection is suggestive of sporotrichosis; however, this pattern is mimicked by atypical mycobacterial infections and, less commonly, by other infections.

- An incisional biopsy or punch biopsy (4 mm at a minimum, preferably 6 mm), bisected, with half being sent for H&E and special staining and half being sent for fungal and acid-fast bacterial cultures, is useful in establishing the diagnosis.

Treatment

- Oral itraconazole (200–400 mg qd for adults) or 3 to 6 mg/kg per day for children), for 3 to 4 months, is the treatment of choice based on efficacy, tolerability, and ease of administration. Some patients may require up to 6 months of therapy.
- Oral terbinafine (500 mg bid) for 3 to 4 months is an alternative treatment.
- Supersaturated potassium iodide (SSKI) has been commonly used, with the primary advantage of affordability. However, administration is inconvenient, and many patients experience side effects. It is typical to begin with five drops SSKI, in orange juice, tid, with increases in the numbers of drops every 1 to 3 days, until a dose of 10 to 20 drops tid is achieved. This treatment should *not* be used in those with thyroid disease.
- Because the organism is heat sensitive, and it sustains irreversible damage at temperatures in excess of 42C (107.6 F), topical heat therapy is sometimes employed. Patients can be treated with hot baths or heating pads in those rare circumstances (e.g., pregnancy) for which oral therapy is not an option.

Clinical Course

Most cases of fixed and lymphocutaneous sporotrichosis will resolve spontaneously, even without treatment, but this can take many months. Also, untreated cutaneous sporotrichosis is always at risk to disseminate, particularly if clinical circumstances lead to diminished immunity.

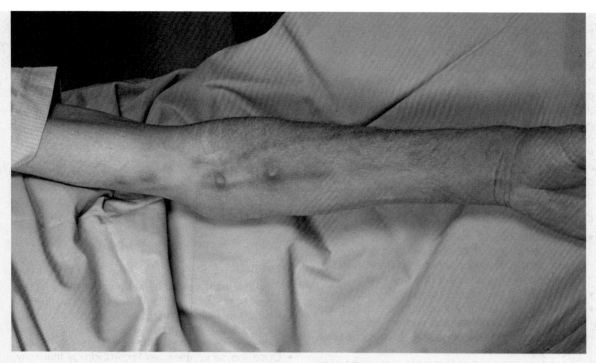

Fig. 18.1. Patient with classic sporotrichosis demonstrating lymphatic abscesses and lymphangitis. The inoculation site on the hand is not visible. (From the Fitzsimons Army Medical Center Collection, Aurora, CO.)

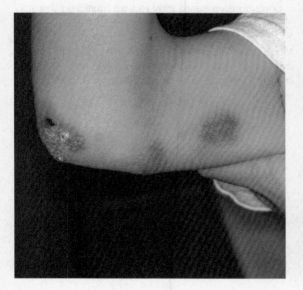

Fig. 18.2. Primary inoculation site on the elbow associated with sporotrichoid lesions of the inner arm. (From the Fitzsimons Army Medical Center Collection, Aurora, CO.)

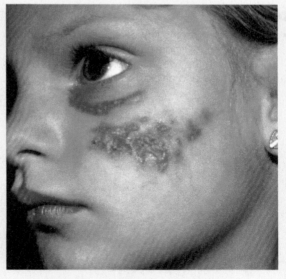

Fig. 18.3. Patient with primary arcuate lesion below the eye from a cat scratch and lymphocutaneous spread to the preauricular lymph node, which was enlarged.

Pathogenesis

Sporotrichoid mycobacterial infections are due to local inoculation of an atypical mycobacterial species into the skin. This produces an inoculation chancre, followed by the development of linear nodules, abscesses, or ulcerations that follow the local lymphatic vessels. Mycobacterial furunculosis, the other common clinical presentation of mycobacterial infection, is discussed in Chapter 13. *Mycobacterium marinum* is most often implicated, but *Mycobacterium chelonae* and *Mycobacterium kansasii* can also produce sporotrichoid lesions.

Clinical Presentation

- Some patients with mycobacterial skin infections may report an injury following water exposure, such as hand trauma while cleaning a fish tank, handling fish, or having a pedicure with a foot bath.
- These infections are usually located on an extremity.
- The primary inoculation chancre appears first and consists of an erythematous nodule, with variable scale, fluctuation, or ulceration. In some cases, there may be more than one inoculation site.
- Secondary sporotrichoid nodules appear later as one or more erythematous or suppurated nodules along the ascending lymphatic drainage (Figs. 18.4 and 18.5). Secondary nodules may also ulcerate.
- Regional lymphadenopathy is variably present.

Diagnosis

- The clinical presentation of sporotrichoid spread along the lymphatic drainage suggests an infectious process, with the two most common causes being sporotrichosis and atypical acid-fast infection.

- Although certain exposures may favor a particular diagnosis, the lesions cannot be distinguished on clinical features alone, and a biopsy is required.
- A punch, incisional, or excisional biopsy should be performed in all cases. If a punch biopsy is used, it should be 4 mm or larger.
- Half of the bisected specimen should be sent for routine histologic examination, but it is important to understand that even with special stains, findings organisms can be difficult. The organisms can be identified in tissue in about 50% of biopsies.
- Therefore, the other half of the bisected specimen should be sent for bacterial and fungal culture. It should be made clear that mycobacterial culture is desired because this requires special media, and many of the species are slow growing.

Treatment

- The treatment of cutaneous mycobacterial infections is not standardized. If the biopsy detects a mycobacterial organism by special stains, oral minocycline (100 mg bid) is a reasonable empiric therapy while awaiting culture and sensitivity results.
- Once the sensitivities are known, drugs that may be used in addition to minocycline include rifampin, clarithromycin, azithromycin, ciprofloxacin, and co-trimoxazole (trimethoprim-sulfamethoxazole [TMP-SMX]), usually for 2 to 4 months. Occasional unresponsive cases may require multidrug therapy.

Clinical Course

Most cases spontaneously resolve without therapy over 2 to 6 months; most treated cases respond more quickly. Rare cases result in disseminated infection.

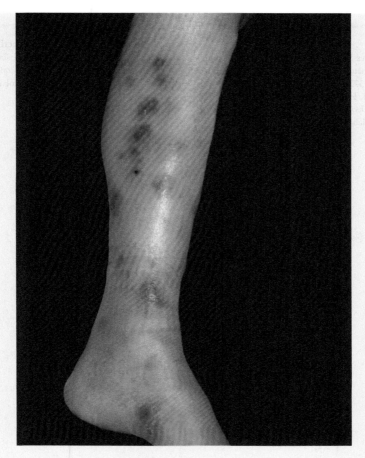

Fig. 18.4. Patient with sporotrichoid mycobacterial infection due to *Mycobacterium chelonae*. Note that the lesions appear to follow more than one lymphatic vessel. (From the Fitzsimons Army Medical Center Collection, Aurora, CO.)

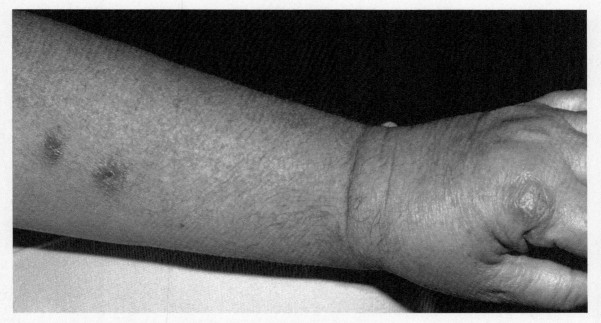

Fig. 18.5. Sporotrichoid mycobacterial infection due to *Mycobacterium marinum*. The primary lesion is on the knuckle, with nodular lymphangitis developing after the primary care provider injected the primary lesion with intralesional triamcinolone to treat a presumed foreign body granuloma. (From the Fitzsimons Army Medical Center Collection, Aurora, CO.)

References

Sporotrichosis
1. Bonifaz A, Saúl A, Paredes-Solis V, et al. Sporotrichosis in childhood: clinical and therapeutic experience in 25 patients. *Pediatr Dermatol*. 2007;24:369-372.
2. Nusbaum BP, Gulbas N, Horwitz SN. Sporotrichosis acquired from a cat. *J Am Acad Dermatol*. 1983;8:386-391.
3. Schechtman RC. Sporotrichosis: part I. *Skinmed*. 2010;8:216-220.

Sporotrichoid Mycobacterial Infections
1. Glickman FS. Sporotrichoid mycobacterial infections. A case report and review. *J Am Acad Dermatol*. 1983;8:703-707.
2. So JK, Paravar T. Sporotrichoid mycobacterial infection. *N Engl J Med*. 2015;373:1761.

Chapter 19
Photosensitive Disorders

Key Terms

Polymorphous Light Eruption
  Polymorphic light eruption
Systemic Lupus Erythematosus
  Bullous systemic lupus
    erythematosus

Discoid lupus erythematosus
  Lupus hair
Discoid Lupus Erythematosus
  Chronic cutaneous lupus
    erythematosus

Hypertrophic discoid lupus
  erythematosus
Dermatomyositis
  Amyopathic dermatomyositis

I t is important to recognize photosensitive disorders because many of these conditions may be ameliorated, or prevented entirely, by sun avoidance and/or withdrawal of a photosensitizing medication. Also, this dermatologic pattern includes some forms of connective tissue disease that may have systemic consequences, including end-organ damage and even death.

Differential Diagnosis of Photosensitive Disorders

- Actinic prurigo
- Chronic actinic dermatitis
- Dermatomyositis
- Erythropoietic protoporphyria
- Lupus erythematosus
- Pellagra
- Photoallergic contact dermatitis
- Photoallergic drug eruptions
- Phototoxic drug eruptions
- Phototoxic contact dermatitis
- Polymorphous light eruption
- Porphyria cutanea tarda
- Solar urticaria
- Sunburn

IMPORTANT HISTORY QUESTIONS

How long have you had a photoaggravated skin condition?

Some photosensitive disorders are acute, such as photoallergic contact dermatitis or photoinduced drug eruptions, whereas other conditions are chronic, such as erythropoietic protoporphyria or pellagra.

Do your lesions itch or burn?

Many photosensitive processes, such as actinic prurigo, chronic actinic dermatitis, and photoinduced drug eruptions, produce pruritus, whereas others may cause pain, such as erythropoietic protoporphyria, phototoxic drug eruptions, and sunburn.

Have you recently started any new medications?

This question is important when considering photoallergic and phototoxic drug eruptions. It could also

be important when investigating drug-induced lupus erythematosus or drug-induced dermatomyositis.

Do you have any other symptoms or recent problems such as muscle pain, joint pain, fever, or other unexplained problems?

This question may reveal overt systemic symptoms, but more in-depth questioning and a complete review of symptoms may be necessary when connective tissue disorders, including lupus erythematosus and dermatomyositis, are specific considerations.

Is there a family history of a similar rash?

Some photodistributed conditions may have a hereditary component, such as actinic prurigo, erythropoietic protoporphyria, and polymorphous light eruption.

IMPORTANT PHYSICAL FINDINGS

Is there any evidence of hair loss?

Systemic lupus erythematosus may be associated with a nonscarring hair loss (so-called lupus hair); discoid lupus erythematosus may demonstrate a scarring alopecia, with characteristic dyspigmented plaques.

What is the distribution of the lesions?

Some disorders manifest a characteristic distribution. For example, systemic lupus erythematosus on the hands usually involves the interphalangeal skin (between joints), whereas dermatomyositis usually involves the skin over the joint spaces (as Gottron papules).

Is a mucosal surface involved?

Although most photosensitive disorders do not have mucosal involvement, discoid lupus, systemic lupus erythematosus, and actinic prurigo are notable exceptions, and all may have oral manifestations.

Does the patient have periungual telangiectasias?

Periungual telangiectasias may be seen in dermatomyositis and systemic lupus erythematosus.

Polymorphous Light Eruption ICD10 code L56.4

Introduction

Polymorphous light eruption (PMLE), also known as a polymorphic light eruption, is the most common photodermatosis, with some studies having shown an incidence that approaches 10% of the population in certain ethnic groups. Familial clustering and a higher incidence in some ethnic groups suggest a genetic predisposition, although the precise pathogenesis is not well understood. It is thought that PMLE represents a form of a delayed-type hypersensitivity process (type IV). PMLE may be precipitated by ultraviolet A (UVA) light (most common), UVB light (Fig. 19.1), or both, depending on the patient.

Clinical Features

- PMLE is more common in women, and it generally presents in the first 3 decades of life.
- Patients with PMLE usually develop a photoexposed eruption in the early spring, with fewer lesions later in the summer (due to hardening) or in the fall, when the UV light intensity wanes.
- The threshold of exposure necessary for the development of lesions may vary from 5 minutes to 3 hours.
- The delay between UV light exposure to the development of lesions is highly variable (30 minutes to 3 days).
- The morphology of PMLE varies widely (hence the term polymorphous) and includes macular erythema (Fig. 19.2), erythematous papules and plaques (Figs. 19.3 and 19.4), and papulovesicles with a dermatitic appearance (Fig. 19.5). In some cases, the lesions may resemble urticaria or erythema multiforme.
- Pruritus is common.

Clinical Diagnosis

- Clinical circumstances, including an affirmative family history, or appropriate ethnic background, may suggest the diagnosis.
- A 3- or 4-mm punch biopsy may be supportive, but the histologic changes are not always diagnostic of only PMLE.
- Screening laboratory studies to consider include antinuclear antibody (ANA) or extractable nuclear antigen antibody (ENA) testing and determination of urine or stool porphyrin levels to exclude porphyria.
- Rare cases may require phototesting (see Fig. 19.1).

Treatment

- Artificial light exposure can be used to harden an individual and decrease observed disease. Narrow-band UVB (NB-UVB) is the preferred modality, followed by PUVA (psoralen plus UVA). Broadband UVB is less effective.
- Oral hydroxychloroquine (200–400 mg qd) is effective for many patients.
- Oral β-carotene (25–50 mg tid) is effective for some patients.
- Oral nicotinamide (1 g tid) induced complete remission in 14 of 25 patients and improved the course of disease in the remaining 11 patients.
- Topical corticosteroids may be helpful, with the strength of the corticosteroid varied according to the amount of disease that is present and the skin affected.
- Sun avoidance behaviors, sun-blocking clothing, and broad-spectrum sunscreens (with UVA and UVB protection) are important strategies to minimize disease activity.

Clinical Course

Lesions of PMLE typically last for 1 to 3 weeks and heal without scarring. The disorder may persist for decades, but the condition usually remits later in life.

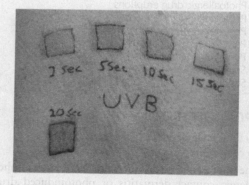

Fig. 19.1. Phototest with red plaques being produced in as little as 2 seconds of UVB exposure.

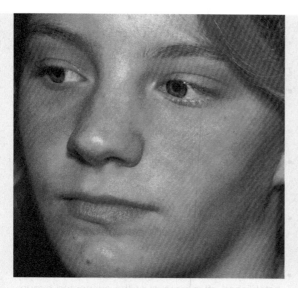

Fig. 19.2. Young lady with macular erythema of the cheeks, nose, and chin that resemble the malar rash of systemic lupus erythematosus. (From the William Weston Collection, Aurora, CO.)

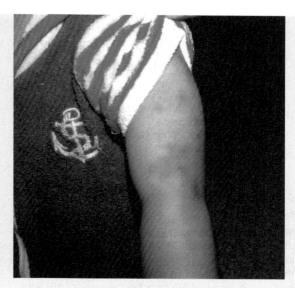

Fig. 19.3. Young child with red indurated plaques confined to the sun-exposed portions of the arm. (From the William Weston Collection, Aurora, CO.)

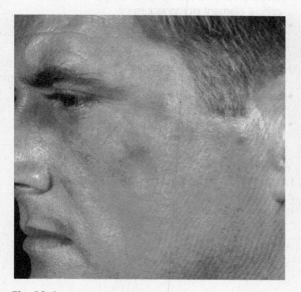

Fig. 19.4. Polymorphous light eruption presenting as plaques of the cheek in a young man. (From the Fitzsimons Army Medical Center Collection, Aurora, CO.)

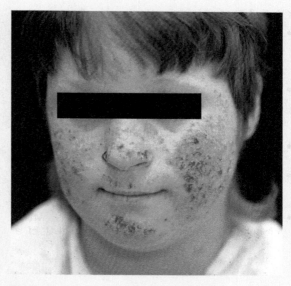

Fig. 19.5. Crusted dermatitic presentation of polymorphous light eruption in a child. (From the William Weston Collection, Aurora, CO.)

Commonly Implicated Drugs in Photoallergic Drug Eruptions

- Celecoxib
- Dapsone
- Furosemide
- Hydrochlorothiazide (very common)
- Hydroxychloroquine
- Pyridoxine hydrochloride (vitamin B_6)
- Trimethoprim-sulfamethoxazole (TMP-SMX)
- St. John's wort

Pathogenesis

Photoallergic drug eruptions are eczematoid tissue reactions that occur after the ingestion of a medication, vitamin, supplement, or even a preservative in food, but the condition requires light exposure for the reaction to transpire. Photoallergic drug reactions can be induced by UVA (most common) or UVB light. Many texts have combined photoallergic and phototoxic drug eruptions into one category of photosensitive drug eruptions, but the processes are distinct, and a separate discussion is warranted.

Clinical Features

- With prior sensitization, photoallergic reactions usually occur 1 day after re-exposure. A new exposure may take up to 3 weeks to foment as a photoallergy.
- The condition causes a photodistributed dermatitis that usually involves the face, posterior neck, upper chest, arms, and hands. There is usually sparing beneath the chin, in a natural shadow area.
- The condition can spread somewhat to non–sun-exposed areas as UV light penetrates clothing.
- Primary lesions vary from macular erythema to indurated eczematous plaques or even, on occasion, vesiculobullous reactions (Figs. 19.6–19.8).
- In contrast to phototoxic drug eruptions, which produce discomfort or pain similar to that of a sunburn, photoallergic drug eruptions are usually pruritic.

Clinical Diagnosis

- A pruritic dermatitis, in a photodistributed or photoaccentuated pattern, and occurring in a patient taking medication(s) or a suspicious exogenous agents, raises concern for a photoallergic drug eruption.
- In some cases, it is difficult to distinguish a photoallergic drug eruption from a contact dermatitis to pollen or sunscreen, which tend to occur on photoexposed portions of the skin.
- Biopsies demonstrate nonspecific features of dermatitis but are only useful in excluding some photosensitive conditions, such as lupus erythematosus, dermatomyositis, or phototoxic drug eruption.
- In many cases, the diagnosis is only definitively established after removal of the suspected exogenous agent, with observed clinical improvement.

Treatment

- Withdrawal of the suspected exogenous agent is a critical element of management.
- Sunlight and allergen avoidance are important to management. Patients should understand that UVA wavelengths, which produce most drug-induced photoallergic drug eruptions, can pass through window glass and produce disease.
- Use of moderate to potent topical corticosteroids is an effective topical treatment.
- Severe cases may require 3 to 14 days of oral prednisone (10–40 mg per day).

Clinical Course

Discontinuing the offending drug usually results in complete resolution in 2 to 3 weeks, although some reactions may persist for a longer duration.

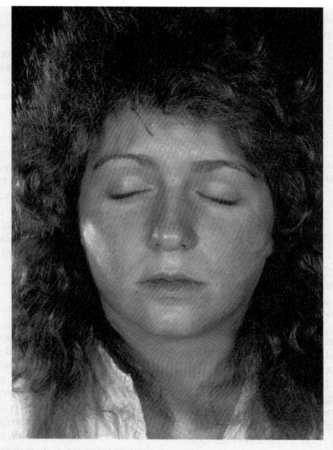

Fig. 19.6. Patient with photoallergic dermatitis manifesting as pruritic erythema on the forehead, malar cheeks, and chin due to cotrimoxazole. (From the Fitzsimons Army Medical Center Collection, Aurora, CO.)

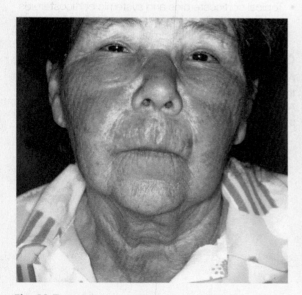

Fig. 19.7. Patient with photoallergic erythema and induration of the malar cheeks and V of the neck caused by hydrochlorothiazide, one of the most common causes of photoallergic drug eruptions.

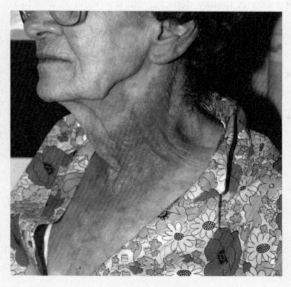

Fig. 19.8. Patient with eczematoid photoallergic erythema of the ears, lateral neck, and V of the neck caused by prochlorperazine, which is a relatively uncommon cause of photoallergy.

Phototoxic Drug Eruption ICD10 code L56.0

Commonly Implicated Drugs and Foods in Phototoxic Eruptions

- Amiodarone
- Capecitabine
- Celery root
- Demeclocycline
- Doxycycline
- 5-Fluorouracil
- Flutamide
- Methotrexate
- Nonsteroidal antiinflammatory drugs (NSAIDs; weak phototoxic drugs)
- Psoralen
- Tetracycline
- Voriconazole

Pathogenesis

Phototoxic drug eruptions are dose-related events. Because the reactions are not immunologically mediated, the condition will occur in any person given enough of the drug and incurring sufficient light exposure. In many cases, phototoxic drug eruptions resemble sunburn, but some drugs produce characteristic reactions, such as the onycholysis observed with tetracyclines or bullous reactions, which resemble porphyria cutaneous tarda caused by naproxen. Rarely, phototoxic eruptions are due to foods (e.g., celery root). Note that oral psoralen, in combination with UVA light (PUVA), is an intentional (iatrogenic) phototoxic drug eruption used to treat dermatologic disease.

Clinical Features

- Patients usually demonstrate erythema in affected areas within hours after light exposure. This is in contrast to photoallergic eruptions, which take 1 day or longer to foment because of dependence on the immune system.
- Erythema develops in a photodistributed pattern (Figs. 19.9 and 19.10) and is often clinically indistinguishable from sunburn.
- Patients experience tender or painful skin that feels like sunburn.

- Severe cases may blister—a second-degree phototoxic drug eruption.
- Patients who continue to receive the drug and are exposed to light may develop variable erythema, which may be intermixed with variable hypopigmentation and hyperpigmentation (Fig. 19.11).

Clinical Diagnosis

- The clinical presentation resembles sunburn. Therefore, when patients present with sunburn-like reactions, clinicians should always review medication lists to include over-the-counter (OTC) medications as potential causes of a phototoxic eruption.
- A shave or punch biopsy can support the diagnosis of a phototoxic drug eruption. It is useful in problematic cases to exclude other photosensitive dermatoses (e.g., lupus), with the exception of sunburn, which is histologically identical.

Treatment

- Withdrawal of the suspected drug is indicated, if clinically feasible. This may not be possible in all cases, such as the patient shown in Fig. 19.11, who was taking flutamide for his prostate cancer.
- Nonspecific treatment measures, such as cool compresses, cool baths, topical cooling agents containing menthol and camphor, and compounds containing aloe vera may provide relief but do not change the natural course of the reaction.
- The use of topical lidocaine-containing agents is controversial but is an option that can be discussed with the patient if he or she is not allergic to such medications.
- Topical corticosteroids and systemic corticosteroids are not particularly effective because the process is not mediated by the immune system.

Clinical Course

Assuming that the patient does not continue to receive the drug, the reaction wanes over 1 to 2 weeks. Affected areas may tan and/or peel but are without permanent sequelae in most cases.

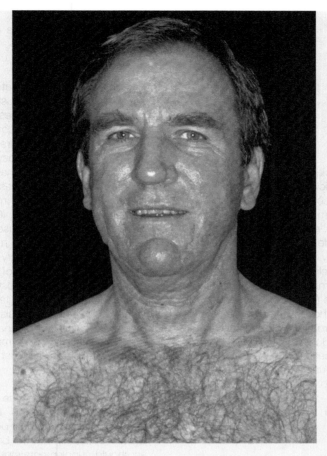

Fig. 19.9. Patient with phototoxic reaction manifesting as erythema of the face, lower neck, and upper chest attributable to tetracycline. (From the Fitzsimons Army Medical Center Collection, Aurora, CO.)

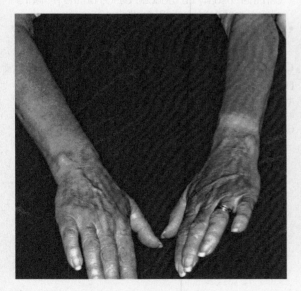

Fig. 19.10. Phototoxic reaction manifesting as erythema of the arms in a patient taking demeclocycline. Note that the area underneath the patient's watchband is not involved. (From the Fitzsimons Army Medical Center Collection, Aurora, CO.)

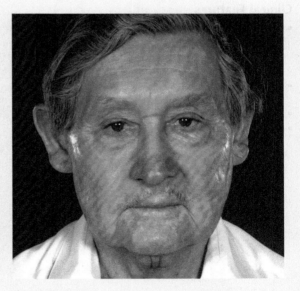

Fig. 19.11. Chronic phototoxic reaction manifesting as low-grade erythema, hypopigmentation, and hyperpigmentation in a patient taking flutamide. (From the Fitzsimons Army Medical Center Collection, Aurora, CO.)

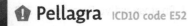

Pellagra ICD10 code E52

NUTRITIONAL DEFICIENCY

Pellagra-Associated Medications
- Anticonvulsants
- Antidepressants
- 5-Fluorouracil
- Isoniazid (INH)
- 6-Mercaptopurine
- Sulfapyridine

Pathogenesis

Pellagra is caused by a niacin (nicotinic acid, vitamin B3) deficiency or by a deficiency in its metabolite, nicotinamide. Nicotinamide comes from the diet or from endogenous synthesis from tryptophan. Because vitamins B_1, B_2, and B_6 are required cofactors for the production of nicotinamide, diets with an insufficient intake of B vitamins may cause pellagra. Niacin is found in many foods, including baker's yeast, liver, and cereals, but not corn. Pellagra is usually seen in those with limited diets (e.g., those dependent on maize alone), alcoholics, those with bowel resections, those with carcinoid syndrome (tryptophan is diverted into excess serotonin production), those with Hartnup syndrome, and in association with certain medications (see box). Although uncommon in industrialized nations, pellagra is probably often missed.

The Four Ds of Pellagra
- **D**ermatitis
- **D**iarrhea
- **D**ementia
- **D**eath

Clinical Features

- Pellagra causes a photodermatitis, with erythema followed by desquamation. The distribution resembles that of other photodistributed eczematous processes (Figs. 19.12 and 19.13).
- Casal necklace is a marginated eruption of the neck that resembles a necklace (Fig. 19.14).
- Angular cheilitis is variably present.
- Systemic manifestations may include fatigue, photophobia, diarrhea (and other gastrointestinal [GI]

symptoms), and dementia (seen in about 4–10% of cases).

Clinical Diagnosis

- Persons with photodermatitis, GI disorders, and psychiatric complaints must be screened for pellagra. In suspicious cases, probative questions regarding diet, alcohol consumption, and other medications should be pursued.
- A 3- or 4-mm punch biopsy may strongly support the diagnosis of a nutritional disorder, but the findings are subtle and are best made by a dermatopathologist with expertise in this area.
- A complete blood count (CBC) may serve as a quick screening test because about 90% of patients with pellagra will have a microcytic hypochromic anemia due to other dietary deficiencies.
- Depressed urine levels of N-methylnicotinamide and 2-pyridone are diagnostic, but many laboratories do not perform these tests.
- In most cases, the diagnosis is established by treatment with niacin or nicotinamide supplementation and observation of the dermatitis because improvement typically occurs in just days.

Treatment

- Topical moisturizers provide some immediate relief.
- Any medications known to aggravate pellagra should be discontinued, if possible.
- Dietary education should be given to the patient, as should supplementation of oral niacin (nicotinic acid) at an initial dose of 50 to 100 mg tid, which can then usually be reduced based on the patient's clinical response over 2–4 weeks.
- Patients often need supplementation of other B vitamins.

Clinical Course

Unrecognized and untreated pellagra has a high fatality rate. In one study, conducted at a mental institution in Alabama in the early 20th century, a fatality rate of 64% was observed.

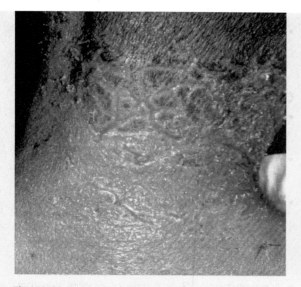

Fig. 19.12. Intense photodistributed eczematoid pellagra in a man being treated with isoniazid. (From the Fitzsimons Army Medical Center Collection, Aurora, CO.)

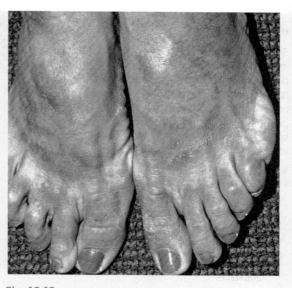

Fig. 19.13. Patient with pellagra presenting as photodistributed erythema and scale on the tops of her feet. The patient also had erythema of her forearms. She had two risk factors, isoniazid therapy and a short bowel syndrome due to surgical resection. (From the Fitzsimons Army Medical Center Collection, Aurora, CO.)

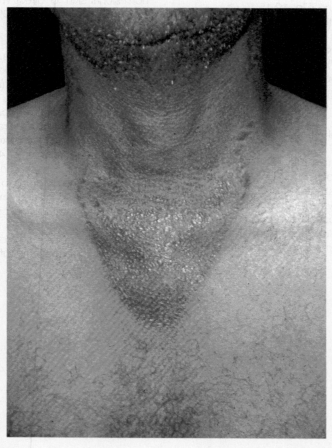

Fig. 19.14. Patient with classic Casal necklace of pellagra presenting as a sharply demarcated dermatitis of the V of the neck.

Systemic Lupus Erythematosus ICD10 code M32.9

Pathogenesis

Systemic lupus erythematosus (SLE), sometimes referred to simply as lupus, is an autoimmune disorder characterized by autoantibodies against various components of nuclear DNA. Subtypes of these antibodies include anti–double-stranded DNA antibodies (anti-dsDNA), anti-Smith antibodies (anti-Sm), and antihistone antibodies. The latter are usually associated with drug-induced lupus (see box).

Commonly Implicated Drugs in Drug-Induced Systemic Lupus Erythematosus

- Hydralazine
- Isoniazid
- Minocycline
- Phenytoin
- Procainamide
- Quinidine

Clinical Features

- SLE usually affects middle-aged adults, with women being affected more often than men.
- Malar erythema of the face (butterfly rash) is the classic cutaneous finding (Fig. 19.15).
- Macular erythema, erythematous papules, or even urticarial lesions can be observed on photoexposed skin of the face, neck, back, chest, arms, and hands (Figs. 19.16 and 19.17).
- When the hands are involved, lesions tend to involve the interphalangeal skin, in contrast to dermatomyositis, which tends to involve skin over the joints (Fig. 19.17).
- Involvement of the oral mucosa is not uncommon (Fig. 19.18).
- Rarely, vesicles or blisters may form (bullous systemic lupus erythematosus).
- About 5% to 10% of patients with SLE may demonstrate discoid lupus erythematosus lesions.
- Diffuse nonscarring alopecia can occur, often with broken-off hairs (so-called lupus hair).
- Constitutional symptoms can include fever and malaise.

- Systemic complications include arthralgias and myalgias, renal disease (≈50%), lymphoreticular complications, cardiac complications, and involvement of the bone marrow or central nervous system.

Clinical Diagnosis

- The appearance of a photodistributed erythema with systemic symptoms should prompt an evaluation for SLE.
- An ANA laboratory test should always be done, with nearly all cases showing ANA positivity, often in high titer.
- Additional laboratory studies include a CBC, determination of the erythrocyte sedimentation rate (ESR) and C-reactive protein (CRP) level (useful to monitor disease activity), urinalysis, renal function tests, liver function tests, and total complement activity (CH50; depressed values correlate with renal disease).
- A punch biopsy (3 or 4 mm) of lesional skin that includes subcutaneous fat will usually be diagnostic of SLE, although it is often not possible to exclude dermatomyositis or other forms of lupus erythematosus completely without clinical details.
- A punch biopsy (3 or 4 mm) from photodistributed nonlesional skin for direct immunofluorescence will highlight a lupus band in 60% to 80% of cases.

Treatment

- Photoprotection (e.g., hats, clothing, sun avoidance, UVA sunscreen) is necessary.
- Drugs that may induce SLE (see box) must be withdrawn or substituted.
- Topical corticosteroids may be tailored to the site and severity of disease. In general, truncal lesions often require moderate to ultrapotent corticosteroids.
- Oral prednisone (starting at 40–60 mg/day) may be used, with a taper based on the response.
- Immunosuppressive drugs to use in a steroid-sparing regimen usually include mycophenolate mofetil, cyclosporine, azathioprine, cyclophosphamide, and rituximab.
- Hydroxychloroquine, chloroquine, or quinacrine may be used to manage cutaneous disease.

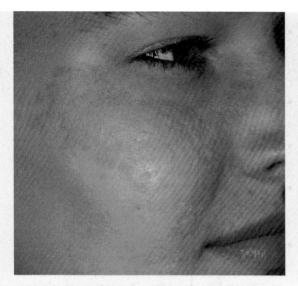

Fig. 19.15. Patient with classic malar erythema (butterfly rash) of systemic lupus erythematosus.

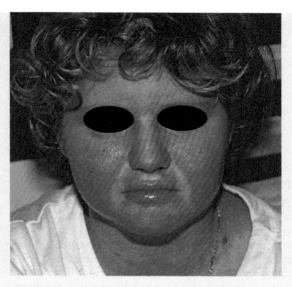

Fig. 19.16. Patient with severe acute lupus erythematosus, with marked erythema in a photodistribution. (From the William Weston Collection, Aurora, CO.)

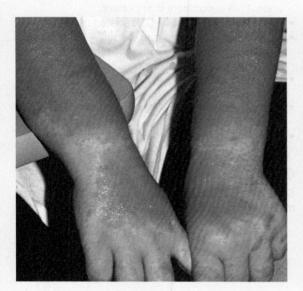

Fig. 19.17. Patient with severe acute lupus erythematosus, with marked erythema on the arms and hands. Note the characteristic interphalangeal involvement of the erythema.

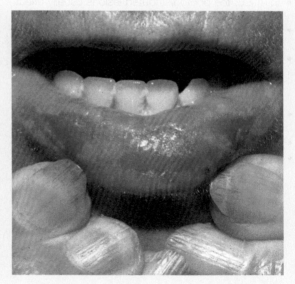

Fig. 19.18. Erosions of the mucosal surface of the lip in a patient with systemic lupus erythematosus. (From the Fitzsimons Army Medical Center Collection, Aurora, CO.)

Subacute Cutaneous Lupus Erythematosus ICD10 code L93.1

AUTOIMMUNE DISORDER

Commonly Implicated Drugs in Drug-Induced Subacute Cutaneous Lupus Erythematosus
- Diltiazem
- Hydrochlorothiazide
- Leflunomide
- Oxprenolol
- Terbinafine
- Ranitidine
- Verapamil

Pathogenesis

Subacute cutaneous lupus erythematosus (SCLE) is a largely cutaneous variant of lupus. As the name implies, the clinical course is usually less severe and less acute than SLE. SCLE is characterized by the presence of anti-Ro (anti-SSA) antibodies and, less often, by anti-La (and SSB) antibodies. Less often, SCLE appears to be triggered by some medications (see box).

Clinical Features

- Middle-aged to elderly women are usually affected.
- In SCLE, the photodistributed lesions usually affect the face, upper chest, arms, and upper back.
- The malar erythema of SCLE may be clinically indistinguishable from that of SLE.
- Erythematous lesions of the arms and trunk may demonstrate annular lesions (Figs. 19.19 and 19.20) or erythematous scaly plaques that may resemble psoriasis (Fig. 19.21). Not all lesions manifest scale.
- The scarring and follicular hyperkeratosis of discoid lupus erythematosus are notably absent.
- Sicca syndrome if often present.
- Systemic symptoms are variable and can be minimal (e.g., low-grade malaise, vague myalgias, arthralgias) to frank impairment of another organ system (e.g., renal or cardiac).

- About 5% to 10% of patients with SCLE have vasculitis at some point during the course of their disease.

Clinical Diagnosis

- The appearance of photodistributed and annular lesions is suggestive of SCLE, particularly in a middle-aged to elderly woman.
- An ANA test is positive in all cases, with anti-Ro (SSS-A) antibodies present in more than 90% of cases.
- A punch biopsy (3 or 4 mm) of lesional skin that includes subcutaneous fat often supports the diagnosis of SCLE, although it is often impossible to exclude dermatomyositis without clinical details.
- A punch biopsy (3 or 4 mm) from photodistributed nonlesional skin for direct immunofluorescence reveals a lupus band or other supportive findings in 60% to 80% of cases. This test is usually only needed in problematic cases.

Treatment

- Photoprotection (e.g., hats, clothing, sun avoidance, UVA sunscreen) is important.
- Drugs that may induce SCLE should be withdrawn.
- Topical corticosteroids can be tailored to the site and severity of disease. In general, truncal lesions require moderate to ultrapotent corticosteroids.
- Oral prednisone (usually 20–40 mg/day) can be used initially and tapered based on the response.
- Hydroxychloroquine (200 mg PO qd or bid) is useful, but it may take 4 to 8 weeks to see improvement.
- Oral isotretinoin may be used as a tertiary agent, 1 to 2 mg/kg per day.

Clinical Course

SCLE is usually relatively easy to control, and patients may go into spontaneous remission.

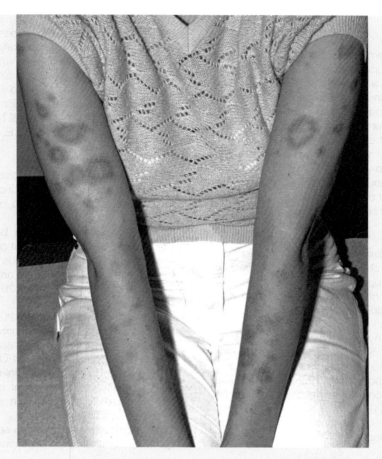

Fig. 19.19. Young woman with subacute cutaneous lupus erythematosus and classic photodistributed red annular lesions on the arms. She also had associated malar erythema. (From the Fitzsimons Army Medical Center Collection, Aurora, CO.)

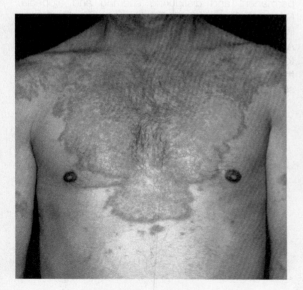

Fig. 19.20. Young man with extensive annular lesions with confluence into plaques on the upper back, outer arms, and V of the chest. (From the Fitzsimons Army Medical Center Collection, Aurora, CO.)

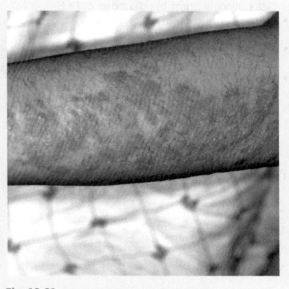

Fig. 19.21. Man with photodistributed slightly indurated papules and plaques, with subtle scale. This pattern is actually more common than the pattern of the more distinctive annular lesions.

Discoid Lupus Erythematosus ICD10 code L93.0

Pathogenesis

Discoid lupus erythematosus (DLE), also known as chronic cutaneous lupus erythematosus, is the most common form of lupus to involve the skin. DLE is nine-fold more common in African American women than in any other population, but white individuals can also be affected. Like other forms of lupus erythematosus, it is considered to be an autoimmune disease, yet only 20% of patients with DLE have a positive ANA response on laboratory testing. About 5% to 10% of patients with cutaneous lesions of DLE have SLE or SCLE. In contrast to other forms of lupus erythematosus, drug-induced cases are uncommon.

Clinical Features

- Photodistributed lesions of DLE often affect the malar face, upper chest, arms, and upper back.
- Primary lesions appear first as an erythematous indurated plaque, often evolving to include hyperkeratosis and dyspigmentation (Figs. 19.22 and 19.23).
- On occasion, the hyperkeratosis can be considerable (hypertrophic discoid lupus erythematosus).
- Involvement of the conchal bowl of the ear is common and distinctive (Fig. 19.24).
- Patients may demonstrate areas of scarring alopecia (see Chapter 24).
- In contrast to SLE, oral lesions are uncommon but can occur occasionally.

Clinical Diagnosis

- Erythematous plaques, with hyperkeratosis, dyspigmentation, and scarring, occurring in a photodistribution, suggest the diagnosis of DLE.
- Conchal bowl involvement or a scarring alopecia are clinical findings that support a diagnosis of DLE.
- A punch biopsy (3–6 mm) of lesional skin is strongly suggestive or even diagnostic of DLE.
- In select cases, a punch biopsy can also be submitted for direct immunofluorescence.

- Recommended laboratory screening is not universally agreed on but should likely include an ANA test (positive in ≈20% of patients), CBC, chemistry profile, and urinalysis. Some also perform complement studies—C3, C4, and CH50. Laboratory screening is important because 5% to 10% of patients with lesions of DLE will have another form of systemic lupus, SCLE or SLE.

Treatment

- Photoprotection (e.g., hats, clothing, sun avoidance, UVA sunscreen) is a critical component of treatment because the disease is driven largely by UV light.
- Topical corticosteroids should be tailored to the site and severity of disease, but generally potent or ultrapotent topical corticosteroids are used to arrest the disease before large scars are formed.
- Intralesional triamcinolone (5–20 mg/mL) can be used for select plaques.
- Oral prednisone (starting dose, 20–40 mg/day) may be used for persons with extensive disease, with a taper based on the treatment response.
- Hydroxychloroquine (200 mg PO qd or bid) is a pillar of care, but it typically takes 4 to 8 weeks before significant improvement is seen. Smoking can increase liver metabolism of the drug and decrease its efficacy.
- Other medications sometimes used include chloroquine, quinacrine, and thalidomide.

Clinical Course

Untreated (or incompletely treated) DLE can cause permanent and disfiguring scarring and alopecia. Rarely, patients with DLE without systemic disease initially will progress to SLE or SCLE at a later point. Although such later progression is unusual, it is useful to screen persons with DLE periodically throughout the course of their illness or if the course of their illness seems to change in some way.

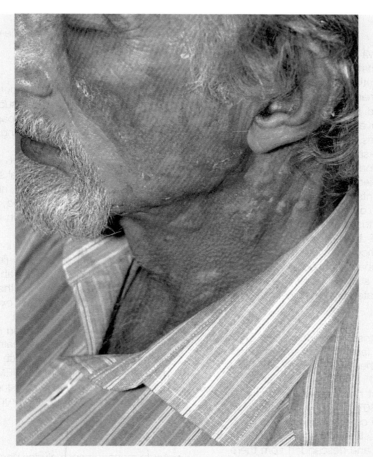

Fig. 19.22. Patient with severe discoid lupus erythematosus, with both atrophic and hypertrophic erythematous to violaceous plaques in a photodistributed pattern. Note the involvement of the conchal bowl.

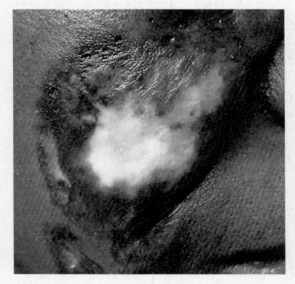

Fig. 19.23. Patient with discoid lupus erythematosus of the right cheek demonstrating follicular hyperkeratosis, scale, atrophy, and severe dyspigmentation.

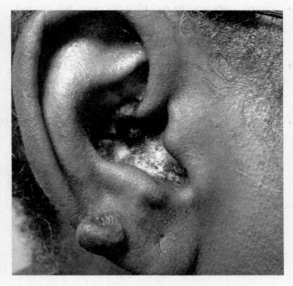

Fig. 19.24. Patient with characteristic erythematous plaque with scale, atrophy, and dyspigmentation of the conchal bowl.

⬤ Dermatomyositis ICD10 code M33.90

Pathogenesis

Dermatomyositis (DM) is an autoimmune disease characterized by genetic predisposition, but also it often has a precipitating event, such as infection, medication, or malignancy. The pathogenesis of DM is not well understood, but about 95% of patients will demonstrate a positive ANA or, less often, antisynthetase autoantibodies. About 40% of patients with DM will have myositis-specific autoantibodies, such as anti-Jo-1, anti-SRP, and anti-Mi-2. Other rare antibodies have been identified on occasion. Approximately 10% to 20% of patients will demonstrate clinical features that overlap with other connective tissue disease (e.g., lupus erythematosus). Depending on the study, anywhere from 4.4% to 60% of cases have been found to be malignancy-associated (paraneoplastic). This wide range is probably caused by variations in the population assessed; suffice it to say that some cases of DM can be associated with malignancy.

Clinical Features

- DM causes a photosensitive dermatitis. Erythema affecting the malar face may resemble the butterfly rash of lupus erythematosus, with variable scale (Fig. 19.25).
- DM may also affect nonphotoexposed skin, especially the scalp (>80%) and bony prominences of the upper back (so-called shawl sign).
- Many patients will state that the condition began with an itchy scalp and descended from there.
- A so-called heliotrope eruption around the eyes consists of periorbital edema and violaceous erythema of the upper eyelids (Figs. 19.25 and 19.26) is common.
- Gottron papules are red to violaceous flat-topped lesions of the dorsal interphalangeal joints (Fig. 19.27). Gottron papules may become atrophic and white in color over time.
- Gottron sign refers to violaceous streaking over the bony prominences of the hands, forearms, and elbows (and possibly the knees). The so-called holster sign refers to similar erythema over the hips.
- There is periungual telangiectasia with variable cuticular hyperkeratosis, also called the Samitz sign (Fig. 19.28).

- Rare cutaneous findings include vasculitis, panniculitis, and acquired ichthyosis.

Diagnosis

- A patient with a photodistributed rash and with suggestive clinical findings, such as a heliotrope rash, Gottron sign, Gottron papules, shawl sign, holster sign, or periungual telangiectasia, should be screened for possible DM.
- Consider performing a 3- to 6-mm punch biopsy (not a shave biopsy) of lesional skin. The histologic findings, although not specific, are usually supportive of the diagnosis. Histologic overlap with SCLE is particularly common, and, in this regard, clinical correlation is important.
- Laboratory screening should include ANA testing and muscle enzyme studies (levels of creatinine kinase and aldolase). The absence of muscle involvement does not exclude the disease, because amyopathic dermatomyositis exists and does not have an associated myopathy.
- Ultimately, the patient will need referral to an internist, dermatologist, or rheumatologist for consideration of magnetic resonance imaging (MRI; or possibly electromyography [EMG]) and muscle biopsy and, based on age, gender, and review of systems, consideration of appropriate screening for malignancy.

Treatment

- Acute management includes photoprotection (UVA, UVB sunscreens) and oral prednisone (0.25–1.0 mg/kg per day, depending on severity of the disease).
- Hydroxychloroquine (200 mg PO, qd or bid) is a common long-term, steroid-sparing agent, but improvement after starting the drug may take 4 to 8 weeks, with maximal improvement occurring up to 6 months after beginning the drug.
- Oral methotrexate (5–30 mg/week) or mycophenolate mofetil are options for unresponsive patients.

Clinical Course

With treatment, about 80% of patients will be free of disease activity within 4 years.

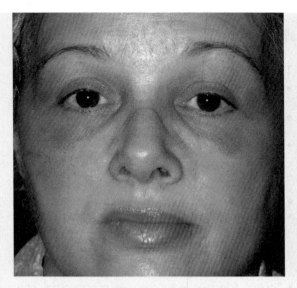

Fig. 19.25. Patient with malar erythema, with red heliotrope rash of the upper eyelids. (From the Fitzsimons Army Medical Center Collection, Aurora, CO.)

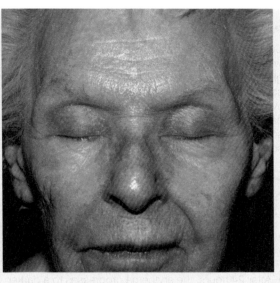

Fig. 19.26. Patient with prominent violaceous heliotrope rash of the upper eyelids. (From the Fitzsimons Army Medical Center Collection, Aurora, CO.)

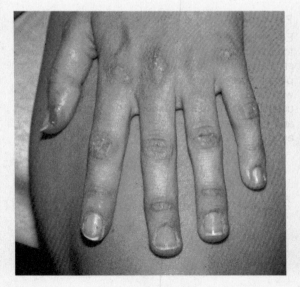

Fig. 19.27. Patient with dermatomyositis with Gottron papules demonstrating erythema and scale over the joint of the hand. (From the William Weston Collection, Aurora, CO.)

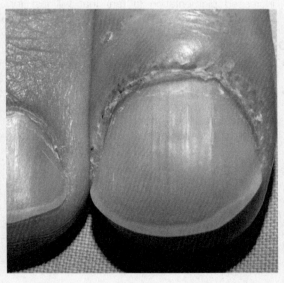

Fig. 19.28. Patient with telangiectasia and hyperkeratosis of the cuticle (Samitz sign), with a normal finger on the left for comparison.

Pathogenesis

Sunburn is caused by excess exposure to UVB light, which represents wavelengths blocked by window glass. To a lesser degree, UVA light produces some solar-induced changes in pigment but is far less effective in producing sunburn. Sunburn can occur from natural sunlight but may be produced by artificial light sources, including tanning beds and therapeutic light sources in a dermatologist's office.

Clinical Features

- Sunburns are photodistributed but, because of clothing or positioning, may produce unusual patterns.
- Erythema usually begins within hours of sun exposure and reaches maximum intensity in 12 to 24 hours (Figs. 19.29 and 19.30).
- After 24 hours, the erythema progresses to a darker hue, followed by desquamation that usually begins 2 to 4 days later, although this is highly variable.
- Severe sunburns may produce a second-degree burn, with superficial blisters (Fig. 19.31).
- Following desquamation, the skin produces increased pigmentation (a tan) that will last for weeks (Fig. 19.32).

Diagnosis

- Clinical presentation and history are usually diagnostic, and the patient generally reports the burn.
- Rare cases may require a shave or punch biopsy to differentiate sunburn from other photosensitive disorders. The histologic findings are usually strongly suggestive of sunburn but will not allow differentiation from drug-induced phototoxic reactions (e.g., reaction to tetracyclines).

Treatment

- No treatment is an option for some sunburns because the condition will resolve without therapy.
- Cool compresses and cool baths are helpful in producing some pain relief.
- Topical cooling agents containing menthol and camphor, or compounds containing aloe vera, may provide some relief but do not change the natural course of the sunburn.
- NSAIDs are used in the first 24 to 48 hours.
- For severe cases, oral indomethacin (50–100 mg PO tid) for the first 24 hours reduces pain and erythema. Indomethacin is a potent prostaglandin inhibitor, but dosing beyond 24 hours after sun exposure does not alter the course of disease.
- Topical lidocaine solutions are controversial and must be used with caution over large areas to prevent lidocaine toxicity. This may be discussed with the patient.
- Topical corticosteroids and systemic corticosteroids are not typically used.

Prevention

Education is important and should include instructions to avoid the midday sun (between 10:00 AM and 2:00 PM), when 60% of the entire day's sunlight strikes the planet. Protective clothing, shade, and sunscreens with a sun protection factor (SPF) of 30 or higher are useful. As demonstrated in Fig. 19.32, tighter weaves and darker shades, or even specially treated fabrics, are more effective in blocking UV light.

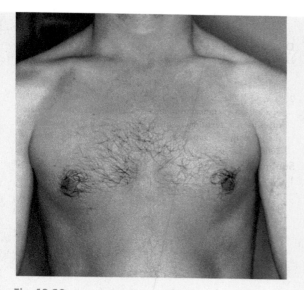

Fig. 19.29. Patient with acute first-degree sunburn acquired at a tanning booth. (From the Fitzsimons Army Medical Center Collection, Aurora, CO.)

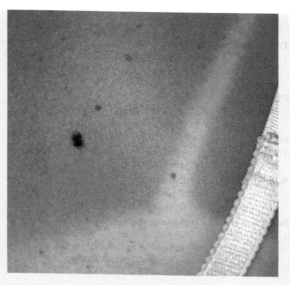

Fig. 19.30. Close-up of a patient with acute first-degree sunburn. The large nevus was an atypical (dysplastic) nevus. The patient needs education regarding sun damage and melanoma!

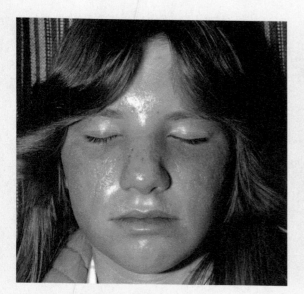

Fig. 19.31. Patient with acute second-degree sunburn with blisters. (From the Fitzsimons Army Medical Center Collection, Aurora, CO.)

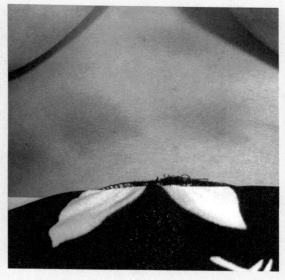

Fig. 19.32. Patient with tanning after sun exposure through white patterns of clothing. The lesson is that UV light will go through some clothing. (From the Fitzsimons Army Medical Center Collection, Aurora, CO.)

References

Polymorphous Light Eruption

1. Jannssens AS, Pavel S, Ling T. Susceptibility to UV-A and UV-B provocation does not correlate with disease severity of polymorphic light eruption. *Arch Dermatol.* 2007;143:599-604.

Photoallergic Drug Eruption

1. Yazici AC, Baz K, Ikizoglue G, et al. Celecoxib-induced photoallergic drug eruption. *Int J Dermatol.* 2004;43:459-461.

Pellagra

1. Wan P, Moat S, Anstey A. Pellagra: a review with emphasis on photosensitivity. *Br J Dermatol.* 2011;164:1188-1200.

Systemic Lupus Erythematosus

1. Jordan N, D'Cruz D. Current and emerging treatment options in the management of lupus. *Immunotargets Ther.* 2016;5:9-20.

Subacute Lupus Erythematosus

1. Callen JP, Hughes AP, Kulp-Shorten C. Subacute cutaneous lupus erythematosus induced or exacerbated by terbinafine. A report of 5 cases. *Arch Dermatol.* 2001;137:1196-1198.

Dermatomyositis

1. Dourmishev LA, Dourmishev AL, Schwartz RA. Dermatomyositis: cutaneous manifestations of its variants. *Int J Dermatol.* 2002;41:625-630.
2. Gerami P, Schope JM, McDonald L, et al. A systematic review of adult-onset clinically amyopathic dermatomyositis (dermatomyositis siné myositis): a missing link within the spectrum of the idiopathic inflammatory myopathies. *J Am Acad Dermatol.* 2006;54:597-613.

Sunburn

1. Monseaue AJ, Reed ZM, Langley KJ, Onks C. Sunburn, thermal, and chemical injuries to the skin. *Prim Care.* 2015;42:591-605.

Chapter 20
Purpuric and Hemorrhagic Disorders

Purpuric and hemorrhagic (P&H) disorders may be caused by systemic illness, potentially fatal infections (e.g. meningococcemia), coagulopathies, vascular occlusive disorders (e.g. cryoglobulinemia), and inflammatory disorders of blood vessels (e.g. vasculitis).

> **Some Purpuric Disorders**
> * Acute bacterial endocarditis
> * Acute hemorrhagic edema
> * Cryofibrinogenemia
> * Cryoglobulinemia
> * Disseminated candidiasis
> * Disseminated gonococcal infection
> * Disseminated staphylococcal infection
> * Henoch-Schönlein purpura
> * Meningococcemia
> * Pityriasis lichenoides et varioliformis acuta
> * Progressive pigmented purpura
> * Purpura fulminans
> * Rocky Mountain spotted fever
> * Solar purpura
> * Traumatic purpura

IMPORTANT HISTORY QUESTIONS

How long have the lesions been present?

Some P&H disorders occur acutely, such as Rocky Mountain spotted fever, whereas other conditions present with a chronic pattern (e.g., progressive pigmented purpura).

Have you had more than one episode?

Some P&H disorders present as a singular event (e.g., meningococcemia, disseminated gonococcal infection), whereas others present as multiple episodes (e.g., pernio, cryofibrinogenemia, Henoch-Schönlein purpura).

What medications do you take?

Some P&H disorders, such as leukocytoclastic (e.g., hypersensitivity) vasculitis and progressive pigmented purpura, may be induced by drugs.

Do you have other known medical conditions?

Collagen vascular disease, in particular, may be associated with leukocytoclastic (hypersensitivity) vasculitis, pernio and chilblains, and cryofibrinogenemia.

Do you or any member of your family have a history of blood clots or a clotting disorder?

Purpura fulminans occurs more often in people with clotting disorders, which can be familial.

Is there a recent history of tick bites or exposure to ticks, especially to a dog with ticks?

This is an important question for establishing a presumptive diagnosis of Rocky Mountain spotted fever.

IMPORTANT PHYSICAL FINDINGS

What is the distribution of the lesions?

This can be an important clue to the diagnosis because some conditions characteristically involve certain anatomic sites. For example, pernio is usually confined to the toes, whereas the rash of Rocky Mountain spotted fever usually begins in acral locations. Some disorders, such as cryoglobulinemia and cryofibrinogenemia, are located at sites exposed to the cold.

Is there any physical evidence of active arthritis or arthralgias?

Some diseases, such as Henoch-Schönlein purpura, cryoglobulinemia, and disseminated gonococcal infection, are often associated with arthritis or arthralgias.

Are there other skin lesions present?

The size and characteristics of the cutaneous hemorrhage may provide clues to the underlying cause. Small nonpalpable purpura (≤4 mm) is usually a noninflammatory event and it is most common in the setting of thrombocytopenia (platelet count <20,000/mm^3) or abnormalities of clotting factors. Small vessel vasculitis usually produces palpable purpura, with elevated papules of up to 10 mm that are surrounded by a rim of erythema, even in addition to the purpura. Large areas of nonpalpable purpura on photo-exposed skin is associated with acquired structural anomalies due to sun damage (e.g., solar purpura). Purpura with a retiform (net-like) pattern is more often associated with vascular occlusion (e.g., calciphylaxis).

Henoch-Schönlein Purpura

Pathogenesis

Henoch-Schönlein purpura (HSP) is a variant of leukocytoclastic vasculitis (LCV) that affects mostly children, but can also affect adults. HSP is a small vessel vasculitis characterized by circulating immunoglobulin A (IgA)-mediated immune complexes that are deposited in vessel walls (Fig. 20.1). This leads to inflammation and vessel damage. Precipitating factors include viral infections (e.g., parvovirus B19, hepatitis B, hepatitis C, human immunodeficiency virus) and bacterial infections (*Streptococcus, Salmonella,* and *Shigella* spp. and *Staphylococcus aureus*). Renal disease is a feared consequence of HSP, but it occurs in a minority of patients.

Clinical Features

- HSP usually affects children between 2 and 10 years of age, but it may also affect younger children, adolescents, and adults.
- HSP is characterized by the rather abrupt onset of symmetrically distributed palpable purpura (Figs. 20.2 and 20.3).
- In about 5% of cases, there may be pustular lesions (Fig. 20.4), hemorrhagic bullae, or ulcerations.
- The legs are most often affected, followed by the buttocks.
- Young children usually demonstrate urticarial lesions, facial edema, and/or scrotal swelling.
- Systemic features include arthritis and arthralgia, headache, nephritis, and gastrointestinal (GI) symptoms, including GI angina and bowel infarction.

Diagnosis

- The occurrence of palpable purpura in a younger child, particularly in association with arthritis and arthralgias, headache, and GI upset, should suggest HSP. Concern is augmented when there is a history of a preceding infection.
- Patients with suspected HSP should have a 3- or 4-mm punch biopsy for routine hematoxylin and eosin (H&E) studies.
- Ideally, an additional punch biopsy, or a portion of a divided punch biopsy, should be submitted for direct immunofluorescent studies (see Fig. 20.1). This specimen can never be placed in formalin.
- A minimal laboratory evaluation should include a complete blood count (CBC) with differential, liver and renal function tests, urinalysis, stool guaiac testing, throat culture, and determination of the streptozyme level.

Treatment

- For patients with renal disease, a number of retrospective or uncontrolled studies have supported the use of pulse methylprednisolone, with or without cyclophosphamide, triple immunosuppressive therapy (prednisolone, cyclophosphamide, and dipyridamole), corticosteroids and azathioprine, plasma exchange, with or without immunosuppressive therapy, and intravenous (IV) immunoglobulin.
- In children with significant or deteriorating renal disease, treatment should consist of high-dose corticosteroid therapy and an immunosuppressive agent (e.g., azathioprine, cyclophosphamide, or mycophenolate mofetil). Consultation with a pediatric nephrologist is important.

Prognosis

In patients who develop renal disease, complete spontaneous remission occurs in about 50%. About 5% of patients with renal disease will develop a progressive course that can include renal failure.

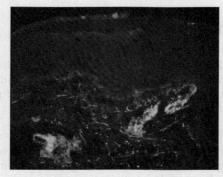

Fig. 20.1. Patient with Henoch-Schönlein purpura, with granular immunoglobulin A in vessels.

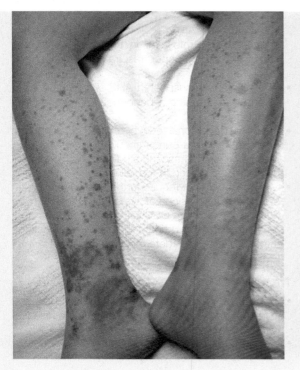

Fig. 20.2. Acute Henoch-Schönlein purpura in a child.

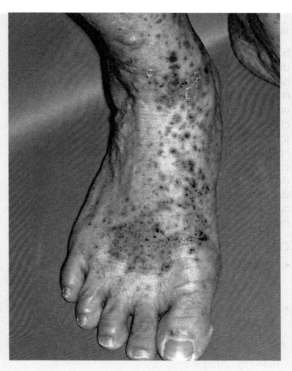

Fig. 20.3. Developed Henoch-Schönlein purpura in a young adult.

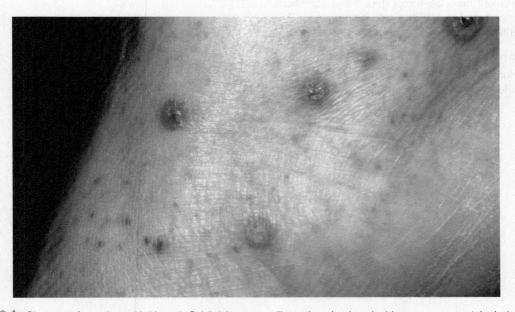

Fig. 20.4. Close-up of a patient with Henoch-Schönlein purpura illustrating classic palpable purpura, a pustular lesion, and older lesions demonstrating early crusting. (From the Fitzsimons Army Medical Center Collection, Aurora, CO.)

Pathogenesis

Some consider acute hemorrhagic edema (AHE) a unique disease, whereas others consider it a variant of HSP. AHE is also referred to as Finkelstein or Seidl-mayer disease. AHE is considered by some to be an entity separate from HSP because of its distinct clinical appearance, the typical lack of systemic symptoms, and the younger ages of affected patients. Like HSP, AHE is a small vessel vasculitis caused by circulating IgA-mediated immune complexes that are deposited in vessel walls. Precipitating factors include viral infections, bacterial infections (e.g., *Streptococcus, Salmonella,* and *Shigella* spp. and *S. aureus*) and, rarely, medications.

Clinical Features

- Classically, AHE affects infants and young children, with most cases occurring in those younger than 2 years. It can rarely affect older children.
- AHE consists of the abrupt onset of symmetrically distributed edematous plaques (Figs. 20.5–20.7) that develop variable hemorrhage (see Figs. 20.6 and 20.7). Sometimes, the hemorrhage is subtle (see Fig. 20.5).
- The face and lower extremities are usually affected, followed by the arms and buttocks. Truncal lesions are uncommon in AHE.
- Although arthritis-arthralgia, nephritis, and GI involvement have been reported, these conditions are uncommon in AHE but are common in HSP.
- Patients with AHE often have a low-grade fever.

Diagnosis

- An infant or young toddler with purpura in fixed urticarial lesions on the face and/or lower extremities should suggest AHE, especially if there is a history of a preceding infection. In Fig. 20.5, the nasal secretions of an upper respiratory infection are readily evident.
- All patients with suspected AHE should have a 3- or 4-mm punch biopsy performed for routine H&E examination.
- Ideally, an additional punch biopsy, or a portion of a larger divided punch should be submitted for direct immunofluorescent studies. This specimen can never be placed in formalin.
- Most cases do not require further evaluation but, in select cases with signs of systemic disease, it may be wise to perform a CBC with differential, liver and renal function tests, urinalysis, stool guaiac testing, throat culture, and determination of streptozyme level.

Treatment

- In the absence of systemic findings, no treatment is necessary, because AHE is a self-limited disease without permanent sequelae.
- In patients with systemic findings, anecdotal cases have responded well to oral corticosteroids.

Prognosis

AHE typically resolves within 2 to 3 weeks, without treatment. There have been case reports of recurrent disease.

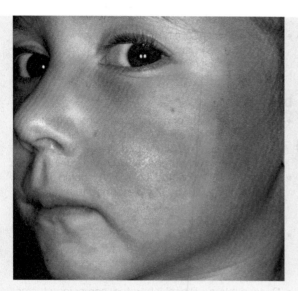

Fig. 20.5. Patient with acute hemorrhagic edema manifesting as an urticarial plaque with subtle hemorrhage. (From the Fitzsimons Army Medical Center Collection, Aurora, CO.)

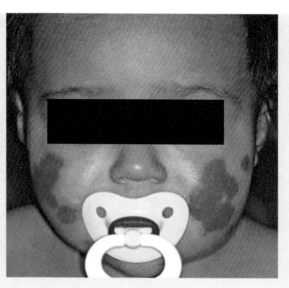

Fig. 20.6. Patient with developed case of acute hemorrhagic edema manifesting as an urticarial plaque with extensive hemorrhage.

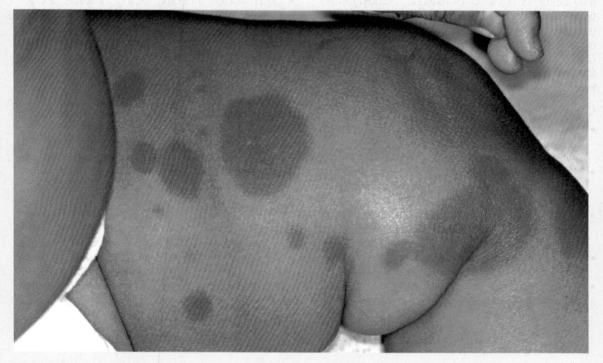

Fig. 20.7. Large urticarial plaques with extensive hemorrhage of the lower extremity in an infant. (From the Joanna Burch Collection, Aurora, CO.)

Drug-Induced Vasculitis

Drugs

- Allopurinol
- Cephalosporin
- Famciclovir
- Gefitinib
- Penicillin
- Phenytoin
- Sirolimus
- Sulfonamide
- Thiazides
- Warfarin

Food and Drug Additives

- Drug dyes
- Sodium benzoate

Pathogenesis

Although LCV is probably the more modern term, the older synonym, "hypersensitivity vasculitis" (HV) emphasizes that this small vessel vasculitis occurs as a reaction to a perturbation in homeostasis. LCV (HV) may occur for a variety of reasons, including infections (streptococcal infections), medication reactions (see box), certain ingestions, and collagen vascular disease. Urticarial vasculitis is another distinct subset of LCV (HV) (see Chapter 5). HV can be IgM-mediated (collagen vascular diseases), IgA-mediated (HSP) or, less often, IgG-mediated.

Clinical Features

- LCV (HV) presents with the abrupt onset of palpable purpura that mainly affects dependent areas of the lower legs, in particular.
- Most individual lesions of LCV (HV) are 1 to 6 mm in size, but larger lesions are not uncommon (Figs. 20.8 and 20.9).
- Clinical variants may include pustules, hemorrhagic vesicles (Fig. 20.10), purpuric lesions with central necrosis, and lesions in a reticulated pattern.
- Lesions may be asymptomatic, or a burning sensation or pain may be reported by some patients.
- Systemic symptoms may include fever, malaise, and arthralgias (the latter is most common).

- Most cases of LCV (HV) in adults are confined to the skin, but any organ system, including the kidneys, GI tract, joints (arthritis), lungs, and heart can be involved.

Diagnosis

- The sudden onset of palpable purpura on the lower extremities of an adult should raise suspicion for LCV (HV), and a history and review of systems should be carried out to identify a potential trigger.
- All cases of suspected LCV (HV) should have a 3- or 4-mm punch biopsy performed to include the subcutaneous fat. If possible, ulcerated or necrotic lesions should be avoided.
- An additional punch biopsy of perilesional skin should be submitted for direct immunofluorescent studies. This specimen cannot be placed in formalin.
- Reasonable additional laboratory screening studies may include a CBC, throat culture (for streptococcal infection), urinalysis (to exclude renal involvement), comprehensive metabolic panel (to include renal function studies and liver enzymes), and stool guaiac testing.
- Other studies, including testing for levels of cryoglobulin, complement (C1q, C3/C4, CH50), rheumatoid factor, antinuclear antibody (ANA), and extractable nuclear antigen antibodies (ENAs), HIV testing, hepatitis B and C studies, and chest x-ray may be ordered in certain cases.

Treatment

- Removal or treatment of the precipitating cause is always the initial step in management.
- Cases of small vessel vasculitis limited to the skin can be treated with prednisone (20–60 mg/day, with a taper over 2 to 3 weeks), colchicine (0.6 to 2.4 mg/day), and dapsone.

Clinical Course

Individual lesions of LCV (HV) heal over 2 to 4 weeks but may leave a reddish-brownish discoloration (hemosiderosis) or scar. Patients may have a single episode of LCV (HV) or multiple recurrent episodes. Rare patients may experience the continued development of new lesions without interruption.

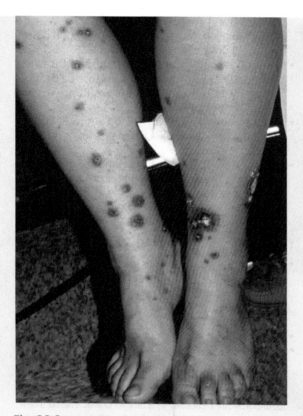

Fig. 20.8. Hydrochlorothiazide-induced adult hypersensitivity vasculitis. The patient had no evidence of systemic involvement. (From the Fitzsimons Army Medical Center Collection, Aurora, CO.)

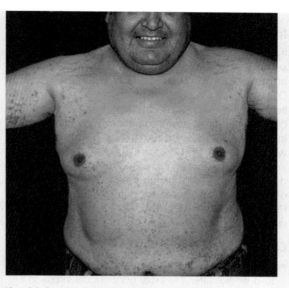

Fig. 20.9. Adult hypersensitivity vasculitis of unknown cause in an adult Hispanic man showing generalized involvement, including the upper arms and torso. The cause was never identified. (From the Fitzsimons Army Medical Center Collection, Aurora, CO.)

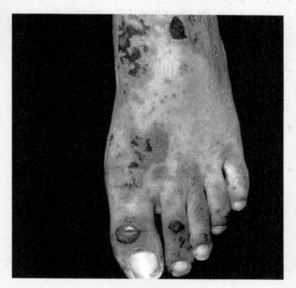

Fig. 20.10. Severe adult hypersensitivity vasculitis in an adult with large hemorrhagic bullous lesions and superficial ulcerations. The patient had arthralgias and mild renal involvement.

Introduction

In 2014, there were more than 350,000 cases of disseminated gonococcal infection (DGI) reported, with an estimated 300,000 additional cases unreported. DGI is due to intravascular septicemia caused by *Neisseria gonorrhoeae*. The bacterium gains access to the bloodstream from asymptomatic or untreated genital infections. DGI develops in 1% to 3% of all patients with gonorrhea, and the vast majority of cases occur in women. There is an increased risk of dissemination during menstruation, during pregnancy, or with pelvic operations or the placement of an intrauterine device. Patients with deficits in the later components of the complement pathway are particularly prone to DGI.

Clinical Presentation

- DGI usually occurs 1 week after menstruation or 2 to 3 weeks after the initial gonococcal infection.
- Cutaneous lesions are present in more than 60% of patients and consist of tender hemorrhagic lesions, usually on the arms and legs (Figs. 20.11–20.13). A pustular component is not uncommon. Cutaneous lesions often present before arthritic symptoms.
- The number of lesions is variable, but, in most cases, there are fewer than 10 lesions.
- A monoarticular arthritis or arthralgia is present in more than 80% of patients and tends to affect larger joints.
- Potential systemic involvement includes tenosynovitis, perihepatitis, meningitis, and endocarditis.

Diagnosis

- Made when there are pustular or pustular-hemorrhagic skin lesions, with arthritic symptoms, in the appropriate social circumstances.
- A recent suspicious sexual contact, history of genitourinary symptoms, and history of past sexually transmitted diseases supports the diagnosis, but DGI must be considered even in the absence of this information. Most patients do not report active urogenital symptoms at the time of a DGI.
- A punch biopsy can be performed but it is often unnecessary. Organisms can sometimes be demonstrated by tissue Gram stain, but tissue cultures are usually negative.
- CBC with an elevated white blood cell (WBC) count supports an infectious process. Leukocytosis is present in most cases.
- Patients with suspected DGI should have polymerase chain reaction (PCR)-based studies of the throat, endocervix (or urethra in men), and anal canal and blood cultures. Blood cultures are positive in about 50% of cases.

Treatment

- Before treatment of DGI is commenced, it is recommended that the Centers for Disease Control and Prevention (CDC) website be checked for the latest treatment guidelines (https://www.cdc.gov/std/gonorrhea/treatment).
- All patients with DGI should be hospitalized.
- Ceftriaxone (1 g IM or IV q24h) plus azithromycin 1 g orally in a single dose represents current first-line therapy. Alternative therapies include cefotaxime (1 g IV q8h) or ceftizoxime (1 g IV q8h) plus azithromycin 1 g orally in a single dose. These treatments are continued for 24 to 48 hours beyond clinical improvement, and then patients are often switched to cefixime (400 mg PO bid) for at least another week of therapy.

Clinical Course

Bacteremia with the development of new cutaneous lesions typically lasts for about the first 3 to 5 days of illness, with joint symptoms predominating after that time. Untreated DGI can cause permanent joint damage.

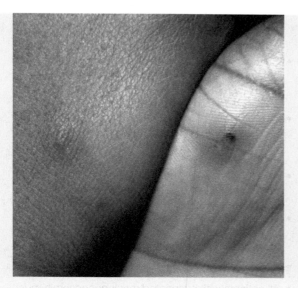

Fig. 20.11. Patient with disseminated gonococcal infection, with pustular and hemorrhagic lesions. (From the Fitzsimons Army Medical Center Collection, Aurora, CO.)

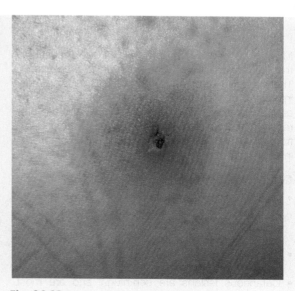

Fig. 20.12. Patient with disseminated gonococcal infection demonstrating papulonecrotic lesion with an intense rim of erythema. (From the Fitzsimons Army Medical Center Collection, Aurora, CO.)

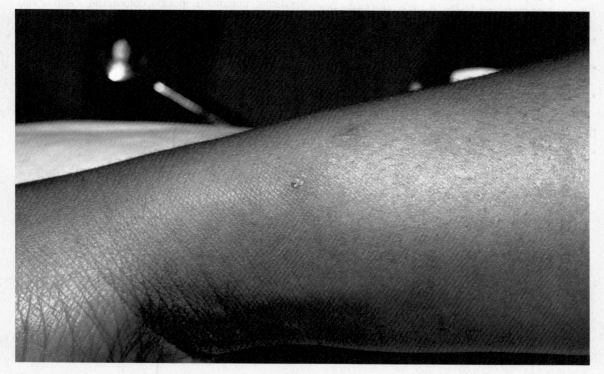

Fig. 20.13. Patient with early papulonecrotic lesion in disseminated gonococcemia associated with joint swelling and pain of the wrist. (From the Fitzsimons Army Medical Center Collection, Aurora, CO.)

Pathogenesis

Meningococcemia is a septicemic infection caused by the gram-negative diplococci, *Neisseria meningitidis*. There are five serotypes, with group B causing most infections in the United States. Transmission is by aerorespiratory spread. The nasopharynx is the only reservoir; carriage rates in the United States range from 5% to 10%. The disease often causes outbreaks in schools and colleges.

Clinical Presentation

- Meningococcemia develops 2 to 10 days after the onset of a nasopharyngeal infection; the latter is usually mild and unnoticed but can involve variable nasal discharge or a sore throat.
- Septicemia usually develops suddenly, with fever, chills, myalgia, arthralgia, and polyarthritis.
- Cutaneous lesions are centrifugal and are most common on the volar wrists, forearms, palms, lower legs, and soles. Unusual cases may involve the trunk and spare acral surfaces.
- Petechiae are seen initially in two-thirds of cases (Figs. 20.14–20.16). Atypical lesions include large ecchymoses, mottled erythema, morbilliform lesions, erythema nodosum, vesicles, pustules, and ulcers.
- Lesions may occur in successive waves, with lesions varying from a handful to several hundred.
- Hypotension and circulatory collapse can occur rapidly, and patients must be closely followed.
- Disseminated infection may occur in almost any organ or organ system.

Diagnosis

- In about 70% of cases, bacteria can be visualized with a Gram stain or Wright stain, using material taken from the buffy coat of peripheral blood or from smears taken from a skin biopsy. Although these tests can be done rapidly, before culture results are available, such techniques are largely a lost skill.
- Cultures of the nasopharynx, blood and skin, and other organs are dictated by the clinical presentation (cerebrospinal fluid in suspected meningitis) and provide evidence of meningococcemia.
- A 3- or 4-mm punch biopsy, which includes subcutaneous tissue, is not often diagnostic because the organism cannot always be visualized, even with a tissue Gram stain.
- A CBC with an elevated WBC count provides presumptive evidence of an infectious process, with most cases demonstrating a leukocytosis.
- A commercially available latex agglutination study is available, but false-positives and false-negatives have been reported with this test.

Treatment

- All patients with suspected meningococcemia must be hospitalized.
- IV penicillin G (300,000 units/kg per day), for a minimum of 7 days, is the treatment of choice. Chloramphenicol can be used in patients allergic to penicillin.
- Other treatments include cefuroxime, ceftriaxone, cefotaxime, and azithromycin. Ciprofloxacin and rifampin are often used as prophylaxis in exposed persons.

Clinical Course

The mortality rate in untreated cases ranges from 70% to 100%, depending on the series. Treated cases have a reported mortality rate of 10% to 15%. A subset of patients with meningococcemia develops disseminated intravascular coagulation (DIC; purpura fulminans). Rarely, patients may develop a chronic meningococcemia variant that produces minimal organ damage.

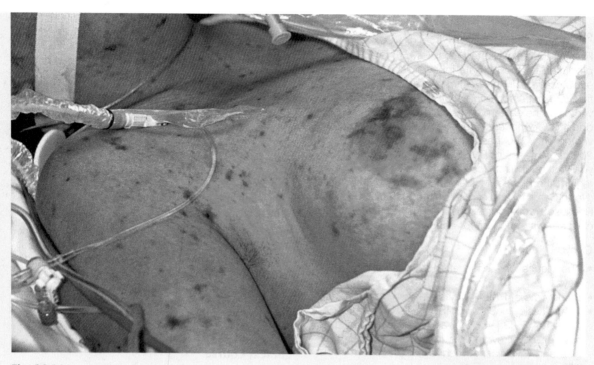

Fig. 20.14. Admixture of petechial and purpuric lesions in a woman hospitalized for meningococcemia. (From the William Weston Collection, Aurora, CO.)

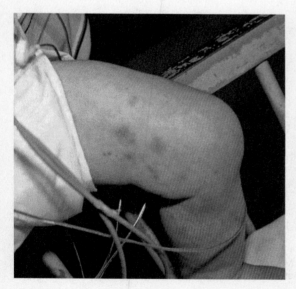

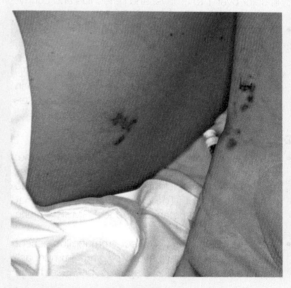

Fig. 20.15. Patient with early lesions of meningococcemia presenting as red papules with subtle hemorrhage. (From the Fitzsimons Army Medical Center Collection, Aurora, CO.)

Fig. 20.16. Close-up of developed petechial lesions in meningococcemia. This case occurred in a college student. (From the Fitzsimons Army Medical Center Collection, Aurora, CO.)

Pathogenesis

Rocky Mountain spotted fever (RMSF) is an infection produced by the obligate intracellular parasite, *Rickettsia rickettsii*. In the western United States, the wood tick *(Dermacentor andersoni)* is the most important vector; in the eastern and southern United States, the dog tick *(Dermacentor variabilis)* is the most important vector. The CDC has estimated that there are about 2000 new cases of RMSF in the United States every year. Although first described in the Rocky Mountain region, the highest incidence is in the south Atlantic (North Carolina) and central United States (Fig. 20.17). Because of outdoor exposure, RMSF usually affects children, who account for about 50% of cases.

Clinical Features

- The incubation period after a tick bite is 2 to 14 days.
- Symptoms of RMSF may be insidious or abrupt.
- The classic triad of RMSF includes rash, fever (100–104°F [38–40°C]), and headache (mild to severe); other symptoms include malaise, arthralgias and myalgias. A rash is not present in about 10% of cases.
- The rash typically begins as pink macules on distal skin—wrists, ankles, palms, soles—with centripetal spread to the trunk and face. The macules deepen in color over 1 to 3 days, and petechiae and ecchymoses develop (Figs. 20.18–20.20).
- Systemic manifestations include GI involvement (e.g., abdominal pain, nausea, vomiting, diarrhea), seen in 30% to 50% of cases, pneumonitis, seen in 12% to 20% of cases, myocarditis, seen in 5% to 25% of cases, skeletal muscle necrosis, seen in 17% to 46% cases, interstitial nephritis, and seizures and coma, seen in 8% to 9% of patients.

Diagnosis

- The classic triad of rash, fever, and headache, occurring in a patient living in an area of high endemicity, or with suspicious exposures, should raise concern for RMSF. The disease is so serious that if the clinical circumstances suggest RMSF, empiric treatment is justified.
- Serologic tests (e.g., indirect immunofluorescent antibody, latex agglutination, enzyme immunoassay) are not useful for diagnosis because these tests do not become positive until 4 to 8 weeks after infection.
- A 3- or 4-mm punch biopsy of lesional skin may demonstrate organisms by immunohistochemical staining, but this special stain is not readily available in most of the country. Immunofluorescent testing on a biopsy has a 30% false-negative rate for detecting the organism.
- Some cases of RMSF require a lumbar puncture to exclude other diseases. Increased lymphocytes or neutrophils in cerebrospinal fluid (CSF) support the diagnosis of RMSF but is not specific.

Treatment

- The treatment of choice for RMSF is doxycycline (100 mg PO bid) for adults and 2.2 mg/kg body weight for children weighing less than 100 pounds. Treatment duration is 7 to 14 days, depending on the response.
- Oral chloramphenicol is an alternative agent for doxycycline-allergic patients and sometimes for pregnant patients.

Clinical Course

Untreated, RMSF has a mortality rate of about 30%, whereas treated disease has a mortality rate of about 4%.

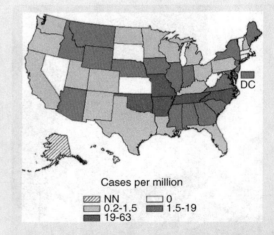

Fig. 20.17. Distribution of reported cases of Rocky Mountain spotted fever. (From https://www.cdc.gov/rmsf/stats.)

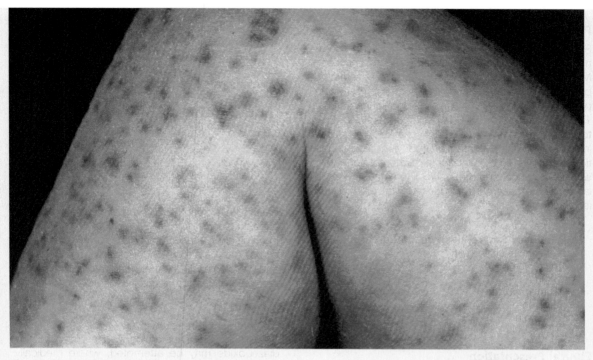

Fig. 20.18. Numerous purpuric papules on the lower thigh and upper calf of a patient with Rocky Mountain spotted fever. (From the Fitzsimons Army Medical Center Collection, Aurora, CO.)

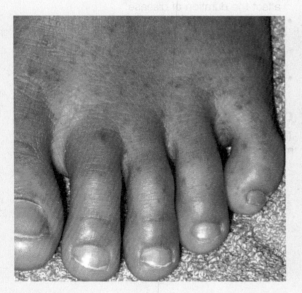

Fig. 20.19. Patient with Rocky Mountain spotted fever presenting as small acral petechiae on the foot. (From the Fitzsimons Army Medical Center Collection, Aurora, CO.)

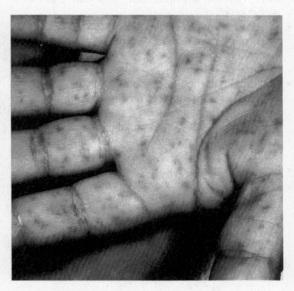

Fig. 20.20. Patient with Rocky Mountain spotted fever manifesting as numerous petechiae on the hand. (From the Fitzsimons Army Medical Center Collection, Aurora, CO.)

Pathogenesis

Progressive pigmented purpura (PPP) is an uncommon disease. There are several variants, including Majocchi purpura, Schamberg purpura, eczematoid purpura (Doucas-Kapetanakis purpura), lichenoid purpura (Gougerot-Blum purpura), and lichen aureus. The pathogenesis of PPP is poorly understood. Histologically, there is a modest perivascular lymphocytic infiltrate, with extravasated erythrocytes. The condition is aggravated by tight-fitting garments, hot baths, saunas, hot tubs, and other stimuli that cause vasodilation. Some cases are associated with medications (see box).

Drug-Induced Progressive Pigmented Purpura

- Acetaminophen
- Amlodipine
- Aspirin
- Chlordiazepoxide
- Interferon-α
- Isotretinoin

Clinical Presentation

- PPP usually affects the lower legs (>90% of cases), but on occasion, it can affect the trunk and upper extremities.
- PPP may be asymptomatic, but some patients report pruritus.
- PPP causes nonpalpable or very minimally palpable pinpoint purpura (usually 1–3 mm in diameter). The color varies from red in active lesions to a golden brown (hemosiderin) in older lesions (Fig. 20.21).
- Schamberg purpura presents with a "cayenne pepper–like" appearance, as if it were sprinkled on the skin, whereas Majocchi purpura presents as vague arcuate or annular configurations. In some cases, the two patterns may be admixed (Figs. 20.22 and 20.23).
- Eczematoid purpura (Doucas-Kapetanakis purpura) is an uncommon variant with a prominent dermatitic

component, including erythema and variable scale, with focal purpura. This variant is more likely to be generalized and pruritic.
- Lichenoid purpura (Gougerot-Blum purpura) is an uncommon variant that may resemble mild lichen planus.
- Lichen aureus is a related entity that causes excessive accumulation of hemosiderin, which causes a golden-yellow or golden-brown color.

Diagnosis

- The clinical presentation of numerous, small, nonpalpable purpuric lesions on the lower extremities, often with a sprinkled or vaguely annular appearance, is diagnostic of PPP.
- In atypical or unusual cases, a 2- or 3-mm punch biopsy can be strongly supportive of the diagnosis and can also exclude other noninflammatory purpuras, vasculitis, and thrombotic disorders.

Treatment

- No treatment is required.
- Discontinuation of acetaminophen, aspirin, or chlordiazepoxide may be attempted, where medically sound, simply to see if this improves the condition.
- Low-potency or moderate-potency topical corticosteroids, applied qd or bid, may be helpful for some patients, but topical corticosteroids do not affect the duration of disease.
- Support hose may decrease the amount of hemorrhage. Discontinuance of hot baths, saunas, and hot tubs, and other causes of vasodilation may make the lesions less pronounced.
- Pentoxifylline (400 mg PO tid) for 4 to 8 weeks has been found useful in anecdotal case reports.

Clinical Course

The clinical course is unpredictable, and the disorder may last for weeks, months, or even years.

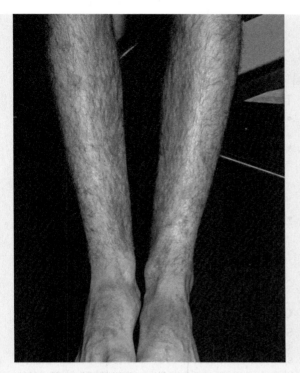

Fig. 20.21. Patient with progressive pigmented purpura with focal hemorrhage and a golden brown color due to hemosiderin deposition.

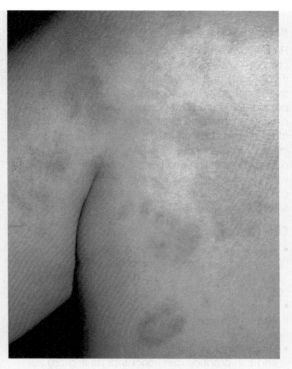

Fig. 20.22. Patient with progressive pigmented purpura, with cayenne pepper hemorrhage.

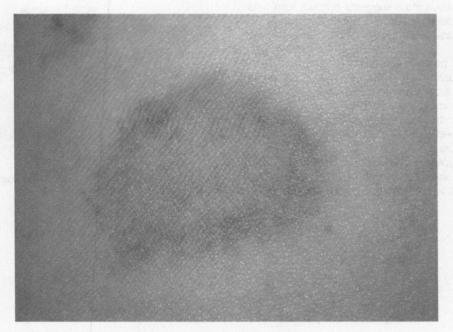

Fig. 20.23. Annular lesion with pinpoint purpura in patient with progressive pigmented purpura.

Pathogenesis

Purpura fulminans is an acute vasculopathy that is characterized by dermal intravascular thrombosis (Fig. 20.24) and DIC. An acquired or inherited clotting abnormality is often present (e.g., homozygous protein C deficiency, homozygous protein S deficiency, antithrombin III disorder). Purpura fulminans is often triggered by an acute infection (e.g., *N. meningitidis, Streptococcus pneumoniae*), or it may occur during the postinfectious convalescent phase (e.g., varicella, scarlet fever). Meningococcemia is the most common cause, but some cases of purpura fulminans are idiopathic.

Clinical Features

- Early lesions consist of painful, well-defined purpura surrounded by a thin erythematous border. Small lesions may resemble the palpable purpura of LCV (Fig. 20.25).
- Lesions progress to vesicles or bullae that may be hemorrhagic and may result in an eschar that is later sloughed.
- Resultant ulcers may extend to muscle and bone and can produce gangrenous digits (Fig. 20.26).

Diagnosis

- The occurrence of unexplained purpura, especially painful purpura, in the setting of acute infection or in a postinfectious state suggests purpura fulminans.
- A CBC, including platelet count, is necessary.
- Blood cultures are necessary to exclude meningococcemia.
- Decreased prothrombin time (PT) and partial prothromboplastin time (PTT), elevated fibrin degradation products, and reduced protein C, protein S, and antithrombin III levels can indicate DIC.
- A 3- or 4-mm punch biopsy of lesional skin should be performed and bisected, with one-half sent for tissue culture.
- Biopsies typically demonstrate dermal and subcutaneous vascular thrombosis, with little inflammation and with secondary hemorrhagic necrosis.

Biopsies are consistent with purpura fulminans but are not diagnostic because other causes of thrombosis cannot be excluded without clinicopathologic correlation.

Treatment

- Immediate respiratory and hemodynamic support are needed.
- Intravenous antibiotics are necessary immediately after blood cultures and tissue cultures are obtained. Ceftriaxone is a common choice, but selection of an antibiotic is dictated by the suspected pathogenesis.
- The patient should be admitted to the hospital for definitive therapy with fresh frozen plasma (10–20 mL/kg q6–12h) and/or protein C concentrate to correct depressed levels of protein S, protein C, and antithrombin III. Fresh-frozen plasma can later be replaced with low molecular weight heparin.

Clinical Course

Some centers have reported mortality rates for purpura fulminans between 25% and 50%. Of patients who survived the disease, over 50% required amputation of one or more digits or even amputation of an entire extremity.

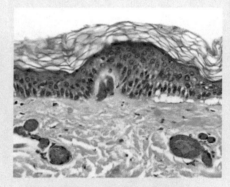

Fig. 20.24. Acute noninflammatory thrombosis in a patient with purpura fulminans.

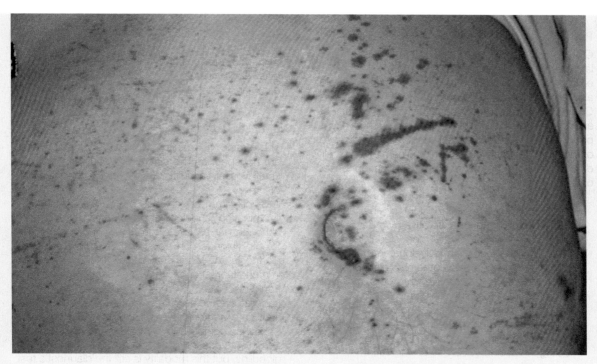

Fig. 20.25. Patient with purpura fulminans demonstrating acute hemorrhagic lesions. (From the Fitzsimons Army Medical Center Collection, Aurora, CO.)

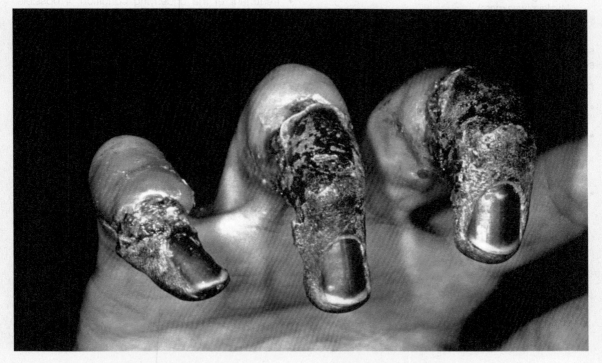

Fig. 20.26. Patient with late-stage purpura fulminans due to meningococcemia. (From the Fitzsimons Army Medical Center Collection, Aurora, CO.)

Pathogenesis

Cryoglobulinemia refers to a disorder caused by circulating single or mixed immunoglobulins that may precipitate in the vasculature of the skin or other organs at a temperature lower than normal body temperature. Cryoglobulins may be essential (idiopathic) or may be associated with an underlying disorder, such as a lymphoproliferative condition, collagen vascular disease, or infection (hepatitis C). Cryoglobulinemia is typically divided into three groups (Brouet classification) based on composition:

- Type I cryoglobulinemia—monoclonal immunoglobulin (IgM, IgG, IgA, light chains). This is caused by a lymphoproliferative disorder.
- Type II cryoglobulinemia—monoclonal immunoglobulin combined with polyclonal immunoglobulin (usually IgM, rarely others). This pattern is seen in lymphoproliferative disorders, collagen vascular diseases, and infection.
- Type III cryoglobulinemia—polyclonal immunoglobulin complexed with another polyclonal immunoglobulin. This pattern is often seen in collagen vascular diseases and infection.

Meltzer Triad
- Palpable purpura
- Arthralgia
- Myalgia (weakness)

Although the Meltzer triad (above) is classically seen in cryoglobulinemia (usually types II and III), similar symptoms can be seen in vasculitis.

Clinical Features

- Cryoglobulinemia usually affects adult and geriatric patients.
- Cryoglobulinemia often yields palpable purpura on the lower extremity (Fig. 20.27). A history of the condition being triggered by cold exposure is not always present.
- Less common cutaneous manifestations include erythematous macules, livedo reticularis (net-like macular lesions), cold-induced urticaria, ulcers, Raynaud phenomenon, acrocyanosis, and pernio-like lesions.
- Systemic manifestations include arthralgias, myalgias, abdominal pain, neuropathy, pulmonary disease, and renal disease, which may vary from mild proteinuria to acute renal failure.

Diagnosis

- The cutaneous manifestations of cryoglobulinemia are nonspecific. The differential diagnosis includes small vessel vasculitis, RMSF, and other purpuric disorders.
- A 3- or 4-mm punch biopsy for routine histologic examination should be done in all cases and, although not usually singularly diagnostic, the histologic findings can be strongly supportive of the diagnosis. An additional punch biopsy for direct immunofluorescence may be useful to exclude frank vasculitis.
- Laboratory studies for rheumatoid factor serve as a surrogate marker for types II and III cryoglobulinemia.
- Serum cryoglobulin levels can be measured. Anticoagulants can interfere with the detection of cryoglobulins, but this modality is still the diagnostic test of choice.

Treatment

- Treatment of the underlying condition, if possible (e.g., hepatitis C, lymphoma), usually improves cryoglobulinemia.
- Nonsteroidal antiinflammatory drugs (NSAIDs) are useful for the symptomatic relief of arthralgias and myalgias.
- Immunosuppressive drugs that decrease immunoglobulin levels (e.g., cyclophosphamide) may be used, and plasmapheresis (Figs. 20.28 and 20.29) or rituximab may be used in severe cases.

Clinical Course

The mortality rate depends on the underlying cause, but fully developed cryoglobulinemic syndrome has a mortality rate of up to 14%.

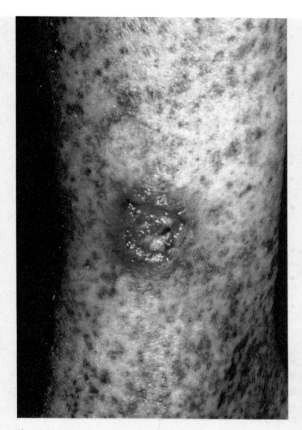

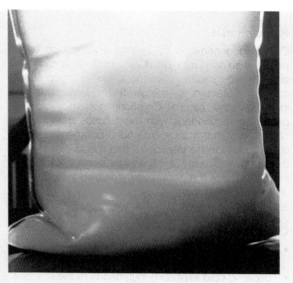

Fig. 20.28. Cryoglobulins removed by plasmapheresis. (From the Fitzsimons Army Medical Center Collection, Aurora, CO.)

Fig. 20.27. Patient with cryoglobulinemia demonstrating palpable purpura and ulcerations. The patient had underlying chronic lymphocytic leukemia that was the cause of the cryoglobulins. (From the Fitzsimons Army Medical Center Collection, Aurora, CO.)

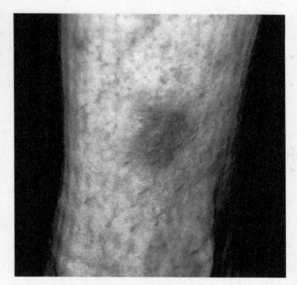

Fig. 20.29. Same location as depicted in Fig. 20.27 demonstrating response to removal of cryoglobulins by plasmapheresis. (From the Fitzsimons Army Medical Center Collection, Aurora, CO.)

Cryofibrinogenemia ICD10 D89.2

Pathogenesis

Cryofibrinogenemia is caused by cryoproteins comprised of an admixture of fibrinogen, fibrin, fibronectin, and fibrin degradation products. These cryoproteins can be detected in refrigerated plasma but not in refrigerated serum. Cryofibrinogenemia can be primary or secondary, with most cases being associated with malignancy, infection, collagen vascular disease, endocrine disorders, and medications (e.g., oral contraceptives). Cryofibrinogens can be detected in about 5% of the population. It is also important to understand that patients may have cryofibrinogens and cryoglobulins.

Clinical Features

- Patients with cryofibrinogenemia may complain of general cold intolerance.
- Following cold exposure, cutaneous manifestations usually consist of petechiae, large areas of purpura (Fig. 20.30), and variable necrosis of the skin (Fig. 20.31).
- Other cutaneous manifestations include Raynaud phenomenon, pernio-like lesions, and livedo reticularis.
- In severe cases, there can be erosions, ulceration, and gangrenous digits that may require amputation.
- Systemic occlusion of vessels in other organ systems (e.g., stroke) can occur. Arthralgias, the second most common complaint, after skin disease, occur in about 30% of patients.

Diagnosis

- Cryofibrinogenemia should be suspected in any patient with a history of cold intolerance and purpuric lesions that are acral or appear cold-induced.

- The diagnosis is based on the demonstration of cryofibrinogens. Testing for cryoglobulins should be commissioned at the same time, because both conditions can be present in the same patient.
- A 3- or 4-mm punch biopsy of lesional skin can demonstrate histologic features consistent with the diagnosis but cannot exclude other causes of vascular thrombosis.

Treatment

- Treatment of the primary disorder (e.g., a malignancy), if possible, may improve cryofibrinogenemia.
- Cold avoidance is useful in all patients, as is removal of other vasoconstricting medications. Cessation of smoking can be helpful.
- Low-dose aspirin is usually recommended, sometimes combined with low-dose oral prednisone.
- Stanozolol (2–4 mg PO qd) has been used anecdotally because of its fibrinolytic properties.
- Severe cases may require the use of immunosuppressive drugs, such as azathioprine and chlorambucil.

Clinical Course

The prognosis in cryofibrinogenemia is usually quite favorable, and many patients will spontaneously go into remission. In one study, the mortality rate was only 5%.

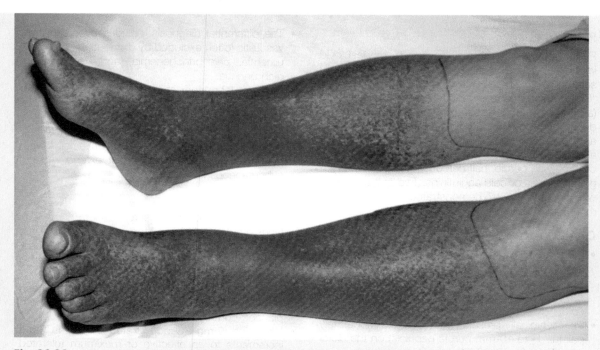

Fig. 20.30. Acute cryofibrinogenemia on the lower legs that occurred with intense cold exposure while the patient was in a wheelchair. (From the Fitzsimons Army Medical Center Collection, Aurora, CO.)

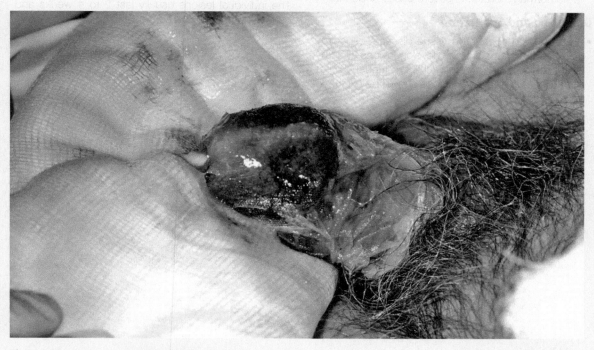

Fig. 20.31. Patient with severe cryofibrinogenemia, with hemorrhage and necrotic changes of the penis. This occurred after passing out in cold weather after an alcoholic binge.

Pernio (Chilblains)

Pathogenesis

Pernio is a distinct clinical reaction to modest cold injury that affects small blood vessels. It is usually seen in cold climates with higher humidity (so-called "English winter") and is not often seen in severely cold (and dry) climates. Histologically, pernio consists of a dense perivascular infiltrate of lymphocytes directed against an unknown antigen. The mechanism for this abnormal reaction is unknown, but in one study of children with pernio, half demonstrated positive cryoglobulin levels or cold agglutinins. Two of the patients with cryoproteins also demonstrated a positive test for rheumatoid factor.

Clinical Features

- Patients usually have a history of recent cold exposure, typically in the past 1 to 7 days. The exposure may seem trivial (e.g., walking the dog on a cold day), but pernio does not have be caused by brutal cold.
- Pernio typically presents with mildly to moderately painful, 1- to 10-mm purple papule(s) on the distal toes (Figs. 20.32–20.34).
- Usually lesions are bilateral; rarely lesions are unilateral.
- The overlying epidermis may yield a blister, or even a hemorrhagic blister, in severe cases of pernio.

Diagnosis and Evaluation

- Patients with connective tissue disease, especially lupus erythematosus, may develop lesions clinically identical to those of pernio (chilblain lupus). Therefore, connective tissue disease should be excluded in all patients with pernio.
- The differential diagnosis includes hypersensitivity vasculitis (often excluded by distribution), cryoglobulinemia, cryofibrinogenemia, and hypergammaglobulinemia.
- Relevant laboratory studies include measurement of cryoglobulins, cryofibrinogens, cold agglutinins, ANA, ENA, and rheumatoid factor levels.
- A biopsy is usually unnecessary, but atypical presentations can be confirmed with a small (3-mm punch) biopsy. The biopsy must extend into the subcutaneous fat.

Treatment

- Prevent or limit cold exposure.
- Nonsteroidal antiinflammatory drugs (NSAIDs) are often used in the treatment of a single episode, although there are no clinical trials demonstrating efficacy.
- Pentoxifylline (400 mg PO tid) for 3 weeks has been shown to be superior to placebo in a double-blind placebo-controlled study.
- Nifedipine (5 mg PO qd), titrated upward in 5-mg increments to an effective or maximum tolerated dose (usually 20–60 mg), is an excellent choice for treating chronic pernio.

Clinical Course

The individual lesions usually last 2 to 4 weeks and heal without scarring. Some patients may have only a single episode of pernio, whereas other patients develop recurring episodes that can be debilitating.

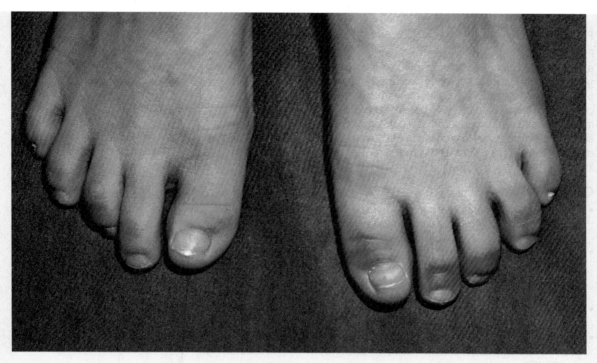

Fig. 20.32. Pernio demonstrating hemorrhagic blisters with brownish tints on the toes of a pediatric patient. (From the Fitzsimons Army Medical Center Collection, Aurora, CO.)

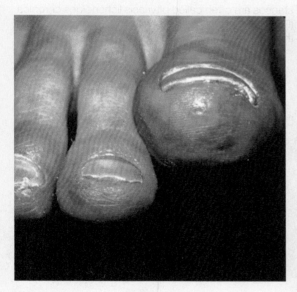

Fig. 20.33. Patient with severe crusted pernio with violaceous tints. (From the Fitzsimons Army Medical Center Collection, Aurora, CO.)

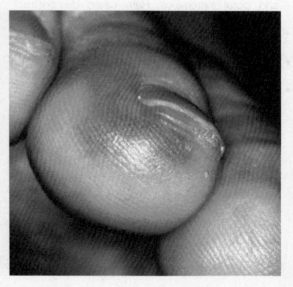

Fig. 20.34. Patient with large hemorrhagic lesion of the distal toe. (From the Fitzsimons Army Medical Center Collection, Aurora, CO.)

Pityriasis Lichenoides et Varioliformis Acuta (Mucha-Habermann Disease) ICD10 code L41.0

Pathogenesis

Pityriasis lichenoides et varioliformis acuta (PLEVA) is a relatively uncommon disorder of unknown pathogenesis. Some studies have demonstrated that up to 57% of cases of PLEVA may demonstrate a monoclonal T-cell population by PCR-based studies. In this regard, it has been proposed that PLEVA is a benign clonal T-cell dyscrasia. Rare cases of PLEVA are associated with HIV, parvovirus B19, and staphylococcal infection.

Clinical Features

- PLEVA usually presents in children, with most cases occurring in those 2 to 14 years of age. Adolescents and young adults may also develop PLEVA.
- Primary lesions are round to oval hemorrhagic papules, from 2 to 10 mm in size (Fig. 20.35). Less often, the lesions appear vesicular during early evolution.
- Multiple skin lesions in different stages of development (crops) are characteristic of PLEVA.
- With time the lesions of PLEVA mature and may become crusted, ulcerated, or scaly (Figs. 20.36 and 20.37).
- The number of lesions is variable, but most patients with PLEVA have 10 to 50 lesions.
- PLEVA usually affects the trunk and proximal extremities, but some cases may involve the face and distal extremities. Rare cases demonstrate nonspecific oral erythema or erosions.
- Symptoms vary from none to mild burning or pruritus.
- Rare cases may present with fever and large ulcerative lesions that cover large areas of the body.
- Ulcerative lesions may scar.

Diagnosis

- A child or young adult with hemorrhagic lesions and eschars, mostly in a central distribution, and with lesions in various stages of development, suggests the possibility of PLEVA. Another consideration, however, is varicella infection.
- Atypical cases or cases in adults should be confirmed with a 3- or 4-mm punch biopsy taken from an early lesion. The histologic findings can be strongly supportive, or in some cases, diagnostic.

Treatment

- PLEVA is usually self-limited, and no treatment is required. There have been no randomized placebo-controlled trials regarding therapy.
- Anecdotal success has been reported with oral antibiotics, including erythromycin and doxycycline. Most case reports and case series employed erythromycin.
- Other treatments include ultraviolet (UV) light therapy (narrow-band UVB, UVA, and psoralen with UVA [PUVA]), oral retinoids, methotrexate, and oral corticosteroids.

Clinical Course

In most cases, the skin lesions of PLEVA disappear in 1 to 10 months, although in some persons the condition may wax and wane for years. These circumstances are often called pityriasis lichenoides chronica (PLC). In general, patients with PLC manifest lesions that are less hemorrhagic but have more scale.

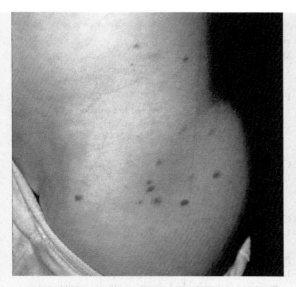

Fig. 20.35. Patient with pityriasis lichenoides et varioliformis acuta demonstrating scattered purpuric lesions. (From the Fitzsimons Army Medical Center Collection, Aurora, CO.)

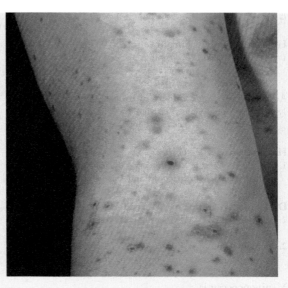

Fig. 20.36. Pityriasis lichenoides et varioliformis acuta in an adult showing purpuric and crusted lesions. (From the Fitzsimons Army Medical Center Collection, Aurora, CO.)

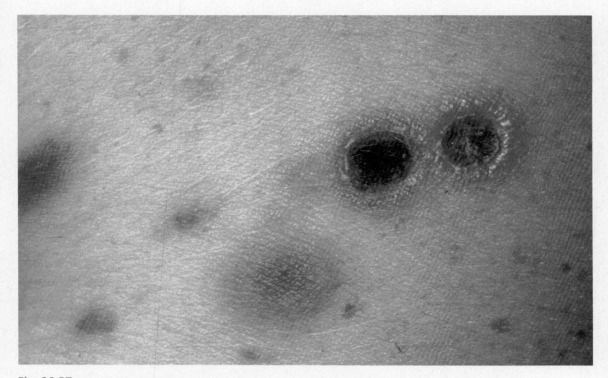

Fig. 20.37. Close-up view demonstrating admixture of hemorrhagic and crusted lesions. (From the Fitzsimons Army Medical Center Collection, Aurora, CO.)

References

Henoch-Schönlein Purpura

1. Modi S, Mohan M, Jennings A. Acute scrotal swelling in Henoch-Schönlein purpura: case report and review of the literature. *Urol Case Rep*. 2016;6:9-11.

Acute Hemorrhagic Edema of Infancy

1. Serra E, Moura Garcia C, Sokolova A, Torre ML, Amaro C. Acute hemorrhagic edema of infancy. *Eur Ann Allergy Clin Immunol*. 2016;48:22-26.

Hypersensitivity Vasculitis

1. Russell JP, Gibson LE. Primary cutaneous small vessel vasculitis: approach to diagnosis and treatment. *Int J Dermatol*. 2006;45:3-13.

Disseminated Gonococcal Infection/Gonococcemia

1. Mehrany K, Kist JM, O'Connor WJ, DiCaudo DJ. Disseminated gonococcemia. *Int J Dermatol*. 2003;42:208-209.
2. Suzaki A, Hayashi K, Kosuge K, et al. Disseminated gonococcal infection in Japan: a case report and literature review. *Intern Med*. 2011;50:2039-2043.

Meningococcemia

1. Takada S, Fujiwara S, Inoue T, et al. Meningococcemia in adults: a review of the literature. *Int Med*. 2016;55:567-572.

Rocky Mountain Spotted Fever

1. Levy C, Burnside J, Tso T, et al. Fatal cases of Rocky Mountain spotted fever in family clusters—three states, 2003. *Arch Dermatol*. 2004;1020:1021.

Progressive Pigmented Purpura (Majocchi-Schamberg Disease)

1. Sardana K, Sarkar R, Sehgal VN. Pigmented purpuric dermatoses: an overview. *Int J Dermatol*. 2004;43:482-488.

Purpura Fulminans

1. David MDP, Dy KM, Nelson S. Presentation and outcome of purpura fulminans associated with peripheral gangrene in 12 patients at Mayo Clinic. *J Am Acad Dermatol*. 2007;57:944-956.

Cryoglobulinemia

1. McGovern TW, Erickson AR, Fitzpatrick JE. Treatment of recalcitrant leg ulcers in cryoglobulinemia types I and II with plasmapheresis. *Arch Dermatol*. 1996;132:498-500.

Cryofibrinogenemia

1. Michaud M, Pourrat J. Cryofibrinogenemia. *J Clin Rheumatol*. 2013;19:142-148.

Pernio (Chilblains)

1. Al-Sudany NK. Treatment of primary perniosis with oral pentoxifylline (a double-blind placebo-controlled randomized therapeutic trial). *Dermatol Ther*. 2016;29:262-268.

Pityriasis Lichenoid et Varioliformis Acuta (Mucha-Habermann Disease)

1. Khachemoune A, Blyumin ML. Pityriasis lichenoides: pathophysiology, classification, and treatment. *Am J Clin Dermatol*. 2007;8:29-36.

Chapter 21
Sclerosing and Fibrosing Disorders

Key Terms

Scleroderma
  Progressive systemic sclerosis

Scleredema
Scleredema adultorum
Scleredema of Buschke

Sclerosing and Fibrosing Disorders: Partial Differential Diagnosis
- Localized scleroderma (morphea)
- Limited scleroderma (CREST syndrome)
- Systemic scleroderma
- Drug-induced sclerosis (e.g., bleomycin)
- Eosinophilic fasciitis
- Graft-versus-host disease
- Mixed connective tissue disease
- Morphea
- Nephrogenic systemic fibrosis
- Porphyria cutanea tarda
- Progressive systemic sclerosis
- Scleredema
- Scleromyxedema

Sclerosing and fibrosing disorders manifest as a hardening or induration of the skin due to the overproduction (fibrosis) and/or thickening (sclerosis) of collagen bundles. Sometimes, organ systems beyond the skin may be affected. Causes include collagen vascular disease and drugs, the latter taken orally or injected.

IMPORTANT HISTORY QUESTIONS

Do you have a history of cold intolerance in your fingers or known Raynaud phenomenon?

This is an important question because systemic scleroderma, limited scleroderma (formerly CREST syndrome [*c*alcinosis, *R*aynaud phenomenon, *e*sophageal dysmotility, *s*clerodactyly, and *t*elangiectasia]), and mixed connective tissue disease (MCTD) can present first in the skin, and the presence of Raynaud phenomenon may be an indication to pursue additional investigation.

Have you noticed swelling in your hands?

Swelling or edema of the hands—puffy hands—can be an early sign of evolving limited or systemic scleroderma or MCTD.

Do you have any difficulty in swallowing solid foods?

Dysphagia can be seen in those with systemic or limited sclerosis or MCTD.

What medications do you take?

This is an important question because some disorders, such as drug-induced sclerosis, eosinophilic fasciitis, and Texier disease, can be drug induced. Texier disease is not discussed in this chapter, but it produces a morphea-like or localized fasciitis-like syndrome at the site of vitamin K injection.

Have you had any recent infections?

Some cases of eosinophilic fasciitis occur after a recent streptococcal or viral infection.

Do you have any other medical conditions?

Other medical conditions of interest include diabetes and multiple myeloma (associated with scleredema). A history of bone marrow transplantation could suggest sclerodermatous graft-versus-host disease.

Have you had any gadolinium-enhanced magnetic resonance imaging (MRI) studies?

Most patients have gadolinium-enhanced MRI studies without consequence, but nephrogenic systemic fibrosis can occur in patients administered these agents in the presence of significant renal disease.

IMPORTANT PHYSICAL FINDINGS

What is the distribution of the fibrosis?

Clinically observed fibrosis or sclerosis can be localized (morphea), confined to limited areas (CREST syndrome, eosinophilic fasciitis), or generalized (systemic scleroderma, generalized morphea, MCTD, or nephrogenic systemic fibrosis).

Are there any other types of skin lesions?

Matlike telangiectasias are often seen on the oral mucosa, face, neck, upper chest, and palms in limited scleroderma (CREST syndrome) but may occur also in systemic scleroderma and MCTD. Also, periungual telangiectasias, often best visualized with an ophthalmoscope, are a feature of limited and systemic scleroderma and MCTD.

Are there any changes in skin color?

Hyperpigmentation of the skin is a feature observed in systemic scleroderma, localized scleroderma (morphea), and eosinophilic fasciitis.

Pathogenesis

Morphea is a localized abnormality of thickened collagen bundles in the dermis and sometimes in the subcutis. In Europe and Japan, *Borrelia burgdorferi* DNA has been detected in some biopsies of morphea, suggesting a possible role in pathogenesis, but this has been disputed, and it is not a feature of most cases in the United States. Importantly, morphea is a cutaneous-limited form of collagen vascular disease. Although some experts have promoted the term *localized scleroderma,* many dermatologists prefer retention of the older term to distinguish it from localized and systemic scleroderma, in which consequences beyond the skin are realized. About one-third of patients with morphea are positive for antinuclear antibody (ANA), usually in low titer. Morphea can also occur in the radiation field after treatment of breast cancer.

Clinical Features

- Morphea is more common in women than men (M : F = 3 : 1) and, although it can occur at any age, it is most common in children, adolescents, and young adults.
- The primary early lesion of morphea is an erythematous to violaceous plaque of variable size, but, in some patients, the inflammatory stage is not observed.
- The trunk and proximal extremities are affected most often.
- Plaque size varies from millimeters to larger than 20 cm.
- As lesions of morphea progress, the center becomes white or yellow-white and indurated, with a violaceous peripheral edge (so-called "lilac ring"; Fig. 21.1).
- Mature lesions lose the lilac ring and, instead, manifest with discoloration, ranging from tan to brown (Figs. 21.2 and 21.3) to white (Fig. 21.4) or even yellow-white.
- Mature lesions may demonstrate depression in relation to the surrounding skin (see Fig. 21.3).
- Most patients are asymptomatic, although mild pruritus may be present.

- Clinical variants include the following:
  - Guttate morphea—multiple to numerous small lesions
  - Linear morphea—linear plaques, often across joint spaces, which may hinder movement
  - Hemifacial atrophy *(coup de sabre)*—a linear form that affects the heads of children or adolescents, yielding facial asymmetry and scarring hair loss
  - Bullous morphea—a rare variant characterized by occasional intermittent blisters
  - Morphea with lichen sclerosus–like changes—the indurated findings of morphea, but with an overlying porcelain white or slightly blue-white color
  - Generalized morphea—involves most of the skin

Diagnosis

- The diagnosis of morphea can usually be made on clinical grounds, with a classic indurated oval or linear plaque, but if an early lesion has a lilac ring, the diagnosis is even more certain.
- Unusual presentations or atypical variants may require a punch biopsy (typically, 4, 5 or 6, mm) or incisional biopsy that includes fat. A shave biopsy is inappropriate to establish the diagnosis of morphea.

Treatment

- No treatment is an option for limited and asymptomatic disease because most cases spontaneously resolve.
- Both psoralen with UVA light (PUVA) or UVA1 phototherapy have limited availability but are probably the treatments of choice.
- If phototherapy is not an option, potent topical corticosteroids, such as clobetasol, or topical calcipotriene 0.005% applied bid, may yield benefit.
- Patients with linear morphea that crosses a joint space should be referred for physical therapy.

Clinical Course

Most patients demonstrate gradual improvement, and even resolution, over a period of 3 to 5 years. Atrophy may not resolve in all cases, even if the inflammation and progression are halted. Patients with localized variants of morphea are not more likely to develop systemic scleroderma.

Fig. 21.1. Patient with early lesion of morphea demonstrating central area of thickened collagen and a lilac rim of discoloration. (From the Fitzsimons Army Medical Center Collection, Aurora, CO.)

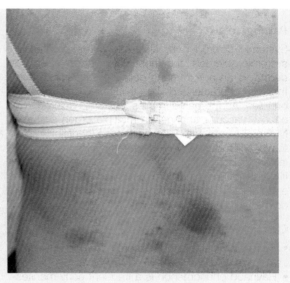

Fig. 21.2. Patient with multiple brownish lesions of morphea on the back. The lesion on the right lower back is brownish-red, indicating an actively inflamed lesion.

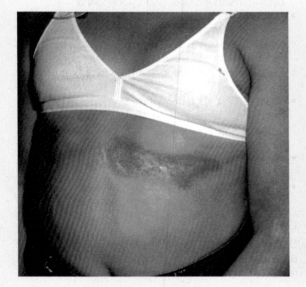

Fig. 21.3. Patient with long-standing brownish indurated plaque that has retracted. The white areas represent lichen sclerosis et atrophicus (LS&A)-like areas. (From the Fitzsimons Army Medical Center Collection, Aurora, CO.)

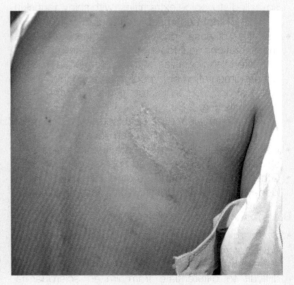

Fig. 21.4. Patient with long-standing morphea with hypopigmented surface reflecting lichen sclerosis et atrophicus (LS&A)-like changes.

❶ Scleroderma ICD10 code M34.0

Pathogenesis

Systemic scleroderma, also known as progressive systemic sclerosis, the most severe form of scleroderma, is an autoimmune collagen vascular disease that is characterized by thickening of collagen bundles. As the name implies, systemic scleroderma causes vascular changes in multiple organ systems. Numerous autoantibodies have been identified in systemic scleroderma, including antinuclear antibodies (anti–topoisomerase I, anti–RNA polymerase I and III), anti–fibrillin I, and autoantibodies directed against endothelial cells. The pathogenesis of systemic scleroderma remains poorly understood.

Clinical Features

- Systemic scleroderma is more common in women than men (M:F = 3:1).
- Raynaud phenomenon is a frequent early manifestation (~70% of patients).
- In early disease, there may be edema of the hands, which can progress into so-called bound-down sclerosis.
- In systemic scleroderma, sclerotic changes eventually involve most of the skin and may produce so-called stovepipe extremities, with shiny, taut skin (Fig. 21.5) that can impair joint mobility.
- As the disease progresses, other cutaneous manifestations include periungual telangiectasias, mat-like telangiectasias of the oral mucosa or skin, hyperpigmentation or hypopigmentation (Fig. 21.6), nail dystrophy, digital infarcts (Fig. 21.7), and calcinosis cutis (Fig. 21.8).
- Patients may also develop ulcers that are most common overlying joints but can develop anywhere.
- Patients usually develop a characteristic facies, with shiny taut skin and restricted opening of the mouth.
- Other organ systems, including the lungs, heart, kidneys, and gastrointestinal tract, may be affected.

Diagnosis

- Systemic scleroderma should be suspected in a patient with Raynaud phenomenon and edema of the extremities (puffy hands). Some cases can be difficult to differentiate from limited scleroderma

(CREST syndrome), diffuse morphea, and mixed connective tissue disease.
- A 3- or 4-mm punch biopsy can be performed on involved skin. The histologic features are usually strongly supportive of the diagnosis.
- A screening ANA test will be positive in about 95% of cases. All cases should have complete panels carried out to look for specific autoantibodies associated with systemic sclerosis.
- Other initial laboratory studies include a complete blood count (CBC) with differential and baseline chemistry studies; these should include renal function, liver function, C-reactive protein, erythrocyte sedimentation rate (ESR), and urinalysis.
- A baseline x-ray of the hands is useful in documenting calcinosis and for later comparison.

Treatment

- The treatment of this systemic disease is beyond the scope of this text. No treatment is uniformly effective in all patients, and some treatments are controversial. Patients should be referred to specialists with expertise in this disease.
- Systemic treatments include D-penicillamine, minocycline, methotrexate, and cyclosporine.
- Calcium channel blockers may be used for Raynaud phenomenon. Antiplatelet drugs (e.g., aspirin) and antiphosphodiesterase inhibitors (e.g., sildenafil, tadalafil) may also be used. Gloves, socks, and avoidance of provocation by cold temperatures are important.
- Vasodilators, such as iloprost, epoprostenol, and treprostinil, or endothelin receptor blockers, such as bosentan and ambrisentan, may be useful for severe disease or systemic compromise.
- Phototherapy, particularly with UVA1 (340–400 nm), may soften affected skin.
- Statins may be of limited benefit due to antiinflammatory and immunomodulatory properties.

Clinical Course

Despite treatment, the 10-year survival rate is only 65% to 80%, with death usually caused by pulmonary, renal, and cardiac complications.

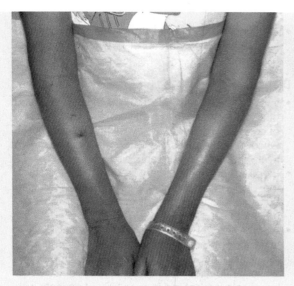

Fig. 21.5. Progressive systemic sclerosis in a young lady demonstrating fibrotic tightly bound-down shiny skin of the arms. (From the Fitzsimons Army Medical Center Collection, Aurora, CO.)

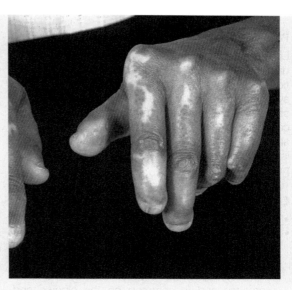

Fig. 21.6. Marked sclerodactyly with nail dystrophy and hypopigmentation in a patient with progressive systemic sclerosis. (From the Fitzsimons Army Medical Center Collection, Aurora, CO.)

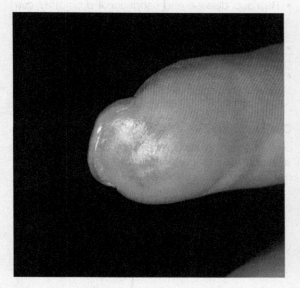

Fig. 21.7. Digital infarcts on the tip of the finger in a patient with progressive systemic sclerosis and severe Raynaud phenomenon. (From the Fitzsimons Army Medical Center Collection, Aurora, CO.)

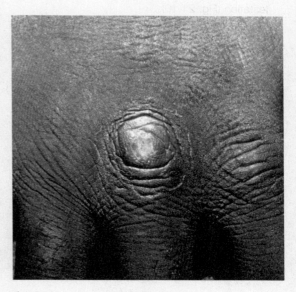

Fig. 21.8. Perforating calcinosis cutis on the knuckle of a patient with progressive systemic sclerosis. (From the Fitzsimons Army Medical Center Collection, Aurora, CO.)

Pathogenesis

Limited scleroderma (formerly known as CREST syndrome) is a collagen vascular disease with a presentation that is slightly less diffuse, and less fulminant, than systemic scleroderma. The term *CREST syndrome* is still preferred by some dermatologists. Patients typically have a positive ANA, with most patients demonstrating anticentromere antibodies (50–90%). There is an association between CREST syndrome and primary biliary cirrhosis.

Clinical Features

- Limited scleroderma typically presents in adults.
- As the CREST acronym implies, limited scleroderma has five main features:
  - Calcinosis cutis—firm, white to yellow-white discrete deposits that occur late in the disease process and is common on the elbows and hands. In some cases, the lesions of calcinosis cutis may erode, ulcerate, or even extrude calcium (Fig. 21.9).
  - Raynaud phenomenon—usually presents early in the disease process and may be the first manifestation (Fig. 21.10).
  - Esophageal dysmotility—difficulty swallowing food, with a sensation of getting stuck, or even with chest discomfort.
  - Sclerodactyly—edematous fingers that may become erythematous, with a tightening of skin over the finger dorsum and limited joint mobility. In severe cases, there may be distal digital infarcts or even infarcted whole digits (Fig. 21.11).
  - Telangiectasias—presents as mats of dilated blood vessels and tend to involve the oral mucosa, face, neck, upper chest, and palmar surfaces of the hands (Fig. 21.12).

- Although most patients do not demonstrate systemic involvement, a subset may develop pulmonary hypertension.

Diagnosis

- In early cases, patients may have only Raynaud phenomenon and hand edema, and a high index of suspicion is needed to investigate the diagnosis. Once all the features of CREST are in place, it is a relatively easy clinical diagnosis to make.
- Biopsies are not usually required to establish the diagnosis; finger biopsies may be ill advised because digits already affected by sclerodactyly may not heal.
- A screening ANA is required, with particular evaluation for anticentromere and anti–topoisomerase I (Scl-70) antibodies. The presence of antitopoisomerase antibodies favors full systemic sclerosis because it is identified in only 10% of patients with limited scleroderma (CREST syndrome).

Treatment

- No treatment is uniformly effective, and the disease tends to be slowly progressive.
- Raynaud disease and esophageal dysmotility can be managed with drugs directed at these symptoms (see earlier, "Scleroderma").
- Calcium deposits that inhibit hand function are usually amenable to removal by a hand surgeon.
- Some patients are treated with oral corticosteroids, D-penicillamine, and methotrexate, but these agents are used for more often systemic scleroderma.

Clinical Course

Limited scleroderma is a chronic but slowly progressive condition. Importantly, patients usually do not usually expire from the disease.

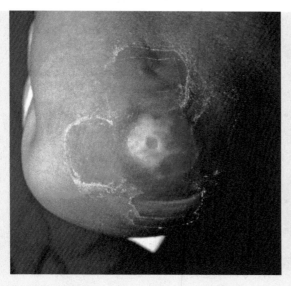

Fig. 21.9. Patient with calcinotic cutis, with eroded hard yellowish-white plaque of dystrophic calcium on the elbow. (From the Fitzsimons Army Medical Center Collection, Aurora, CO.)

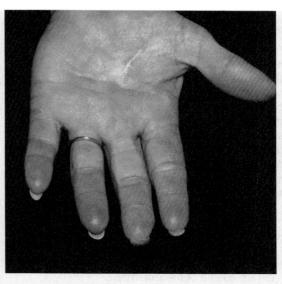

Fig. 21.10. Severe cyanosis from Raynaud phenomenon. The patient was seen smoking outside the clinic after this visit. (From the Fitzsimons Army Medical Center Collection, Aurora, CO.)

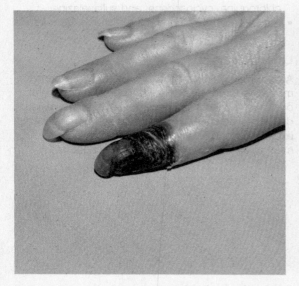

Fig. 21.11. Patient with severe sclerodactyly and a partially gangrenous digit, which had to be amputated. (From the Fitzsimons Army Medical Center Collection, Aurora, CO.)

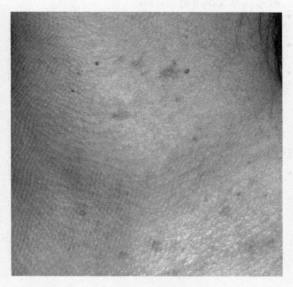

Fig. 21.12. Matlike telangiectasia on the neck and upper chest in a patient with CREST syndrome. (From the Fitzsimons Army Medical Center Collection, Aurora, CO.)

Pathogenesis

Eosinophilic fasciitis (EF) is a disorder characterized by inflammation and thickening of the collagen bundles of the superficial fascia overlying muscle, with variable extension of the process into the fibrous septae of the lower subcutaneous tissue. The pathogenesis is poorly understood although, in some patients, the process is precipitated by exertion. An epidemic of an eosinophilic fasciitis–like syndrome (eosinophilia-myalgia syndrome) was linked to the oral intake of L-tryptophan with unknown trace contaminants and also to contaminated rapeseed oil.

Clinical Features

- EF can involve persons of any age but is most common in 40- to 50-year-olds.
- Initial manifestations of EF include increased and diffuse edema of the extremities.
- As EF matures, a *peau d'orange* appearance and marked induration of affected areas ensues.
- Brawny induration usually spares the areas around superficial veins, producing a so-called groove sign or superhero sign, with exaggerated definition of muscle groups (Fig. 21.13).
- Variable focal hyperpigmentation can develop in EF during its later stages (Fig. 21.14).
- Rare patients with EF may develop focal morphea-like changes that confound the diagnosis.
- Most EF patients do not demonstrate systemic manifestations, but noncutaneous consequences can include joint contracture (Fig. 21.15), carpal tunnel syndrome, muscle weakness, arthralgias, arthritis, and pulmonary symptoms.

Diagnosis

- Edema, *peau d'orange* changes to the skin, and woody induration confined to the extremities, without Raynaud phenomenon, should suggest EF. The ability to pinch overlying skin easily is a feature of eosinophilic fasciitis that is not seen in systemic scleroderma or diffuse morphea. The presence of a "groove sign" or "superhero sign" also supports the diagnosis of EF.
- To be useful in diagnosis, an incisional biopsy must extend to the superficial muscle. Biopsies that are too superficial are not uncommon. Hence, when EF is suspected, the biopsy should be done by a clinician who is comfortable doing biopsies that extend into muscle.
- MRI can be used to detect fascial thickening and may even suggest a high-yield area for biopsy.
- Laboratory studies that support the diagnosis include a CBC (will usually demonstrate peripheral eosinophilia in 60% of cases), elevated ESR, and hypergammaglobulinemia (seen in 50% of cases).

Treatment

- Oral prednisone (20–60 mg/day for at least 1 month) is often used and is gradually tapered based on the clinical response.
- Other steroid-sparing agents include oral hydroxychloroquine, cyclosporine, and sulfasalazine.
- Patients with joint contractures should be referred to physical therapy.

Clinical Course

Approximately 80% of patients with EF will experience moderate to considerable improvement with therapy, but most patients continue to have some residual disease, even after effective treatment. Some patients experience only slight improvement, or no improvement at all, even with aggressive management.

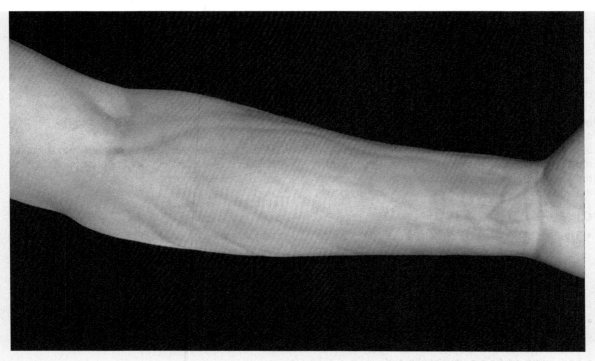

Fig. 21.13. Eosinophilic fasciitis in a 30-year-old soldier that developed after strenuous physical activity. In addition to induration, this case demonstrates the groove sign. (From the Fitzsimons Army Medical Center Collection, Aurora, CO.)

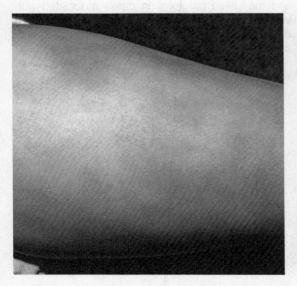

Fig. 21.14. Patient with late-stage eosinophilic fasciitis showing a woody indurated thigh, with focal faint hyperpigmentation.

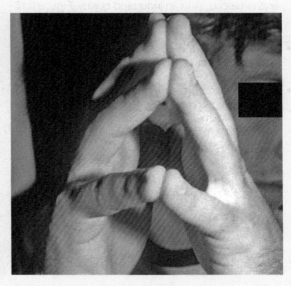

Fig. 21.15. Loss of joint flexibility in a patient with eosinophilic fasciitis. (From the Fitzsimons Army Medical Center Collection, Aurora, CO.)

Scleredema ICD10 code M34.9

Pathogenesis

Scleredema, also known as scleredema of Buschke and scleredema adultorum, is a rare disorder characterized by thickening of the collagen and variable mucin deposition in the skin or other organs. The condition usually occurs in adults with diabetes, but it may also occur after an infection (including streptococcal and viral infections). This infection-associated variant is more common in children and young adults. Scleredema can also be associated with malignancy, or it may be idiopathic. The mechanism(s) that produces these distinctive changes in the dermis are unknown.

Clinical Features

- The neck and upper back are usually affected in diabetes-associated cases, and this form is most common in obese men. In such cases, type 2 diabetes has usually been present for years, or even decades, and the patient is usually insulin-dependent.
- In cases associated with infections, the onset is usually more abrupt, and disease is more likely to involve the face, neck, and upper chest. Children and young adults are usually affected.
- Rarely, a generalized variant that involves most of the body can occur.
- The skin is usually normally colored, or mildly erythematous, with an indurated quality (Figs. 21.16 and 21.17). The overlying skin usually cannot be pinched.
- In some cases, the skin demonstrates a puckered appearance, and this is especially common on the extremities or in the pelvic region.
- Some patients may report difficulty swallowing or protruding the tongue, which is thought to be related to restriction of muscle movement by thickened collagen.

Diagnosis

- The diagnosis is usually established based on clinical findings, particularly in the diabetes-related variant common in adults.
- In select cases, a 4- to 6-mm punch biopsy or incisional biopsy, to fat, may be necessary. Characteristically, if scleredema is present, it is difficult to suture the wound.
- Because some cases are associated with multiple myeloma, serum protein electrophoresis should be considered as a screening modality.

Treatment

- No treatment is uniformly effective in all patients. If the patient is not troubled by the condition, treatment is not required.
- Both PUVA or UVA1 phototherapy can be partially effective in some cases.
- Electron beam therapy has been used successfully in severe cases, but there are many long-term side effects to consider before using this modality.
- Patients with lesions that impair joints should be referred to physical therapy.

Clinical Course

In most cases, and particularly with the variant associated with diabetes, scleredema may last indefinitely and may even progress. In cases associated with infection, some patients will spontaneously improve over a period of months to years. In patients with scleredema associated with multiple myeloma, treatment of the plasma cell dyscrasia can yield significant improvement.

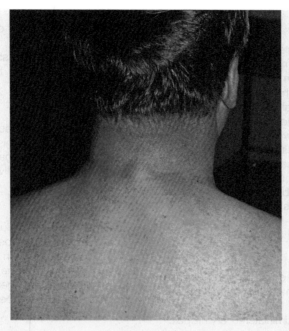

Fig. 21.16. Man with type 2 diabetes and markedly erythematous, firm, indurated plaque of the neck and upper back. (From the Fitzsimons Army Medical Center Collection, Aurora, CO.)

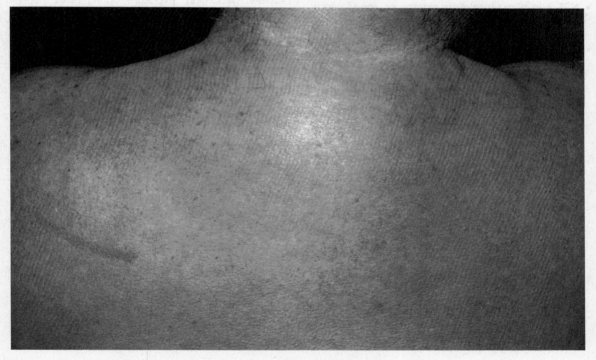

Fig. 21.17. Man with type 2 diabetes who presented for evaluation of pruritus. An excoriation is present on the left side of his back. The patient was obese and had not noted the erythema and marked induration of his neck and upper back until it was pointed out to him during the initial visit. (From the Fitzsimons Army Medical Center Collection, Aurora, CO.)

Pathogenesis

Nephrogenic systemic fibrosis (NSF) is a condition that was first identified in hemodialysis patients, with cutaneous lesions that resembled scleromyxedema clinically and histologically. Although the patient population affected (those with renal failure) was well recognized, the cause of the condition was unknown. It was discovered in 2006, through work done in part by one of the authors (WAH). Gadolinium, derived from materials used in contrast-enhanced MRI, was deposited in the tissue of persons with NSF. The deposition of this material is considered to be involved in the development of NSF, which causes indurated fibrotic skin, joint contractures, and even fibrosis of other organ systems, leading to morbidity and death.

Clinical Features

- NSF occurs in patients with significant renal disease and exposure to gadolinium-based contrast materials used in MRI.
- Hyperphosphatemia, co-administered erythropoietin, or iron supplementation, and even the particular chelating agent used in a specific brand of gadolinium contrast, are all probable cofactors in the development of NSF, but exposure to gadolinium is a common requisite element.
- NSF can begin weeks to months or, rarely, years after exposure to the contrast agent during a period of renal insufficiency.
- The skin develops a fibrotic indurated texture, a *peau d'orange* or pebbled appearance to the skin may ensue (Fig. 21.18), and the patient develops joint contractures and stooped posture and may even become wheelchair bound (Fig. 21.19).

- Fibrotic plaques may develop in some patients (Fig. 21.20).
- Some patients demonstrate characteristic yellow-white concretions in the sclera of their eyes (Fig. 21.21).

Diagnosis

- The diagnosis is based on clinical presentation, appropriate exposure history (gadolinium exposure during a period of renal insufficiency), and characteristic and supportive histologic changes on biopsy.

Treatment

- Treatment is difficult. Supportive measures for the joint contractures and loss of mobility are important.
- Antifibrotic agents, such as imatinib mesylate, have proven effective in some persons.
- Immunosuppressive agents are of limited use.
- Physical therapy may be useful for those with joint contractures.

Clinical Course

In 2006, the discovery of gadolinium in the tissue of persons with NSF marked a turning point in disease incidence. With recognition of the strong association between gadolinium exposure during renal insufficiency and the development of NSF and the improved screening for renal insufficiency prior to dosing these agents, the incidence of NSF decreased from about 40 to about 6 persons per 100,000 contrast-enhanced MRI examinations. The condition is now rarely seen as long as exposure to gadolinium-based agents is avoided in persons at risk of developing NSF.

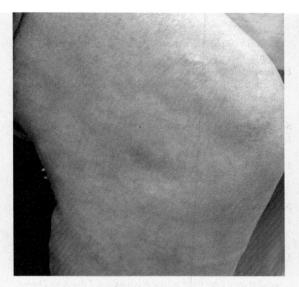

Fig. 21.18. Patient with nephrogenic systemic fibrosis with marked induration of the leg, with a pebbled appearance.

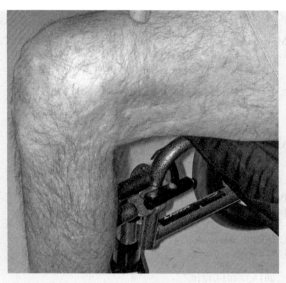

Fig. 21.19. Severe induration of the leg resulting in the patient with nephrogenic systemic fibrosis becoming wheelchair-bound.

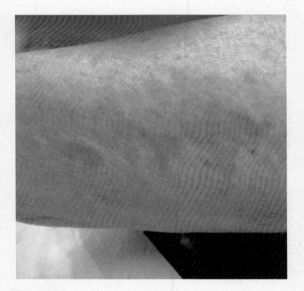

Fig. 21.20. Patient with lightly pigmented defined plaques of nephrogenic systemic fibrosis on an extremity.

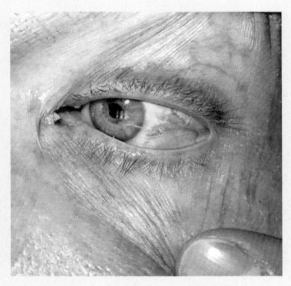

Fig. 21.21. Patient with characteristic yellowish scleral plaques of nephrogenic systemic fibrosis.

References

Morphea

1. Christen-Zaich S, Hakim MD, Afsar FS, Paller AS. Pediatric morphea (localized scleroderma): review of 136 patients. *J Am Acad Dermatol.* 2008;59:385-396.
2. David DA, Cohen PR, McNeese MD, Duvic M. Localized scleroderma in breast cancer patients treated with supervoltage external beam radiation: radiation port scleroderma. *J Am Acad Dermatol.* 1996;35:923-927.
3. Dharamsi JW, Victor S, Aguwa N, et al. Morphea in adults and children cohort III. Nest case-control study—the clinical significant of autoantibodies in morphea. *JAMA Dermatol.* 2013;149:1159-1165.

Progressive Systemic Sclerosis

1. Hachulla E, Launday D. Diagnosis and classification of systemic sclerosis. *Clin Rev Allergy Immunol.* 2011;40:78-83.

CREST Syndrome

1. Merlino G, German S, Carlucci S. Surgical management of digital calcinosis in CREST syndrome. *Aesthetic Plast Surg.* 2013;37:1214-1219.
2. Nishimagi E, Kawaguchi Y, Terai C, et al. Progressive interstitial renal fibrosis due to Chinese herbs in a patient with calcinosis Raynaud esophageal sclerodactyly telangiectasia (CREST) syndrome. *Intern Med.* 2001;40:1059-1063.

Eosinophilic Fasciitis

1. Bischoff L, Derk CT. Eosinophilic fasciitis: demographics, disease pattern and response to treatment: report of 12 cases and review of the literature. *Int J Dermatol.* 2008;47:29-35.

Scleredema

1. Jung S-E, Kim YC. Scleredema of Buschke following streptococcal infection. *Ann Dermatol.* 2015;27:478-480.
2. Rongieoletti F, Kaiser F, Cinotti E, et al. Scleredema. A multicentre study of characteristics, comorbidities, course and therapy in 44 patients. *J Eur Acad Dermatol Venereol.* 2015;29:2399-2404.

Nephrogeneic Systemic Fibrosis

1. Girardi M, Kay J, Elston DM, et al. Nephrogenic systemic fibrosis: clinicopathological definition and workup recommendations. *J Am Acad Dermatol.* 2011;65:1095-1106.
2. High WA, Ranville JF, Brown M, et al. Gadolinium deposition in nephrogenic systemic fibrosis: an examination of tissue using synchrotron x-ray fluorescence spectroscopy. *J Am Acad Dermatol.* 2010;62:38-44.

Atrophic Disorders: Partial Differential Diagnosis

- Acrodermatitis chronica atrophicans
- Anetoderma
- Aging—extrinsic (photoaging)
- Aging—intrinsic
- Aplasia cutis congenita
- Atrophic lichen planus
- Atrophic scar
- Atrophoderma of Pasini and Pierini
- Corticosteroid atrophy
- Focal dermal hypoplasia
- Follicular atrophoderma
- Lichen sclerosus et atrophicus (Chapter 27)
- Lipodystrophies
- Poikiloderma atrophicans vasculare
- Postinjection lipoatrophy
- Striae distensae

Atrophic disorders are a group of heterogeneous diseases characterized by an atrophic (thinned) epidermis, dermis, or subcutis. Some atrophic diseases affect the epidermis (e.g., photoaging, topical corticosteroid overuse), whereas others affect the dermis (atrophoderma from intralesional steroid injections). Although the term *atrophy* implies that the skin was once normal, some disorders in this disease group (see box) are actually congenital and are caused by hypoplasia (focal dermal hypoplasia), in which the skin is less fully formed, or by aplasia (aplasia cutis congenita), in which a particular layer of the skin was never formed.

IMPORTANT HISTORY QUESTIONS

When was this change in your skin noted?

This question is designed to distinguish congenital disorders (e.g., aplasia cutis congenita, focal dermal hypoplasia) from acquired disorders (e.g., photoaging, lichen sclerosus).

Over what period of time did these changes occur?

Some atrophic conditions foment quickly (e.g., striae distensae, anetoderma due to steroid injections) whereas others may develop over months, years, or decades (e.g., poikiloderma atrophicans vasculare, intrinsic aging, photoaging).

Have you used any steroids in the area, or have you had steroid injections or taken steroid pills?

Topical corticosteroids, especially potent forms, may thin the skin or produce striae. Localized atrophy may be caused by corticosteroid injections (intradermal or intramuscular). Even oral glucocorticosteroids, when taken in a higher dose and/or for extended durations, may lead to skin thinning and striae.

Have you been given any other injections in the area?

Injections of insulin, vaccines, antibiotics, of other injectable agents of any type may cause atrophy, especially if injected in the same area, for an extended duration, or with a suboptimal technique.

Do you have any other medical conditions?

Other medical conditions of interest include *Borrelia* infection (e.g., acrodermatitis chronica atrophicans, atrophoderma of Pasini and Pierini) and collagen vascular disease or cutaneous T cell lymphoma.

IMPORTANT PHYSICAL FINDINGS

What is the distribution of the atrophy?

Many atrophic disorders have a characteristic distribution. For example, striae distensae (stretch marks) usually involve the axillae, abdomen, and upper thighs, whereas postinjection atrophy involves regions of the body where injections are delivered (e.g., upper arms, upper buttock, abdomen).

How large are the areas of atrophy, and how are they shaped?

Some forms of atrophy yield large lesions (e.g., atrophoderma of Pasini and Pierini), or cover large areas (e.g., photoaging). Other forms of atrophy are localized (e.g., postinjection atrophy).

Are there any changes in skin color?

Hypopigmentation may be seen in lichen sclerosus et atrophicus, atrophic scars, striae distensae, and atrophy due to corticosteroid injections; hyperpigmentation is more common in atrophoderma of Pasini and Pierini. Disorders with a hypoplastic or aplastic dermis may appear yellow due to visible fat.

Pathogenesis

Striae, also known as striae distensae or stretch marks, are linear atrophic areas of skin that are characterized by an absence of elastic fibers and altered collagen bundles. The pathogenesis has not been fully elucidated, but associations with rapid weight gain and steroid use suggest that more than one factor may be involved. Histologic evaluation and electron microscopy used on early lesions have demonstrated an inflammatory element, with mast cells and other inflammatory cells elaborating elastase and altering elastic fibers. Striae are seen with increased frequency in adolescents with rapid weight gain, pregnancy (striae gravidarum), and disorders with elevated systemic adrenocorticoid levels (Cushing disease) and with systemically administered corticosteroids. Striae may also be induced by topical corticosteroids.

Clinical Features

- Most striae occur in adolescents with rapid weight gain, during pregnancy, with administration of systemic corticosteroids, or with use of topical corticosteroids.
- The most frequently affected sites include the axilla, upper thighs, and lower back.
- Striae may be elevated, rather than depressed, and are often red in color (striae rubra) (Fig. 22.1). As any associated inflammation subsides, the lesions may become violaceous (Fig. 22.2) and may eventually develop a white color (striae alba; Fig. 22.3).
- Mature striae are linear, depressed, and may demonstrate a wrinkled cigarette paper–like surface.
- Striae gravidarum usually develop during the sixth and seventh months of pregnancy and often affect the lower abdomen (Fig. 22.4) and breasts. Incidence rates in pregnant women vary from 50% to 90%.

Cocoa Butter: Does It Prevent Striae?

No. Although studies have shown that more than 60% of pregnant women use cocoa butter or other so-called bio-oils to prevent stretch marks, there is no medical evidence that this works. In fact, in a large (210 women), double-blinded, randomized, placebo-controlled trial, cocoa butter did not prevent stretch marks.

Diagnosis

- The clinical diagnosis of striae is usually made easily and is often assessed by the patient.
- Rare spontaneous cases may require an endocrine evaluation to exclude Cushing disease or another disorder of excess adrenocorticoids.
- Biopsies do not have a role in the assessment of striae.

Treatment

- No specific treatment for striae is particularly effective.
- Iatrogenic cases are managed with withdrawal or reduction of topical or systemic corticosteroids.
- In early disease (striae rubra), some therapies may improve cosmesis, such as topical 0.1% tretinoin, but should not be used in pregnant or breastfeeding patients, mesotherapy (hyaluronic acid injected with a mesogun), microdermabrasion, and lasers (Nd:YAG).
- In select cases, surgical excision of isolated lesions may improve cosmesis.

Clinical Course

For most patients, once striae develop, they are permanent, because the skin has no way to reattach the disrupted elastic fibers. In the setting of striae induced by topical corticosteroid overuse, some patients may notice varied improvement with prompt removal of the offending agent(s).

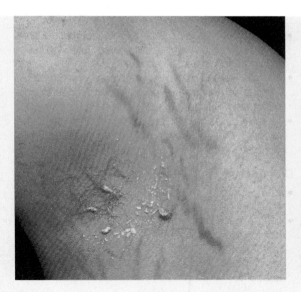

Fig. 22.1. Acute onset of red striae in an adolescent with recent weight gain. (From the William Weston Collection, Aurora, CO.)

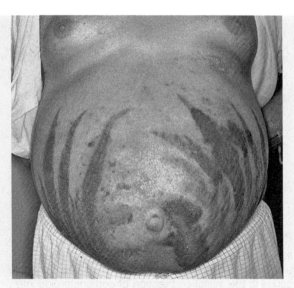

Fig. 22.2. Patient with massive violaceous striae due to oral corticosteroids and rapid weight gain. (From the Fitzsimons Army Medical Center Collection, Aurora, CO.)

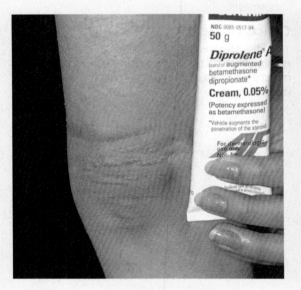

Fig. 22.3. Patient with older striae with white and violaceous colors. This case was produced by a potent topical corticosteroid. (From the William Weston Collection, Aurora, CO.)

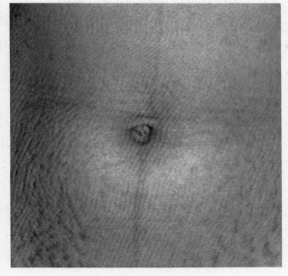

Fig. 22.4. Patient with striae gravidarum. Note the associated linea nigra of pregnancy.

Postinjection Lipoatrophy ICD10 code L90.8

Causes of Postinjection Lipoatrophy

Common Causes

- Benzathine penicillin
- Corticosteroids
- Insulin

Uncommon Causes

- Copolymer I
- Diphtheria, tetanus, and acellular pertussis (DTaP) vaccine
- Human growth hormone
- Iron dextran
- Methotrexate
- Vasopressin

Pathogenesis

Injection-related atrophy of the subcutaneous tissue is a well-recognized adverse reaction. The most common cause is the mistaken injection of corticosteroids into the subcutaneous tissue, rather than into the dermis or muscle. Other less frequent causes are listed in the box. In some cases, lipocytes are damaged by trauma and/or a host response to another injected material (e.g., insulin), whereas corticosteroids cause atrophy due to direct catabolic and metabolic effects.

Clinical Features

- Lipoatrophy usually develops 4 to 8 weeks after injection.
- Postinjection lipoatrophy usually occurs on the upper arms (Fig. 22.5), upper lateral buttock (Fig. 22.6), and abdomen, which corresponds with areas often used for medical injections.

- The primary lesion consists of a depressed area of skin, with loss of subcutaneous fat. Significant inflammation is usually absent.
- The depression may be skin-colored (see Fig. 22.6) or may demonstrate hypopigmentation due to corticosteroid injection (Fig. 22.7; see Fig. 22.6).
- In rare cases, when the skin is pulled taut, the injected corticosteroid may be identified as white concretions (see Fig. 22.7).

Diagnosis

- In most cases, the diagnosis is made clinically via a history of an injection at the site.
- In rare cases, where the corresponding history is not forthcoming, or history of an injection is denied (see Fig. 22.7), a 4-mm punch biopsy may demonstrate material consistent with corticosteroid in the subcutis.

Treatment

- No treatment for postinjection atrophy is consistently effective.
- In rare cases, surgical fat transfer may improve cosmesis.

Clinical Course

The clinical course is unpredictable. Some patients demonstrate partial or even complete resolution over months or years, but for some patients the damage is permanent.

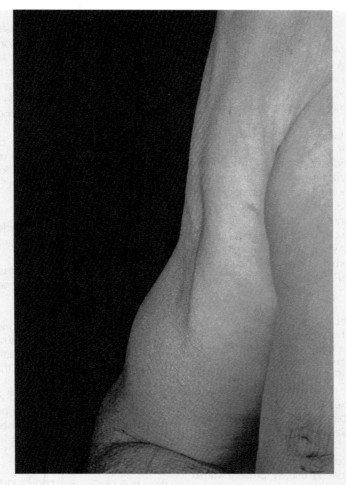

Fig. 22.5. Patient with multiple areas of depression due to atrophy of the subcutaneous fat caused by repetitive insulin injections.

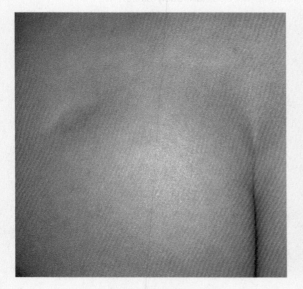

Fig. 22.6. Patient with subcutaneous atrophy and hypopigmentation due to injected triamcinolone. This was supposed to be an intramuscular injection, but the triamcinolone was injected into the fat.

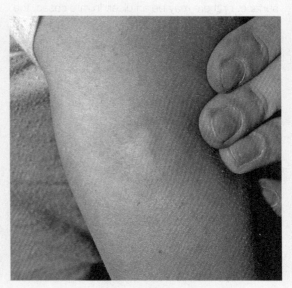

Fig. 22.7. Patient with subcutaneous atrophy and hypopigmentation due to injected triamcinolone. With the skin pulled taut, whitish triamcinolone could be visualized in the center of the lesion. (From the Fitzsimons Army Medical Center Collection, Aurora, CO.)

Aplasia Cutis Congenita ICD10 code Q48.8

Pathogenesis

Aplasia cutis congenita (APC) is an uncommon disorder (~3 cases/100,000 births) but is the most common cause of a congenital scarring alopecia. The mechanism is poorly understood, but the presence of familial cases of APC—autosomal dominant and autosomal recessive variants exist—suggests a genetic basis (OMIM 10760). In one family, the defect was linked to a mutation in the *BMS1* gene on chromosome 10. APC is also a component of several syndromes, including Johanson-Blizzard syndrome, Adams-Oliver syndrome, Wolf-Hirschhorn syndrome, epidermolysis bullosa, and trisomy 13. Intrauterine infection with herpes simplex virus and varicella-zoster virus has been implicated in some cases. Certain drugs, including cocaine, marijuana, valproic acid, methimazole, carbimazole, and misoprostol, have also been linked to the development of APC.

Clinical Features

- APC is present at birth.
- Most cases involve the vertex of the scalp (Figs. 22.8–22.10), usually just lateral to the midline (~70% of cases). Other sites less often involved include the back and extremities (Fig. 22.11).
- APC may be a solitary condition (70% of cases), or lesions may be multiple (30% of cases).
- Lesions of APC may be round or oval and linear or stellate and range in size from 0.5 cm to more than 10 cm.
- There may be absence of all skin or simply partial loss. Complete hair loss is usually present within atrophic areas.
- The surface may be shiny, with a thinned or scaly surface, or there may be an ulcer. In rare cases, the surface may appear bullous.

- Some lesions may demonstrate a so-called hair collar sign, with a ring of longer, darker hair that surrounds the area of hair loss (see Fig. 22.10). Patients with a hair collar sign are more likely to have underlying defects of bone or neurologic abnormalities (e.g., meningomyelocele, porencephaly).
- Patients may have underlying bony or neurologic defects.
- Some cases of APC have been associated with fetus papyraceus (so-called vanishing twin).
- Complications of APC include hemorrhage into the skin, bleeding, and infection.

Diagnosis

- The diagnosis is usually made on clinical grounds, with observation of focal scarring, devoid of hair, on the vertex of a newborn.
- Select cases should have imaging studies to evaluate for underlying bony or neural defects.

Treatment

- No treatment is required. Conservative intervention, particularly to promote healing when ulceration is present, includes topical petrolatum, silver sulfadiazine cream, or dressings that contain epidermal growth factor.
- Select cases can be treated with surgical intervention. Cases with underlying bone defects are best managed by a multidisciplinary team of neurosurgeons and plastic surgeons.

Clinical Course

APC is a permanent condition that will demonstrate mature scar with time. In most cases, any bone defects will spontaneously close.

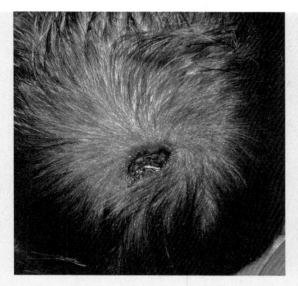

Fig. 22.8. Patient with solitary lesion of ulcerated aplasia cutis congenita. (From the William Weston Collection, Aurora, CO.)

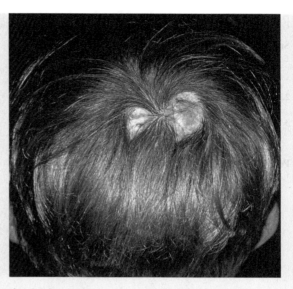

Fig. 22.9. Two lesions of aplasia cutis congenita on the scalp of an older child with the appearance of a scaly scar. (From the Fitzsimons Army Medical Center Collection, Aurora, CO.)

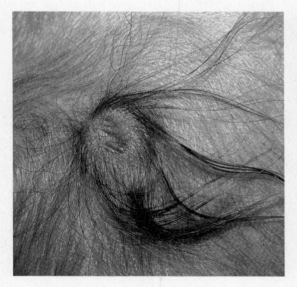

Fig. 22.10. Close-up of aplasia cutis congenita on the scalp of a patient demonstrating a hair collar sign. (From the William Weston Collection, Aurora, CO.)

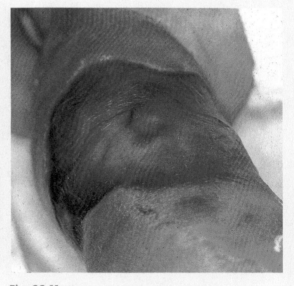

Fig. 22.11. Patient with large lesion of aplasia cutis congenita on the leg. (From the William Weston Collection, Aurora, CO.)

References

Striae

1. Brennan M, Clarke M, Devane D. The use of anti-stretch marks products by women in pregnancy: a descriptive, cross-sectional survey. *BMC Pregnancy Childbirth.* 2016;16:276.
2. Karia UK, Padhiar BB, Shah BJ. Evaluation of various therapeutic measures in striae rubra. *J Cutan Aesthet Surg.* 2016;9:101-105.
3. Osman H, Usta IM, Rubeiz N, et al. Cocoa butter lotion for prevention of striae gravidarum: a double-blind, randomized and placebo-controlled trial. *BJOG.* 2008;115:1138-1142.

Postinjection Lipoatrophy

1. Chantelau EA, Prätor R, Prätor J. Insulin-induced localized lipoatrophy preceded by shingles (herpes zoster): a case report. *J Med Case Rep.* 2014;8:223.

2. Sardana K, Garg VK, Bhushan P, et al. DPT vaccine-induced lipoatrophy: an observational study. *Int J Dermatol.* 2007;46:1050-1054.

Aplasia Cutis Congenita

1. Duan X, Yang GE, Yu D, et al. Aplasia cutis congenita: a case report and literature review. *Exp Ther Med.* 2015;10:1083-1085.
2. Winston KR, Ketchh LL. Aplasia cutis congenita of the scalp, composite type: the criticality and inseparability of neurosurgical and plastic surgical management. *Pediatr Neurosurg.* 2016;51:11-120.

Chapter 23
Follicular Disorders

Selected Follicular Disorders
Common
- Acne vulgaris
- Dermatophytic folliculitis
- Drug-induced acneiform disorders
- Keratosis pilaris
- Neonatal acne
- *Pityrosporum* folliculitis
- Rosacea
- Staphylococcal folliculitis

Uncommon
- Eosinophilic folliculitis
- Follicular atopic dermatitis
- Follicular mycosis fungoides
- Lichen spinulosus
- Perioral dermatitis
- Pseudomonal folliculitis
- Viral folliculitis

Follicular disorders represent pathologic processes that alter or otherwise inflame the pilosebaceous (follicular) unit. Alopecias are also follicular disorders but are considered elsewhere in this text. Numerous disorders can affect the follicle, including infections, disorders of keratinization, some neoplasms (e.g., follicular mycosis fungoides), genodermatoses, and other inflammatory disorders. The following questions are important to ask during the evaluation of follicular disorders.

IMPORTANT HISTORY QUESTIONS

How long has the follicular alteration been present?

It is helpful to determine if the condition is acute or chronic. For example, acne vulgaris, keratosis pilaris, and follicular atopic dermatitis are typically chronic disorders, whereas drug-induced acneiform eruptions and pseudomonal folliculitis are acute events.

Have you started any new medications in the past month?

This question is most relevant to drug-induced acneiform eruptions. Oral corticosteroids, androgens, isoniazid, lithium, and some birth control medications can cause medication-induced acne.

Are you putting anything on the skin of the affected area?

Many patients use home remedies, over-the-counter remedies, or even prescription remedies, which can worsen follicular disorders. For example, some patients with acne use comedogenic cosmetic products that aggravate the condition. Mistaken or misguided use of topical corticosteroids can also aggravate acne vulgaris and rosacea, cause perioral dermatitis, or complicate dermatophyte infections.

Have you recently used a hot tub or hot springs pool or had some other immersive water exposure?

This question is pertinent when the clinical differential diagnosis includes *Pseudomonas* folliculitis.

IMPORTANT PHYSICAL FINDINGS

What is the distribution of the follicular disorder?

Some follicular disorders have characteristic distributions. Acne vulgaris usually involves the face and upper trunk, whereas rosacea is typically confined only to the face. *Pseudomonas* folliculitis is almost always truncal and is most prevalent beneath areas that were covered by a bathing suit.

Is there a distinct pattern to the dermatitis?

Some follicular disorders are grouped (e.g., lichen spinulosus) or dermatomal. Grouped erythematous follicle-situated papules or vesicles, in a dermatomal pattern, lead to consideration of herpes zoster.

Are other mucocutaneous findings present?

Some follicular disorders have other cutaneous findings that suggest the diagnosis. For example, rosacea often has background erythema, telangiectasias, or ocular findings, whereas pseudomonal folliculitis may be associated with mastitis, conjunctivitis, otitis externa, or pharyngitis.

Is a pustular component present?

Some follicular disorders, such as lichen spinulosus or follicular eczema, are almost never pustular, whereas staphylococcal folliculitis or pseudomonal folliculitis often demonstrate follicle-centered pustules.

Pathogenesis

Acne is a multifactorial disorder. Abnormal follicular maturation, in response to an altered hormonal milieu, leads to follicular plugging and retained sebum. This results in the overgrowth of a commensal bacteria called *Propionibacterium acnes*. The bacterium elaborates proinflammatory mediators, and follicular rupture leads to the liberation of proinflammatory free fatty acids into the dermis. The result is a classic "zit." Follicular plugging alone causes comedones (blackheads, whiteheads). This concept of acne as a multifactorial disorder is important because treatment may be directed against any of these contributing factors. Ergot, agents that prevent comedone formation, reduce sebum production, decrease bacterial growth, or blunt the proinflammatory response, may improve the condition.

Clinical Features

- Acne typically begins during puberty (after andrenarche).
- Acne is usually distributed on the face (most common site), neck, and upper chest or back.
- Acne typically causes the following:
  - Comedones (blocked pores), which may be open (blackheads; Fig. 23.1) or closed (whiteheads)
  - Erythematous follicle-based papules
  - Follicle-based pustules and nodules
  - Acneiform epidermoid cysts (see Fig. 34.2)
  - Scarring may develop at sites of marked follicular inflammation or follicular rupture; this may result in substantial residual pigmentary changes, particularly in persons with darker skin.

Diagnosis

- Acne is almost always a clinical diagnosis; often it has already been diagnosed by the patient.
- Women with male pattern hair growth on the face or genitals, early-onset alopecia, cliteromegaly, severe acne, and other signs of hirsutism warrant an endocrine evaluation.

Treatment

- Mild acne (primarily comedonal acne)
  - Mild comedonal acne can be treated with a topical retinoid or azelaic or salicylic acid.
  - Mild inflammatory acne with papular and/or pustular elements can be treated with a topical retinoid and topical benzoyl peroxide.
- Moderate acne (substantial comedones and/or a papular or pustular component)
  - This can be treated with topical retinoid plus benzoyl peroxide and/or a topical antibiotic (including combination agents with benzoyl peroxide and erythromycin or clindamycin).
  - This can be treated with a topical retinoid plus topical benzoyl peroxide plus an oral antibiotic. Topical or oral antibiotic monotherapy is not recommended for more than 12 weeks to prevent the development of bacterial resistance.
- Severe acne (nodulocystic, with scarring or the potential to scar; see Fig. 23.2)
  - Systemic isotretinoin
  - Hormonal therapy in women
- Antibiotic selection depends on a number of variables, including cost. Although most dermatologists consider minocycline to be superior to doxycycline due to better penetration into the sebaceous unit, it is generally more expensive and sometimes associated with drug-induced lupus. Minocycline and doxycycline are both considered superior to simple tetracycline.

Clinical Course

The clinical course of acne is capricious. Some adolescents have mild disease that resolves quickly, whereas others progress to severe acne with scarring. Acne may persist for years or decades, especially in women. Acne is generally not a problem of late middle or older age, and occurrence in this age group should prompt investigation for an instigating agent (e.g., endocrine abnormality, drug effect).

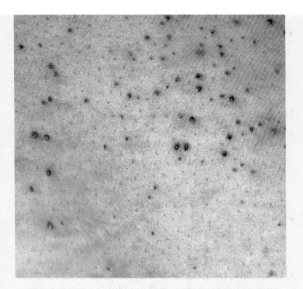

Fig. 23.1. Open comedones (blackheads) on the back of an adolescent male with acne.

Face Washing—Myth or Helpful?
A single-blinded, randomized, controlled clinical trial of 27 men was carried out for 6 weeks using a foaming facial cleanser that had no active antiacne properties. They were randomized to groups that washed once, twice, or four times daily. At the end of the study, no statistically significant differences among the three groups were realized, although the group that washed twice daily subjectively demonstrated slight improvement. The authors concluded that there is some evidence for washing the face twice daily.

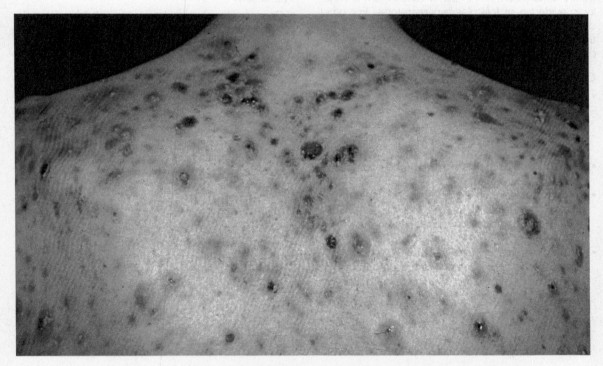

Fig. 23.2. Patient with severe acne with follicular papules, follicular pustules, and acneiform cysts. This will produce permanent scarring, and the patient is a strong candidate for systemic isotretinoin. (From the Fitzsimons Army Medical Center Collection, Aurora, CO.)

Drug-Induced Acneiform Reactions

Acneiform Drug Eruptions: Selected Drugs
- Androgens
- Bromides
- Cetuximab
- Corticosteroids
- Erlotinib
- Iodides
- Isoniazid
- Lithium
- Phenytoin
- Sirolimus
- Vitamin B_{12}

Pathogenesis

The common causes of drug-induced acneiform reactions are systemic corticosteroids and other androgens (steroid acne), but more than 200 drugs have been reported to cause or worsen acne. For many drugs, the mechanism whereby acne is caused is poorly understood, but in some cases there is histologic evidence of follicular hyperkeratosis. For other drugs, it has been speculated that follicular concentration or excretion results in irritation and inflammation of the pilosebaceous unit.

Clinical Features

- Acneiform eruptions are typically abrupt, especially when induced by systemic medications. However, there are exceptions, and some patients may experience an insidious onset, especially if the condition is caused by topical corticosteroids.
- Drug-induced acne is usually monomorphic in appearance.
- The primary lesion is a follicle-based erythematous papule or pustule (Figs. 23.3 and 23.4). Rare patients can demonstrate follicular hemorrhage (Fig. 23.5).
- Comedones are generally absent in early drug-induced acne and, if present, are usually the result of coexisting simple acne vulgaris or a chronic drug-induced process.

- Patients treated with certain drugs (e.g., bromides) may demonstrate background erythema (Fig. 23.6) or erythema with scale that can resemble dermatitis or seborrheic dermatitis (epidermal growth factor [EGF] receptor inhibitors).

Diagnosis

- The diagnosis is typically based on the appearance and history of recent use of a drug known to cause acne. The monomorphic appearance, absence of comedones, abnormal distribution (compared to acne vulgaris), and severe degree of involvement should suggest drug-induced acne.
- A 2- or 3-mm punch biopsy may be performed to exclude other disorders in the differential. However, the findings in acne not usually singularly diagnostic but may be supportive of the clinical assessment.
- Unusual presentations may require a culture of unroofed pustules to exclude staphylococcal folliculitis and pseudomonal folliculitis.

Treatment

- Because drug-induced acne is a self-limited condition, which will resolve with discontinuance of the drug, expectant resolution is often a reasonable approach to the condition.
- If the offending agent cannot be discontinued (e.g., EGF receptor inhibitors in cancer), mild drug-induced acne can be treated with benzoyl peroxide and/or topical antibiotics, such as clindamycin and erythromycin.
- More severe drug-induced acne can be treated with oral antibiotics, such as minocycline and doxycycline. Rare severe cases may require oral isotretinoin.

Clinical Course

Most drug-induced acneiform eruptions will spontaneously resolve, over a period of weeks to months, once the drug is removed and without permanent sequelae. Rare cases may persist for longer periods of time.

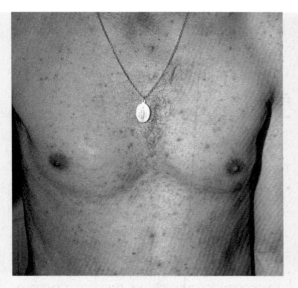

Fig. 23.3. Patient with generalized acneiform eruption due to isoniazid, a common cause of this reaction. (From the John Aeling Collection, Aurora, CO.)

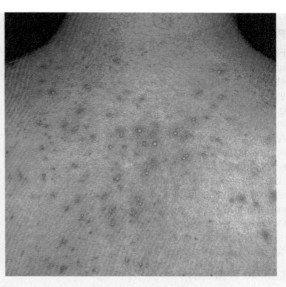

Fig. 23.4. Patient with acneiform eruption with follicle-based papules and pustules due to oral corticosteroids. (From the Walter Reed Army Medical Center Collection, Washington, DC.)

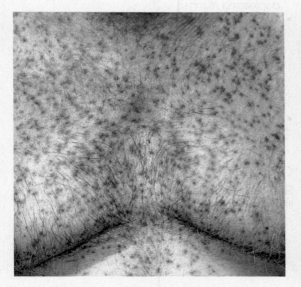

Fig. 23.5. Patient with a hemorrhagic acneiform eruption due to trametinib, an MEK1 and MEK2 inhibitor used to treat melanoma.

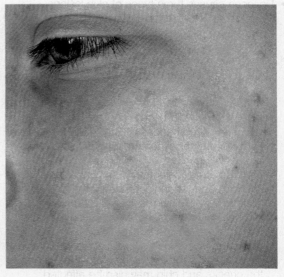

Fig. 23.6. Patient with acneiform eruption with background erythema resembling rosacea. This case was caused by the bromine component of dextromethorphan hydrobromide, the active ingredient in Pertussin. (From the Fitzsimons Army Medical Center Collection, Aurora, CO.)

Rosacea ICD10 code L71.8

Pathogenesis

Rosacea is a common disorder, with about 14 million affected Americans, but the cause is poorly understood. Genetic factors probably play a role because the condition is common in persons of certain ethnic groups (e.g., Northern Europeans) and uncommon in persons of other ethnic groups (e.g., African Americans). Proposed theories include an abnormal response to microorganisms of the skin (e.g., bacterial, yeast, *Demodex* mites), or certain ingestions, solar damage, vascular anomalies, and dermal matrix abnormalities. It is well recognized that triggers are important in rosacea, such as sunlight, alcohol, caffeine, and tomato-based products, but these triggers may vary among individuals. Topical corticosteroids can aggravate rosacea.

Clinical Features

- Rosacea can affect persons of a wide age range, from adolescence to the elderly.
- Rosacea affects the face, particularly the forehead, nose, cheeks, and chin.
- Extrafacial rosacea (upper chest, scalp) can occur but is uncommon.
- Rosacea causes three types of skin lesions:
  1. Erythema with telangiectasias
  2. Acneiform papules and pustules
  3. Sebaceous gland hypertrophy

Presentations may vary, and patients may demonstrate a combination of these elements:

- Papulopustular rosacea (classic rosacea)—erythema and variable telangiectasias of the face, with follicle-based papules and pustules but without comedones (Figs. 23.7–23.9). This subtype may also demonstrate variable flushing and facial edema.
- Erythromatotelangiectatic rosacea—prominent flushing and telangiectasias, with or without edema. The flushing is typically brought on by alcohol, spicy foods, hot beverages, or exertion.
- Rhinophyma (phymatous rosacea)—irregular surface nodularity due to sebaceous gland overgrowth that is most prominent on the nose, but the cheeks and chin may also be affected.

- Ocular rosacea—50% to 90% of patients with rosacea may have some degree of ocular involvement that typically manifests as blepharitis, conjunctivitis, or conjunctival erythema.

Diagnosis

- The diagnosis of rosacea is usually established on clinical grounds, but rare cases may require a biopsy to exclude other disorders (e.g., lupus).

Treatment

- Topical treatments for rosacea include metronidazole, 0.75% lotion, gel, or cream (applied bid), metronidazole, 1% cream (applied qd), azelaic acid, 15% gel or 20% cream (applied bid), sodium sulfacetamide, 10% lotion or cream (applied bid), or ivermectin, 1% cream (applied qd).
- Brimonidine, 0.33% gel (applied qd), is a topical vasoconstrictor available for diminishing redness, but a small number of patients may experience rebound worsening when the drug wears off.
- Topical tretinoin, 0.025% to 0.1% cream or gel, may be useful for some patients with rosacea, but, in other patients, it may increase erythema in a displeasing manner.
- Systemic treatments for rosacea include doxycycline or minocycline (50–100 mg PO every other day, qd, bid) or even subantimicrobial dosing of 40 mg of doxycycline (30 mg immediate release, 10 mg delayed release) have been shown to improve rosacea. Systemic medications can also treat ocular rosacea.
- Other treatment options include intense pulsed light therapy, topical tacrolimus ointment, and topical pimecrolimus cream.

Clinical Course

Rosacea can be improved with therapy, but it is a lifelong condition that is not "cured" in the strict sense.

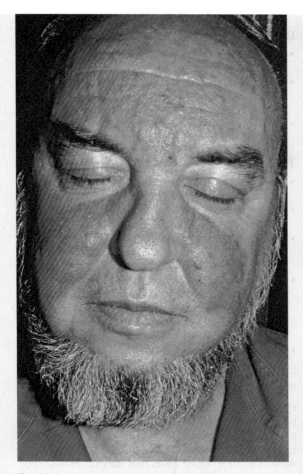

Fig. 23.7. Patient with severe rosacea with follicular papules and erythema. Note the photosensitive distribution. Some patients improve with sunscreen use. (From the Fitzsimons Army Medical Center Collection, Aurora, CO.)

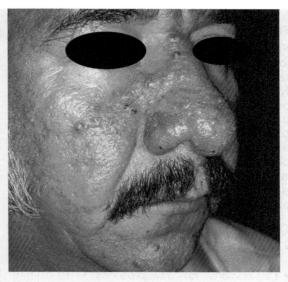

Fig. 23.8. Severe rosacea with follicular papules, erythema, pustules, and rhinophyma in a Hispanic man. (From the Fitzsimons Army Medical Center Collection, Aurora, CO.)

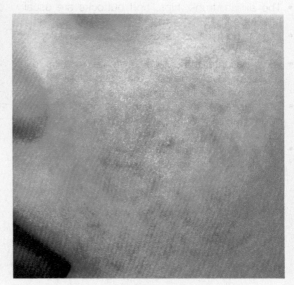

Fig. 23.9. Patient with steroid rosacea due to topical corticosteroid use. (From the William Weston Collection, Aurora, CO.)

Pseudomonas Folliculitis ICD10 code L73.9

Pathogenesis

Pseudomonas folliculitis, sometimes called hot tub folliculitis, is caused by infection of the follicular apparatus with *Pseudomonas aeruginosa*, especially serotype O:11, which is acquired from exposure to water, particularly that of heated pools, whirlpools, and hot tubs. Bacterial overgrowth in these water sources occurs when the pH is high, chlorine levels are low, and there is high usage and/or less frequent draining of the pool/tub. Less often, pseudomonal folliculitis is acquired from sponges, wet suits, and epilation. A similar but uncommon follicular infection is produced by *Aeromonas hydrophila*.

Clinical Features

- Pseudomonal folliculitis usually presents 1 to 3 days after exposure to a contaminated water source.
- Pseudomonal folliculitis produces 1- to 10-mm erythematous follicle-based papules, usually on the trunk and particularly on skin that is covered by the bathing suit (Figs. 23.10 and 23.11).
- Some erythematous papules may develop a central pinpoint pustule.
- The axillae, trunk, hips, and buttocks are usually affected.
- Larger nodules or abscesses may develop on occasion.
- Rare patients may develop acute mastitis (Fig. 23.12) or involvement of the palmoplantar sweat glands (so-called hot hand-foot syndrome).
- Otitis externa, conjunctivitis, or pharyngitis can develop if the head is immersed in contaminated water.
- Systemic symptoms are usually absent, but occasional patients develop malaise and low-grade fever.

Diagnosis

- The clinical presentation, when combined with an appropriate exposure history, is typically diagnostic.
- Culture of a pustule is confirmatory, or culture of the suspected water source can provide further support for the diagnosis.
- Biopsy usually demonstrates only a nonspecific folliculitis because the bacteria are difficult to visualize.

Treatment

- Pseudomonal folliculitis is self-limited in most healthy persons, and generally no treatment is required.
- Acetic acid, 5% compresses (applied for 20 minutes tid tor qid), may be used.
- Severe cases may benefit from oral ciprofloxacin, 500 mg PO tid for 5 to 7 days, but this has not been rigorously studied.
- It is important to educate the patient about the cause of the folliculitis and encourage preventive measures, such as draining and cleaning the hot tub, improved chlorination, and maintenance of proper pH.
- If the hot tub or pool is a public facility, the appropriate health authorities must be contacted.

Clinical Course

Pseudomonal folliculitis usually resolves without treatment in 1 to 2 weeks. Occasional patients may become carriers and continue to develop new pustules and abscesses for months. Lesions are more likely to occur in moist areas that support *Pseudomonas* carriage, such as the axillae, groin, and perianal area.

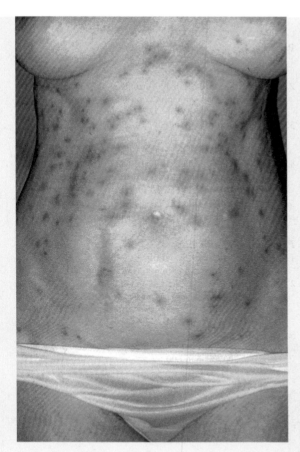

Fig. 23.10. Patient with numerous follicle-based, intensely red papules on pustules. (From the Fitzsimons Army Medical Center Collection, Aurora, CO.)

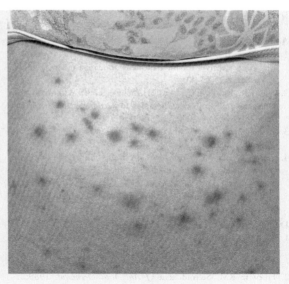

Fig. 23.11. Close-up of pseudomonal folliculitis. (From the Fitzsimons Army Medical Center Collection, Aurora, CO.)

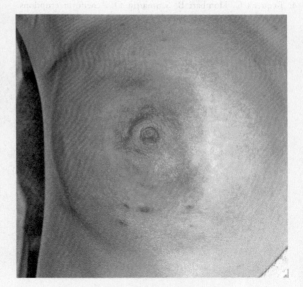

Fig. 23.12. Patient with tender swollen breast with lymphangitis and small numbers of follicular papules confined to the area beneath the top part of the bathing suit of this febrile patient. She was hospitalized for systemic antibiotics. (From the Fitzsimons Army Medical Center Collection, Aurora, CO.)

References

Acne Vulgaris

1. Arrington EA, Patel NS, Geranger K, Feldman SR. Combined oral contraceptives for the treatment of acne: a practical guide. *Cutis.* 2012;90:83-90.
2. Amin K, Riddle CC, Aires DJ, Schweiger ES. Common and alternate oral antibiotic therapies for acne vulgaris: a review. *J Drugs Dermatol.* 2007;6:873-880.
3. Bowe WP, Joshi SS, Shalita AR. Diet and acne. *J Am Acad Dermatol.* 2010;63:124-141.
4. Choi JM, Lew VK, Kimball AB. A single-blinded, randomized, controlled clinical trial evaluating the effect of face washing in acne vulgaris. *Pediatr Dermatol.* 2006;23:421-427.
5. Gold LS. Topical treatments in acne vulgaris: guidance for the busy dermatologist. *J Drugs Dermatol.* 2015;14:567-572.

Drug-Induced Acneiform Eruptions

1. DeWitt CA, Siroy AE, Stone SP. Acneiform eruptions associated with epidermal growth factor receptor-targeted chemotherapy. *J Am Acad Dermatol.* 2007;56:500-505.
2. Hurwitz RM. Steroid acne. *J Am Acad Dermatol.* 1989;21: 1179-1181.
3. Patrizi A, Binachi F, Neri I. Rosaceiform eruption induced by erlotinib. *Dermatol Ther.* 2008;21:543-545.
4. Requena C, Llombart B, Sanmartin O. Acneiform eruptions induced by epidermal growth factor receptor inhibitors: treatment with oral isotretinoin. *Cutis.* 2012;90:77-80.

Rosacea

1. Bikowski JB, Goldman MP. Rosacea: where are we now? *J Drugs Dermatol.* 2004;3:251-261.
2. Conde JF, Yelverton CB, Balkrishnan R, et al. Managing rosacea: a review of the use of metronidazole alone and in combination with oral antibiotics. *J Drugs Dermatol.* 2007;6:495-498.
3. Liu RH, Smith MK, Basta SA, Farmer ER. Azelaic acid in the treatment of papulopustular rosacea. A systematic review of randomized controlled trials. *Arch Dermatol.* 2006;142:1047-1052.
4. Two AM, Wu W, Gallo RL, Hata TR. Rosacea. Part I. Introduction, categorization, histology, pathogenesis and risk factors. *J Am Acad Dermatol.* 2015;72:749-758.
5. Two AM, Wu W, Gallo RL, Hata TR. Rosacea. Part II. Topical and systemic therapies in the treatment of rosacea. *J Am Acad Dermatol.* 2015;72:761-770.

Pseudomonas Folliculitis

1. Bergere RS, Siefert MR. Whirlpool folliculitis: a review of its cause, treatment, and prevention. *Cutis.* 1990;45:97-98.
2. Manresa MJ, Villa AV, Giralt AG, González-Enseñat MA. *Aeromonas hydrophila* folliculitis associated with an inflatable swimming pool: mimicking *Pseudomonas aeruginosa* infection. *Pediatr Dermatol.* 2009;26:601-603.
3. Yu Y, Cheng AS, Wang L, et al. Hot tub folliculitis or hot hand-foot syndrome caused by *Pseudomonas aeruginosa*. *J Am Acad Dermatol.* 2007;57:596-600.

Chapter 24
Alopecia

Alopecia (hair loss) is one of the ten most common causes of skin-related visits to physicians in the United States. Alopecia can be classified as scarring or nonscarring, and, although this is an important categorization, it is important to note that some alopecia can be both nonscarring and scarring, depending on the clinical circumstances (e.g., tinea capitis with kerion formation).

Classification of Alopecia

Nonscarring Alopecia
- Alopecia areata
- Anagen effluvium
- Androgenetic alopecia
- Syphilitic alopecia
- Telogen effluvium
- Tinea capitis (rarely scarring)
- Traction alopecia (can scar)

Scarring Alopecia
- Central centrifugal scarring alopecia
- Discoid lupus erythematosus
- Folliculitis decalvans
- Frontal fibrosing alopecia

IMPORTANT HISTORY QUESTIONS

When did you first notice that you were losing hair?

Sudden diffuse hair loss favors telogen effluvium, anagen effluvium, or diffuse alopecia areata, whereas most other types of alopecia are insidious in onset (e.g., androgenic alopecia).

What products do you put on your hair?

Harsh chemicals that straighten hair (relaxers) or curl hair (perms) can damage it, yielding an alopecia.

Do you have any other known medical conditions?

Lupus erythematosus, secondary syphilis, thyroid disease, or chronic anemia may be associated with alopecia.

Have there been recent changes in your health?

A recent and significant physical stressor (e.g., pregnancy, marked weight loss, sustained high fever, major surgery, significant blood loss) can induce telogen effluvium.

What medications are you taking, and are any of these new?

Some medications can occasionally cause telogen effluvium (e.g., anticoagulants, oral retinoids, beta blockers, lithium), or anagen effluvium (e.g., chemotherapeutic agents).

Do you find yourself pulling on your hair under stress?

Trichotillomania is an alopecia caused by mechanical pulling of the hair. Some patients will openly admit to pulling at their hair, whereas others will hide such behavior.

IMPORTANT PHYSICAL FINDINGS

What is the distribution of hair loss?

The distribution of hair loss is important because it may be discrete (e.g., alopecia areata), patchy (syphilitic so-called moth-eaten alopecia), patterned (e.g., male-female pattern alopecia), or diffuse (e.g., telogen effluvium).

Is there evidence of inflammation or pustules?

Pustules may be indicative of folliculitis decalvans, dissecting cellulitis, or dermatophyte infection.

Is there evidence of epidermal changes in addition to the alopecia?

Epidermal changes, such as scale and crusting, may be seen in discoid lupus erythematosus or lichen planus, whereas many other forms of alopecia, such as alopecia areata, manifest little epidermal pathology.

Is there any scarring?

Alopecia may be divided into scarring (e.g., lupus erythematosus) and nonscarring forms (e.g., alopecia areata), so the presence of scar is significant. Some alopecias may be scarring or nonscarring (e.g., tinea capitis).

Is there hair loss in other hairy areas?

Involved eyebrows or eyelashes may favor trichotillomania, alopecia areata, or syphilitic alopecia.

Are there nail changes?

Beau lines may suggest telogen effluvium, whereas rough nails may suggest alopecia areata, and the formation of pterygium (e.g., split nails, often with a triangular lunula) may favor lichen planus.

Androgenic Alopecia ICD10 codes L64.9

GENETIC DISORDER

Pathogenesis

Androgenic (androgenetic) alopecia is the most common cause of hair loss in men and women. By age 50 years, about 50% of men will demonstrate significant androgenic alopecia and, at age 60 years, 50% of women will demonstrate this same condition. There is a definitive genetic component, with mutations in the androgen receptor gene playing a role. Androgenic alopecia is a result of increased follicular activity of 5α-reductase in men and increased dehydrogenase enzyme levels in women. In women, other mechanisms may also be important; thus, some authorities prefer the term *female pattern hair loss*. The increased enzymatic activity causes a short anagen (growing) stage in hair follicles, resulting in small, non-pigmented (miniaturized) hairs that are barely visible.

Clinical Features

- Women demonstrate a pattern of diffuse thinning on the vertex scalp, with general preservation of the front hairline.
- Although female pattern hair loss is most noticeable around the time of menopause, the thinning develops earlier in some women (Fig. 24.1).
- Men demonstrate recession of the bilateral temporal hairline, with or without thinning of the crown (Figs. 24.2–24.4).
- Severe cases in men demonstrate only a residual rim of hair around the posterior hairline.

Diagnosis

- The clinical presentation is usually diagnostic, but early-onset androgenic alopecia, which can occur as early as adolescence, can be difficult to diagnose and difficult for the patient to accept.
- Biopsy (with a 4-mm or larger punch) may not be diagnostic for only androgenic alopecia, but it can exclude a scarring and/or inflammatory alopecia. Miniaturization of hairs and increased sebaceous gland activity is compatible with androgenic alopecia. In general, the skillful evaluation of alopecia usually requires evaluation by a dermatopathologist rather than a general pathologist.
- In difficult cases, some dermatologists will perform a trichogram (so-called hair pluck), in which 50 to 100 hairs are pulled and examined to determine the ratio of anagen, catagen, and telogen hairs. This test is painful and requires expertise for interpretation. It is not recommended in the urgent care setting.

Treatment

- For men, finasteride (1 mg PO qd) produces improved hair counts of about 9% at 1 year and 15% at 2 years. It is most successful in early-onset androgenic alopecia. It is not nearly as efficacious in older women and should never be used in any woman who can become pregnant.
- Topical minoxidil solution (to the scalp, bid) is efficacious. Topical 5% minoxidil has been found to be statistically superior to topical 2% minoxidil in men and women.
- Cyproterone acetate is an antiandrogenic agent used in women with androgenic alopecia due hyperandrogenic states.
- There is weak evidence that concomitant seborrheic dermatitis may worsen androgenic alopecia, and treatment with 1% pyrithione zinc shampoo or a ketoconazole-based shampoo may decrease hair loss.
- Spironolactone (100–200 mg po qd) competitively inhibits androgen receptor binding. The drug does not reverse hair loss but may slow progression. Because of its side effect profile, it can only be used in women and cannot be used by women who may become pregnant because it may feminize a male fetus.
- As a last resort, hair transplantation is an option for some patients. However, a hair transplant is a time-consuming, painful, and expensive procedure, with the results being dependent on the skill of the surgeon.

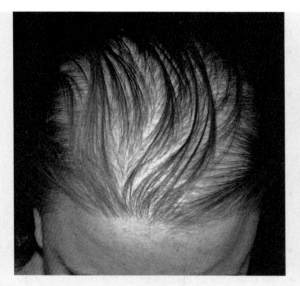

Fig. 24.1. Typical diffuse pattern of hair loss on the vertex of the scalp in a woman.

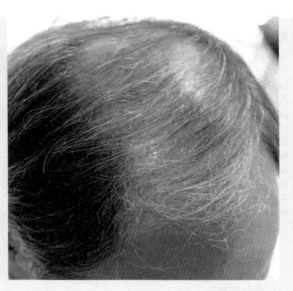

Fig. 24.2. Moderately severe thinning of the frontoparietal area and crown in a man.

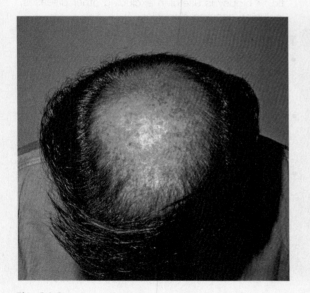

Fig. 24.3. Severe androgenic alopecia of the crown in a man.

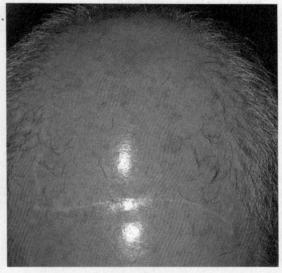

Fig. 24.4. Almost complete loss of hair in the frontoparietal area and crown in a man. Note the scar from excision of a skin cancer.

Pathogenesis

Telogen effluvium results from abnormal synchronization of a normal random hair growth cycle. In normal persons, 90% to 95% of the scalp hairs are in anagen (the growth phase), 1% are in catagen (a regressive phase), and 5% to 10% are in telogen phase (a rest phase). In telogen effluvium, a major physical stressor, such as childbirth, marked weight loss, sustained high fever, or a similar event, induces a large number of hairs to transition from anagen to catagen and telogen simultaneously. Hence, there is marked hair loss 2 to 4 months after the physical insult because many hairs enter telogen at the same time.

Precipitating Causes of Telogen Effluvium

- Childbirth
- Endocrinologic changes
- High fever
- Idiopathic (no cause found in one-third of cases)
- Malabsorption syndromes
- Medication changes
- Surgery (usually major surgery)
- Trauma (car wreck with injury)
- Weight loss (typically crash diet)

Clinical Features

- Telogen effluvium causes an abrupt diffuse hair loss (Fig. 24.5). Patients have described hair as "falling out by its roots."
- The hair loss usually occurs 2 to 4 months after a precipitating event (Figs. 24.6–24.8).
- Typically, less than one-third of all hairs are lost.
- The scalp appears normal, without erythema or scale, unless a second skin disorder is also present (e.g., seborrheic dermatitis).
- Examination of the nails may demonstrate horizontal lines (Beau lines) from the same stressful event that has interrupted nail growth.

Diagnosis

- The history of a precipitating cause is important to the diagnosis, but, in some cases, the patient may not report an identifiable event.
- If no precipitating event is identified, the patient's medications should be reviewed. Drugs usually implicated in inducing telogen effluvium include hormone and thyroid replacement drugs, nonsteroidal antiinflammatory drugs (NSAIDs), anticoagulants, beta blockers, systemic retinoids, and some antihyperlipidemia agents.
- In cases without a readily identifiable cause, a complete blood count (CBC), serum ferritin level (to rule out iron deficiency), and thyroid function studies should be ordered.
- Hair loss should be diffuse, with less than one-third of the hair lost and with a normal scalp.
- The presence of Beau lines of the nails is strongly supportive of a diagnosis of telogen effluvium.
- A biopsy (4-mm punch biopsy to fat) may suggest the diagnosis, but the result is usually nondiagnostic. A biopsy is useful in excluding other diseases, including scarring alopecia.

Treatment

- No treatment other than reassurance is reasonable because most cases are self-limited. Over time, the hair will return to a random growth pattern, and the condition will resolve.
- Patients with telogen effluvium due to various systemic perturbations, such as thyroid disease, malnutrition, or anemia, may demonstrate persistent alopecia unless those conditions are rectified.
- Rare patients, especially middle-aged women, may develop a chronic telogen effluvium that continues for years. There are few data on the treatment of this rare and persistent variant, but topical minoxidil is the most reasonable treatment approach because it promotes and prolongs the anagen phase.

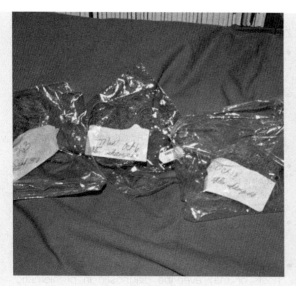

Fig. 24.5. Telogen effluvium daily hair counts demonstrating loss of more than 200 hairs/day. (From the Fitzsimons Army Medical Center Collection, Aurora, CO.)

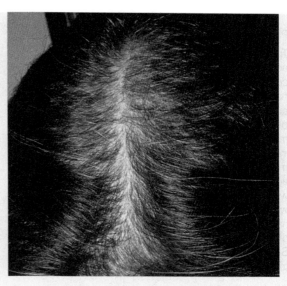

Fig. 24.6. Moderate telogen effluvium demonstrating accentuation of the part. (From the Fitzsimons Army Medical Center Collection, Aurora, CO.)

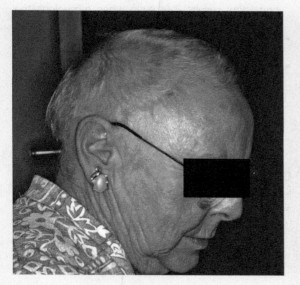

Fig. 24.7. Woman with severe telogen effluvium. (From the Fitzsimons Army Medical Center Collection, Aurora, CO.)

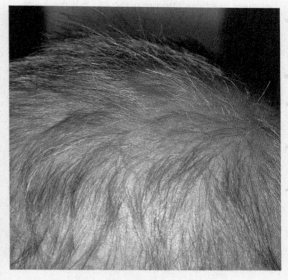

Fig. 24.8. Severe telogen effluvium due to hypothyroidism.

Trichotillomania ICD10 code F63.3

Pathogenesis

Trichotillomania is a neuropsychiatric condition characterized by a compulsion to pull out one's hair. The compulsion may range from a mild, stress-relieving habit, similar to thumb sucking, to a near maniac and psychotic compulsion that is comorbid with other psychiatric issues. The incidence of trichotillomania is unknown, but the condition is more common in young children and adolescents and in females more than males. Two patterns are recognized—automatic, where hair is pulled nearly inadvertently while the person is engaged in another activity (e.g., watching television, studying), and focused, where hair pulling is the only activity at the time. About 50% of patients play with or chew their hair after pulling it. Some patients swallow the hair, leading to a gastric trichobezoar.

Clinical Features

- Irregular patches of nonscarring alopecia may occur anywhere but are most common on the vertex scalp. Some patients may demonstrate scarring from repetitive pulling or from additional psychotic behavior, such as attempting to dig out the hairs.
- An important clinical clue is hairs of different lengths in a single area of perceived loss. This results from patients pulling hairs individually, over time, with partial regrowth (Figs. 24.9 and 24.10).
- If the hair loss is unilateral, it tends to occur on the same side as the dominant hand.
- Rare cases may demonstrate hemorrhage or erosion (Fig. 24.11), particularly in patients who pull out larger patches of hair at one time.
- Less often, hair of other body sites is affected, such as the eyebrows (40%), eyelashes (50%; Fig. 24.12), and pubic hair (15%).
- Trichobezoars can be a complication because about 10% of patients eat the hair (trichophagy).

Diagnosis

- A history of other psychiatric disorders (e.g., anorexia, bulimia, obsessive-compulsive disorder) is also supportive of trichotillomania.
- Some patients will admit to hair pulling. Many affected patients describe a feeling of tension before pulling the hair, with some release of this tension after pulling. The patient may also report a feeling of elation, gratification, or pleasure after pulling the hair.
- If other family members are present, asking if the patient unconsciously tugs at his or her hair is less threatening than asking if the hair is being pulled out.
- Occluding an area of alopecia, with a bandage or dressing, so that the patient cannot pull those hairs out, will result in regrowth (so-called Band-Aid sign).
- A 4- to 6-mm punch biopsy can support the diagnosis or may even be diagnostic in problematic cases.

Treatment

- Selective serotonin reuptake inhibitors (SSRIs), such as oral fluoxetine (40–80 mg PO qd), produce inconsistent results, but even when efficacious the results are limited (11% improvement in one study).
- Tricyclic antidepressants, such as clomipramine, produce only marginal improvement.
- In adults, a randomized trial demonstrated that behavior modification therapy (e.g., diary entries, sensory aids to make the patient conscious of pulling, postponement interventions, response consequences involving undesirable tasks) was more effective than SSRIs, with 64% of patients showing improvement.

Clinical Course

In children, trichotillomania is often self-limited, but, in adults, it is often chronic or relapsing.

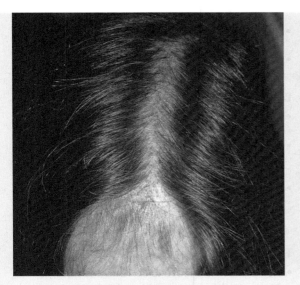

Fig. 24.9. Trichotillomania in an adolescent girl demonstrating hairs of variable lengths. (From the Fitzsimons Army Medical Center Collection, Aurora, CO.)

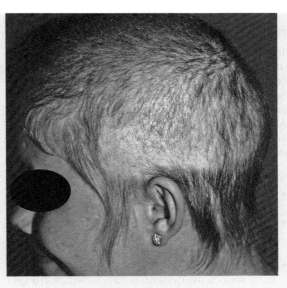

Fig. 24.10. Severe trichotillomania in a woman with hairs of variable lengths. (From the William Weston Collection, Aurora, CO.)

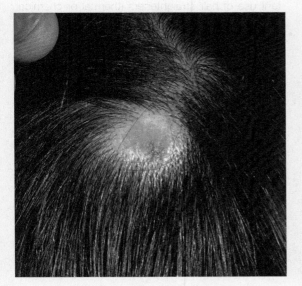

Fig. 24.11. Focal trichotillomania in a woman, with evidence of recent trauma. (From the Fitzsimons Army Medical Center Collection, Aurora, CO.)

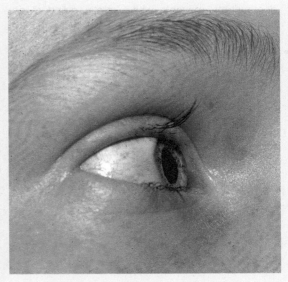

Fig. 24.12. Patient with trichotillomania of the eyelashes. (From the William Weston Collection, Aurora, CO.)

Traction Alopecia ICD10 code L65.8

Pathogenesis

Traction alopecia is a mechanically induced alopecia usually caused by a particular method of styling the hair (e.g., hair rollers that produce traction on the hair bulb, use of barrettes) or a particular hairstyle (e.g., cornrows, chignon, tight ponytails, tight pigtails). Although typically considered a nonscarring alopecia, in severe cases there may be some focal scarring and permanent loss of hair.

Clinical Features

- The condition can occur at any age and is much more common in women.
- The pattern is dependent on the hairstyle used (e.g., tight braids, tight ponytail, hair weaves) or by prolonged use of curlers in one area.
- Marginal traction alopecia of the frontal and temporal scalp is the most common presentation (Figs. 24.13 and 24.14).
- Chignon traction alopecia affects the occipital scalp and is caused by twisting the hair to maintain the bun.
- Examination of the hair with a hand lens may demonstrate movable white keratin cylinders on the hair shaft (peripilar casts), follicular erythema, and even pustules.
- The remainder of the scalp exam is typically normal.

- Acute and subacute cases may demonstrate broken hairs and vellus hairs in areas of alopecia.
- Chronic cases may demonstrate perifollicular scarring, with complete loss of hair.

Diagnosis

- The diagnosis is usually made based on the clinical presentation.
- Examination of adjacent hair under the microscope may demonstrate breakage (trichorrhexis nodosa), especially if a straightening product is being used.
- Biopsy with a 4-mm or larger punch may be diagnostic of traction alopecia, but it is usually nondiagnostic. However, it allows for an inflammatory alopecia to be excluded.

Treatment

- Some patients choose to continue the hairstyle that produced the alopecia, and no treatment is desired.
- Patients willing to change their hairstyle should select a new style that does not place tension on the hair, and usually there will be some regrowth.
- Hair loss that is further aggravated by a concomitant use of hair straighteners (thermal or chemical straightening) should be discontinued.
- In chronic cases, with resultant scar, the only option is hair transplantation.

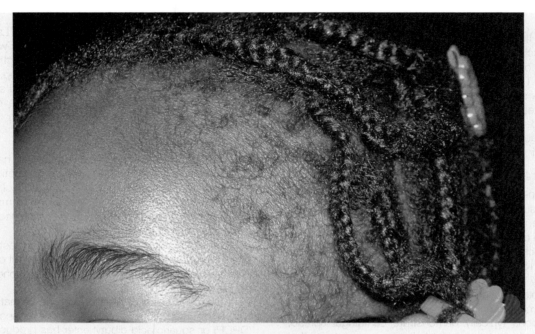

Fig. 24.13. Girl with traction alopecia associated with a cornrow braiding hairstyle.

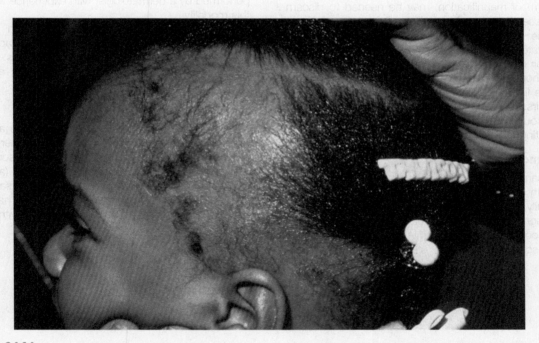

Fig. 24.14. Severe traction alopecia. Note new growth in the anterior areas. (From the Fitzsimons Army Medical Center Collection, Aurora, CO.)

Pathogenesis

Alopecia areata is a form of hair loss that is the direct result of an autoimmune attack on the hair bulb by T cells. The antigen triggering this misguided immune response is unknown. However, persons with alopecia areata are more likely to have other autoimmune disorders, especially vitiligo. From 1% to 2% of all individuals will develop alopecia areata at some point in their lives.

Clinical Features

- Alopecia areata can affect persons of any age, but it usually affects those between 20 and 40 years.
- The scalp is usually affected, but any hair-bearing site may be involved.
- Patches of discrete hair loss are common (Figs. 24.15 and 24.16), but, on occasion, a diffuse form may affect the entire scalp (Fig. 24.17).
- In older patients, there is often preferential loss of pigmented hairs, with preservation of gray hairs.
- Lesions typically demonstrate centrifugal spread, with exclamation point hairs (broken-off hairs that are wider at the top than the bottom) at the peripheral edge (see Fig. 24.15). A hand lens, or other form of magnification, may be needed to discern these changes.
- The skin, although usually normal, may demonstrate subtle erythema in early lesions.
- Hair regrowth may develop in the center of lesions, although this may consist of vellus hairs or hairs that are finer and less pigmented than normal terminal hairs.
- About 10% of patients will also have subtle nail pitting, yielding a roughly textured nail.

Diagnosis

- Sharply circumscribed, usually annular, hair loss, with a smooth and normal-appearing scalp, especially if exclamation point hairs are present, is usually diagnostic of alopecia areata.
- Secondary syphilis may mimic alopecia areata, and a screening serologic study (e.g., rapid plasma reagin [RPR] test, Venereal Disease Research Laboratory [VDRL] test) is reasonable for persons who are sexually active or were recently sexually active.
- A biopsy (4-mm or larger punch) can be diagnostic of alopecia areata when T cells are visualized surrounding the hair bulb—dermatopathologists call this a swarm of bees pattern.

Treatment

- For patients who are unconcerned and/or have limited disease, no treatment is a reasonable option.
- Potent topical corticosteroids (e.g., clobetasol) is a first-line therapy, but often the treatment must be continued for a long period, and spontaneous resolution confounds any claims of efficacy.
- Intralesional triamcinolone (2.5–5 mg/mL) injected into the active peripheral edge is often used but can lead to some scalp atrophy, particularly if a stronger concentration is administered.
- Purposeful induction of allergic contact dermatitis with the application of diphenylcyclopropenone (DPCP) or squaric acid dibutyl ester has produced modest success, and occasionally spectacular results, but this complex treatment plan is best performed by a dermatologist with experience with this modality.
- Light therapy, using a towel soaked in 8-methoxypsoralen, followed by ultraviolet A radiation, has produced modest to excellent results.
- Topical minoxidil produces variable success and has few side effects.

Clinical Course

The course of alopecia areata is highly variable and unpredictable. Most affected patients experience spontaneous resolution over months, but some patients will progress and lose all their scalp hair (alopecia totalis) or all their body hair (alopecia universalis; see Fig. 24.17). Moreover, many patients will have reactivation of disease at some later point, with a waxing and waning clinical course, over time.

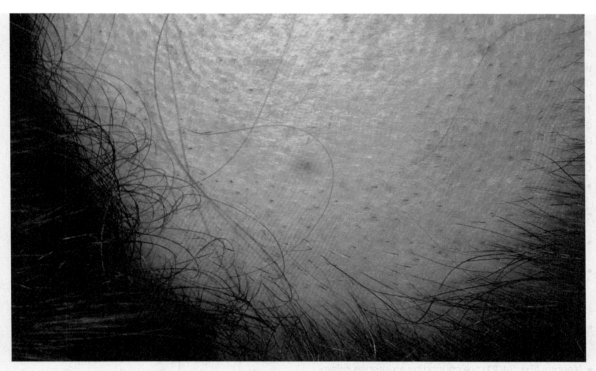

Fig. 24.15. Close-up of active lesions of alopecia areata demonstrating exclamation point hairs along the periphery of the hair loss. (From the Fitzsimons Army Medical Center Collection, Aurora, CO.)

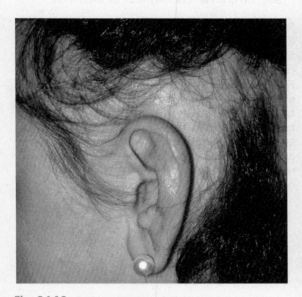

Fig. 24.16. Patient with alopecia areata that involves the hairline (ophiasis) is often associated with progressive disease areas. (From the Fitzsimons Army Medical Center Collection, Aurora, CO.)

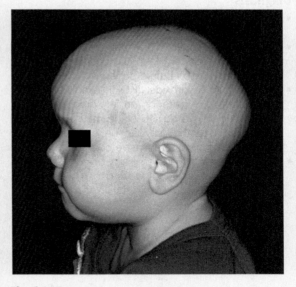

Fig. 24.17. Patient with alopecia universalis demonstrating total loss of hair areas. (From the Fitzsimons Army Medical Center Collection, Aurora, CO.)

Tinea Capitis ICD10 code B35.0

Pathogenesis

Tinea capitis is a fungal infection caused by species that can use follicular keratin as a food source. The most common species in North America are *Trichophyton tonsurans,* followed by *Microsporum canis.* The prevalence of tinea capitis is unknown, but one study has found a 4% incidence in a pediatric population.

Clinical Features

- Tinea capitis preferentially affects the occipital and parietal scalps.
- Solitary patches of alopecia may be present, or two distinct areas of alopecia may merge.
- The patches of alopecia are well defined but may be round, oval, or irregular.
- Broken hairs in the area of alopecia may be enlarged (so-called black dot ringworm; Fig. 24.18), or acute folliculitis with purulence may be apparent (Fig. 24.19).
- The skin surface may demonstrate variable scale and scattered broken hairs. These infections may resemble seborrheic dermatitis (Fig. 24.20).
- Kerions (Fig. 24.21) are caused by an intense inflammatory host response, resulting in boggy purulent masses of hair loss (see Chapter 13).

Diagnosis

- A high index of suspicion should exist in any child with hair loss and/or a scaling scalp.
- Consider tinea capitis in any prepubertal child diagnosed with seborrheic dermatitis because that condition is uncommon before puberty.
- A potassium hydroxide (KOH) examination on plucked broken hairs or on a scraping across broken hair with a no. 15 blade may confirm the diagnosis. A toothbrush can be used to collect broken hairs from apprehensive children.
- Fungal cultures of broken hairs or scrapings are typically positive in 1 to 4 weeks.

- A punch biopsy (3–4 mm) is the least preferable method for diagnosis because it is invasive and difficult to do in children.
- Wood light will demonstrate fluorescence in 5% to 10% of cases—those caused by *Microsporum* spp.

Treatment

- The most widely used treatment is micronized griseofulvin (20–25 mg/kg per day) or ultramicronized griseofulvin (10–15 mg/kg per day), given as a single daily dose with a fat-containing meal for 6 to 12 weeks.
- Unless there is cause for concern (e.g., hepatitis), griseofulvin therapy lasting less than 3 months does not require laboratory monitoring (CBC, liver function tests [LFTs]).
- Itraconazole (3–5 mg/kg per day for 2–6 weeks) may be used as an alternative to griseofulvin.
- Terbinafine (3–10 mg/kg per day for 4–8 weeks) is effective for *T. tonsurans* infections, but cases caused by *M. canis* may require higher doses and extended durations (6–10 mg/kg per day for 8–12 weeks).
- Topical antifungal shampoos lessen fungal shedding.
- Routinely examine other children in the family because they are at high risk for infection. Adults have a lower risk of acquiring the disease from affected children but may also be examined.

Comment

It is the position of the American Academy of Dermatology and American Academy of Pediatrics that a child should not miss school because of tinea capitis. Fungal shedding can be addressed with selenium sulfide or ketoconazole shampoo. Once children begin systemic and topical therapy, they may return to school. Affected children should not share hats, combs, or brushes with others. Routine cases of tinea capitis do not result in permanent alopecia. Kerions result in permanent hair loss in about one-third of cases.

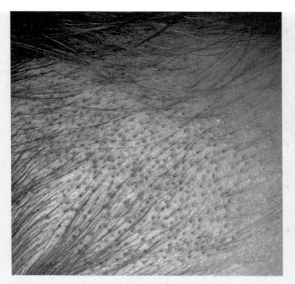

Fig. 24.18. Patient with black dot ringworm demonstrating prominent broken hairs. (From the Fitzsimons Army Medical Center Collection, Aurora, CO.)

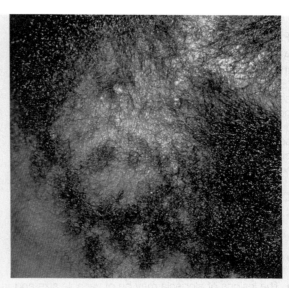

Fig. 24.19. Patient with black dot ringworm with alopecia and acute folliculitis.

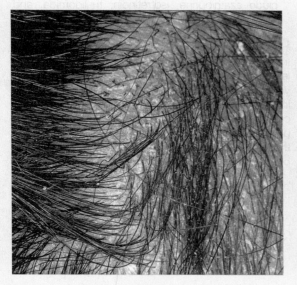

Fig. 24.20. Patient with alopecia with broken hair shafts and diffuse scaling resembling seborrheic dermatitis. This case was due to *Microsporum canis*.

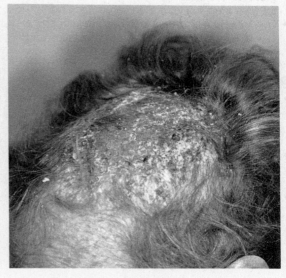

Fig. 24.21. Highly inflammatory tinea capitis (kerion) in an 80-year-old woman. Although tinea capitis is most common in prepubertal children, it can occur at any age.

Pathogenesis

A scarring alopecia can accompany discoid lupus erythematosus (DLE) or systemic lupus erythematosus (SLE). Up to 35% of patients with DLE will develop scalp involvement. Patients with SLE can develop a nonscarring alopecia affecting hairs in the frontal scalp (lupus hairs), or, less commonly, they can develop a scarring alopecia. Microscopically, the scarring alopecia of all forms of lupus are mediated by a destructive lymphoid infiltrate.

Clinical Features

- Patients may have other findings of DLE (e.g., involvement of the conchal bowl) or SLE (e.g., malar erythema).
- Areas of alopecia may be solitary or multiple and may involve any area of the scalp.
- The lesions of alopecia may be of variable size and shape but are often round (discoid). Lesions may continue to enlarge and become confluent.
- Early lesions consist of plaques of hair loss, with variable erythema (Figs. 24.22 and 24.23) that progress to the development of adherent scale and follicular plugging (so-called carpet tack sign).
- Fully developed lesions demonstrate atrophy and variable dyspigmentation (hypopigmentation and/or hyperpigmentation; Figs. 24.24 and 24.25).

Diagnosis

- The clinical presentation is often diagnostic, and an associated history and/or appropriate clinical findings of DLE (see Fig. 24.25) or SLE would strongly support the diagnosis.
- A punch biopsy (3–6 mm) of an active edge is usually diagnostic, whereas biopsies taken from central scarred areas are not usually diagnostic.
- Direct immunofluorescence studies may also be of value, with a lupus band being present in most cases.

- Recommended screening studies include an antinuclear antibody (ANA) test, positive in about 20% of patients, CBC, comprehensive metabolic panel (to include liver enzymes), and possibly total hemolytic complement studies. These studies are important because some patients will have SLE.

Treatment

- Photoprotection is important and should include sun avoidance, hats and other protective clothing, and a broad-spectrum sunscreen.
- For localized cases, a potent topical corticosteroid (clobetasol cream or ointment) is applied to active lesions bid.
- Intralesional triamcinolone (5–10 mg/mL) may be used for patients unresponsive to topical corticosteroids. Oral prednisone is also effective, but a steroid-sparing agent will then be necessary.
- Hydroxychloroquine (200 mg PO bid) is the most widely used oral therapy. The onset of action is slow, and patients typically require 2 to 3 months of use before its efficacy can be assessed.
- Second-line steroid-sparing systemic agents include azathioprine, isotretinoin, thalidomide, and mycophenolate mofetil.

Clinical Course

In scarred areas, hair loss is permanent. In early lesions, where there is active inflammation, but not yet fully developed scar, aggressive therapy may result in some regrowth. On rare occasions, squamous cell carcinoma can arise in long-standing scarred plaques (Marjolin ulcer). Any new papule or nodule that develops in a plaque of DLE on the scalp should be biopsied.

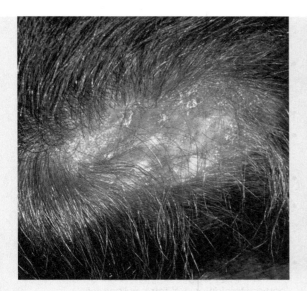

Fig. 24.22. Solitary patch of scarring alopecia with erythema in a patient with discoid lupus erythematosus.

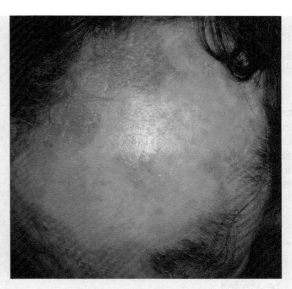

Fig. 24.23. Patient with large confluent patches of scarring alopecia. Patches of erythema represent active sites of inflammation.

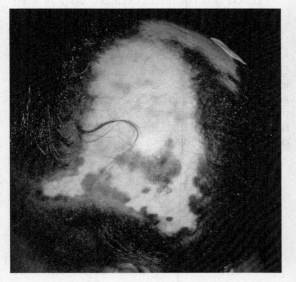

Fig. 24.24. Patient with scarring alopecia due to discoid lupus erythematosus, with prominent hypopigmentation.

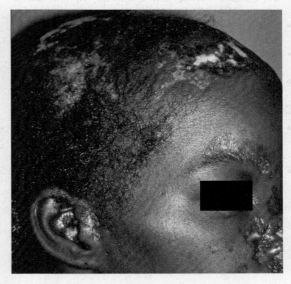

Fig. 24.25. Patient with multiple areas of scarring alopecia with hypopigmentation and hyperpigmentation. Note discoid lupus erythematosus in the ears and on the face. (From the Fitzsimons Army Medical Center Collection, Aurora, CO.)

Pathogenesis

Central centrifugal cicatricial alopecia (CCCA), formerly called hot comb alopecia or follicular degeneration syndrome, is a scarring alopecia of unknown cause. There is a controversial relationship between CCCA and pseudopelade of Brocq. Despite attempts to implicate hair products (e.g., relaxers) and hairstyling behaviors (e.g., hot combs, traction), the pathogenesis is still not well understood. Histologically, CCA is a folliculocentric, lymphocyte-mediated disorder that leads to destruction of the upper third of the hair follicle and a permanent scarring hair loss.

Clinical Features

- CCCA typically affects young to middle-aged women, with most patients being of African American heritage, but men and other ethnic groups may be affected.
- The disease usually affects the crown and vertex scalp and progresses slowly in a centrifugal pattern.
- Patches of scarring alopecia, without follicular plugging and with minimal scale or erythema, arise; the condition is typically ill defined, without sharp borders (Figs. 24.26–24.28).
- Some cases demonstrate multiple hair shafts emanating from a single follicular orifice (see Fig. 24.27).
- Symptoms vary from none to a mild or moderate pruritus.
- Other hair on the body is not affected.

Diagnosis

- A scarring alopecia that predominantly affects the crown and vertex scalp of an African American woman is particularly suspicious for CCCA.
- A 4- to 6-mm punch biopsy of the active edge often manifests supportive or even diagnostic findings.

Biopsies taken from scarred areas will only demonstrate scar.
- Negative direct immunofluorescence results are useful in excluding lichen planopilaris and discoid lupus erythematosus.

Treatment

- Potent topical corticosteroids (e.g., clobetasol) should be applied to the active edge, but treating scarred areas is unnecessary.
- Oral doxycycline or minocycline at standard dosages may be combined with topical corticosteroids.
- Intralesional triamcinolone (5–10 mg/mL), injected every 4 weeks for 6 months, is often used if topical corticosteroids fail. This treatment can also be used in combination with oral tetracyclines.
- Oral hydroxychloroquine (200 mg PO bid) for 6 months or longer is often used if intralesional corticosteroids or oral tetracyclines fail.
- Methotrexate (5–25 mg/week) or mycophenolate mofetil (1.5–2.5 g/day in divided doses) is reserved for severe cases.
- Surgical options for the scarred areas include scalp reduction and hair transplantation. Surgical intervention is not typically done until the disease has become quiescent.

Clinical Course

CCCA is a progressive scarring alopecia that may last for decades before spontaneous remission transpires. Although disease progression may be arrested with the treatments specified, no controlled clinical trial has demonstrated that any treatment modality can definitively modify the disease course.

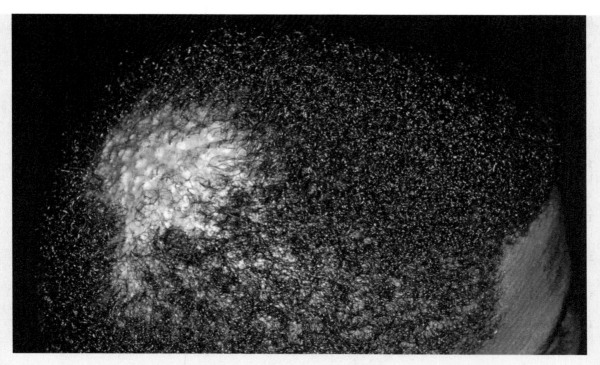

Fig. 24.26. Patient with central centrifugal cicatricial alopecia on the vertex of the scalp, the most common site. This case demonstrates an ill-defined scarring alopecia, with a perifollicular scar. (From the Fitzsimons Army Medical Center Collection, Aurora, CO.)

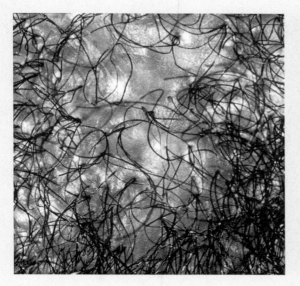

Fig. 24.27. Close-up of central centrifugal cicatricial alopecia demonstrating a perifollicular scar and multiple hairs emanating from dilated orifices. (From the Fitzsimons Army Medical Center Collection, Aurora, CO.)

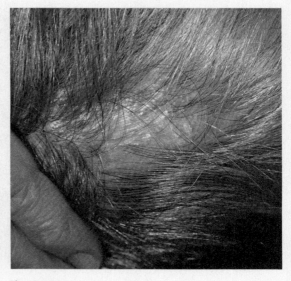

Fig. 24.28. Patient with early central centrifugal cicatricial alopecia on the central scalp demonstrating an ill-defined cicatricial alopecia. (From the Fitzsimons Army Medical Center Collection, Aurora, CO.)

References

Androgenetic Alopecia

1. Sehgal VN, Aggarwal AK, Srivastava G, Rajput P. Male pattern androgenetic alopecia. *Skinmed*. 2006;5:128-135.
2. Olsen EA, Dunlap FE, Funicella T, et al. A randomized clinical trial of 5% topical minoxidil versus 2% topical minoxidil and placebo in the treatment of androgenetic alopecia in men. *J Am Acad Dermatol*. 2002;47:377-385.
3. Rogers NF, Avram MR. Medical treatments for male and female pattern hair loss. *J Am Acad Dermatol*. 2008;59:547-566.

Telogen Effluvium

1. Whiting DA. Chronic telogen effluvium: increased scalp hair shedding in middle-aged women. *J Am Acad Dermatol*. 1996;35:899-906.

Trichotillomania

1. Nuss MA, Carlisle D, Hall M, et al. Trichotillomania: a review and case report. *Cutis*. 2003;72:191-196.
2. Prather HB, Kundu RV, Mahlberg MJ. The Band-Aid sign of trichotillomania: a helpful diagnostic technique in the setting of hair loss. *Arch Dermatol*. 2010;9:1052-1053.
3. Sah DE, Koo J, Price VH. Trichotillomania. *Dermatol Ther*. 2008;21:13-21.

Traction Alopecia

1. Hantash BM, Schwartz RA. Traction alopecia in children. *Cutis*. 2003;71:18-20.

2. Khumalo NP, Jessop S, Gumedze F, Erlich R. Determinants of marginal traction alopecia in African girls and women. *J Am Acad Dermatol*. 2008;59:432-438.

Alopecia Areata

1. Alkhalifah A, Alsantali A, Wang E, et al. Alopecia areata update. Part I. Clinical picture, histopathology, and pathogenesis. *J Am Acad Dermatol*. 2010;62:177-188.
2. Alkhalifah A, Alsantali A, Wang E, et al. Alopecia areata update. Part II. Treatment. *J Am Acad Dermatol*. 2010;62:191-202.

Tinea Capitis

1. Ginter-Hanselmayer G, Smolle J, Gupta A. Itraconazole in the treatment of tinea capitis caused by *Microsporum canis*: experience in a large cohort. *Pediatr Dermatol*. 2004;21:499-502.
2. Kakourou T, Uksal U. Guidelines for the management of tinea capitis in children. *Pediatr Dermatol*. 2010;27:226-228.

Lupus Erythematosus

1. Hordinsky M. Cicatricial alopecia: discoid lupus erythematosus. *Dermatol Ther*. 2008;21:245-248.

Central Centrifugal Scarring Alopecia

1. Whiting DA, Olsen EA. Central centrifugal cicatricial alopecia. *Dermatol Ther*. 2008;21:268-278.

Key Terms

Paronychia	Chronic paronychia	Onychauxis	Trachyonychia
Acute paronychia	Onychomycosis	Thick hyperkeratotic	Twenty-nail dystrophy
	Leukonychia mycotica	nails	

N ail disorders are often encountered as "Oh, by the way…" issues, meaning that the patient brings up the concern during an evaluation for some other medical ailment. Even for dermatologists, the evaluation of nail disorders can be daunting because of the challenging terminology and sheer number of conditions that can affect the nail. Many dermatologists have one or more nail books in their personal reference library for this reason.

Nail Glossary
- Anonychia—absence of the nail
- Brachyonychia—short nails
- Chromonychia—discolored nails
- Koilonychia—spoon nails
- Leukonychia—white nails
- Micronychia—small nails
- Onychauxis—thick nails
- Onychocryptosis—ingrown nails
- Onycholysis—separation of the nail from the bed
- Onychomadesis—nail shedding
- Onychorrhexis—longitudinal nail ridging
- Onychoschizia—split nails
- Paronychia—nail fold inflammation
- Trachyonychia—rough nails

IMPORTANT HISTORY QUESTIONS

How long have your nails been abnormal?

Nail disorders can be congenital or acquired. Infections are more likely to have an acute onset.

Is there any family history of a similar disorder?

Most nail disorders are acquired, but some conditions, such as pachyonychia congenita and Darier disease, are inherited in an autosomal dominant manner. In psoriasis, which has a strong familial element, this question will elicit a positive response in less than half of cases.

Has there been any trauma, and are the nails continuing to change?

Nail trauma can lead to subungual hemorrhage, but even this should be limited to a point in time—the nail discoloration will grow out distally and, eventually, will be sloughed. Ongoing and persistent change, or even worsening disease, is more concerning and could even be a sign of a malignant process.

IMPORTANT PHYSICAL FINDINGS

How many nails are involved?

Some disorders of the nail suggest a systemic disturbance, particularly when multiple nails, or even all the nails, are involved. Other disorders usually involve just one nail, such as onycholysis caused by *Pseudomonas* infection.

Which portion(s) of the nail are affected by the disease?

Some disorders affect the entire nail plate, whereas other conditions affect only the lunula (argyria) or the distal nail (most forms of onychomycosis). If the nail is thickened, it is important to determine how much of the nail plate is affected. Onychomycosis usually involves just the subungual area; psoriasis usually involves all layers of the nail plate.

If tan, brown, or black pigment is present in the nail, in a linear fashion, what is the shape of this pigmented area?

Nails are formed in the matrix and move forth as dead keratin. Therefore, the nail provides a 6- to 12-month window into the history of nail health. As shown in Fig. 25.1, the shape of the pigment deposited provides a clue as to whether the process is growing over time (a widening streak), or if it is a stable process (no widening over time). Longitudinal bands of 4 mm or more in width are more likely to be malignant.

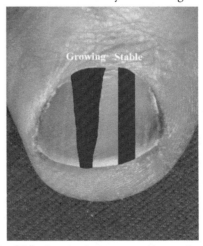

Growing Stable

Fig. 25.1. Growing lesions are wider proximally.

Paronychia ICD10 code L03.0

Pathogenesis

Acute paronychia is usually caused by bacterial infection, including *Pseudomonas* spp., *Staphylococcus aureus*, and β-hemolytic streptococci. Acute paronychia may also be caused by foreign body reactions (ingrown toenails). Chronic paronychia is more often due to infection with *Candida albicans*. Risk factors for paronychia include frequent gardening, dishwashing, or occupational food handling (one of the authors developed chronic paronychia tending bar). Excessive hand washing (including those in health care) or exposure to solvents and glues may also predispose one to paronychia. Excessive cosmetic removal of the cuticle can result in a space between the nail plate and nail fold that allows for the buildup of irritants (soaps) or for the overgrowth of bacteria *(Pseudomonas)* and yeast *(Candida)*.

Clinical Features

- Acute paronychia is an abrupt inflammatory disorder affecting the proximal nail fold, characterized by pain and erythema. Many cases will drain pus with pressure, or even spontaneously, which may indicate development of an abscess (Fig. 25.2).
- Chronic paronychia is a persistent inflammatory disorder of the proximal nail fold. It affects chiefly women, but both genders and any age group may be affected. It presents as erythema and edema of the proximal nail fold, with loss of the cuticle (Figs. 25.3 and 25.4). The nails may be normal but often demonstrate excessive ridges (Beau lines), variable onycholysis, other nail irregularities, or even a green-blue discoloration due to *Pseudomonas* infection.

Diagnosis

- Acute, chronic, or recurrent erythema and swelling of the proximal nail folds associated with pain

suggest the diagnosis; the physical examination is typically diagnostic.

Treatment

Acute Paronychia

- Acute paronychia with abscesses, as seen in Fig. 25.3, should be incised with a no. 11 scalpel blade (usually incised where the skin meets the nail fold or where the nail fold meets the nails). The contents should be cultured.
- The most commonly used oral antibiotics are directed against *Staphylococcus aureus;* options include oral dicloxacillin, cephalexin, and clindamycin if methicillin-resistant *S. aureus* (MRSA) is a concern.

Chronic Paronychia

- Use hand protection (gloves) from potential irritants and water.
- Discourage removal of cuticle during a manicure. Explain to the patient that the cuticle is a normal structure necessary to ensure that the nail fold attaches to the nail plate. The absence of this structure results in a space that collects food, soap, bacteria, and yeast.
- Discourage the use of antibacterial soaps that result in loss of the normal gram-positive skin flora, resulting in increased gram-negative skin flora (i.e., *Pseudomonas*) and yeast overgrowth.
- The mainstay of therapy is use of a medium (e.g., triamcinolone) to potent (e.g., clobetasol) topical corticosteroid cream or ointment for 2 to 4 weeks. Approximately 85% of cases will be improved or in complete remission at 4 weeks. However, a high percentage of cases will relapse.
- Rare cases may benefit from the addition of a systemic antifungal agent directed against *Candida* spp. (e.g., itraconazole, 200 mg/day for 4–6 weeks).

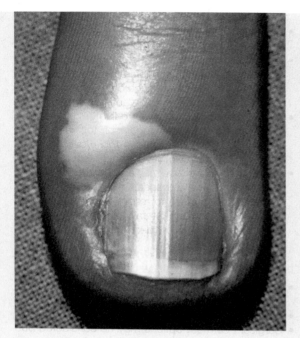

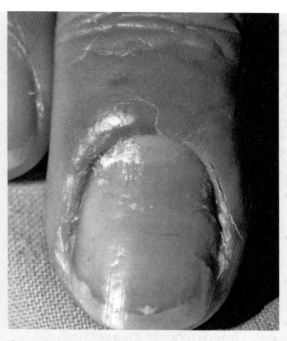

Fig. 25.2. Patient with acute paronychia, with abscess and marked erythema. (From the Fitzsimons Army Medical Center Collection, Aurora, CO.)

Fig. 25.3. Patient with chronic paronychia, with dystrophic nail. (From the Fitzsimons Army Medical Center Collection, Aurora, CO.)

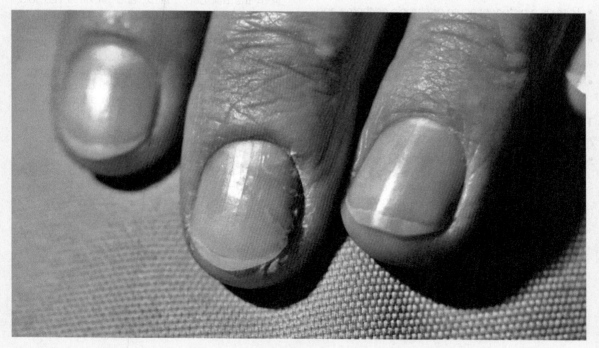

Fig. 25.4. Patient with chronic paronychia, with superficial peeling (onychoschizia) of nails. (From the Fitzsimons Army Medical Center Collection, Aurora, CO.)

Pathogenesis

Onychocryptosis is due to an overcurved nail plate that is wider than the nail bed. In many cases, the cause cannot be elucidated, although in some cases it is due tight-fitting shoes, maceration of the lateral nail groove, or cutting the distal nail plate too short. The increased incidence in patients with misalignments of the great toe or wide feet suggests that other mechanical factors are important.

Clinical Features

- It may occur in any age group, including neonates, but is most common in adolescents and young adults.
- The great toenail is usually affected, but other or multiple toenails may be involved. Less commonly, the nails of the hand can be involved.
- Early in the course, erythema, edema, and pain on pressure of the lateral nail groove are present (Fig. 25.5).
- In addition to erythema and edema, developed lesions may demonstrate abscess formation.
- Chronic lesions demonstrate granulation tissue and hypertrophy of the lateral nail fold (Fig. 25.6).

Diagnosis

- There is a history of acute or chronic erythema and pain of the lateral nail fold.
- The physical appearance demonstrates variable edema and erythema that is most pronounced on the distal lateral nail fold.
- Compression of the lateral nail fold toward the nail plate will almost invariably produce pain.

Treatment

Acute Ingrown Toenail

- Neonatal ingrown toenails can usually be treated by soaking the nail in warm water, followed by gentle massaging of the distal nail plate and lateral nail fold and then the application of petrolatum.

- Adult nails can also be treated with soaking the nail in warm water (with or without Epsom salts).
- A wisp of cotton can be gently inserted between the distal lateral nail and lateral nail fold to reduce contact. This can be replaced daily. The cotton can also be impregnated with an antiseptic.
- The topical application of a medium (e.g., triamcinolone) to potent (e.g., clobetasol) topical corticosteroid cream or ointment for 1 to 2 weeks is useful for reducing the inflammatory host response.
- A strip of adhesive tape may also be attached to the lateral nail fold, pulled beneath the toe, and adhered to the plantar surface to relieve the pressure point between the nail and lateral nail groove. This can be repeated daily, as needed, until the inflammation improves.

Developed Ingrown Toenails With Abscesses

- Conservative measures, as outlined for acute ingrown toenails, can be used.
- An abscess should be drained for immediate relief.
- Surgical treatment options may be considered but require local anesthesia, with a proximal block.
- Although many surgical treatments have been described, the most common technique involves using a septum elevator to free the lateral nail fold from the nail bed, matrix, and proximal nail fold, followed by longitudinally splitting the nail (using an English anvil nail splitter) to the matrix and removing a portion of the lateral nail (typically, ≈2 mm wide). This is followed by cauterization of the lateral matrix with 90% phenol for 2 to 3 minutes (some authorities prefer three separate 30-second applications), followed by flushing the area with alcohol to neutralize the phenol.

Chronic Ingrown Toenails With Granulation Tissue and Hypertrophy

- Surgical treatment is required in some cases. This should be done by a clinician with experience.

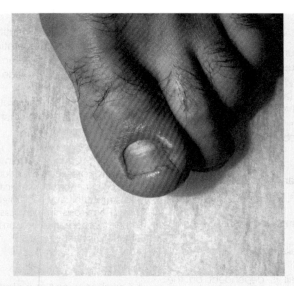

Fig. 25.5. Onychocryptosis of the big toenail in an adult demonstrating marked erythema, induration, and crust of the medial nail fold.

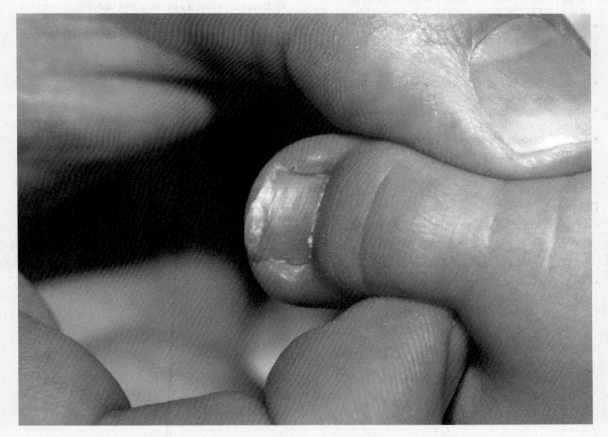

Fig. 25.6. Chronic pediatric bilateral onychocryptosis in a young child. Note that the nail demonstrates more than normal curvature, a frequent clinical finding. (From the William Weston Collection, Aurora, CO.)

Pathogenesis

Onychomycosis (tinea unguium) is a fungal infection of the nail that is usually caused by infection with a dermatophyte, with *Trichophyton rubrum* accounting for the vast majority of cases (>70%). Less commonly, nondermatophytes including *Candida* spp. (≈10%), *Scopulariopsis brevicaulis* (≈10%), *Fusarium* spp., and others may produce disease.

Clinical Features

- Although it may occur at any age, the prevalence increases with older age and is most common in the elderly.
- Although any nail may be infected, usually toenails are preferentially involved.
- The number of infected nails is variable, one to all nails.
- The appearance of the nail is dependent on the degree of infection. Typically, the dorsum of the nail plate is normal, and the underlying subungual area is affected with hyperkeratotic crumbly keratin, which may produce a yellow-white discoloration of the nail (Fig. 25.7).
- The distal portion of the nail is typically involved, and the proximal area near the skin is spared.
- Associated findings consistent with tinea pedis are often present (Fig. 25.8).
- Less commonly, the nail may demonstrate onycholysis (loss of adhesion).
- The nail plate may be normal or dystrophic; very rarely, the nail demonstrate full-thickness infection.
- Leukonychia mycotica is a less common variant characterized by a white discoloration on the surface of the nail. This is produced when the dermatophyte has infected the surface of the nail.

Diagnosis

- In regard to the clinical presentation, onychomycosis is in the differential diagnosis in any nail disorder demonstrating subungual discoloration or onycholysis.
- The diagnosis can be confirmed by sampling the subungual debris with a small curette or scalpel blade (no. 14) and identifying hyphae with a potassium hydroxide preparation (see Chapter 2).
- Material for culture can be obtained by a small curette or scalpel blade or by clipping or cutting the nail.
- For biopsy, the nail plate can be clipped or cut and sent to a pathologist or dermatopathologist for special staining.

Role of Surgical Avulsion

Although prospective randomized trials have not been performed, surgical avulsion of nails as a monotherapy has a high recurrence rate in onychomycosis. In those cases in which it needs to be done for mechanical reasons, concomitant antifungal therapy is needed.

Treatment

- Onychomycosis is a chronic and often progressive infection that does not spontaneously resolve.
- No treatment is an option because the treatment is not always successful; however, patients with diabetes or a history of recurrent cellulitis should be considered for treatment to reduce the chance of developing recurring cellulitis. Patients with painful onychomycoses are also candidates for therapy.
- Topical treatments include ciclopirox olamine, 8% lacquer, or efinaconazole, 10% topical solution. Both treatments are applied once daily to the nail for 1 year. The cure rate is around 10%.
- Oral terbinafine, which has a cure rate of about 60% to 70%, is the treatment of choice. Fingernails are treated at a dose of 250 mg/day for 6 weeks; toenails are usually treated with 250 mg/day for 12 weeks.
- Oral itraconazole and oral fluconazole are alternative options in patients who are not able to take terbinafine; however, the cure rate is lower for both drugs.
- Laser ablation followed by topical therapy is an option for select patients who cannot take oral drugs. Approximately 50% of patients demonstrate a complete response with this treatment.

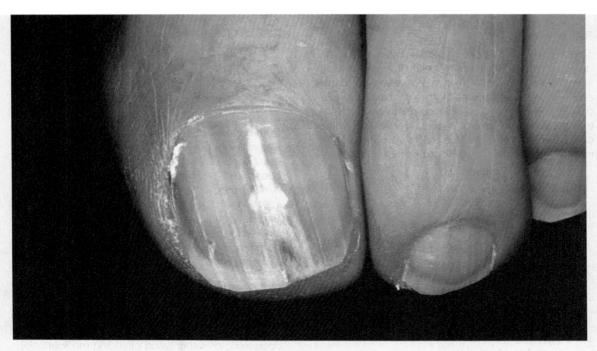

Fig. 25.7. Patient with onychomycosis demonstrating a yellowish-white subungual infection. (From the Fitzsimons Army Medical Center Collection, Aurora, CO.)

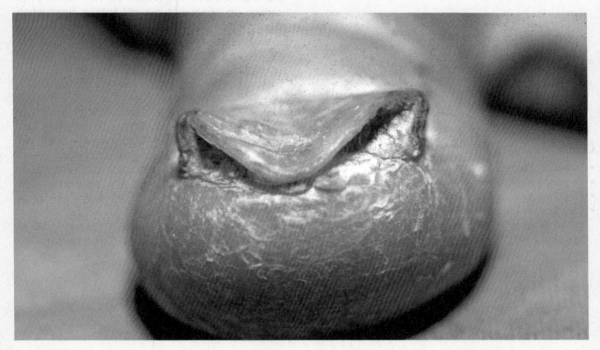

Fig. 25.8. Patient with dry scaly tinea pedis, with development of subungual onychomycosis. (From the Fitzsimons Army Medical Center Collection, Aurora, CO.)

Onycholysis ICD10 code L60.1

Pathogenesis

Onycholysis is not a specific disease but is a term that describes separation of the nail plate from the underlying nail bed. Numerous disease processes may cause onycholysis, including infection (e.g., fungus), medications (e.g., tetracycline-induced photo-onycholysis), trauma (e.g., immersing fingers in scalding water, self-induced), endocrine disorders (e.g., hyperthyroidism), and primary skin disorders (e.g., psoriasis).

Causes of Onycholysis

Infection
- *Candida* spp.
- Dermatophyte
- *Pseudomonas* spp.
- Internal disorders
- Anemia
- Hypothyroidism and hyperthyroidism
- Scleroderma

Medications
- Chemotherapy
- Doxycycline
- Oral contraceptives
- Fluoroquinolones
- Tetracycline

Idiopathic

Neoplasia
- Glomus tumor
- Squamous cell carcinoma

Skin Disorders
- Dermatitis
- Psoriasis

Traumatic

Clinical Features

- Onycholysis can occur at any age.
- Onycholysis may involve one nail or multiple nails.
- Onycholysis may be asymptomatic or painful.
- Onycholysis usually affects the distal nail, but proximal onycholysis may occur, particularly with chemotherapy.

- The lytic (separated) portion of the nail is usually white or yellow-white in color (Figs. 25.9–25.12).
- Subungual hemorrhage may be present.

Diagnosis

- Onycholysis is usually easily recognized, with observation of a white nail and loss of normal attachment to the underlying nail bed.
- Determining the cause of onycholysis is more difficult because multiple disease processes must be considered (see box).
- A KOH prep or fungal culture can exclude fungal infection.
- Biopsies are usually not performed but may be considered to exclude malignancy, particularly if there is a single onycholytic nail of chronic duration.
- In some cases, no cause is ever ascertained (idiopathic).

Treatment

- Treatment of the underlying disorder causing onycholysis is the most effective therapy (e.g., decreasing or withdrawing offending medication[s], treatment of infection). It is important to explain to the patient that onycholysis can be permanent.
- Unless specific patient behaviors are contributing to the problem, the nails should be trimmed back to reduce the chance of external trauma aggravating the condition.
- Repetitive trauma, such as typing or drumming or tapping the nails, should be avoided, where possible.
- Prolonged immersion of the nails in water should be avoided, where possible.
- Bacterial colonization can be a contributing factor—*Pseudomonas* produces proteolytic enzymes that aggravate the separation—and yeast can overgrow in the lytic space. Therefore, topical thymol, 3% to 4% in alcohol, applied underneath the nail plate bid for 6 to 12 weeks, is useful. This solution can be formulated by compounding pharmacies or may be purchased via the Internet.
- A topical imidazole solution (e.g., clotrimazole) is useful if secondary candidiasis is a concern.

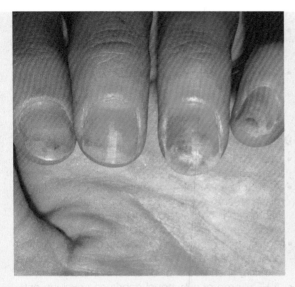

Fig. 25.9. Acute photo-onycholysis due to tetracycline that occurred when the patient was reading a book at the pool. (From the Fitzsimons Army Medical Center Collection, Aurora, CO.)

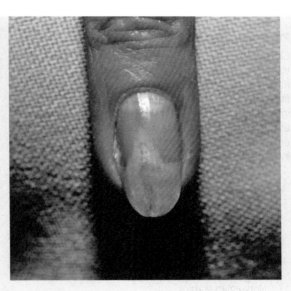

Fig. 25.10. Patient with chronic onycholysis due to repeated trauma of long nails. (From the Fitzsimons Army Medical Center Collection, Aurora, CO.)

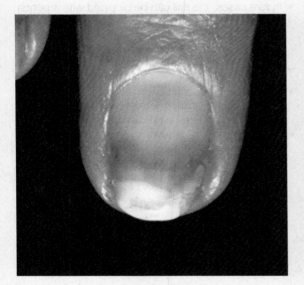

Fig. 25.11. Patient with onycholysis due to excessive use of topical nail hardeners. (From the Fitzsimons Army Medical Center Collection, Aurora, CO.)

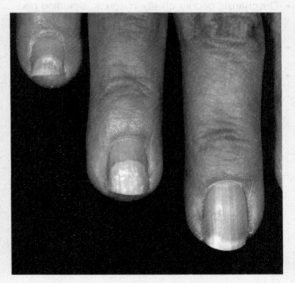

Fig. 25.12. Patient with iatrogenically induced onycholysis due to excessive thyroid supplementation. (From the Fitzsimons Army Medical Center Collection, Aurora, CO.)

Pathogenesis

Onychauxis is a descriptive medical term that refers to thick hyperkeratotic nails caused by a buildup of keratin. The most common cause is a dermatophyte (fungal) infection, which is discussed in greater detail in this chapter (see "Onychomycosis"). Psoriasis is another common cause that can be difficult to differentiate from onychomycosis. Other causes are listed in the box.

Causes of Onychauxis

Common
- Onychomycosis
- Onychogryphosis
- Psoriasis

Uncommon
- Darier disease
- Norwegian scabies
- Pachyonychia congenita
- Reactive arthritis (Reiter disease)

Clinical Features

- Onychauxis occurs chiefly in adults, including geriatric patients. Children are infrequently affected unless the cause is a genodermatosis.
- The condition may affect one or more nails (Figs. 25.13 and 25.14).
- Keratin buildup may be confined to the subungual area or may affect the entire nail. For example, in pachyonychia congenita and onychomycosis, only the subungual region is affected, whereas in psoriasis (Fig. 25.13) and crusted scabies (see Fig. 25.14), the entire nail plate is often affected.

- Elderly patients, particularly those unable to groom themselves well, may develop thick nails with hyperkeratosis in addition to other nail abnormalities.
- Other signs of cutaneous disease that can affect the nail should be sought. For example, evidence of psoriasis, scabies, reactive arthritis, or tinea pedis may be associated with onychauxis.

Diagnosis

- The clinical presentation may or may not be diagnostic.
- A history of a genodermatosis, such as Darier disease and pachyonychia congenita, is helpful information, but lack of a family history does not exclude a spontaneous mutation.
- A history or physical presence of a preexisting acquired skin disorder, such as psoriasis, reactive arthritis, tinea pedis, or scabies, is important.
- A KOH prep of subungual debris can exclude onychomycosis, particularly because it can be difficult in some cases to distinguish psoriasis confined to the nails from dermatophyte infection. A generous clipping of the dystrophic nail may also be sent for histologic examination to exclude fungal infection.
- In rare cases, the nail can be biopsied with a punch and submitted for histologic examination. Evaluation of nail plates can be challenging, and there is preference for review by a dermatopathologist.

Treatment

- There are no specific treatments for thick hyperkeratotic nails. Treatment focuses on identifying and treating any underlying primary disorder, if possible.
- Clearly, patients with onychauxis due to an inherited disorder cannot be cured.

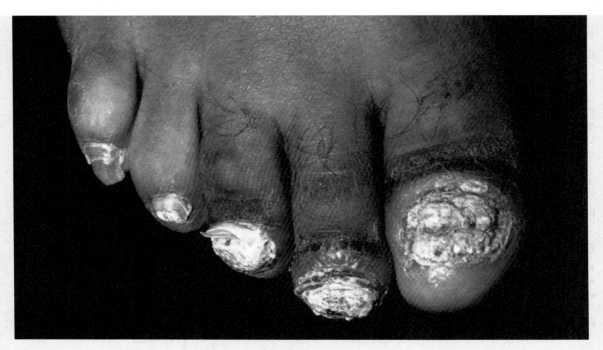

Fig. 25.13. Psoriatic nails without other cutaneous evidence of cutaneous psoriasis. This patient was erroneously treated for more than 1 year as suffering from onychomycosis. (From the Fitzsimons Army Medical Center Collection, Aurora, CO.)

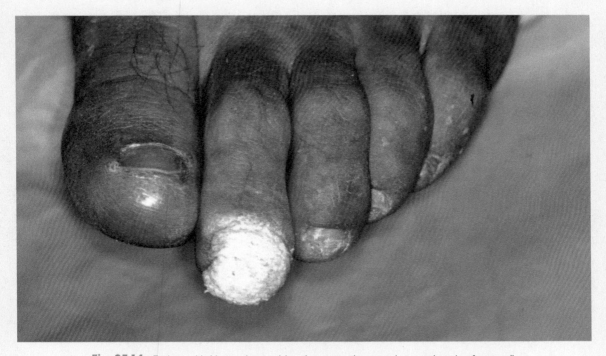

Fig. 25.14. Patient with Norwegian scabies demonstrating massive onychauxis of one nail.

Onychoschizia (Lamellar Dystrophy) ICD10 code L60.3

EXTERNAL ETIOLOGY

Pathogenesis

Onychoschizia, also known as lamellar dystrophy, or brittle nails by patients, is usually a result of aging, and the condition is common in the elderly. Brittle nails usually demonstrate associated longitudinal ridging, roughness to the nail (trachyonychia), and horizontal splitting of the distal nail plate (lamellar dystrophy). Other common causes include repetitive hydration and dehydration of the nail plate from repeated water immersion and damage from the use of nail enamel, nail polish remover, and chemical cuticle removers. Trauma and previous surgical procedures can also produce lamellar dystrophy.

Clinical Features

- Increased longitudinal ridging of nails
- Rough nails also frequently present
- Increased distal horizontal splitting of nails (Figs. 25.15 and 25.16)
- Increased distal vertical splitting of nails

Diagnosis

- The clinical presentation is usually diagnostic.

Treatment

- Elimination or minimization of exogenous damage (e.g., harsh nail products, repeated water immersion, unnecessary nail trauma) is important in management.
- Another therapy consists of purposeful soaking of the nails in tap water for 10 to 15 minutes once daily (best done in the evening), followed by direct application of 12% ammonium lactate lotion containing moisturizers.
- Oral biotin (vitamin B_7), 2500 μg (2.5 mg)/day has shown modest improvement in nail health in about two-thirds of patients in limited studies. The rationale for the use of biotin to treat thin or brittle nails is that oral biotin has been used to increase the thickness of hoofs in farm animals. A large, well-controlled, blinded trial in humans has never been performed.

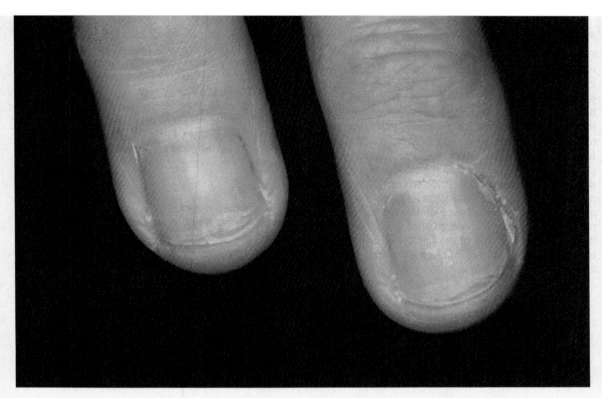

Fig. 25.15. Patient with onychoschizia manifesting as horizontal splitting of the distal nail. (From the Fitzsimons Army Medical Center Collection, Aurora, CO.)

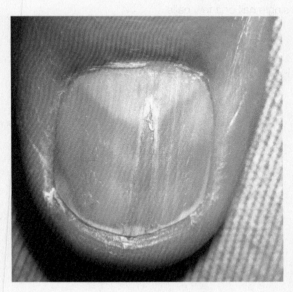

Fig. 25.16. Patient with severe linear onychoschizia secondary to severe trauma of the nail bed. (From the Fitzsimons Army Medical Center Collection, Aurora, CO.)

Beau Lines ICD10 code L60.4

Pathogenesis

Beau lines represent stunted or arrested growth of the nail, usually due to a systemic insult or less commonly localized trauma. Examples of primary events that can induce Beau lines include high fever, drug reactions, major surgery, new medication (particularly chemotherapeutic agents), and other significant insults to the patient. Some patients may have associated telogen effluvium for similar reasons. Severe insults produce deep indentations; minor insults produce subtle transverse lines. Similarly, a single event may produce a narrow line, whereas a longer lasting insult produces a wider line. Based on the location on the nail, the approximate time of the nail insult, relative to the normal growth time of the nail (3–6 months), can be estimated by measuring from the proximal nail fold to the line.

Fingernail Growth

The average adult's fingernail grows about 3 mm/month. When examining a patient with Beau lines, the approximate time of the insult can be estimated. However, it is also important to know that the rate of fingernail growth slows down as an individual ages, a factor that also needs to be considered.

Clinical Features

- Beau lines can occur in any age group.
- If the insult was relatively minor or localized, Beau lines may present in only a single nail or a few nails.

If the insult was severe or systemic, Beau lines are present in all the nails of the hands and feet.

- The primary lesion is a transverse line or depression in the nail plate, of varied width and depth (Fig. 25.17). In severe cases (e.g., with chemotherapy), the nails demonstrate wide bands of stunted growth, or the nails may even be shed (Fig. 25.18).
- As the nails grow, the involved area near the distal edge of the nail plate may manifest increased brittleness or flaking.

Diagnosis

- The clinical presentation is diagnostic, and additional testing is not required.
- Identifying a precipitating event may involve measuring the distance from the proximal nail fold to the Beau line. Because the nail grows about 3 mm/month, it is possible to estimate the date of any precipitating event and compare this to the patient's recollection or history.

Treatment

- There is no effective treatment for Beau lines, but, with removal of the insult, the line will eventually be displaced from the nail with normal growth.

Clinical Course

If the insult is removed, the Beau line will grow out and be shed, without permanent sequelae.

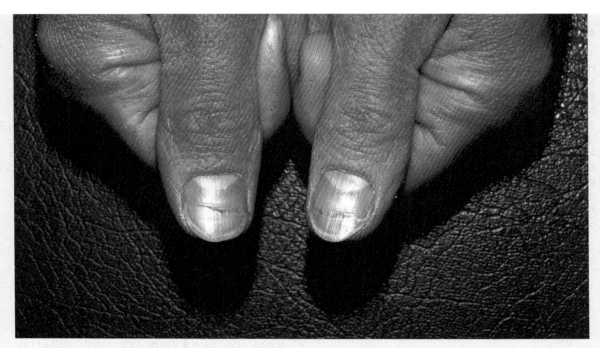

Fig. 25.17. Patient with sharply demarcated Beau lines that were secondary to an episode of toxic shock syndrome.

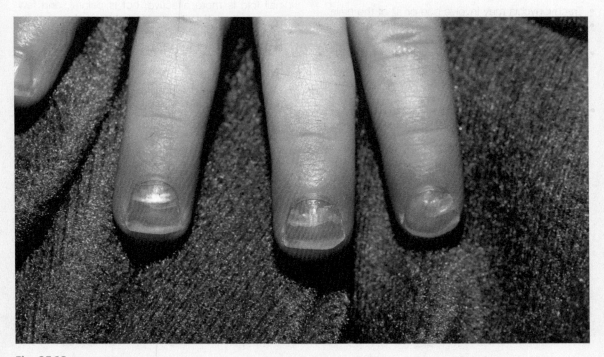

Fig. 25.18. Child with severe Beau lines due to chemotherapy that is bordering on becoming a shedding of nails (onychomadesis).

Trachyonychia (Rough Nails, Nail Pitting) ICD10 code L60.3

Pathogenesis

Trachyonychia is a broad term used to describe rough nails. It usually implies that the entire nail is involved. Nail pitting is a limited form of trachyonychia, in which the changes are focal. *Twenty-nail dystrophy* is the term used when essentially all the nails are affected; the condition occurs chiefly in children. It is thought that most cases of twenty-nail dystrophy represent lichen planus or alopecia areata, although in some cases an underlying condition cannot be established. In sum, twenty-nail dystrophy is not thought to be a specific disease, but the name is still often used in dermatology, even when the underlying cause is unknown.

Causes of Rough Nails and Pitting
- Alopecia areata
- Dermatitis
- Lichen planus
- Psoriasis
- Trauma
- Twenty-nail dystrophy
- Vitiligo

Clinical Features
- Trachyonychia may involve one or all of the nails.
- Trachyonychia may involve any portion of the nail plate.
- Nail pitting is a minimal form of trachyonychia, in which there are small pits present in the nail; this condition is often associated with psoriasis (Fig. 25.19).
- Changes may be focal and minimal or diffuse and severe, in which case the entire nail may be rough (Figs. 25.20 and 25.21).

- In rough nails in patients with dermatitis or trauma, there are often other irregularities of the nail plate, such as ribbing.

Diagnosis
- The diagnosis is usually established by clinical examination of the nail and correlation with a history of another skin disorder, such as alopecia areata, lichen planus, or psoriasis.
- In rare cases, a punch biopsy can be performed through the nail plate, with the specimen submitted for histologic analysis.

Treatment
- Trachyonychia is difficult to treat. Because it does not affect the patient's overall health, no treatment is required unless the patient desires it. If an underlying condition is present (e.g., alopecia areata, lichen planus, psoriasis), often the best therapy involves treatment of the underlying condition.
- For patients with rough nails secondary to alopecia areata, dermatitis, or psoriasis, use of a potent topical corticosteroid (e.g., clobetasol), applied qd or bid to the proximal nail fold, may occasionally be helpful. Intralesional triamcinolone into the proximal nail fold is more effective, but is painful, and few patients think that the discomfort is worth the result.
- In a double-blind randomized trial of patients with nail pitting due to psoriasis, tazarotene, 0.1% gel, applied nightly for 6 months, was shown to improve the condition.
- For patients with rough nails due to self-inflicted trauma, behavior modification therapy is useful.

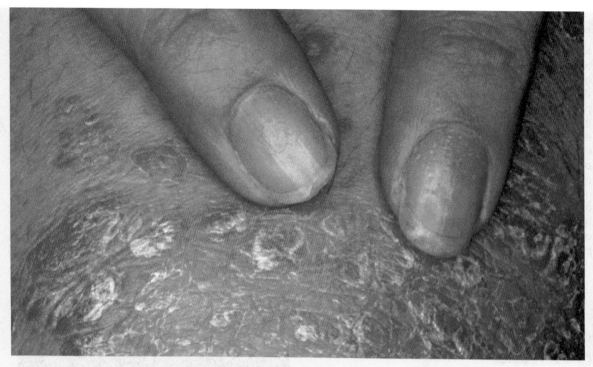

Fig. 25.19. Patient with classic plaque psoriasis, with numerous nail pits. (From the Fitzsimons Army Medical Center Collection, Aurora, CO.)

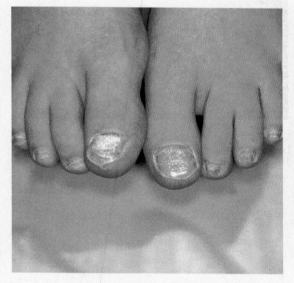

Fig. 25.20. Trachyonychia that involved all the nails in a child with twenty-nail dystrophy.

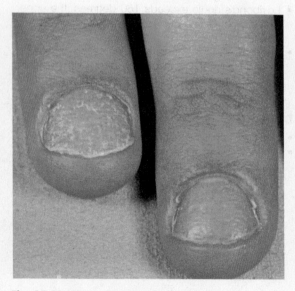

Fig. 25.21. Severe trachyonychia in a patient with alopecia areata.

Pathogenesis

Nail clubbing is caused by overgrowth of the soft tissue of the fingertip, resulting in increased curvature of the nail plate in the horizontal and longitudinal axes. When viewed from the side, the angle between the nail plate and proximal nail fold (Lovibond angle) is greater than 160 degrees (the upper limit of normal) and often exceeds 180 degrees. The mechanism of this process is unknown. Although some cases can be inherited or idiopathic, acquired nail clubbing can be a sign of systemic disease, especially pulmonary disease (e.g., malignancy, pneumonia, bronchiectasis, emphysema) or, less often, cardiovascular disease (e.g., congestive heart failure, congenital heart defects, atrial myxoma) or gastrointestinal disease (e.g., ulcerative colitis, primary biliary cirrhosis).

Classification of Nail Clubbing
- Inherited
- Acquired
- Idiopathic

Clinical Features

- Nail clubbing usually affects all the digits of the hands and feet.
- There is an overgrowth of soft tissue of the pulp of the distal digit.
- Lovibond's angle exceeds 160 degrees (the upper limit of normal) and often exceeds 180 degrees (Fig. 25.22).
- The nail plate demonstrates increased curvature, longitudinally and horizontally, often with the longitudinal curvature being the most dramatic (see Fig. 25.22).

Diagnosis

- The clinical presentation is diagnostic.
- When clubbing is discovered, the history should be expanded to determine if the condition is lifelong or if there is a family history of similar-appearing nails (Figs. 25.23A and 25.24).
- A complete review of systems should be performed on all patients with nail clubbing to direct any additional evaluation.
- A chest x-ray is recommended for all persons with acquired nail clubbing (see Fig. 25.23B).

Treatment

- There is no effective treatment for nail clubbing, but any underlying condition that is discovered should be managed.

Clinical Course

Treatment or removal of the cause of acquired clubbing may improve the condition (partially), but once considerable soft tissue overgrowth of the distal digits has occurred, there is no complete resolution.

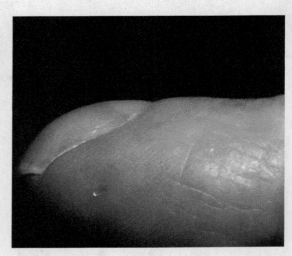

Fig. 25.22. Lateral view of nail clubbing, with a Lovibond's angle that exceeds the normal upper limit of 160 degrees.

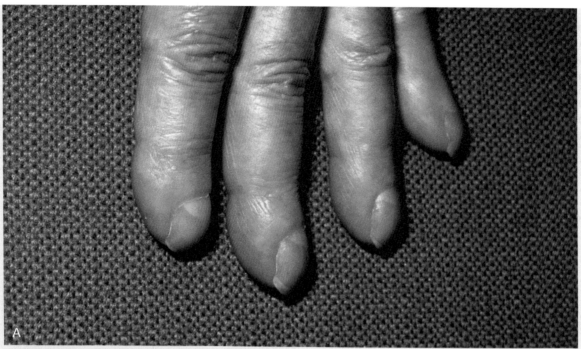

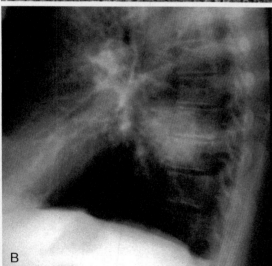

Fig. 25.23. (A) Acquired nail clubbing in a woman who presented with shortness of breath due to carcinoma of the lung as shown below left. (B) Chest x-ray of a patient who presented with digital clubbing. (From the Fitzsimons Army Medical Center Collection, Aurora, CO.)

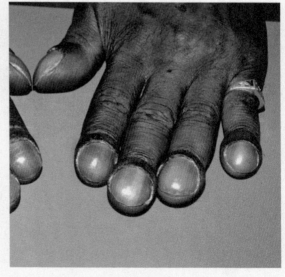

Fig. 25.24. Familial clubbing in a 20-year-old man. His father had identical nail changes. (From the Fitzsimons Army Medical Center Collection, Aurora, CO.)

Habit Tic Deformity (Onychotillomania) ICD10 code F95.0

Pathogenesis

A so-called habit tic deformity of the nail, less often referred to as onychotillomania, is a common nail abnormality that occurs in persons with a repetitive habit of pushing the nail cuticle back and/or picking at the nail itself. It is this mechanical insult that produces a characteristic deformity of the nail(s).

Clinical Features

- Patients are usually adults and have usually had the nail condition for years or even decades.
- The thumbnails are usually affected, with dystrophic changes being unilateral or bilateral.
- The cuticle is often pushed back, exposing an enlarged lunula. The cuticle may also be hyperkeratotic.
- The characteristic finding is central nail dystrophy that manifests as multiple transverse ridges of variable size, giving a washboard appearance to the nails (Figs. 25.25–25.27).
- In some patients with habit tic, the grooves in the nail may be discolored.

Diagnosis

- In an adult, the clinical presentation of washboard nails, with variable damage to the cuticle, is essentially diagnostic (see Figs. 25.25 and 25.26).
- The only other nail condition that is difficult to differentiate is so-called median nail dystrophy (Heller disease), which is a rare acquired nail dystrophy characterized by a thin longitudinal split or deep groove with smaller transverse ridges, yielding a fir tree pattern of one or both thumbnails (see Fig. 25.27). It is very important to realize that although some dermatologists consider this a separate disease (a unique condition), other dermatologists simply consider this to be subset of habit tic deformity.

Treatment

- The condition is benign, and no treatment is required. A candid discussion of the cause may produce behavior modification, with improvement, but the success rate is low.
- Having the patient cover the affected nail(s) with tape (or bandages) may reduce or eliminate the repetitive trauma, but this requires a motivated and compliant patient.
- An alternative topical approach is application of cyanoacrylate glue once or twice a week at the proximal nail plate and cuticle, again with the goal being to interrupt the damage caused by the repetitive behavior. However, this may also serve as a nidus for additional picking.
- Oral selective serotonin reuptake inhibitors (SSRIs) have been used with success, but, given the relatively minimal nature of this disorder, it is not recommended unless there are other conditions responsive to such drugs (e.g., anxiety disorder, depression).

Clinical Course

If the habit tic can be controlled or interrupted, the nail will usually regrow, without permanent sequelae.

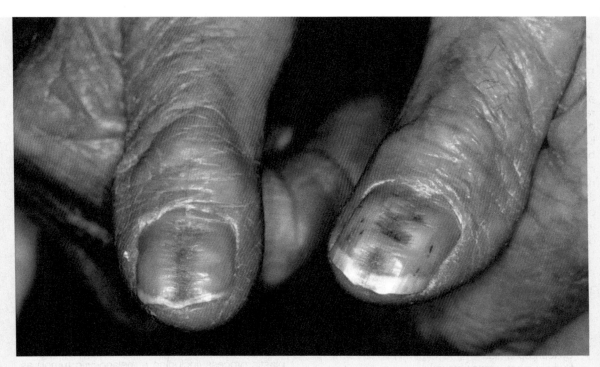

Fig. 25.25. Patient with bilateral habit tic deformity with washboard nails that are discolored from debris, chemicals, and/or other external agents. (From the Fitzsimons Army Medical Center Collection, Aurora, CO.)

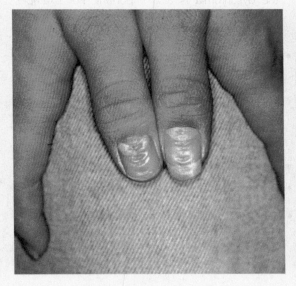

Fig. 25.26. Patient with bilateral habit tic deformity, with prominent lunula.

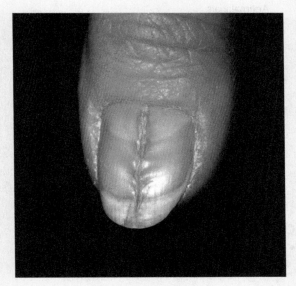

Fig. 25.27. Patient with characteristic fir tree dystrophy of the thumbnail in a median nail dystrophy. (From the Fitzsimons Army Medical Center Collection, Aurora, CO.)

Nail Discoloration ICD10 codes (numerous)

Pathogenesis

Discolored nails can result from external (e.g., nail polish, topical medications) or internal sources (e.g., oral silver ingestion, melanin). Moreover, nail discoloration can occur in all nail components of the nail apparatus, including the nail plate, nail bed, and cuticle, or only in portions of the nail apparatus, such as the lunula or nail plate. Color changes may be induced by a variety of compounds and/or structural abnormalities, including melanin, parakeratosis (retained nail plate causing a white color), serum (retained in the nail plate and causing a yellow color), vascular changes in the nail bed, or exposure to carotenoids and medications. There are hundreds of causes of nail discoloration; the adjacent box is only a partial list.

Causes of Nail Discoloration

Black Nails
- Melanoma
- Subungual hematoma

Brown Nails
- Azidothymidine (AZT; zidovudine)
- Cyclophosphamide
- Hydroquinone (orange-brown)
- Normal variation
- Melanocytic tumors

Blue-Gray Nails
- Antimalarials
- Tetracycline antibiotics
- Silver (argyria)
- Wilson disease

Green Nails
- *Pseudomonas* infection

White Nails
- Leukonychia mycotica
- Mees lines
- Muehrcke lines
- Punctate leukonychia
- Terry nails

Yellow Nails
- Yellow nail syndrome

Clinical Features

- Nail discolorations may affect those in any age group.

- Depending on the cause, one or more nails may be affected.
- Color changes include brown (Figs. 25.28–25.31), black (Fig. 25.32), purple-black (Fig. 25.33), white (Fig. 25.34), blue-gray (Figs. 25.35 and 25.36), green, or yellow (Fig. 25.37) and any variation thereof.
- Nail discoloration may occur on the surface, in the nail plate itself, or beneath the nail plate in the nail bed.
- Nail discolorations are asymptomatic.
- Some nail discolorations can occur with other nail abnormalities. Melanoma may cause discoloration of the nail plate, with extension of pigment onto the proximal nail fold (Hutchinson sign). Similarly, the green color of a *Pseudomonas* infection may be associated with onycholysis.

Diagnosis

- The diagnosis is established via a medication history, exposure to topical agents, and history of other known systemic diseases. Patients with a solitary discolored nail are more likely to have an infectious process, trauma-related process, or neoplastic process (including a melanocytic tumor) as the cause, whereas patients with multiple involved nails are more likely to have a systemic cause.
- In addition to the color involved, the location of the dyschromia is also important. For example, excessive silver ingestion (argyria) typically affects the lunula, whereas the use of AZT for HIV/AIDS usually produces transverse brown bands.
- In cases in which the pigment lies on on the surface of the nail, it can be removed by shaving the top of the nail plate with a scalpel. For example, the brown color induced by topical hydroquinone and iodine compounds and the white color of leukonychia mycotica are removed (in whole or in part) when scraped with a scalpel blade.

Treatment

- Treatment is dependent on identification and avoidance of the cause.
- Resolution will occur as the stimulus is removed and normal nail growth displaces the affected nail. At present, there is no way to bleach the nail effectively to return it to its original color.

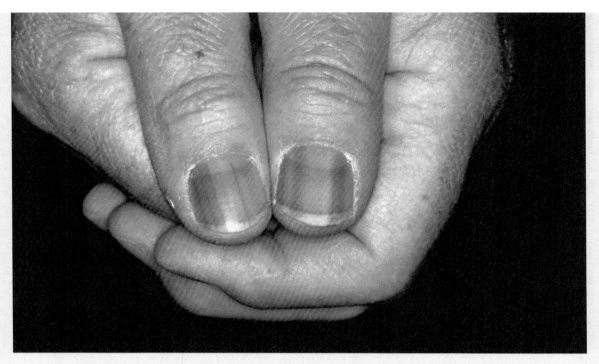

Fig. 25.28. Brown nails in addition to brown streaking can be a normal variant in nail coloration.

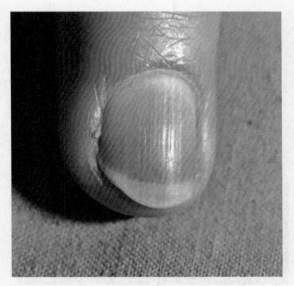

Fig. 25.29. Patient with brown nails due to repeated exposure to topical hydroquinone. (From the Fitzsimons Army Medical Center Collection, Aurora, CO.)

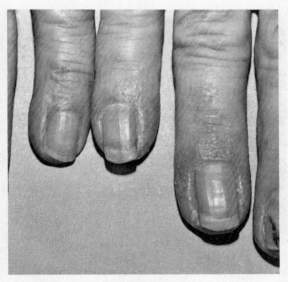

Fig. 25.30. Patient with yellow-brown discoloration from repeated exposure to an iodine-containing topical preparation. (From the Fitzsimons Army Medical Center Collection, Aurora, CO.)

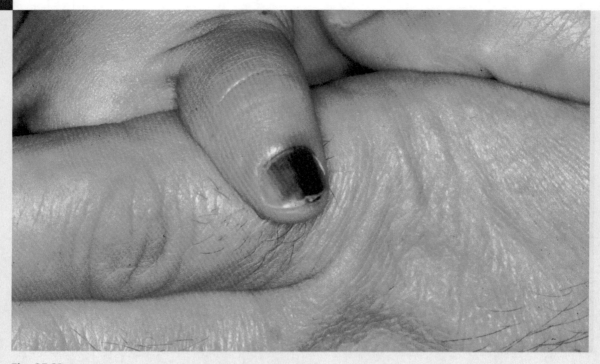

Fig. 25.31. Marked dark brown melanonychia striata (nail lentigo) in a child. Note that the edge is straight, suggesting that this lesion is stable in size. (From the William Weston Collection, Aurora, CO.)

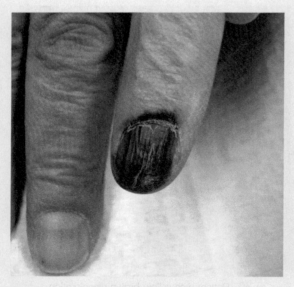

Fig. 25.32. Patient with acral lentiginous melanoma arising in a nail, with a positive Hutchinson sign (discoloration of the proximal nail fold).

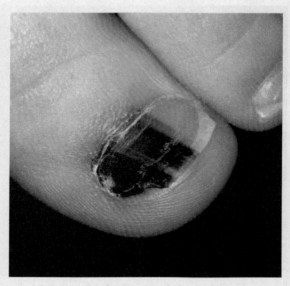

Fig. 25.33. Patient with a subungual hematoma demonstrating a purple-black discoloration. (Courtesy Dr. Joseph Morelli.)

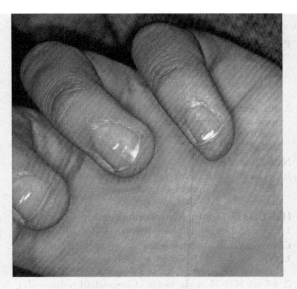

Fig. 25.34. Patient with punctate leukonychia, the most common cause of white discoloration.

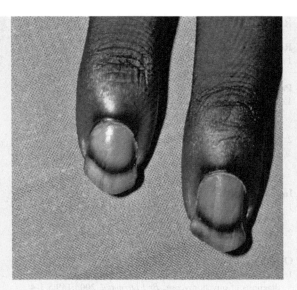

Fig. 25.35. Patient with admixture of gray and brown bands of the nail produced by treatment with AZT. (From the Fitzsimons Army Medical Center Collection, Aurora, CO.)

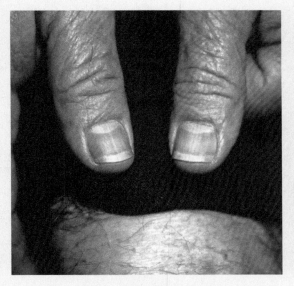

Fig. 25.36. Patient with blue-gray discoloration of the nail secondary to minocycline. (From the Fitzsimons Army Medical Center Collection, Aurora, CO.)

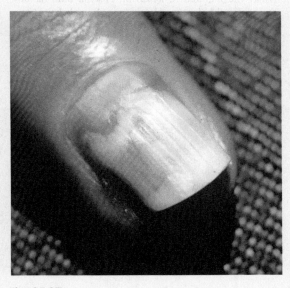

Fig. 25.37. Patient with onycholytic nail with yellow-green color due to *Pseudomonas*. (From the Fitzsimons Army Medical Center Collection, Aurora, CO.)

References

Review

1. Fawcett RS, Linford S, Stulberg D. Nail abnormalities: clues to systemic disease. *Am Fam Physician*. 2004;69:1417-1424.

Paronychia

1. Durdu M, Ruocco V. Clinical and cytologic features of antibiotic-resistant acute paronychia. *J Am Acad Dermatol*. 2014;70:120-126.
2. Tosti A, Piraccini BM, Ghetti E, Colombo D. Topical steroids versus systemic antifungals in the treatment of chronic paronychia: an open, randomized double-blind and double dummy study. *J Am Acad Dermatol*. 2002;47:73-76.

Ingrown Nails

1. Daniel CR III, Iorizzo M, Tosti A, Piraccini BM. Ingrown toenails. *Cutis*. 2006;78:407-408.
2. Haneke E. Ingrown and pincer nails: evaluation and treatment. *Dermatol Ther*. 2002;15:148-158.

Onychomycosis

1. Faergemann J, Baran R. Epidemiology, clinical presentation and diagnosis of onychomycosis. *Br J Dermatol*. 2003;149:S-1-4.
2. Rosen T, Friedlander SF, Kircik L, et al. Onychomycosis: Epidemiology, diagnosis, and treatment in a changing landscape. *J Drugs Dermatol*. 2015;14:223-228.

Onycholysis

1. Daniel CR 3rd, Tosti A, Iorizzo M, Piraccini BM. The disappearing nail bed: a possible outcome of onycholysis. *Cutis*. 2005;76:325-327.

Psoriatic Nails

1. Jiaravuthisan MM, Sasseville D, Vender RB, et al. Psoriasis of the nail: anatomy, pathology and clinical presentation, and a review of the literature on therapy. *J Am Acad Dermatol*. 2007;57:1-27.
2. Rigopoulos AD, Gregoriou S, Katsambas A. Treatment of psoriatic nails with tazarotene cream 0.1% vs. clobetasol propionate 0.05% cream: a double-blind study. *Acta Derm Venereol*. 2007;87:167-168.

Nail Clubbing

1. Spicknall KE, Zirwas MJ, English JC 3rd. Clubbing: an update on diagnosis, differential diagnosis, pathophysiology, and clinical relevance. *J Am Acad Dermatol*. 2005;53:1020-1028.

Habit Tic Deformity (Onychotillomania)

1. Perrin AJ, Lam JM. Habit-tic deformity. *CMAJ*. 2014;186:371.

Chromonychia

1. Braun RP, Baran R, Le Gal FA, et al. Diagnosis and management of nail pigmentations. *J Am Acad Dermatol*. 2007;56:835-847.
2. Jellinek N. Nail matrix biopsy of longitudinal melanonychia: diagnostic algorithm including the matrix shave biopsy. *J Am Acad Dermatol*. 2007;56:803-810.

Chapter 26
Infestations, Stings, and Bites

Numerous arthropods can produce infestations, stings, and bites (see box). In addition to infestations, like scabies, arthropods can produce pruritic bites and local envenomation reactions that can result in tissue necrosis and ulceration. Moreover, some arthropods, such as ticks, mosquitoes, and flies, can be vectors of viral, rickettsial, bacterial, and protozoan infections that can cause skin disease or even systemic disease.

Arthropod Reactions: Selected Causes

Insects
- Ants (see Chapters 6 and 12)
- Bees
- Bedbugs (see Chapter 6)
- Fleas (see Online Chapter)
- Flies (see Chapter 13 and Online Chapter)
- Mosquitoes
- Sandflies (see Chapter 36)
- Wasps
- Yellowjackets

Arachnids
- Mites (see Chapters 6 and 12)
- Scorpions
- Spiders (also see Chapter 14)
- Ticks

IMPORTANT HISTORY QUESTIONS

Did you see what bit or stung you?

For arthropods that cause skin injury, rather than an infestation, the answer to this question, in an observant and reliable patient, establishes the diagnosis. However, one must not be misled because there is tendency for patients to assume an exogenous explanation, such as a spider bite, when another disease process is actually the cause. For example, in one study of 600 skin injuries attributed to "spider bites" by patients, 20% ultimately had some other disease process at play.

Did you capture, kill, or photograph the "bug" that bit or stung you?

Patients only rarely bring in the arthropod, but increasingly patients have used smartphones to document the offending arthropod.

Does anyone else that you know have a similar problem?

An affirmative response favors some infestation. A child with head lice may have siblings, playmates, or classmates with a similar problem. Head lice can also be transmitted by shared hats, combs, hairbrushes, and other fomites. Scabies is another infestation that often affects multiple persons in a household.

Are you sexually active?

This question is important in the assessment of pubic louse and scabies infestations. The answer may be useful in establishing the diagnosis, but the answer is even more important in identifying others who require treatment. It is also important to realize that pubic louse infestations are not always sexually acquired, and the condition may be passed from those simply in close contact with an infested individual.

Does the lesion itch, or is it painful?

Most arthropod reactions are pruritic, but if pain is reported, this raises the possibility of a spider bite, reduviid bug bite, sting reaction (e.g., bees, wasps, yellowjackets, scorpions), or infected arthropod bite.

How do you feel?

Systemic symptoms are important in some severe envenomation reactions, such as those of the black widow spider, or with multiple bee stings, or in any bite causing anaphylaxis.

IMPORTANT PHYSICAL FINDINGS

What is the distribution of the lesions?

Some arthropod reactions are more likely to involve specific body regions. For example, head lice involve the scalp and upper neck, whereas pubic lice involve the genital areas or, rarely, the eyelashes. Tick bites often involve the scalp, neck, or intertriginous skin folds.

What does the bite site look like?

Spider bites often demonstrate two closely apposed fang marks, whereas other arthropod reactions cause red papules, often without a visible punctum. Skin necrosis should prompt consideration of brown recluse spider bite, particularly if the tissue damage is relentlessly expanding.

Pediculosis Capitis ICD10 code B85.0

Pathogenesis

Pediculosis capitis is caused by infestation with the human head louse, *Pediculus humanus* var. *capitis* (Fig. 26.1). Head louse infestations are seen mostly in children, with 6 to 12 million new cases in the United States each year. The condition is least common in African American children.

Clinical Features

- Pruritus is variable, ranging from negligible to severe.
- Primary skin lesions consist of macular erythema or erythematous papules on the scalp. The posterior auricular scalp is often most affected (Fig. 26.2). Lymphadenopathy and a morbilliform eruption (pediculid) may be present.
- Secondary skin findings include excoriations and crusts.
- Lice are difficult to locate because the organisms rapidly relocate when the hair is disturbed. However, nits (louse eggs) are affixed to hair shafts and are usually easy to locate (Fig. 26.3).

Diagnosis

- Any dermatitis on the scalp of a young child prompts concern for head louse infestation.
- Posterior auricular or cervical lymphadenopathy should raise the index of suspicion further.
- The diagnosis is established by the visualization of nits on scalp hair (see Fig. 26.3) or by combing the hair with a fine-toothed comb (so-called nit comb) to extract the eggs or lice (Fig. 26.4).

Treatment

- Permethrin, 1% shampoo, has been a long-standing treatment, and it is available over the counter (OTC). However, as of 2015, resistance to permethrin was reported in 25 states. Also, permethrin is not ovicidal, so nits must be removed manually, and a second treatment with permethrin must be applied, 7 to 10 days after first use.
- Malathion, 0.5% lotion (Ovide), kills lice and eggs rapidly, although resistance has been reported. It can be used in children 6 years of age and older. Malathion lotion is flammable and expensive.
- Pyrethrins with piperonyl butoxide are available OTC and can be used in children 2 years of age and older. Some resistance has been reported in the

United States. A second treatment is needed 7 to 10 days later.

- Ivermectin may be used as a 0.5% lotion or as a single-dose oral treatment (200 µg/kg). It is not ovicidal. A second treatment is recommended, 7 to 10 days after the first, to kill late-hatching organisms.
- Benzyl alcohol, 5% lotion, kills lice but is not ovicidal, and a second treatment is needed 7 days after the first treatment to kill late-hatching lice organisms. It can be irritating to the skin.
- Lindane 1% (Kwell), formerly a first-line agent, is now a second-line agent because of toxicity; use is advocated only when other treatments have failed.
- Lice require hair to complete their life cycle, and shaving of the scalp is an alternative therapy. Nit removal with combs (wet combing) is a useful adjunctive measure. Diluted vinegar, 8% formic acid, and a specially formulated enzymatic cream rinse may be helping in removing nits.

Clinical Course

The American Academy of Pediatrics (AAP) and the National Association of School Nurses (NASN) are opposed to so-called no-nit policies, and the presence of nits should not bar a child from returning to school.

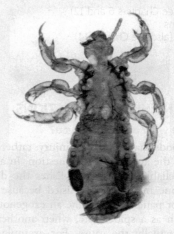

Fig. 26.1. Human head louse. It is indistinguishable from the body louse. (From the Fitzsimons Army Medical Center Collection, Aurora, CO.)

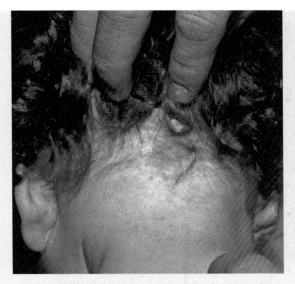

Fig. 26.2. Patient with posterior scalp dermatitis due to head lice infestation. Nits were difficult to find. (From the Fitzsimons Army Medical Center Collection, Aurora, CO.)

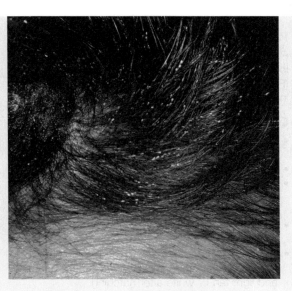

Fig. 26.3. Patient with extensive infestation by numerous nits. Nits are red-brown before hatching and light tan or white after hatching. (From the Fitzsimons Army Medical Center Collection, Aurora, CO.)

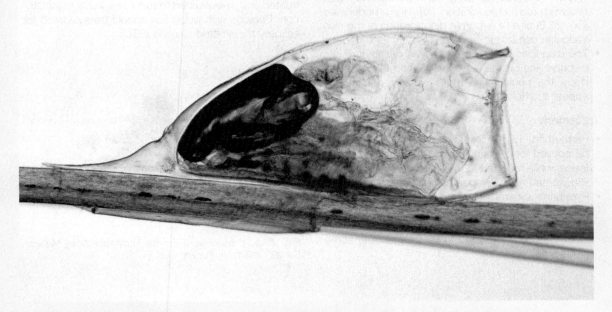

Fig. 26.4. Microscopic appearance of an empty egg casing. Suspected nits should be examined microscopically to differentiate from white hair casts that surround hair shafts.

Pathogenesis

Pediculosis pubis is due to infestation with the pubic louse, *Pthirus pubis*, also known as the "crab" louse (Fig. 26.5). Pubic louse infestations are seen primarily in sexually active young adults.

Clinical Features

- The infestation usually affects pubic hair. Less often, it affects the eyelashes or scalp of black children.
- Pruritus is variable, ranging from negligible to severe.
- Primary skin lesions, if present, consist of macular erythema or erythematous papules in the genital region.
- Secondary skin findings include excoriations and crusts.
- Nits (eggs) vary from a few to many in number (Fig. 26.6). The nits appear red-brown before hatching and light tan or white after hatching.
- Typically, the lice are easily found, and are located at the base of the hair shafts. The lice appear as tan, crablike, flattened insects, with three pairs of legs and large pincer claws (Fig. 26.7).

Diagnosis

- Dermatitis in the genital area of sexually active adults should raise concern for pubic louse infestation.
- Severe infestations may be associated with brownish-red discoloration of the underwear (Fig. 26.8) or a blue-purple discoloration of the skin (maculae ceruleae).
- The diagnosis is established by visualization of nits or pubic lice on the pubic hair. When taken off the body, the pubic louse moves slowly, and it may appear to shake.

Treatment

- Permethrin, 1.0% (Nix), is available OTC. It should be applied for 10 minutes and then rinsed. Resistance, while reported in the United States, is not as widespread as resistance among head lice.
- Pyrethrins synergized with pyrethrins (e.g., A-200 Shampoo, Clear Lice System, RID Mousse, RID Shampoo, Pronto) are available OTC. Again, resistance has been reported to these agents in some areas.

- Malathion, 0.5% (Ovide), is a second-line treatment that kills lice rapidly, including permethrin-resistant strains, but it has not been formally approved by the US Food And Drug Administration (FDA) for the treatment of pubic lice.
- Topical and single-dose oral ivermectin (200 μ/kg) has been reported to be effective against pubic lice infestations, but it is not ovicidal and treatment must be repeated in 7 to 10 days to kill late-hatching lice. It has not been formally approved by the FDA for the treatment of pubic lice.
- Shaving of pubic hair is an effective alternative or adjunctive therapy.
- Lindane, 1% (Kwell), the former treatment of choice, is now a second-line drug because of toxicity and is only recommended when other treatments have failed.
- Involvement of the eyelashes must not be treated with anything oculotoxic. Typically, eyelash involvement is treated only with ophthalmic-grade white petrolatum to smother the organisms.

Clinical Follow-up

All sex partners in the past 30 days should be informed that they are at risk for infestation, and they should be treated. Sexual contact should be avoided until the patient and sex partners have been successfully treated and re-evaluated to rule out persistent infestation. Persons with pubic lice should be evaluated for sexually transmitted disease (STD).

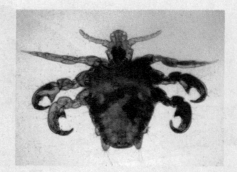

Fig. 26.5. Crab louse. (From the Fitzsimons Army Medical Center Collection, Aurora, CO.)

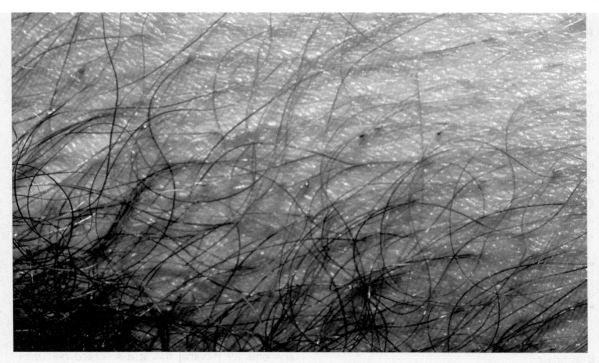

Fig. 26.6. Patient with numerous tan to brownish nits attached to hair shafts of the pubic area. (From the Fitzsimons Army Medical Center Collection, Aurora, CO.)

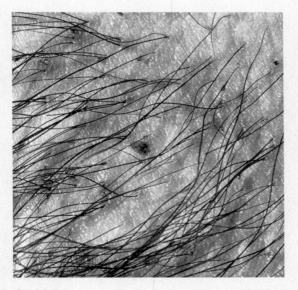

Fig. 26.7. Close-up of a crab louse attached to hair shafts of a patient. Several brown nits are also present. (From the Fitzsimons Army Medical Center Collection, Aurora, CO.)

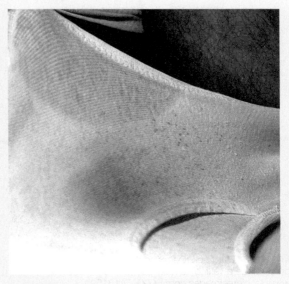

Fig. 26.8. Patient with massive crab louse infestation causing brownish discoloration of the underwear. (From the Fitzsimons Army Medical Center Collection, Aurora, CO.)

Pathogenesis

There are more than 800 species of hard ticks (Fig. 26.9) that feed by attaching to skin. Relevant species vary throughout the country. Ticks attach by inserting a long mouth part, called a hypostome, into the skin. The hypostome (Fig. 26.10) is covered with barbs to resist removal. Some species of ticks, such as *Dermacentor*, secrete a cement-like material that further solidifies attachment to the host. Ticks are responsible for the transmission of numerous vector-borne diseases, including Lyme disease (Fig. 26.11).

Clinical Features

- Tick bites usually occur in the spring and summer.
- Ticks may attach to any skin site but prefer protected areas, such as body folds and the scalp.
- Ticks produce an anesthetic-like substance to keep the feeding site asymptomatic, but, once the tick drops off, the site often becomes pruritic.
- In addition to a puncture site, the surrounding area demonstrates variable redness and swelling (Fig. 26.12).

Diagnosis

- In most cases, the diagnosis is established easily and simply based upon the clinical appearance.

- Rare cases may be mistaken for thrombosed acrochordons or pedunculated nevi, and the diagnosis can be established by doing a deep shave or punch biopsy.

Treatment

- Optimal removal is accomplished by grasping the tick mouth parts with tweezers and gently pulling the tick straight out, in the reverse direction that the hypostome was inserted into the skin (Fig. 26.13). Steady backward pulling works best. In most cases, the tick can be removed intact.
- If the hypostome breaks off and remains in the skin, it should be treated as a foreign body and should be removed as such, just as a wood splinter would be removed. This may include simply punch-excising the area.
- In endemic areas, prophylactic treatment of Lyme disease may be indicated.

Clinical Course

Most tick bites resolve spontaneously over a period of weeks, but rare cases may demonstrate residual erythema for months; this is a so-called persistent tick bite reaction.

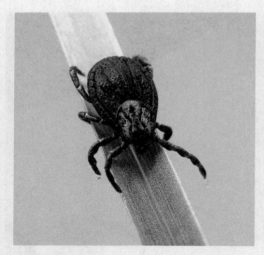

Fig. 26.9. Hard tick (Dermacentor species) tick on grass blade awaiting its next victim. (From https://www.stockfreeimages.com/000005418159.)

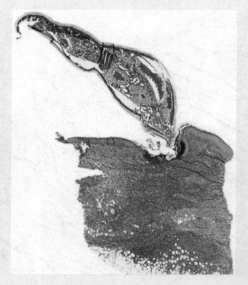

Fig. 26.10. Biopsy of an attached tick with hypostome embedded in the dermis (H&E; 20×). (From the Fitzsimons Army Medical Center Collection, Aurora, CO.)

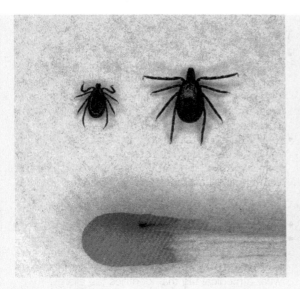

Fig. 26.11. Immature and mature forms of hard ticks (Ixodes species), which are the most common vectors of Lyme disease. (From the Fitzsimons Army Medical Center Collection, Aurora, CO.)

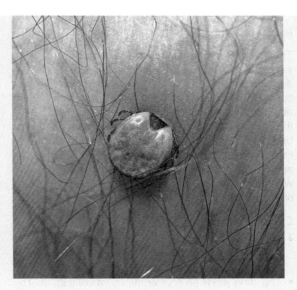

Fig. 26.12. Patient with attached, partially engorged hard body tick, with inflammatory host response. (From the Fitzsimons Army Medical Center Collection, Aurora, CO.)

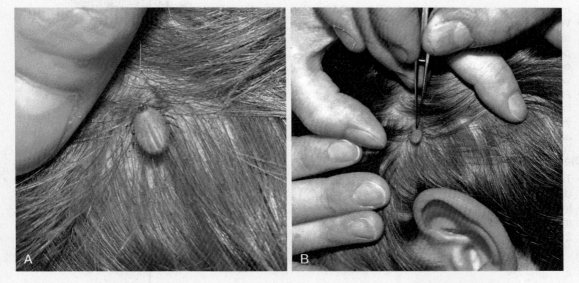

Fig. 26.13. A, Attached partially engorged tick on the scalp of a child, with an inflammatory host response. B, Proper removal of tick by grasping the head with forceps and gently pulling on the tick until it releases. (From the William Weston Collection, Aurora, CO.)

Pathogenesis

The order Hymenoptera contains a number of stinging insects including bees, hornets, wasps, and harvester and fire ants. The stinging apparatus varies with the species, but in general, it consists of a barbed stinger attached to a venom sac. With bee stings (Fig. 26.14), the stinger remains attached to the skin, and the bee dies after stinging. Hornets and wasps can sting multiple times with the same stinger because barbs are not present. Biting ants anchor themselves to skin with their mandibles and then pivot, stinging multiple times around a central anchor point.

Clinical Features

- Stings from Hymenoptera can be singular or multiple and produce immediate pain, followed by variable burning and pruritus.
- The sting yields an erythematous wheal (Fig. 26.15) that may have central blanching and a punctum at the site of penetration.
- Most stings subside over hours, but variable erythema and edema can persist for up to 7 days in some patients. Rarely, considerable massive edema may produce a bullous appearance (Fig. 26.16).
- With a large number of stings (>50), systemic reactions can develop due to vasoactive amines, peptides, and enzymes. The median lethal dose is estimated to be about 19 strings/kg body weight, which is about 500 stings in an average adult.
- Anaphylaxis can occur within minutes or, rarely, as late as 72 hours after a sting. At least 50 deaths/year in the United States have been attributed to an anaphylactic reaction to Hymenoptera stings.

Diagnosis

- The clinical presentation and history are usually diagnostic.
- In rare cases, a patient will bring in a photo or the actual insect for identification (Figs. 26.17 and 26.18).

Treatment

- Anaphylaxis is a medical emergency. In adults, it should be treated with 0.3–0.5 mL of subcutaneous epinephrine (1:1000 solution). Half-strength dilutions are used in children. Antihistamines, corticosteroids, bronchodilators, vasopressors, intravenous fluid, and oxygen may also be necessary.
- In the case of bee stings, the stinger should be removed as soon as possible. The venom sac continues to pump through the stinger apparatus but empties in about 1 minute. Stingers can be removed by flicking with a credit card or something similar to avoid squeezing the sac.
- Cool compresses can alleviate discomfort.
- Patients with anaphylaxis should be given education and a prescription for self-administered epinephrine (e.g., EpiPen). These patients should also wear a medical tag that identifies the allergy.

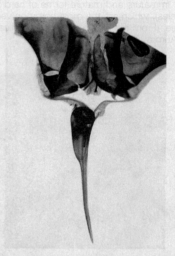

Fig. 26.14. Bee stinger removed from the skin. Barbs located at the end were sheared off during removal. (From the Fitzsimons Army Medical Center Collection, Aurora, CO.)

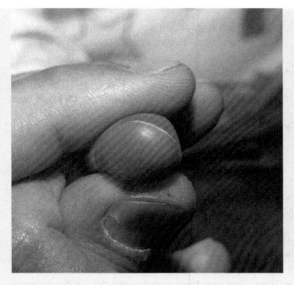

Fig. 26.15. Marked erythema at the site of a bee sting. The sting apparatus depicted in Fig. 26.14 was removed from this site. (From the Fitzsimons Army Medical Center Collection, Aurora, CO.)

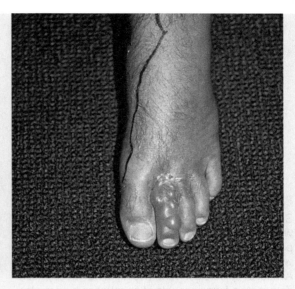

Fig. 26.16. Patient with bee sting of the toe, with massive edema resembling a bullous reaction. (From the Fitzsimons Army Medical Center Collection, Aurora, CO.)

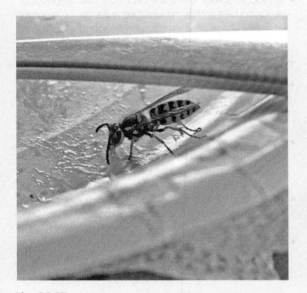

Fig. 26.17. Western yellowjacket *(Vespula pennsylvanica)* eating at a picnic table. Yellowjackets are aggressive and account for up to 90% of all stings in some parts of the United States.

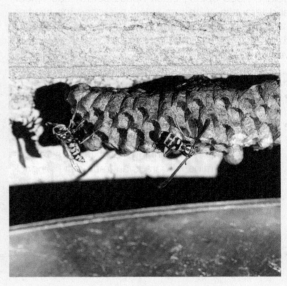

Fig. 26.18. European paper wasp *(Polistes dominulus)* in Colorado, another common cause of stings. Although not aggressive as yellow jackets, these wasps will sting to protect a nest.

The Brown Widow Spider

The brown widow spider has been expanding its range into the southeastern states and California. Despite being slightly smaller, the brown widow spider will kill and replace the black widow spider in the environment.

The venom of the brown widow spider is identical to that of the black widow spider, but the injected amount is less, and most bites produce only local reactions.

Pathogenesis

Spiders are arachnids, with four pairs of legs and no wings, and most have a silk-spinning apparatus at the posterior end. There are more than 20,000 species worldwide and over 3000 species in the United States. Almost all spiders use venom to hunt, but most spiders do not have fangs capable of penetrating human skin. About 50 spider species can produce skin reactions in humans, with the most important being the black widow spider (Fig. 26.19), brown widow spider (Fig. 26.20), brown recluse spider (see Chapter 14), wolf spider, hobo spider, black house spider, sac spider, and tarantula. With tarantulas, it is often the stinging hairs and not the bite that cause a skin reaction. More than 2600 black widow spider bites are reported each year in the United States.

Clinical Features

- The clinical presentation of a spider bite varies with the species and amount of venom injected.
- Black widow and brown widow spiders inject α-latrotoxin, which results in depletion of acetylcholine at motor nerve endings and triggers release of catecholamines. There is an immediate pinprick sensation and, later, dull pain. In cases of severe envenomation, patients can develop muscle rigidity and fasciculation, headache, weakness, abdominal pain, salivation, respiratory paralysis, seizures, and, rarely, death.
- Brown recluse spider bites contain at least eight components, but sphingomyelinase D is the agent responsible for the characteristic expanding tissue necrosis, which may necessitate surgical intervention.
- Most other venomous spiders in the United States produce only local tissue reactions. On close inspection, spider bites may be seen to have two puncture marks from the spider fangs.
- In contrast to most other arthropod reactions, spider bites are often painful rather than pruritic. However, some species that inject histamine, such as the hobo spider, can cause pruritus at the bite site.
- A necrotic center may result from fusion of the two puncture sites caused by the fangs (Fig. 26.21).

Diagnosis

- The complete clinical presentation of a black widow spider bite is typically diagnostic.
- Bites from less toxic species are difficult to differentiate from furuncles and other insect bites.
- Patients may have seen the spider or may bring in a dead spider, and the diagnosis can then be established.
- Although spider bites are probably overdiagnosed, a painful bite with two puncture wounds, or an older lesion with an elongated necrotic center, suggests the diagnosis.

Treatment

- Black and brown widow spider bites are best treated in an emergency room with antivenom. Adjunctive treatments include calcium gluconate for hypocalcemia, benzodiazepines, and opioids.
- Brown recluse spider bites may require surgical intervention. To date, no well-controlled human studies have shown dapsone to affect the clinical outcome of a brown recluse spider bite.
- For minor spider bites, the site can be cleaned and treated with cool compresses and pain medication.
- For all spider bites, a tetanus booster may be prudent, and the site should be monitored for signs of infection (Fig. 26.22).

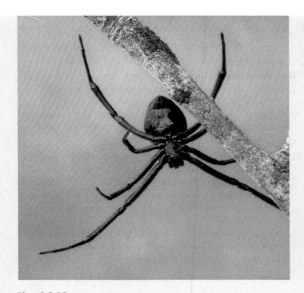

Fig. 26.19. The infamous female black widow spider demonstrating the characteristic red hourglass on the ventral surface. (From https://www.stockfreeimages .com/4421414.)

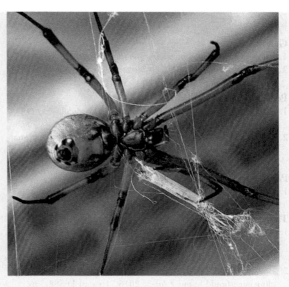

Fig. 26.20. The lesser known female brown widow spider that is primarily found in the southeastern United States and California. This one was photographed in Alabama.

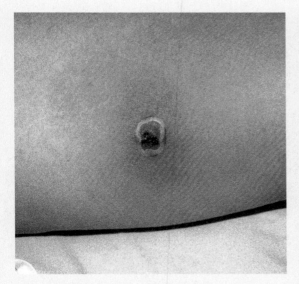

Fig. 26.21. Patient with painful necrotic irregular bite site surrounded by marked erythema and induration. Based on the description of the spider, this may have been due to a sac spider. (From the Fitzsimons Army Medical Center Collection, Aurora, CO.)

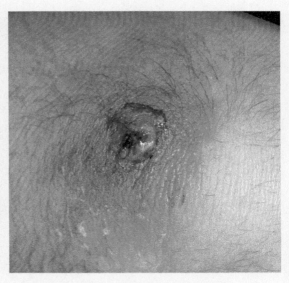

Fig. 26.22. Patient with presumed spider bite with secondary staphylococcal infection. In the absence of a spider or good description, this type of lesion is hard to differentiate from a furuncle. (From the Fitzsimons Army Medical Center Collection, Aurora, CO.)

References

General

1. Juckett G. Arthropod bites. *Am Fam Physician*. 2013;88:841-847.
2. Steen CJ, Carbonaro PA, Schwartz RA. Arthropods in dermatology. *J Am Acad Dermatol*. 2004;50:819-842.

Pediculosis Capitis (Head Lice)

1. Elston DM. Drugs used in the treatment of pediculosis. *J Drugs Dermatol*. 2005;4:207-211.
2. Mumcuoglu KY, Barker SC, Burgess IG, et al. International guidelines for effective control of head louse infestations. *J Drugs Dermatol*. 2007;6:409-414.

Pediculosis Pubis (Crab Lice)

1. Galiczynski EM Jr, Elston DM. What's eating you? Pubic lice *(Pthirus pubis)*. *Cutis*. 2008;81:109-114.

Tick Bites

1. Akin Belli A, Dervis E, Kar S, et al. Revisiting detachment techniques in human-biting ticks. *J Am Acad Dermatol*. 2016;75:393-397.
2. Buckingham SC. Tick-borne diseases of the USA: ten things clinicians should know. *J Infect*. 2015;71(suppl 1):S88-S96.

3. Ogden NH, Lindsay LR, Schofield SW. Methods to prevent tick bites and Lyme disease. *Clin Lab Med*. 2015;35:883-899.

Bee, Wasp, and Yellowjacket Stings

1. Bacelieri RE, Elston DM. What's eating you? Vespids. *Cutis*. 2004;73:157-160.
2. Lewis FS, Smith LJ. What's eating you? Bees, part 1: characteristics, reactions, and management. *Cutis*. 2007;79:439-444.

Spider Bites

1. Elston DM. What's eating you? Tarantulas (Theraphosidae). *Cutis*. 2002;70:182-183.
2. Monte AA, Bucher-Bartelson B, Heard KJ. A US perspective of symptomatic *Latrodectus* spp. envenomation and treatment: a National Poison Data System review. *Ann Pharmacother*. 2011;45:1491-1498.
3. Prongay R, Kelsberg G, Safranek S. Clinical inquiry: which treatments relieve painful muscle spasms from a black widow spider bite? *J Fam Pract*. 2012;61:694-695.

Chapter 27
Discolorations of the Skin

Discolorations of the skin include disorders of hypopigmentation (lightening), disorders of hyperpigmentation (darkening), and disorders caused by abnormal deposition of any pigment that alters skin color. The abnormal pigmentation can be endogenous (e.g., iron in hemochromatosis) or exogenous (e.g., a medication, such as minocycline) in origin.

Selected Causes of Skin Discoloration

Depigmentation
- Albinism
- Piebaldism
- Vitiligo

Hypopigmentation
- Nevus depigmentosus
- Pityriasis alba
- Postinflammatory hypopigmentation
- Tinea versicolor

Hyperpigmentation
- Acanthosis nigricans
- Addison disease
- Confluent and reticulated papillomatosis
- Melasma (chloasma)
- Postinflammatory hyperpigmentation
- Tinea versicolor

Yellow Discoloration
- Carotenoderma
- Jaundice
- Quinacrine

Blue-Gray Discoloration
- Amiodarone
- Argyria (silver)
- Chloroquine
- Chlorpromazine
- Hydroxychloroquine
- Minocycline

IMPORTANT HISTORY QUESTIONS

How long has the abnormal color been present?

Some discolorations are congenital (e.g., albinism, nevus depigmentosus), but most are acquired (e.g., vitiligo).

How are you treating this discoloration?

Many patients use over-the-counter (OTC) or prescription remedies that may alter the clinical appearance.

Is the color change stable, progressive, or resolving?

Some disorders, such as pityriasis alba on the face of a young child, are waxing and waning. Other conditions, such as albinism, are largely stable. Still yet, other conditions are progressive. For example, dyspigmentation from minocycline worsens until discontinuation.

Do you have photos of the affected area, taken at an earlier time, when the pigmentation was not present?

Although not always the case, sometimes discoloration may be better appreciated with a prior frame of reference.

What medications are you taking?

Numerous drugs can alter skin color, with some common drugs listed in the box.

IMPORTANT PHYSICAL FINDINGS

What is the color of the abnormal skin?

This is a critical physical finding because it will determine what questions regarding the history will be necessary.

What is the distribution of the color change?

Some discoloration is unilateral (e.g., segmental vitiligo) or localized to certain areas (e.g., pityriasis alba affects the face), whereas other conditions are generalized (e.g., jaundice, albinism).

Is the change in pigmentation sharply demarcated?

Some forms of dyspigmentation or depigmentation (e.g., vitiligo) have sharp demarcation, whereas other forms (e.g., postinflammatory hypopigmentation) are more poorly demarcated.

If it is not clear whether something is hypopigmented or depigmented, use your Wood light.

Use of a Wood lamp is discussed in more detail in Chapter 2. In general, disorders with true depigmentation (e.g., vitiligo, piebaldism) accentuate greatly with use of a Wood lamp, whereas disorders of lesser hypopigmentation (e.g., postinflammatory hypopigmentation) accentuate to a lesser degree.

Vitiligo   ICD10 code L80

Pathogenesis

Vitiligo is an autoimmune disease characterized by the destruction of melanocytes that produce melanin pigmentation for the skin. It is widely thought that vitiligo is an autoimmune disease, but other mechanisms of melanocyte death have been postulated by some authors. There is likely also a hereditary component because 8% of adults with vitiligo have similarly affected family members. Vitiligo is relatively common, with about 1% to 2% of the population affected. The condition is more noticeable in those with darker skin. The condition is associated with autoimmune disorders of other tissues and organ systems, such as Graves disease, Addison disease, Hashimoto thyroiditis, and alopecia areata.

Clinical Features

- Vitiligo can present at any age, but most cases of vitiligo occur before 20 years of age.
- Early lesions of vitiligo may demonstrate a faint rim of erythema or an eczematous border (Fig. 27.1).
- The primary lesion is a depigmented macule, with a sharply demarcated border that may be scalloped.
- Lesions may be symmetric (Fig. 27.2), focal, linear (Fig. 27.3), or generalized (e.g., vitiligo universalis).
- Vitiligo can involve mucosal surfaces, such as the lips or genitalia (Fig. 27.4).

Diagnosis

- The clinical presentation of macular depigmentation in characteristic anatomic locations is usually diagnostic.
- Wood lamp examination is useful because it accentuates true depigmentation and thereby distinguishes vitiligo from other conditions of hypopigmentation, with lesser accentuation.
- Early lesions may require a biopsy. It is useful to take 3-mm or larger punch biopsies from lesional and normal skin so that the dermatopathologist can compare the pigment (this often requires a special stain for melanin) and judge melanocyte density (this requires an immunohistochemical stain for

melanocytes) between affected and unaffected sites.

Treatment

- Vitiligo is a chronic disease that is not typically managed in an acute care environment. Any response to therapy is slow and incomplete.
- Initial care recommendations in an acute setting may include sunscreen use to protect the area from sunburn and to diminish differences between the adjacent tanned skin and depigmented skin, a medium-potency topical corticosteroid (0.1% triamcinolone) for affected areas of the trunk and extremities, or 0.1% hydrocortisone valerate for facial lesions.
- The patient should be referred to a dermatologist who may continue topical therapy (perhaps with alterations in corticosteroid strength), or who may employ ultraviolet (UV) light therapy. Psoralen plus UVA or narrow-band UVB therapy may be initiated. In one randomized, double-blind study, it was found that narrow-band UVB therapy is superior to PUVA therapy, but there are certain cases that do not respond well to any modality.
- Topical tacrolimus (0.03%–0.1% ointment bid) is an alternative to topical corticosteroid therapy.
- Topical pimecrolimus (1% cream bid) for at least 3 months is also an alternative to topical corticosteroids.
- Rare cases are treated surgically (e.g., melanocyte transplantation), but this is the domain of the specialist.

Clinical Course

Vitiligo cannot be cured. Many patients continue to develop new lesions of vitiligo over their lifetime. In general, about 70% of patients with vitiligo improve with therapy. A systematic review of the literature, combined with the results of patient questionnaires, suggested that topical corticosteroids are the best therapy for localized disease, and that narrow-band UVB is the best therapy for generalized disease.

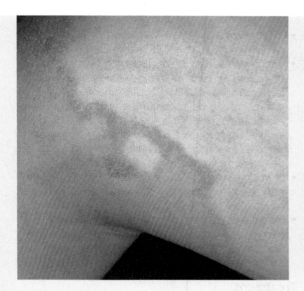

Fig. 27.1. Patient with early vitiligo demonstrating erythema and scale at the advancing edge. This degree of inflammation is unusual. (From the Joanna Burch Collection, Aurora, CO.)

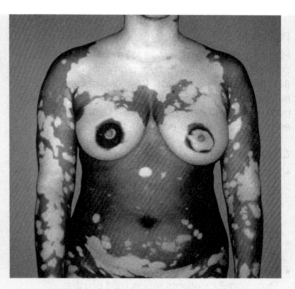

Fig. 27.2. Patient with severe vitiligo demonstrating the tendency for a symmetric distribution. (From the Walter Reed Army Medical Center Collection, Washington, DC.)

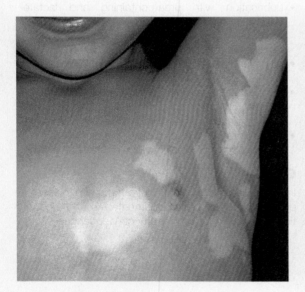

Fig. 27.3. Segmental vitiligo in a young child affecting the lateral thorax and arm.

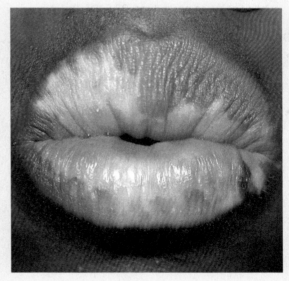

Fig. 27.4. Patient with vitiligo of the mucosal surfaces of the lip demonstrating a sharp demarcation between depigmented areas and normal skin.

Pathogenesis

Pityriasis alba is a low-grade form of eczema that presents, by definition, as hypopigmentation. Although the pathogenesis is not fully understood, studies suggest it is a variant of atopic dermatitis. Photoexposure accentuates the condition because light preferentially tans normal adjacent skin.

Clinical Features

- Pityriasis alba usually affects children between the ages of 6 and 12 years of age. In most series, 90% of patients are within this age range. Less often, the condition affects younger children or older adolescents.
- Pityriasis alba is more noticeable in children with darker skin.
- The condition is asymptomatic in most cases. Occasionally, patients report mild pruritus.
- The face, especially the cheeks, is most often affected. Less often, it affects the upper extremities.
- Early lesions consist of round to oval areas of subtle erythema, with variable fine white scale.
- Mature lesions demonstrate ill-defined patchy hypopigmentation with round to oval areas, with a subtle fine white scale (Figs. 27.5–27.7).

Diagnosis

- The clinical presentation is diagnostic in most cases. A history of atopic dermatitis or an atopic diathesis (see Fig. 27.6) in the patient or in family members supports the diagnosis.
- The differential diagnosis includes tinea versicolor, early vitiligo, postinflammatory hypopigmentation, and nevus depigmentosus. Hypopigmented mycosis fungoides is also in the differential diagnosis, but this is an extremely rare condition (less than one case per 4 million persons per year). Moreover, it is unusual for hypopigmented mycosis fungoides to occur exclusively on the face.

- Tinea versicolor may be excluded by performing a potassium hydroxide (KOH) examination.
- Vitiligo can usually be excluded on clinical grounds because it results in depigmented skin, whereas pityriasis alba results in hypopigmented skin. This difference can be accentuated with a Wood lamp examination (see Chapter 2). Also, the primary lesions of vitiligo are usually sharply demarcated, whereas pityriasis alba manifests a gradual transition to normal skin at the edges of lesions.
- Nevus depigmentosus can usually be excluded because it is solitary, sharply demarcated, and lacks any scale.
- Rare cases may require a 3-mm punch biopsy. Histologic examination usually demonstrates a low-grade spongiotic dermatitis with variable scale that is consistent with pityriasis alba.

Treatment

- The condition is benign and self-limited, and reassurance alone is a reasonable option.
- Broad-spectrum sunscreens lessen visible differences between the hypopigmented macules and adjacent tanned skin.
- Lubrication with urea-containing and lactate-containing moisturizers is an often employed treatment, but it typically takes weeks to months of use to observe a response.
- All patients should be switched to a mild facial soap, such as Dove, Cetaphil, or Aveeno.
- A low-potency topical corticosteroid, such as 1% hydrocortisone cream or 0.05% desonide cream may be beneficial in some cases.
- Topical tretinoin and topical pimecrolimus have been reported to be efficacious but are more costly.

Clinical Course

Individual lesions typically last from months to years—up to 7 years has been documented—but the condition is benign and without any consequences.

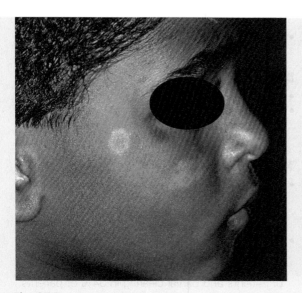

Fig. 27.5. Pityriasis alba demonstrating hypopigmented macules on the face. (From the Joanna Burch Collection, Aurora, CO.)

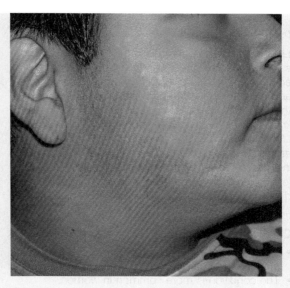

Fig. 27.6. Pityriasis alba on fair skin is usually more subtle. This patient also has background erythema from his atopic dermatitis.

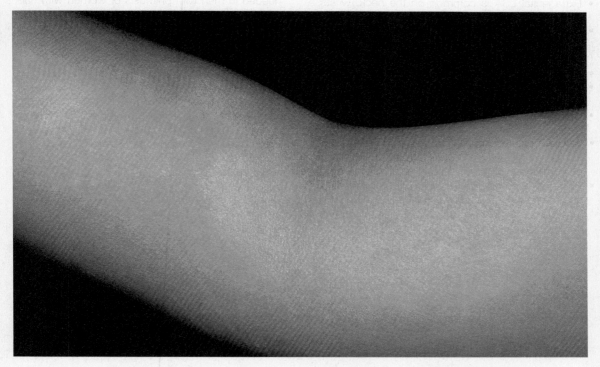

Fig. 27.7. Patient with pityriasis alba of the arms. This is often confused with hypopigmented tinea versicolor.

Lichen Sclerosus et Atrophicus ICD10 code L90.0 (nongenital)

Pathogenesis

Lichen sclerosus et atrophicus (LSA) or, simply, lichen sclerosus, is a disorder characterized by an atrophic epidermis, altered collagen in the superficial dermis, and an overlying white or white-blue appearance to the skin. The terms *balanitis xerotica obliterans* and *kraurosis vulvae* have been applied to genital lesions of LSA in men and women, respectively. The pathogenesis of LSA is poorly understood, but the increased incidence of LSA with other autoimmune diseases (e.g., morphea) and the presence of autoantibodies directed against extracellular matrix protein 1 suggest LSA is an autoimmune disorder.

Clinical Features

- LSA may present at any age, from pediatric to geriatric age groups.
- The condition is more common in women.
- The anogenital region alone is affected in about 50% of cases, anogenital and extragenital disease is present in about 25% of cases, and only extragenital areas are affected in about 25% of cases.
- Extragenital LSA is common on the neck, wrists, and inframammary areas.
- Anogenital LSA in girls and women often demonstrates an hourglass-like or figure-eight configuration that surrounds the genitalia and anal region.
- Early LSA may be pruritic or asymptomatic.
- Primary lesions quickly evolve into white atrophic areas (Fig. 27.8), with variable telangiectasias.
- Some cases demonstrate surrounding brown hyperpigmentation.
- Variable features include hyperkeratosis and follicular plugging, fissures, blister formation (Fig. 27.9), hemorrhage (Fig. 27.10), and ulceration.
- Phimosis is a complication in uncircumcised men, and urethral stricture may also occur.

- Squamous cell carcinoma is a rare complication with chronic genital LSA.

Diagnosis

- The clinical presentation is usually diagnostic.
- A deep shave biopsy or punch biopsy (preferred) is useful in established lesions. Sampling early disease, with erythema alone, may not be diagnostic.

Treatment

- Potent topical corticosteroids, such as clobetasol, 0.5% ointment (applied qd or bid), is generally used initially, followed by a taper to less potent steroids as the condition improves.
- In a study of 85 pediatric and adult patients with LSA, topical tacrolimus, 0.1% ointment (applied bid for 16 weeks), produced complete clearing in 43% of patients and partial clearing in 34% of patients. This drug is an alternative for patients who do not wish to use topical corticosteroids. Tacrolimus does cause a burning feeling in about 20% of users.
- Surgical intervention and/or dilation are sometimes needed in men with phimosis or women with narrowing of the vaginal introitus.
- Systemic immunosuppression may be used in those with severe or recalcitrant LSA, but this is the domain of experts.

Clinical Course

In children, long-term follow-up data are limited. In the most insightful studies, about 50% of children had complete clearing by puberty, with the other 50% having disease that was better, stable, or worse. In adults, the disease is usually chronic, and the condition is sometimes progressive.

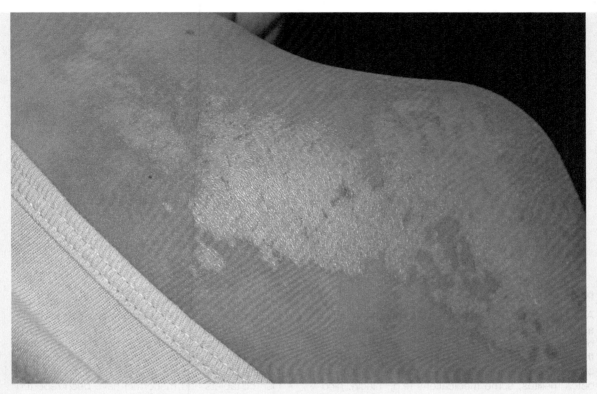

Fig. 27.8. Patient with classic truncal lichen sclerosus et atrophicus demonstrating an atrophic wrinkled epidermis, with a white color.

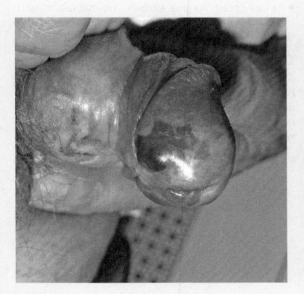

Fig. 27.9. Patient with lichen sclerosus et atrophicus of the penis demonstrating a hemorrhagic blister and white atrophic skin. (From the Fitzsimons Army Medical Center Collection, Aurora, CO.)

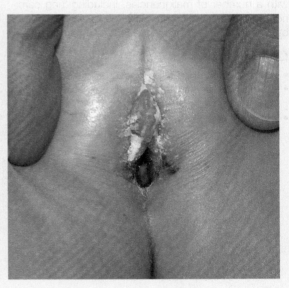

Fig. 27.10. Lichen sclerosus et atrophicus in a young girl demonstrating white atrophic skin and focal hemorrhage.

Acanthosis Nigricans ICD10 code L83

Selected Causes of Acanthosis Nigricans
- Obesity (most common)
- Malignancy
  - Adenocarcinoma of the gastrointestinal (GI) tract
- Endocrine disorders
  - Acromegaly
  - Cushing syndrome
  - Diabetes mellitus
  - Stein-Leventhal syndrome
- Drug-induced
  - Corticosteroids
  - Niacin
  - Nicotinamide
- Syndrome-associated
  - Bloom syndrome
  - Rud syndrome

Pathogenesis

Although acanthosis nigricans (AN) may seem to be a pigmentary disorder, because the skin appears brown, it is actually caused by subtle thickening of the stratum corneum with papillomatous hyperplasia of the epidermis. AN is associated with obesity, diabetes mellitus, some medications (e.g., niacin, nicotinamide), malignancy (as a paraneoplastic condition), and a number of rare genetic syndromes. Paraneoplastic (or malignant) AN can be seen in association with a number of malignancies, including lung carcinoma, breast carcinoma, and testicular carcinoma, but most cases are associated with GI carcinomas.

Clinical Features

- AN most often occurs in obese children.
- AN usually affects the skin of the axillae, neck, and other body folds (Figs. 27.11 and 27.12).
- AN may affect the dorsal hands and feet (acral acanthotic anomaly) and areola (Fig. 27.13).

- Mucosal involvement is seen only in paraneoplastic forms of AN.
- Affected skin appears velvety and hyperpigmented.
- Patients may complain that the affected skin appears dirty, even despite vigorous cleansing.
- AN may be associated with numerous acrochordons (see Fig. 27.12).

Diagnosis

- The clinical presentation, appearance, and associated conditions are usually diagnostic of AN.
- Rare cases may require a shave biopsy or 3- or 4-mm punch biopsy (preferred).

Treatment

- Treatment of the underlying condition is the best management. For example, in cases associated with obesity, the attainment of an ideal body weight may result in complete resolution.
- Topical 12% ammonium lactate lotion, available OTC and by prescription, may make the condition less noticeable.
- Topical tretinoin cream and glycolic acid lotion, both applied qd, are other options; some patients may tolerate use bid.
- Fish oil tablets and metformin have been reported to be of benefit in the literature, but this evidence is largely anecdotal and has not been subjected to vigorous trials.
- In rare cases, surgical excision, dermabrasion, and electrofulguration have been used, although the latter modality produces variable scarring.

Clinical Course

Acanthosis nigricans is typically a chronic condition, but if the driving force(s) can be removed or substantially improved (e.g., obesity, diabetes), AN will often resolve and/or substantially improve, typically over weeks to months.

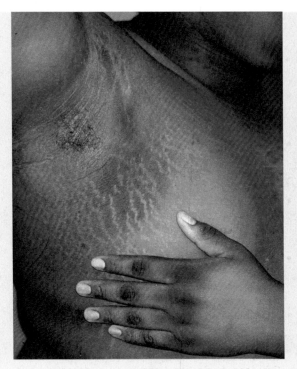

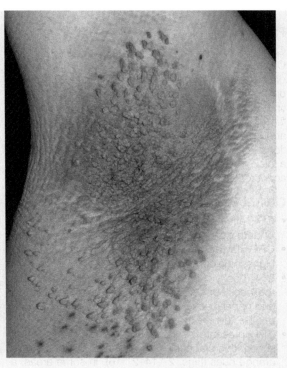

Fig. 27.11. Patient with acanthosis nigricans of the neck, axillae, and dorsum of the hands.

Fig. 27.12. Patient with acanthosis nigricans of the axilla, with numerous acrochordons.

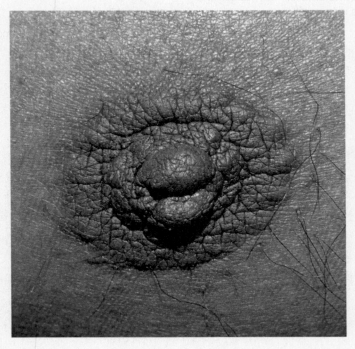

Fig. 27.13. Close-up of a patient with acanthosis nigricans of the nipple and areola that clearly demonstrates the papillomatous nature of this condition. (From the Fitzsimons Army Medical Center Collection, Aurora, CO.)

Pathogenesis

Confluent and reticulated papillomatosis of Gougerot-Carteaud (CRP) is an uncommon disorder with a distinctive clinical appearance. The cause of CRP is unknown, but it is thought to be a disorder of keratinization, perhaps precipitated by yeast (*Malassezia furfur*), bacteria (*Dietzia papillomatosis*), endocrine abnormalities (insulin resistance), or functional mutations in keratin 16. Histologically, CRP demonstrates a thickened stratum corneum (hyperkeratosis), with an acanthotic and elongated epidermal rete.

Clinical Features

- CRP affects chiefly adolescents and young adults of both genders (mean age, 15 years).
- CRP may affect any racial or ethnic group, with the highest incidence in whites.
- CRP has a characteristic distribution that includes the neck, upper trunk, and axillae. The midchest and upper back are also often involved. Few cases of CRP involve the face or extremities.
- CRP presents as tan to brown hyperpigmented, subtle, thin plaques, with varied yellow, light red, or orange hues (Figs. 27.14–27.16). In some areas, a reticulated pattern may become confluent. Close examination of lesions demonstrates subtle scale (see Fig. 27.16B).
- CRP is usually asymptomatic, but occasional patients report some mild pruritus.

Diagnosis

- In most situations, the diagnosis may be established on clinical grounds, based upon the patient's age, the distribution, and the distinctive reticular pattern of scale and discoloration.
- The differential diagnosis includes an unusual presentation of tinea versicolor (pityriasis versicolor), which is also characterized by tan, slightly scaly macules and plaques. However, a KOH examination will be positive in tinea versicolor and can help to distinguish between the two conditions.
- Rare cases may require a shave or punch biopsy to substantiate the diagnosis.

Treatment

- CRP is a condition without serious consequences, and reassurance alone is reasonable if the patient is unconcerned. Many patients desire treatment because of the cosmetic appearance of the rash.
- Controlled studies in CRP are lacking, but oral antibiotics, such as minocycline (50–100 mg PO bid for 6 weeks), are often used. Azithromycin and clarithromycin represent alternative agents.
- Topical tretinoin and salicylic acid–containing products desquamate the skin. Ammonium or sodium lactate–containing moisturizers may be used for the same reason.
- Oral isotretinoin has been used successfully, but with its serious side effects and teratogenic consequences, it is not often used for CRP unless there is also severe acne.

Clinical Course

Untreated, CRP typically last months or even years before spontaneous resolution.

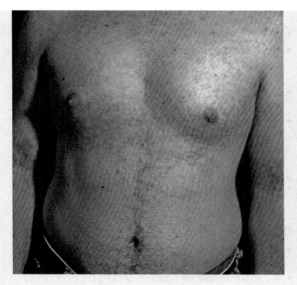

Fig. 27.14. Patient with confluent and reticulated papillomatosis of Gougerot-Carteaud, with light reddish-brown reticulated lesions. (From the Fitzsimons Army Medical Center Collection, Aurora, CO.)

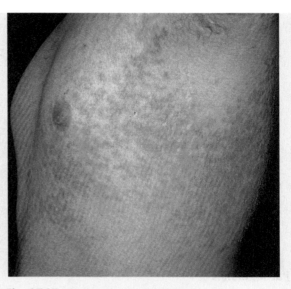

Fig. 27.15. Patient with confluent and reticulated papillomatosis of Gougerot-Carteaud, with yellowish-brown reticulated lesions of the thorax. (From the Fitzsimons Army Medical Center Collection, Aurora, CO.)

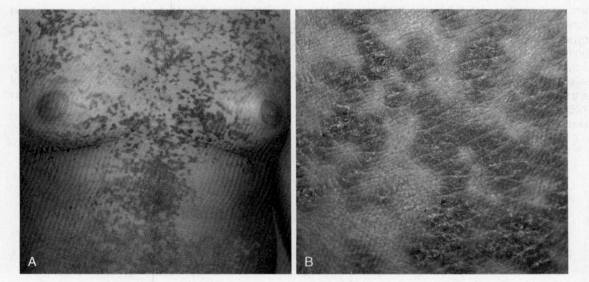

Fig. 27.16. A, Dramatic confluent and reticulated papillomatosis of Gougerot-Carteaud, with dark brown reticulated lesions on an adolescent. B, Closer view demonstrates that the pigment is due to subtle papillomatous hyperplasia.

Mechanisms for Addison Disease

- Destruction of adrenal glands
  - Autoimmune
  - Deposition disorders (e.g., amyloidosis)
  - Hemorrhage, infarction (e.g., Waterhouse-Friderichsen syndrome, antiphospholipid syndrome)
  - Infections (e.g., tuberculosis)
  - Metastatic disease in the gland
- Adrenal dysgenesis
  - Rare genetic syndromes
- Impaired steroid production
  - Genetic enzymatic deficiencies
  - Medications (e.g., azoles, rifampin, phenytoin)

Pathogenesis

Addison disease, or adrenal insufficiency, is an endocrine disorder caused by insufficient production of steroid hormones by the adrenal cortex. The condition is divided into primary adrenal insufficiency (destruction or impairment of the adrenal cortex), secondary adrenal insufficiency (reduced secretion of adrenocorticotropic hormone [ACTH] by the pituitary), and tertiary adrenal insufficiency (reduction in the area of the hypothalamus that produces corticotropin-releasing hormone). Hyperpigmentation of the skin occurs only in primary adrenal insufficiency, due to elevated levels of ACTH or related peptide fragments, which are closely related to melanocyte-stimulating hormone (MSH). The result is overproduction of melanin in the skin.

Clinical Features

- Addison disease may affect persons of any age, but the condition is most common in middle-aged women.
- Manifestations include diffuse hyperpigmentation that is not photodistributed (Fig. 27.17).
- Hyperpigmentation is accentuated in the palmar creases (Fig. 27.18A), on the gingiva (see Fig. 27.18B) and buccal mucosa, on the areola, and at sites of friction, including trauma and scars.
- Systemic symptoms include fatigue, muscle weakness, fever, weight loss, anxiety, nausea, diarrhea, and headache.

Diagnosis

- Diffuse progressive hyperpigmentation should raise concern for primary Addison disease.
- A careful review of systems should be performed.
- For confirmation, ACTH and cortisol levels should be determined.

Treatment

- Patients should be referred to an endocrinologist for appropriate studies and management.
- Corticosteroid replacement must be commenced under the guidance of the endocrinologist.

Clinical Course

With proper management and replacement therapy, most patients with adrenal insufficiency have a normal life span. With replacement therapy, skin pigmentation will return to normal.

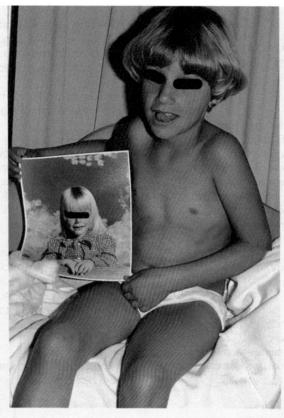

Fig. 27.17. Young child who presented with unexplained diffuse darkening of her skin. Compare her skin color to the skin color in a photograph taken several years earlier. (From the Fitzsimons Army Medical Center Collection, Aurora, CO.)

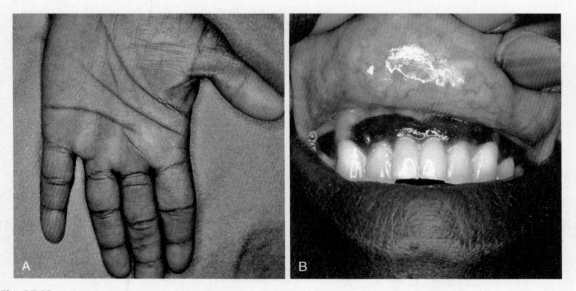

Fig. 27.18. A, Patient with hyperpigmentation of the palmar creases. B, Marked hyperpigmentation of the gingiva in the same patient.

Jaundice

Origins

The word *jaundice* is derived from the word *jaune*, a French word that means "yellow."

Pathogenesis

Jaundice is a systemic disorder caused by elevated levels of bilirubin in the blood. Bilirubin is a breakdown product of red blood cells that is normally removed by the liver. Bilirubin can occur in conjugated and unconjugated forms. There are many causes of jaundice, but hepatocellular injury and biliary obstruction are the two most common causes. Hyperbilirubinemia precedes the development of clinical jaundice by several days. Adults demonstrate clinically detectable jaundice when bilirubin levels reach 2.5 to 3 mg/dL; infants may require levels as high as 6 to 8 mg/dL to produce appreciable jaundice.

Clinical Features

- Jaundice may affect persons of any age, from infants to geriatric populations.
- The entire mucocutaneous surface is affected, but the soft palate and sublingual areas are the sites where jaundice can first be appreciated.

- The skin discoloration varies from yellow to yellow-green in hue (Figs. 27.19–27.22).
- In contrast to carotenoderma, the scleral conjunctiva is affected in jaundice (scleral icterus; see Figs. 27.20–27.22).
- Patients frequently complain of pruritus, and the urine may be darker than normal.

Diagnosis

- The occurrence of yellow to yellow-green discoloration of the skin with scleral icterus is diagnostic.
- Liver function testing, serum bilirubin levels, and a complete blood count (CBC) are initial studies that should be performed in all cases.

Treatment

- Treatment of the primary disorder producing the elevated levels of bilirubin is key.
- There is no specific treatment of jaundice, with the exception of neonatal jaundice, for which ultraviolet light therapy is used to prevent irreversible brain damage.

Clinical Course

After the bilirubin levels are normalized, tissue-bound bilirubin dissipates over several days to a week.

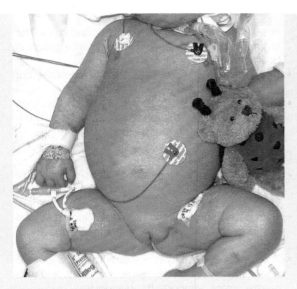

Fig. 27.19. Patient with modest jaundice secondary to drug-induced hepatitis (DRESS syndrome). Note the associated macular erythema due to the drug eruption.

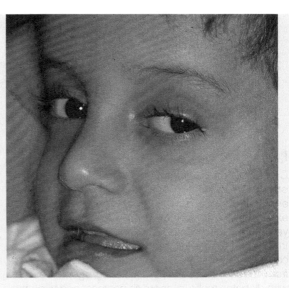

Fig. 27.20. Patient with modest jaundice and scleral icterus due to Alagille syndrome, a rare liver disorder. (From the William Weston Collection, Aurora, CO.)

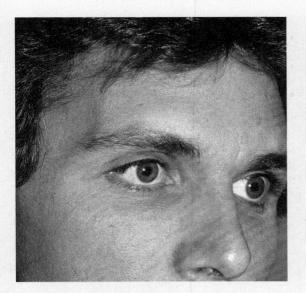

Fig. 27.21. Patient with jaundice, with yellow-green discoloration of skin and marked scleral icterus.

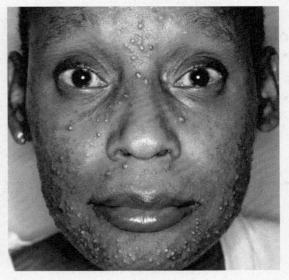

Fig. 27.22. Patient with jaundice and marked scleral icterus due to primary biliary cirrhosis. The papules are eruptive xanthoma. (From the Fitzsimons Army Medical Center Collection, Aurora, CO.)

Carotenoderma ICD10 code L81.9

Origins

Carotenoids are found in the stratum corneum of normal skin and contribute to normal skin color and UV protection.

So-called tanning pills can contain canthaxanthin, a carotenoid, which, if consumed in large quantities, produces an orange-brown color in the skin.

Pathogenesis

Carotenoderma is the cutaneous manifestation of carotenemia, which is in turn caused by excess carotenoids in the blood. This usually occurs because of excess intake of carrots, but excess intake of other yellow vegetables (e.g., sweet potatoes) and yellow fruits (e.g., mangoes, cantaloupe, apricots) can also cause the condition. Carotene can also be acquired from foods that use it as a coloring agent. Patients with diabetes mellitus, anorexia nervosa, and hypothyroidism are prone to this disorder because of abnormal metabolism of carotenoids. Patients with renal dysfunction can develop this condition due to diminished excretion. A similar disorder is associated with excess intake of lycopene, another carotenoid, found in high amounts in tomatoes.

Clinical Features

- Carotenoderma may affect persons of any age, from infants to geriatric populations, but it is usually found in children and in vegetarians.
- Diffuse yellow (Fig. 27.23) or yellow-orange pigmentation (Fig. 27.24) of the skin occurs. The color change may be subtle and is best appreciated in comparison to normal skin (see Fig. 27.24). In patients with high lycopene intake, a deeper orange hue can be appreciated.
- The discoloration is most obvious in areas with higher concentrations of sweat glands and a thick stratum corneum, such as the palms and soles. The tip of the nose, forehead, chin, nasolabial fold, and behind the ears are also often affected.
- Discoloration may rarely affect the hard palate, but the sclera are spared.
- Patients lack the systemic symptoms and findings of liver disease and jaundice—notably fever, pruritus, nausea, vomiting, and stool color changes.

Diagnosis

- A dietary history is important to identify sources of excess carotenoid intake. Most patients can quickly identify the source once the condition is explained.
- Rare patients with eating disorders, such as those with anorexia nervosa, may evade questions about diet.
- The clinical presentation of yellow to yellow-orange skin, accentuated on the palms and soles, and with normal sclera, supports the diagnosis.
- The diagnosis can be confirmed with laboratory testing, including liver function testing and determination of beta-carotene levels.
- Skin biopsies are of no value.

Treatment

- Carotenoderma is a benign condition that does not require treatment.
- For patients with cosmetic concerns, excess carotenoid intake must be reduced.
- High beta-carotene levels will not result in hypervitaminosis A because the body acts to reduce the conversion of beta-carotene to vitamin A.

Clinical Course

If excess carotenoid intake is moderated effectively, the skin will return to normal color in 1 to 3 months.

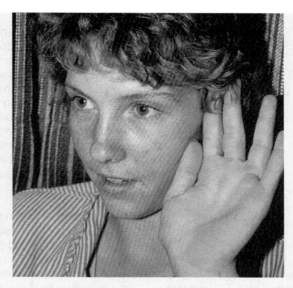

Fig. 27.23. Patient with carotenoderma due to a vegetarian diet that included large numbers of carrots and squash. Note the accentuation of the yellow color on the palms and normal sclera, both characteristic features of this condition. This patient was admitted from the emergency room to the hospital for so-called jaundice. (From the Fitzsimons Army Medical Center Collection, Aurora, CO.)

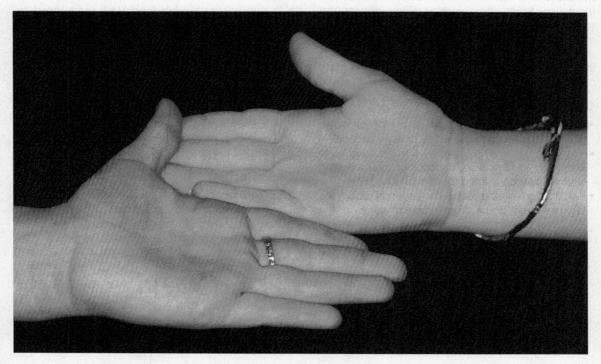

Fig. 27.24. Iatrogenic carotenoderma with a yellow-orange color in a patient with erythropoietic protoporphyria being treated with beta-carotene. Note the comparison to a normal palm.

Drug-Induced Blue-Gray Discoloration ICD10 code L81.9

Causes of Drug-Induced Blue-Gray Skin Discoloration
- Amiodarone
- Amodiaquine
- Argyria (silver)
- Chloroquine
- Chlorpromazine
- Chrysiasis (gold)
- Clofazimine
- Hydroxychloroquine
- Iron
- Minocycline

Pathogenesis

Numerous ingested drugs may produce a blue-gray discoloration of the skin (see box above). Some drugs produce this coloration via direct deposition in the skin (e.g., silver in argyria), some form complexes with other compounds (e.g., melanin-chloroquine complexes), and others stimulate endogenous pigmentation (e.g., lipofuscin in clofazimine-induced pigmentation). Some drugs, such as minocycline, appear to induce dyspigmentation by more than one mechanism. Common implicated drugs include antimalarial drugs and minocycline. The incidence of argyria has increased due to self-directed use of silver in many naturopathic remedies.

Clinical Features

- In most cases, patients have taken the offending medications for months, years, or even decades.
- The discoloration is variable, from slate-gray to blue-gray to dark blue, depending upon the drug and amount consumed (or deposited).
- Localization of the deposits depends upon the drug involved. Some drugs preferentially deposit in certain anatomic sites. Classic deposition patterns for some of the medications are as follows:

- Deposition in scars—minocycline (Fig. 27.25)
- Deposition in stasis dermatitis—minocycline (Fig. 27.26)
- Deposition on photoexposed skin—amiodarone (Fig. 27.27), chlorpromazine, gold (Fig. 27.28)
- Deposition in skin overlying bone—antimalarials
- Deposition over the hard palate—antimalarials
- Deposition in skin over the buttocks—iron (from an intramuscular injection)
- Deposition in the lunula of the nails—silver
- Deposition in the cartilage of the ear—minocycline

Diagnosis

- The diagnosis is contingent upon recognizing the abnormal blue-gray or slate-gray color is present.
- Prescriptions, past and present, must be carefully reviewed.
- Naturopathic medications must be scrutinized, as iron and silver can be present in these agents.
- If a cause cannot be established, a 3- or 4-mm punch biopsy from the darkest area should be performed. In some cases, the histologic findings are diagnostic, whereas in others it may simply be supportive.
- In rare cases, a specialized facility may need to perform electron microscopy or other advanced analytic techniques, but these technologies are expensive and difficult to employ.

Treatment

- Discontinuation of the offending medication is essential.
- In cases that are photoaccentuated, a broad-spectrum sunscreen, blocking UVA and UVB, may be useful.

Clinical Course

Even with discontinuance of the offending medication, it may take months or years for improvement or resolution of the dyspigmentation. Pigmentation caused by argyria (silver deposition) is often permanent.

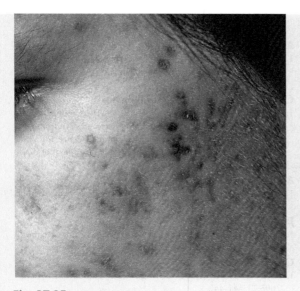

Fig. 27.25. Patient with minocycline-induced blue-gray discoloration in acne scars. (From the Fitzsimons Army Medical Center Collection, Aurora, CO.)

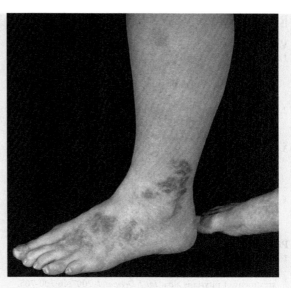

Fig. 27.26. Patient with minocycline-induced dyspigmentation in stasis dermatitis. (From the Fitzsimons Army Medical Center Collection, Aurora, CO.)

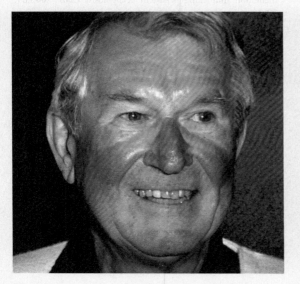

Fig. 27.27. Patient with photoaccentuated blue-gray discoloration from amiodarone. (From the Fitzsimons Army Medical Center Collection, Aurora, CO.)

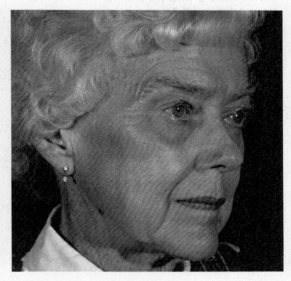

Fig. 27.28. Patient with subtle, photoaccentuated, slate-gray discoloration secondary to gold. (From the Fitzsimons Army Medical Center Collection, Aurora, CO.)

References

Vitiligo

1. Alikhan A, Felstein LM, Daly M, et al. Vitiligo: a comprehensive review. Part I. Introduction, epidemiology, quality of life, diagnosis, differential diagnosis, associations, histopathology, etiology, and work-up. *J Am Acad Dermatol.* 2011;65:473-491.
2. Felsten LM, Alikhan A, Petronic-Bosic V. Vitiligo: a comprehensive review. Part II: Treatment options and approach to treatment. *J Am Acad Dermatol.* 2011;65:493-514.
3. Mazereeuw-Hautier J, Bezio S, Mahe E. Segmental and non-segmental childhood vitiligo has distinct clinical characteristics: a retrospective observational study. *J Am Acad Dermatol.* 2010;62:945-949.
4. Yones SS, Der D, Palmer RA. Randomized double-blind trial of treatment of vitiligo. Efficacy of psoralen-UV-A vs narrowband-UV-B therapy. *Arch Dermatol.* 2007;143:578-584.

Pityriasis Alba

1. Fujita WH, McCormick CL, Parneix-Spake A. An exploratory study to evaluate the efficacy of pimecrolimus cream 1% for the treatment of pityriasis alba. *Int J Dermatol.* 2007;46:700-705.
2. Line RL, Janninger CK. Pityriasis alba. *Cutis.* 2005;76: 21-24.

Lichen Sclerosus et Atrophicus

1. Smith SD, Fischer G. Childhood onset vulvar lichen sclerosus does not resolve at puberty: a prospective case series. *Pediatr Dermatol.* 2009;26:725-729.

Acanthosis Nigricans

1. Brickman WJ, Binns HJ, Jovanovic BD, et al. Acanthosis nigricans: a common finding in overweight youth. *Pediatric Dermatol.* 2007;24:601-606.

Confluent and Reticulate Papillomatosis

1. Davis MDP, Weenig RH, Camilleri MJ. Confluent and reticulate papillomatosis (Gougerot-Carteaud syndrome: a minocycline-responsive dermatosis without evidence for yeast in pathogenesis. A study of 39 patients and a proposal of diagnostic criteria. *Br J Dermatol.* 2006;154:287-293.

Addison Disease

1. Kumar R, Kumari S, Ranabijudi PK. Generalized pigmentation in Addison disease. *Dermatol Online J.* 2008;14:13.

Jaundice

1. Haught JM, Patel S, English JC 3rd. Xanthoderma: a clinical review. *J Am Acad Dermatol.* 2007;57:1051-1058.

Carotenoderma

1. Arya V, Grzybowski J, Schwartz RA. Carotenemia. *Cutis.* 2003;71:441-442.

Drug-Induced Blue-Gray Discolorations

1. McKenna JK, Hull CM, Zone JJ. Argyria associated with colloidal silver supplementation. *Int J Dermatol.* 2003;42:549.
2. Youssef S, Langevin KK, Young LC. Minocycline-induced pigmentation mimicking persistent ecchymosis. *Cutis.* 2003;84: 22-26.

Chapter 28
Papillomatous and Verrucous Lesions

Key Terms

Verrucae Vulgaris
  Myrmecia
  Verrucae palmaris
  Verrucae plantaris
  Warts
Verrucae Plana
  Epidermodysplasia
    verruciformis
  Flat warts

Condyloma Acuminatum
  Anogenital warts
  Venereal warts
Seborrheic Keratosis
  Dermatosis papulosa nigra
  Inflamed seborrheic keratoses
  Melanoacanthoma
  Sign of Leser-Trélat
  Stucco keratosis

Acrochordon
  Fibroepithelial polyps
  Skin tags
  Soft fibromas
North American Blastomycosis
  Gilchrist disease
Verrucous Carcinoma
  Ackerman tumor
  Buschke-Löwenstein tumor
  Epithelioma cuniculatum

Papillomatous and verrucous lesions of the skin include viral infections (e.g., warts, molluscum), deep fungal infections (e.g., blastomycosis), and benign and malignant neoplasms. Papillomas are pedunculated or sessile, chiefly epidermal growths, often with a cauliflower-like appearance. Similarly, the term *verrucous,* as the name implies, suggests an exophytic lesion, like a wart, often with spirelike, outward projections of the epidermis. The linear presentation of papillomatous lesions has been addressed in Chapter 17.

Differential Diagnosis of Verrucous and Papillomatous Lesions

Common	Uncommon
• Acrochordons	• Deep fungal infections
• Condyloma acuminatum	• Epidermal nevus
• Dermatosis papulosa nigra	• Inflamed linear verrucous epidermal nevus
• Papillomatous intradermal nevi	• Verrucous carcinoma
• Seborrheic keratosis	• Verrucous incontinentia pigmenti
• Stucco keratosis	
• Verrucae plana	
• Verrucae vulgaris	

IMPORTANT HISTORY QUESTIONS

When did this lesion(s) develop?

The temporal course is important. Some lesions develop acutely (e.g., condylomata acuminata), whereas others are insidious, but can last for decades (e.g., acrochordons, seborrheic keratoses, verrucous carcinoma). Still yet, other conditions may be congenital in nature (e.g., epidermal nevus).

Has the lesion changed?

Many malignant tumors, such verrucous carcinoma, demonstrate relentless and progressive growth, whereas a benign lesion is more likely to remain stable.

Where have you visited or lived in the past few years?

Some infections, like verrucous cutaneous blastomycosis (see Fig. 28.20), are more common in certain geographic areas. Infections may also be acquired from travel to endemic areas.

IMPORTANT PHYSICAL FINDINGS

How many verrucous or papillomatous lesions are present?

Some verrucous and/or papillomatous processes are typically multiple (e.g., acrochordons, condylomata, dermatosis papulosa nigra, seborrheic/stucco keratosis), whereas others are most often solitary (e.g., epidermal nevus, verrucous carcinoma).

What is the distribution of the lesions?

Many verrucous and/or papillomatous processes have characteristic distributions. Acrochordons are often found on flexural surfaces, such as the neck, axilla, and inguinal folds. Condylomata acuminata (genital warts) are usually found in or near the genitalia. Dermatosis papulosa nigricans is found around the eyes and cheeks of persons of color. Verrucous carcinoma is usually found in the oral cavity (Ackerman tumor), anogenital area, or on the feet (epithelioma cuniculatum).

What is the arrangement of the lesions?

Some papillomas may be linear (e.g., epidermal nevus, verruca plana), whereas others are widely distributed.

What is the size of the lesions?

Some papillomas are usually small (e.g., acrochordons, stucco keratosis, verrucae plana), whereas others vary in size (e.g., seborrheic keratoses). Some may be usually large (e.g., epidermal nevus, verrucous carcinoma).

Verrucae Vulgaris ICD10 code B07.8

Pathogenesis

Verrucae (warts) are cutaneous and/or mucocutaneous infections of keratinocytes caused by human papillomavirus (HPV). There are more than 100 subtypes of HPV, with some subtypes affecting characteristic skin locations. In most cases, the infection follows direct inoculation of the skin by HPV, presumably through minor (imperceptible) skin breaks. In the United States, the lifetime risk of developing a clinically-relevant HPV infection has been estimated to be about 80%.

Clinical Features

- Verrucae can occur in any age group but are most common in young children.
- Verrucae can affect any cutaneous site and, occasionally, mucosal surfaces.
- Lesions present as skin-colored verrucous papules or plaques (Figs. 28.1 and 28.2), often with overlying scale, which can disrupt normal skin lines (dermatoglyphs). There may be black dots that represent thrombosed capillaries, and this phenomenon can be called "seed warts" by patients.
- Verrucae often occur on the hands (verrucae palmaris) or feet (verrucae plantaris; Fig. 28.3).
- Myrmecia (Greek for "ant") represent endophytic verrucae caused by HPV1 that occur upon the feet (common) or hands (less common). Myrmecia may be painful.
- Destructive modalities may spread a wart in peripheral fashion, causing a so-called "fairy ring" of lesions (Fig. 28.4). Still, these treatment modalities are widely used, and the risk is often tolerated.

Diagnosis

- The diagnosis is often based chiefly upon the clinical appearance of the lesion.
- It can be difficult to distinguish plantar warts from corns and callosities because both cause overlying scale. Lesions may be removed from this overlying keratin with a scalpel blade to examine the base.

Plantar warts demonstrate a loss of normal skin lines (dermatoglyphs), whereas corns and callosities retain such markings.
- Problematic cases can be sampled by a deep shave and submitted for histologic examination.

Treatment

- Over-the-counter treatments are usually based on topical salicylic acid, with or without other additives, such as lactic acid. The response rate is from 40% to 84% (average, 61%). Other topical therapies used include cantharidin (so-called "blister beetle juice"), imiquimod, tretinoin, and 5-fluorouracil.
- Liquid nitrogen (LN$_2$) cryotherapy is a destructive therapy often used by health care providers. In published studies, the cure rate of LN$_2$ is between 26% and 96%. Optimal results are achieved with treatment every 2 to 3 weeks. Plantar warts respond better if excess keratin is pared before LN2 treatment and if two freeze-thaw cycles are employed.
- Occlusion with duct tape was widely reported in the lay press a number of years ago. Medical evidence suggests the efficacy of duct tape is highly variable.
- Immunotherapy includes topical sensitization with diphencyprone or squaric acid dibutylester or the intralesional injection of Candida antigen.
- Systemic therapies for recalcitrant warts include oral cimetidine and oral retinoids. The efficacy of these modalities, particularly cimetidine, is dubious.
- Laser therapy is usually performed with a carbon dioxide laser or flashlamp pulsed dye laser. The first is an ablative laser, whereas the latter targets the increased blood supply that is present in verruca.
- Intralesional therapies include bleomycin, interferon, and formic acid, but these modalities are usually reserved for the most recalcitrant verruca.

Clinical Course

About 40% to 70% of verrucae resolve spontaneously, usually in about 2 years.

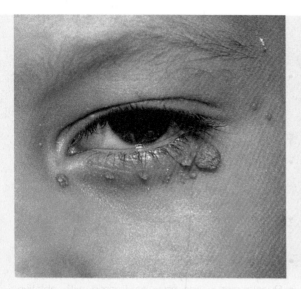

Fig. 28.1. Multiple periocular verrucae in a child, always a therapeutic challenge. (From the William Weston Collection, Aurora, CO.)

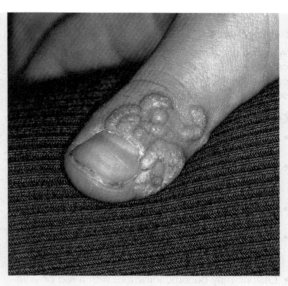

Fig. 28.2. Patient with multiple periungual warts. The periungual and subungual regions are particularly challenging to treat. (From the William Weston Collection, Aurora, CO.)

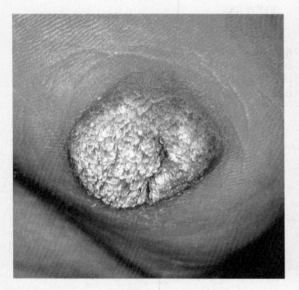

Fig. 28.3. Patient with plantar wart. (From the Fitzsimons Army Medical Center Collection, Aurora, CO.)

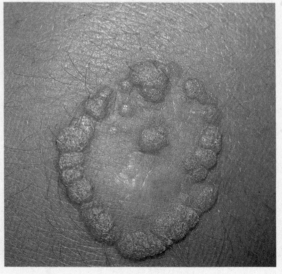

Fig. 28.4. Patient with the frustrating fairy ring wart that occurred after cryotherapy. The wart has recurred in the margins of the blister, plus the patient now also has a scar from the therapy.

Pathogenesis

Verrucae plana, also known as flat warts, are usually caused by HPV3. Because of differences in the clinical presentation and management, it is useful to discuss separately verrucae plana.

Clinical Features

- Verrucae plana are more common in children and young adults but can affect any age group.
- Verrucae plana usually occur on the face and dorsal hands but can also affect the trunk and lower extremities.
- Lesions are typically numerous and may number in the hundreds.
- The primary lesion is a skin-colored to tan to light brown small papilloma that rarely exceeds 3 mm in diameter (Figs. 28.5 and 28.6).
- Lesions may become inflamed, with a red or violaceous color (Fig. 28.7).
- Lesions may appear in a linear configuration due to autoinoculation (see Fig. 28.7).
- Variations include a so-called "intermediate wart," which has features of both a flat and common wart.
- Epidermodysplasia verruciformis (EV) is a genetic predisposition to extensive flat warts caused by HPV5, HPV8, HPV14, or HPV17. Lesions of EV may mimic other neoplasms or inflammatory conditions (Fig. 28.8). Lesions of EV have some oncogenic potential, and squamous cell carcinoma can arise in some cases.

Diagnosis

- In most cases, the occurrence of multiple, small, uniform skin-colored to brownish papillomas is diagnostic. In some cases, it may be difficult to distinguish verrucae plana from other papillomatous conditions, such as seborrheic keratosis.
- Problematic cases, including lesions in adults, truncal lesions, and inflamed lesions, should be biopsied to clarify the diagnosis. The findings are often specific (koilocytosis).

Treatment

- Verrucae plana can be difficult to treat, and if the lesions are few in number and are not bothersome, therapy is not required. Treating numerous lesions may be challenging.
- If treatment is desired, nonscarring modalities, such as topical tretinoin gel (0.025%–0.1% applied qd), is a reasonable option.
- Topical imiquimod cream (applied three times/week for up to 16 weeks) is also a reasonable choice.
- Recalcitrant cases may be treated with ablative lasers.
- Destructive modalities (e.g., LN_2, electrodessication) may be utilized but can cause scarring, and for this reason, such modalities are often avoided on the face.

Clinical Course

Most verrucae plana will resolve without treatment, usually over 2 to 3 years. EV often persists longer and also has the potential to eventuate into squamous cell carcinoma, on occasion.

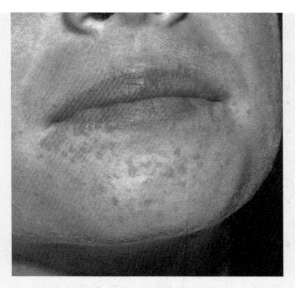

Fig. 28.5. Patient with numerous small tan papillomas in a perioral distribution of focal coalescence into a small plaque. (From the William Weston Collection, Aurora, CO.)

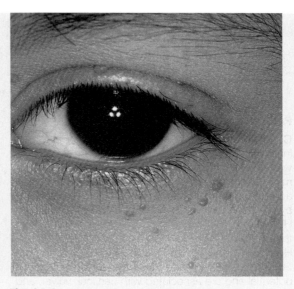

Fig. 28.6. Patient with numerous small tan, flat warts that are clinically difficult to distinguish from small seborrheic keratoses.

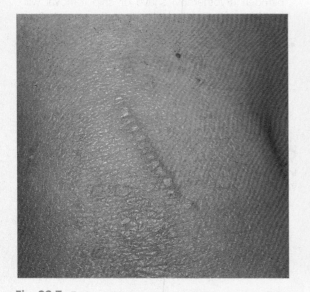

Fig. 28.7. Patient with verrucae plana with autoinoculation at a site of a superficial injury. These lesions are violaceous in color due to inflammation.

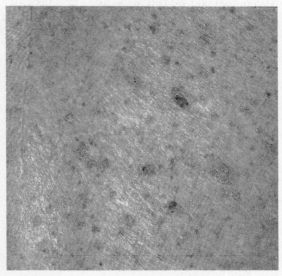

Fig. 28.8. Numerous inflamed red flat papillomas on the trunk in a patient with epidermodysplasia verruciformis.

Condylomata Acuminata and the Toilet Seat

Although it is difficult to disprove transmission of HPV via fomites, such as a toilet seat, there are no documented cases in which this has happened.

Pathogenesis

Condylomata acuminata (singular, condyloma acuminatum), also called anogenital warts or venereal warts, represent the most common sexually transmitted infection in the United States. Lesions may be acquired in utero, via ascension up the birth canal, or by the neonate, as it passes through the birth canal. HPV6 and HPV11 cause 90% of genital warts, and these strains have low oncogenic potential. Some HPV subtypes—16, 18, 31, 33, 35, 39, 45, 51, 52, 56, 58, 59, 68, 73, and 82—have a high oncogenic potential and are associated with cervical, vulvar, and penile carcinoma. Each year, in the United States, there are about 5 million new cases of genital warts.

Clinical Features

- Genital warts are most common in sexually active young men and women, especially those persons with multiple partners.
- In women, lesions occur most often on the labia majora, labia minora, and perianal area. Less often lesions occur on the skin of the clitoris, inguinal region, abdomen, and thighs.
- In men, lesions are usually found on the penis (glans, shaft, and urinary meatus) and perianal area, with lesions less often on the skin of the inguinal region, abdomen, or thighs.
- Genital warts range from skin-colored to tan to brown to black vegetations that may appear moist and usually have less scale than common warts (Figs. 28.9–28.12).
- The size of genital warts is also variable, with some lesions as small as 1 mm and other lesions 5 cm or more in size, resembling cauliflower. Large lesions are more common in immunocompromised patients.

Diagnosis

- The clinical presentation of genital warts is diagnostic in most cases.
- Some cases may require a shave biopsy and perhaps HPV subtyping to determine if an oncogenic strain is present.

Treatment

- The CDC maintains an updated website with recommendations regarding treatment and counseling (http://www.cdc.gov/std/treatment).
- At present, no single therapy is uniformly superior. Selection of a treatment modality is impacted by the clinical situation, patient expectations, and clinician's personal experience and practice style.
- Topical medications that can be applied at home include imiquimod 5% cream, podofilox 0.5% solution or gel, and sinecatechins 15% ointment.
- Destructive and surgical interventions include liquid nitrogen cryotherapy, shave or snip removal with surgical scissors, electrofulguration, and laser destruction.
- In children, anogenital warts may cause concern for potential sexual abuse (see Fig. 28.12). However, a Canadian study of 72 children suggested that even the presence of sexually-related subtypes of HPV is not predictive of sexual abuse. A careful history and appropriate investigation remain the optimal ways to include or exclude sexual abuse.

Clinical Course

In one study, a spontaneous clearance rate of about 70% was observed over a 12-month period.

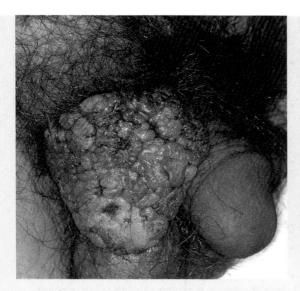

Fig. 28.9. Patient with gigantic, cauliflower-like, condyloma acuminatum, with variegation in color.

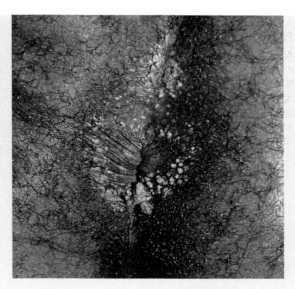

Fig. 28.10. Patient with numerous small perianal condylomata. Many but not all perianal infections are due to receptive anal intercourse. (From the Fitzsimons Army Medical Center Collection, Aurora, CO.)

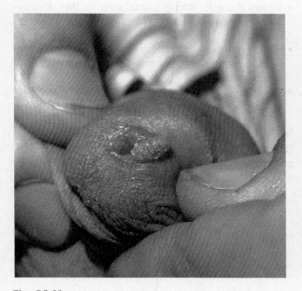

Fig. 28.11. Patient with genital warts affecting the urethral meatus, a common site in men.

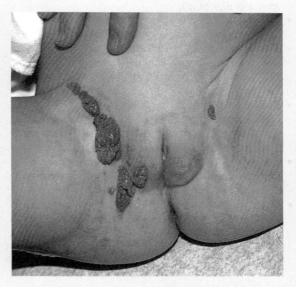

Fig. 28.12. Large cauliflower-like genital warts in an infant, a presentation that may or may not be sexually acquired. (From the William Weston Collection, Aurora, CO.)

Pathogenesis

A seborrheic keratosis (SK) is a benign epithelial tumor composed of keratinocytes. The pathogenesis of SKs is poorly understood, but in one study, *FGFR3* mutations were identified in more than half of all lesions examined. SKs are common in some ethnic groups, and the prevalence of SKs exceeds 90% by 65 years of age.

Warning! Be Careful!

Whereas most often SKs may be confidently diagnosed on simple visual inspection, all dermatologists have biopsied a presumed SK that was actually a melanoma, when analyzed under the microscope. Therefore, even in a patient with numerous SKs, if there is a so-called "ugly duckling," or a lesion that appears and/or behaves differently from the others, it should be biopsied and sent for histologic examination.

Clinical Features

- SKs can present in adolescence, but most occur after the age of 50.
- SKs are common on the face, back, and chest but can occur anywhere, except the palms and soles.
- SKs present as a stuck-on waxy or scaly papule, with color that ranges from near-white to yellow (Fig. 28.13) to tan to brown (Fig. 28.14) to black (Fig. 28.15).
- SKs near skin folds, such as the periocular area, neck, axilla and groin, are more likely to be papillomatous, with a narrow stalk (Fig. 28.14). This variant can be difficult to differentiate from an acrochordon.
- Dermatosis papulosa nigra (DPN) is a variant with multiple small dark black SKs around the eyes and cheeks of persons with darker skin (Fig. 28.16).
- Melanoacanthoma is an SK with a particularly dark black color due to abundant melanin in the lesion.

This variant can be clinically difficult to differentiate from a nodular melanoma (see Fig. 28.15).
- Stucco keratosis is a variant with multiple small near-white hyperkeratotic SKs that presents on the distal aspects of the extremities.
- The sign of Leser-Trélat is the explosive onset of innumerable SKs in association with an underlying malignancy, especially gastrointestinal cancer, and with some lymphomas.
- Inflamed seborrheic keratoses (see Chapter 29), as the name implies, are often pruritic and demonstrate varying degrees of erythema and scale, with an underlying inflammatory response.

Diagnosis

- In most cases, the diagnosis is based upon the clinical appearance.
- Suspicious lesions should sampled by shave biopsy, with the tissue submitted for histologic analysis.

Treatment

- In most cases, reassurance (without treatment) is appropriate, because SKs are benign.
- When there is strong confidence in the diagnosis, SKs can be destroyed with LN_2 cryotherapy or curettage.
- Shave removal, or snip removal for pedunculated lesions, will allow for histologic analysis to confirm the diagnosis.
- Chemical peels can be used for those with multiple small lesions, such as dermatosis papulosa nigra.

Clinical Course

SKs may occasionally disappear due to inflammation or trauma, but in most cases, SKs enlarge slowly, and new lesions continue to appear with age.

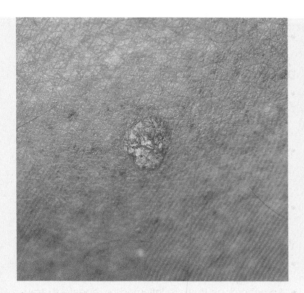

Fig. 28.13. Close-up of typical small, stuck-on seborrheic keratosis.

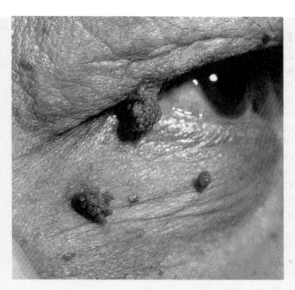

Fig. 28.14. Close-up of multiple seborrheic keratoses, with some being very exophytic.

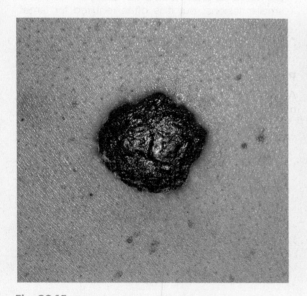

Fig. 28.15. Close-up of a darkly pigmented stuck-on seborrheic keratosis (melanoacanthoma), which could be confused with a melanoma. (From the Joanna Burch Collection, Aurora, CO.)

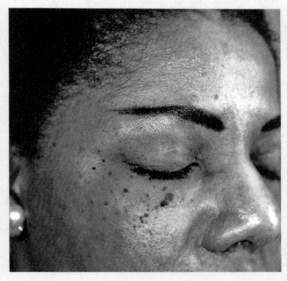

Fig. 28.16. Patient with dermatosis papulose nigricans, a clinical variant of seborrheic keratosis.

Acrochordon (Soft Fibroma) ICD10 code L91.8

Pathogenesis

Acrochordons, also known as skin tags, are benign exophytic neoplasms that consist of an unremarkable epidermis, with a normal collagenous core of papillary dermis. Larger lesions, with abundant dermis, or even fat, are often called soft fibromas or fibroepithelial polyps. The pathogenesis of acrochordons is poorly understood. Associations with obesity, diabetes, pregnancy, and acromegaly support a hormonal influence. A genetic influence is also likely because acrochordons have been seen with increased frequency in Birt-Hogg-Dubé and Beare-Stevenson syndromes, and may even be present from birth.

Clinical Features

- Most acrochordons are found in middle-aged or geriatric populations, but acrochordons can occur at any age.
- Acrochordons vary from a single lesion to hundreds of lesions.
- Common locations include the neck, axillae, groin, and eyelids. Other sites of lesser involvement include the trunk and proximal extremities.
- The primary lesion is soft, fleshy, baglike exophytic lesion with a narrow stalk. Most lesions are between 1 and 10 mm in size. The color varies from skin-colored to light brown (Figs. 28.17 and 28.18).
- Larger lesions (soft fibromas) are usually solitary and may be larger than 3 cm (Fig. 28.19).

- Occasional acrochordons are traumatized or strangulated, leading to hemorrhage or necrosis.

Diagnosis

- The diagnosis is usually made based upon the clinical appearance and the involvement of characteristic anatomic locations. The presence of multiple acrochordons, all with similar features, is reassuring.
- The clinical appearance of acrochordons may be mimicked by papillomatous or pedunculated nevi or neurofibromas, other benign fibromas, and papillomatous or pedunculated SKs.
- A snip or shave biopsy is often curative and diagnostic.

Treatment

- No treatment is necessary because acrochordons are benign lesions.
- Acrochordons that are inflamed or repeatedly traumatized may be removed by snipping the base of the stalk with sharp surgical scissors (see Fig. 28.18). Local anesthesia is not always required for smaller lesions, but it is often required for larger lesions.
- Other treatment options include cryotherapy (to the stalk) and electrodessication.

Prognosis

Acrochordons are benign lesions without any malignant potential.

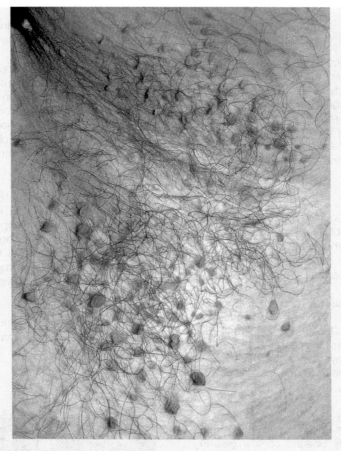

Fig. 28.17. Numerous acrochordons in an obese man, with subtle findings of acanthosis nigricans. (From the Fitzsimons Army Medical Center Collection, Aurora, CO.)

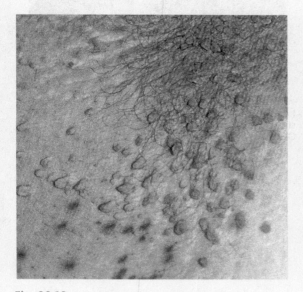

Fig. 28.18. Close-up of numerous soft, baglike acrochordons. Note the red scars at the bottom, where some of these had been previously taken off by snip removal. It is a real herculean task to remove all these skin tags.

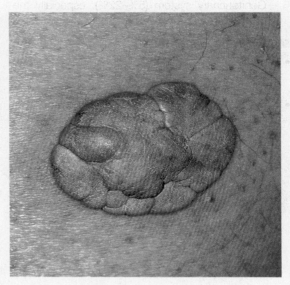

Fig. 28.19. Close-up of large flattened soft fibroma on the buttock.

☝ North American Blastomycosis ICD10 code B40.9

Pathogenesis

North American blastomycosis (Gilchrist disease) is a deep fungal infection produced by the soil saprophyte, *Blastomyces dermatitidis*. This dimorphic fungus exists as yeast in the body, but it has a mycelial phase in soil. Infections are acquired via an aerorespiratory route and are most common in the Ohio-Mississippi-Lawrence river basins (Fig. 28.20). The fungus can also be seen in parts of Africa, the Middle East, and Central and South America.

Clinical Features

- Primary blastomycosis infections are divided into pulmonary and cutaneous disease:
  - Primary pulmonary blastomycosis (which can be associated with erythema nodosum)
  - Primary cutaneous inoculation blastomycosis (rare; confined to laboratory accidents and dog bites)
- Systemic blastomycosis, caused by hematogenous spread from the lungs, is divided into two forms:
  - Chronic localized blastomycosis (the most common with skin involvement)
  - Generalized blastomycosis
- Chronic localized blastomycosis can affect any organ system, but the tissues usually affected are as follows:
  - Skin (50%)—usually begins as a papule that becomes verrucous (Figs. 28.21 and 28.22). Chronic lesions may ulcerate or scar (see Fig. 28.22).
  - Bone (25%–50%)
  - Genitourinary system (5%–22%), especially the prostate

Diagnosis

- The clinical presentation of a chronic verrucous lesion, particularly occurring in an area of high endemicity, can be diagnostic.
- A potassium hydroxide (KOH) examination of skin or sputum (from pulmonary disease) is positive in 60% of skin lesions.

- A skin biopsy (punch or incisional specimen) is usually diagnostic if the organism can be identified (Fig. 28.23).
- A fungal culture of a skin biopsy is positive in about 80% of cases, but results may take 1 to 4 weeks.
- Serologic tests, including an immunodiffusion test (positive in 80% of cases) and complement fixation test (positive in 50% of cases), are commercially available, but a definitive diagnosis still requires demonstration of the organism by culture or biopsy.

Treatment

- Chronic localized disease is usually treated with itraconazole (200–400 PO mg qd) for 6 to 12 months. The cure rate is approximately 90%.
- Severe disease (e.g., meningeal disease, cases in immunocompromised or AIDS patients) is usually treated with intravenous amphotericin B, with an oral azole antifungal for maintenance.

Clinical Course

The overall mortality rate in immunocompetent patients is about 2% but approaches 30% in immunocompromised patients.

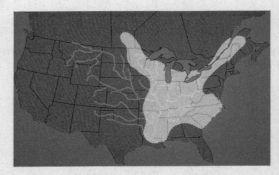

Fig. 28.20. Highly endemic areas of blastomycosis shaded in *yellow*. (From the Fitzsimons Army Medical Center Collection, Aurora, CO.)

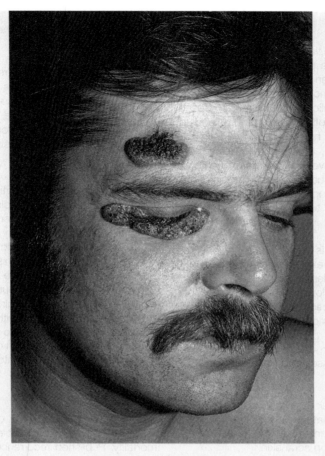

Fig. 28.21. Acute onset of verrucous lesions of the forehead and around the eye in a case acquired in Colorado. (From the Fitzsimons Army Medical Center Collection, Aurora, CO.)

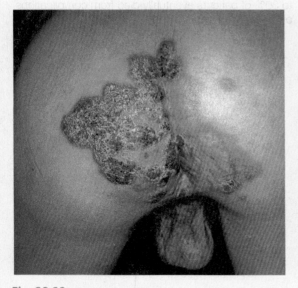

Fig. 28.22. Patient with chronic cutaneous blastomycosis of the perianal and buttock areas, with both verrucous lesions and scarring.

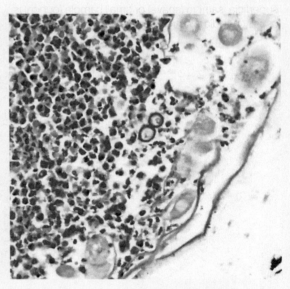

Fig. 28.23. Characteristic thick-walled yeast in an infection acquired in Colorado. The organisms are typically 8 to 15 μm in size and demonstrate broad-based budding when replicating (periodic acid–Schiff–diastase stain; 400×).

Pathogenesis

Verrucous carcinoma is a variant of well-differentiated squamous cell carcinoma that most often occurs in the oral cavity (Ackerman tumor), on the genitalia (Buschke-Löwenstein tumor), and on acral skin, particularly the foot (epithelioma cuniculatum). Cases of verrucous carcinoma often arise in long-standing warts. Molecular studies have identified HPV in the tumor, with subtypes 1, 2, 11, 16, and 18 being most common. Other cases have arisen in areas of chronic trauma or inflammation, such as scars, chronic draining fistulas, dystrophic epidermolysis bullosa, and lupus vulgaris (cutaneous tuberculosis).

Clinical Features

- Verrucous carcinoma is more common in older patients, with the only exception being cases that arise in dystrophic epidermolysis bullosa.
- Lesions are typically slow-growing and are composed of hyperkeratotic papillomatous or verrucous plaques or tumors of variable size (Figs. 28.24–28.26).
- The tumor may contain crypts of keratin that can lead to draining abscesses and fistulas.

Diagnosis

- A high degree of suspicion is required for large verrucous and/or papillomatous lesions that manifest aggressive behavior, particularly in the oral cavity, on anogenital area, or on acral skin.
- The diagnosis is established via deep incisional biopsy. The examining pathologist should be told of the clinical concern for verrucous carcinoma. A superficial sample (shave) or small sample (punch) is usually not diagnostic because the examiner needs to be able to evaluate the growth pattern. HPV subtyping may be helpful.
- Verrucous carcinoma can be a difficult histologic diagnosis to make. If a first sampling results in a benign diagnosis, such as pseudoepitheliomatous hyperplasia, but if clinical concern for verrucous carcinoma persists at the site, a larger second biopsy should be performed, and/or the case should be discussed with the pathologist or dermatopathologist.

Treatment

- Complete surgical extirpation is the treatment of choice for verrucous carcinoma. Because of the typical large size, the surgery may be difficult. Local recurrence rates are high, perhaps over 50% in some studies. Micrographic surgery (Mohs surgery) should be considered, if this technique is available.
- LN_2 cryosurgery might be considered for lesions that cannot be resected, but this destructive modality does not allow for margin control, and it must be performed by someone with expertise in this area.
- Radiation therapy can also be performed in cases that are inoperable, but, on occasion, this treatment can transform the tumor into a higher grade form of squamous cell carcinoma.

Clinical Course

The clinical course is that of a locally aggressive malignancy, with considerable morbidity and lesser mortality. Published recurrence rates in the literature vary, but in some studies the local recurrence rate has exceeded 50% (Fig. 28.27). The tumor only rarely becomes metastatic, but, in some studies, about 20% to 30% of patients eventually died from complications of the malignancy.

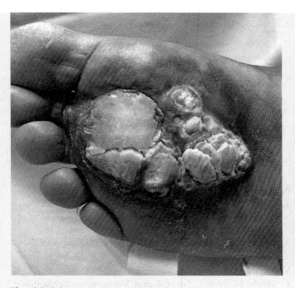

Fig. 28.24. Patient with large eroded verrucous carcinoma of the plantar surface of the foot that demonstrates verrucous hyperplasia punctuated by keratinous crypts.

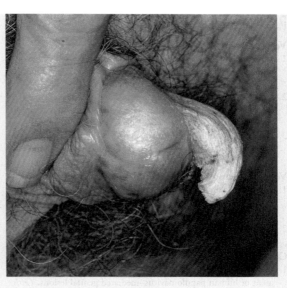

Fig. 28.25. Patient with early verrucous carcinoma of the penis, with an overlying cutaneous horn.

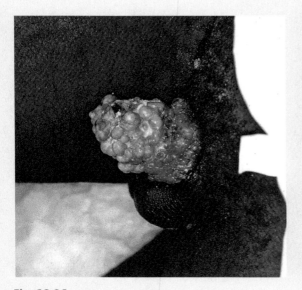

Fig. 28.26. Patient with an advanced verrucous carcinoma that has almost totally replaced the penis.

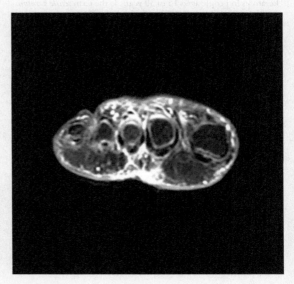

Fig. 28.27. Cross-sectional magnetic resonance imaging (MRI) scan of the forefoot demonstrating a recurrent verrucous carcinoma *(white areas)*. These were initially treated with Mohs surgery but recurred and penetrated through the foot to the dorsum.

References

Verrucae Vulgaris (Warts)

1. Kuykendall-Ivy TD, Johnson SM. Evidence-based review of management of nongenital cutaneous warts. *Cutis.* 2003;71:213-222.
2. Manz LA, Pelachyk JM. Bleomycin-lidocaine mixture reduces pain of intralesional injection in the treatment of recalcitrant verrucae. *J Am Acad Dermatol.* 1991;25:524-526.
3. Parsad D, Pandhi R, Juneja A, Negi KS. Cimetidine and levamisole versus cimetidine alone for recalcitrant warts in children. *Pediatr Dermatol.* 2001;18:349-352.

Verrucae Plana and Epidermodysplasia Verruciformis

1. Balevi A, Üstüner P, Özdemir M. Use of Er:YAG for the treatment of recalcitrant facial verruca plana. *J Dermatolog Treat.* 2016;1-15.
2. Hunzeker CM, Soldano AC, Prystowsky S. Epidermodysplasia verruciformis. *Dermatol Online J.* 2008;14:2.

Condyloma Accuminatum

1. Brodell LA, Mercurio MG, Brodell RT. The diagnosis and treatment of human papillomavirus–mediated genital lesions. *Cutis.* 2007;79(suppl 4):5-10.
2. Marcoux D, Nadeau K, McCauig C, et al. Pediatric anogenital warts: a 7-year review of children referred to a tertiary-care hospital in Montreal, Canada. *Pediatr Dermatol.* 2006;23:199-207.

Seborrheic Keratosis

1. Gill D, Dorevitch A, Marks R. The prevalence of seborrheic keratoses in people aged 15 to 30 years. Is the term *senile keratosis* redundant? *Arch Dermatol.* 2000;136:759-762.

2. Hafner C, Hartmann A, Real FX, et al. Spectrum of *FGFR3* mutations in multiple intraindividual seborrheic keratoses. *J Invest Dermatol.* 2007;127:1883-1885.
3. Lupo MP. Dermatosis papulosis nigra: treatment options. *J Drugs Dermatol.* 2007;6:29-30.

Acrochordon (Skin Tag)

1. Garg S, Bavejua S. Giant acrochordons of the labia majora: an uncommon manifestation of a common disease. *J Cutan Aesthet Surg.* 2015;8:119-120.
2. Lee JA, Khodaeee M. Enlarging pedunculated skin lesion. Acrochordon. *Am Fam Physician.* 2012;85:1191-1192.

North American Blastomycosis

1. Brick KE, Drolet BA, Lyon VB, Galbraith SS. Cutaneous and disseminated blastomycosis: a pediatric case series. *Pediatr Dermatol.* 2013;30:23-28.
2. Castillo CG, Kauffman CA, Micelli MH. Blastomycosis. *Infect Dis Clin North Am.* 2016;30:247-264.

Verrucous Carcinoma

1. Ahsaini M, Tahiri Y, Tazi NM, et al. Verrucous carcinoma arising in an extended giant condyloma acuminatum (Buschke-Löwenstein tumor): case report and review of the literature. *J Med Case Rep.* 2013;7:273.
2. Penera KE, Maji KA, Craig AB, et al. Atypical presentation of verrucous carcinoma: a case study and review of the literature. *Foot Ankle Spec.* 2013;6:318-322.

Chapter 29
Tumors With Scale

Key Terms

Squamous Cell Carcinoma in Situ
  Bowen disease
  Erythroplasia of Queyrat

Keratoacanthoma
  Keratoacanthoma centrifugum
    marginatum

Benign Lichenoid Keratosis
  Lichen planus–like keratosis

Tumors with scale are common and represent a heterogeneous group of epithelial neoplasms. This group of important skin tumors includes benign conditions, in situ malignancies (those confined to the epidermis), and frankly invasive cancers. Although the conditions covered in this chapter usually have scale present on the surface, exceptions exist. There may be lesser scale in early or evolving lesions, or, if the tumor is ulcerated, scale may be absent.

> **Differential Diagnosis of Tumors With Scale**
>
> Common
> - Benign lichenoid keratoses
> - Inflamed seborrheic keratosis
> - Keratoacanthoma
> - Squamous cell carcinoma
> - Squamous cell carcinoma in situ
>
> Uncommon
> - Acantholytic acanthoma
> - Epidermolytic acanthoma
> - Warty dyskeratoma

IMPORTANT HISTORY QUESTIONS

How long has this lesion been present?

The temporal course may suggest a benign or malignant process. A lesion present for years, or even decades, is less likely to be malignant than a lesion that arises quickly, over weeks or months.

Has the lesion recently changed?

Benign lesions can become inflamed (e.g., an inflamed seborrheic keratosis, a lichenoid keratosis arising in a solar lentigo), but a history of evolution sometimes suggests a malignant process.

Is this lesion growing rapidly?

Some malignant processes arise quickly (e.g., keratoacanthoma type of squamous cell carcinoma, aggressive forms of squamous cell carcinoma). Any rapid growth should be noted.

Has the lesion bled?

Any skin lesion, benign or malignant, can bleed when traumatized, particularly if the lesion is exophytic. However, an affirmative response to this question could suggest malignant qualities. A conservative approach is to consider biopsy of any lesion that has bled.

Have you had a previous skin cancer?

Persons with sufficient sun exposure to develop a nonmelanoma skin cancer of any type are at increased risk for a second such neoplasm. Once a person has one nonmelanoma skin cancer, he or she has a 50% chance of having another in the next 3 to 5 years. Skin cancer risk is also affected by chronic immunosuppression, exposure to radiation or arsenic, or infection with oncogenic forms of human papilloma-virus (HPV).

IMPORTAN PHYSICAL FINDINGS

What is the location of the lesion or lesions?

Certain scaling tumors may be associated with characteristic locations. For example, seborrheic keratoses occur often on the face, chest, and proximal extremities. Squamous cell carcinoma in situ and squamous cell carcinoma occur on sun-damaged skin or the genitalia.

What type of skin does the patient have?

Assessment of patient skin type (Fitzpatrick I–VI) may assist in predicting the risk of kertainocyte derived skin cancer. Persons with fair skin and light eyes are more likely to develop cutaneous malignancies. In particular, persons with red hair and blue eyes are among those at highest risk.

What does the lesion feel like on palpation?

Palpation to identify dermal extension, although imperfect, is useful in differentiating a benign or in situ malignant process from a deeply invasive form of skin cancer.

Pathogenesis

Squamous cell carcinoma in situ (SCCIS), also known as *Bowen disease,* is intraepidermal form of squamous cell carcinoma. SCCIS can occur on the skin (Fig. 29.1) and mucous membranes. Multiple causative factors are associated with SCCIS, including ultraviolet light, arsenic ingestion, and infection with oncogenic strains of HPV. SCCIS is more common in immunocompromised persons.

Clinical Features

- Most SCCIS arises on sun-exposed skin or genitalia of middle-aged to elderly persons.
- Patients typically report a persistent lesion, with progressive horizontal expansion. Sometimes, there may be a history of bleeding.
- The primary lesion consists of a sharply defined scaly papule or plaque, with variable erosion or ulceration (Figs. 29.2–29.4). There may be inflammation and erythema due to the host response.
- Some SCCIS may be papillomatous, resembling a wart (Fig. 29.5). Other forms are hyperkeratotic. On occasion, there may even be an overlying cutaneous horn of hyperkeratosis.
- *Erythroplasia of Queyrat* is a term used for HPV-induced squamous cell carcinoma of the genitalia.

Diagnosis

- The history and observation of an expanding scaly and/or eroded papule or plaque on sun-damaged skin is important to the diagnosis. Similarly, an expansive lesion located in the anogenital area is concerning for SCCIS.
- The diagnosis must be established by biopsy. A deep shave, large punch (depending on the size of the lesion), or incisional or excisional biopsy may be employed depending on the clinical situation. The latter technique has the potential advantage of providing uninvolved margins, if expressly commented on by the pathologist, thereby providing definitive management.

Treatment

- Excision provides for assessment of the surgical margins and exclusion of dermal invasion.
- A deep shave biopsy, followed by curettage and electrodessication, is another treatment option. Although this treatment does not require suturing, it precludes margin assessment. Appropriate serial surveillance is necessary to ensure local eradication.
- Cryosurgery is less often used, but it does have an adequate cure rate in experienced hands.
- Topical 5-fluorouracil may be used, and various products and strengths are available (2% and 5% solutions and 0.5%, 1%, and 5% creams). Typical use is qd or bid for at least 6 to 8 weeks.
- Topical imiquimod applied two to three times per week for 16 weeks is an option for some patients.

Clinical Course

SCCIS can grow slowly and insidiously for many years, before later becoming invasive. The risk of progression for SCCIS to frankly invasive squamous cell carcinoma (SCC) is from 5% to 15% per year.

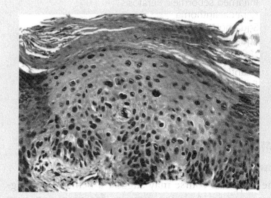

Fig. 29.1. Patient with small squamous cell carcinoma in situ demonstrating full-thickness atypia of the keratinocytes.

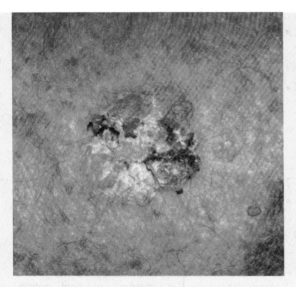

Fig. 29.2. Patient with squamous cell carcinoma in situ presenting as a scaly nodule with variable colors, including white, red, and dark purple. (From the Fitzsimons Army Medical Center Collection, Aurora, CO.)

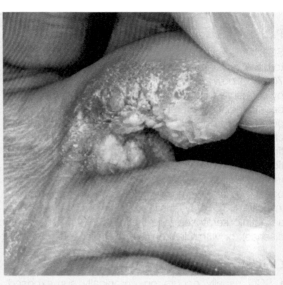

Fig. 29.3. Patient with large squamous cell carcinoma in situ presenting as a large scaly plaque between the toes, with marked scale. (From the Fitzsimons Army Medical Center Collection, Aurora, CO.)

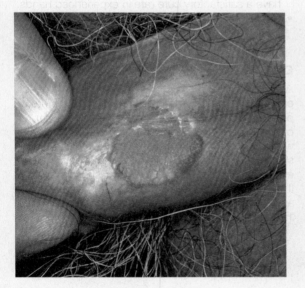

Fig. 29.4. Patient with human papillomavirus–induced squamous cell carcinoma in situ of the penis. This variant was formerly termed *erythroplasia of Queyrat*. (From the Fitzsimons Army Medical Center Collection, Aurora, CO.)

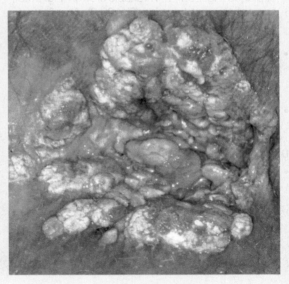

Fig. 29.5. Large papillomatous squamous cell carcinoma in situ of the anus that was human papillomavirus–induced in a man who was HIV-positive.

Pathogenesis

SCC is the second most common skin cancer, second to basal cell carcinoma, with an estimated 200,000 to 700,000 new cases per year. Most SCC is caused by exposure to ultraviolet light (outdoors or in tanning beds), radiation therapy, arsenic ingestion, or some petroleum products. SCC can also occur at sites of chronic injury, including burn scars, chronic skin infections, chronic ulcers, and chronic inflammatory conditions (e.g., lichen sclerosus). Importantly, SCC occurs more often in immunocompromised patients and may behave in an aggressive fashion in this population. Invasive SCC may arise in precursor lesions, such as actinic keratoses (see Fig. 29.5), SCCIS (Bowen disease), or within leukoplakia on mucosal surfaces.

Clinical Features

- SCC usually occurs on chronically sun-exposed skin of middle-aged or elderly persons.
- SCC often presents as a persistent lesion with progressive enlargement, possibly with bleeding.
- The clinical presentation is variable, but most often SCC consists of a scaly papule (Fig. 29.6), nodule, or plaque (Fig. 29.7) with variable erosion (Fig. 29.8), hemorrhage, or ulceration (Fig. 29.9). An inflammatory host response, such as surrounding erythema, is often observed.
- Verrucous carcinoma is caused by HPV, and it often has a papillomatous appearance. Ulcerated SCC may resemble the classic, so-called rat bite ulcer of basal cell carcinoma.
- Some invasive SCC may arise in contiguity with an actinic keratosis (see Fig. 29.6) or with SCCIS.

Diagnosis

- The clinical presentation of a rapidly growing papule or nodule, occurring on chronically sun-exposed skin, and in a patient with moderate to severe solar damage, is important.

- Immunosuppressed patients are more likely to have SCC. In this population, SCC may behave in an aggressive fashion. The threshold for performing a biopsy should be low in these persons.
- The diagnosis of SCC must be established by biopsy. Options include a deep shave biopsy, large punch (depending on the size of the lesion), and an incisional or excisional biopsy. An excisional biopsy allows for evaluation of margin status and may be curative (assuming the margins are uninvolved).

Treatment

- SCC is a malignant process, and it must be completely removed from the body. Surgical excision is usually used. Micrographically controlled (Mohs) surgery may be used for higher risk lesions or for tissue conservation.
- A deep shave biopsy, followed by curettage and electrodessication, is another treatment option. Although this treatment does not require suturing, it precludes margin assessment, and appropriate serial surveillance is necessary to ensure local eradication.
- Cryosurgery is less often employed, but it does have a satisfactory cure rate in experienced hands.
- Radiation therapy may be utilized, particularly in those who are not surgical candidates, or in elderly persons, sometimes for a variety of reasons.

Clinical Course

Aggressive SCC may occur at specific sites (e.g., lip, ear) and may be of lesser differentiation (moderate or poorly differentiated), deeply invasive (>3–4 mm), or of larger size. A fatal outcome is more likely in SCC with a diameter greater than 4 cm, perineural invasion, origin on a mucocutaneous junction, or deep extension into the subcutaneous tissue or beyond. It is estimated that cutaneous SCC, in general, has approximately a 4% rate of nodal metastasis and 1.5% rate of disease-specific death.

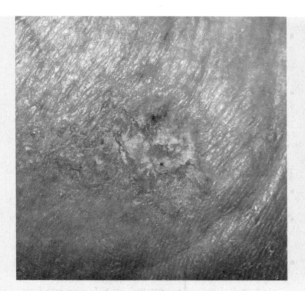

Fig. 29.6. Patient with early squamous cell carcinoma, with superficial invasion arising in an actinic keratosis. (From the Fitzsimons Army Medical Center Collection, Aurora, CO.)

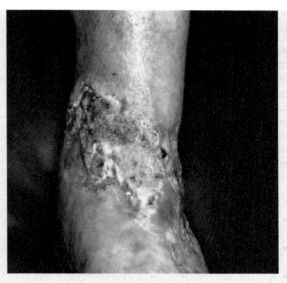

Fig. 29.7. Patient with neglected large squamous cell carcinoma, with marked scale. (From the Fitzsimons Army Medical Center Collection, Aurora, CO.)

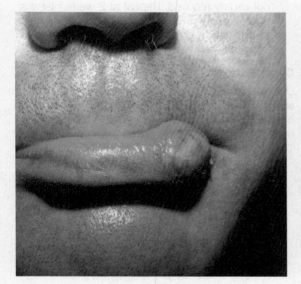

Fig. 29.8. Eroded squamous cell carcinoma (SCC) of the mucocutaneous margin of a 25-year-old man that was metastatic to a regional lymph node. SCCs of mucocutaneous junctions are very aggressive. (From the Fitzsimons Army Medical Center Collection, Aurora, CO.)

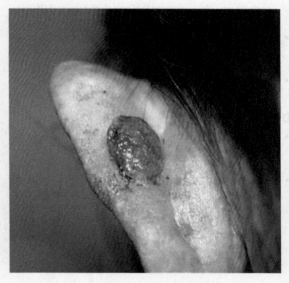

Fig. 29.9. Ulcerated nodule on the ear of an elderly patient that was a poorly differentiated squamous cell carcinoma. The clinical differential diagnosis includes many different cutaneous malignancies. (From the Fitzsimons Army Medical Center Collection, Aurora, CO.)

Pathogenesis

Keratoacanthoma (KA) is a low-grade form of SCC that arises from the follicular infundibulum. It is more common on heavily sun-damaged skin, and it has been estimated that there are about 200,000 new cases per year in the United States. Some KAs arise at sites of trauma, even repeatedly after surgery. Historically, KA was not considered a malignancy because many of the lesions spontaneously involuted, but it is now the modern trend to consider KA to be a form of squamous cell carcinoma.

Clinical Features

- KA usually presents as a rapidly evolving lesion on sun-exposed skin or at sites of trauma.
- The condition is largely limited to the sun-exposed skin of middle-aged or elderly persons.
- KA usually presents as a dome-shaped, crateri-form papule, with a central hyperkeratotic plug that widens as the lesion matures (Figs. 29.10–29.12).
- Size of KA varies from smaller than 0.5 cm to 5 cm or larger (see Fig. 29.12).
- Keratoacanthoma centrifugum marginatum is a rare variant with relentless lateral expansion that can produce roughly annular lesions that exceed 30 cm in size.
- Rare patients may have multiple KAs. Multiple KAs often occur at sites of trauma and may recur at sites of surgery (Fig. 29.13).
- KAs are more common in persons with Muir-Torre syndrome and xeroderma pigmentosum.

Diagnosis

- The history of a rapidly growing papule or nodule on the sun-exposed skin of a middle-aged to elderly person with solar damage strongly suggests KA.
- Observation of a crateriform papule or nodule with central hyperkeratotic debris augments this concern.

- The diagnosis of KA must be established by biopsy. Options include a deep shave biopsy or incisional or excisional biopsy. An excision allows for evaluation of margin status and potentially may be curative.
- In many cases, the pathologist or dermatopathologist may render the diagnosis of a well-differentiated SCC, without mention of KA-like features, particularly if this suspicion is not conveyed in the accession information.

Treatment

- Complete surgical excision is the most widely utilized management.
- A deep shave followed by curettage and electrodessication may also be employed. A 5% to 10% recurrence rate should be anticipated with this modality.
- Intralesional therapy may be successfully used:
  - 5-Fluorouracil (FU): 0.1 mL injected sublesionally; 0.1 to 0.4 mL of 50 mg/mL of 5-FU injected circumferentially. This may be repeated at 1-week intervals, with most lesions responding in two to four treatment sessions.
  - Methotrexate: infiltrate the tumor with 0.4 to 1.5 mL, 12.5 to 25 mg/mL. Local anesthesia is not usually required. Repeat at 2-week intervals. Some patients may require a second treatment. In one study of nine patients, a mean of 1.7 injections was required for resolution.

Clinical Course

Untreated, most KAs will spontaneously involute over about 3 to 6 months. However, about 6% to 10% of KAs will persist and may behave in a manner like other forms of SCC. This includes a risk of metastasis. Therefore, all KAs should be treated.

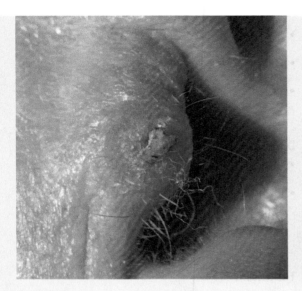

Fig. 29.10. Patient with developing keratoacanthoma demonstrating a red nodule, with a central keratotic plug. (From the Fitzsimons Army Medical Center Collection, Aurora, CO.)

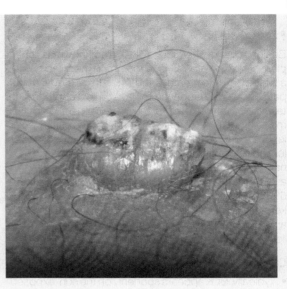

Fig. 29.11. Side view of a developed keratoacanthoma demonstrating a large keratotic plug. (From the Fitzsimons Army Medical Center Collection, Aurora, CO.)

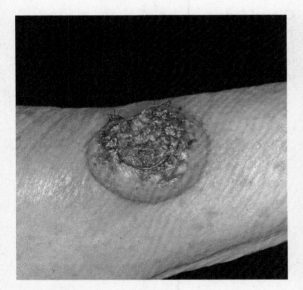

Fig. 29.12. Patient with giant keratoacanthoma of the forearm exceeding 4 cm in diameter. (From the Fitzsimons Army Medical Center Collection, Aurora, CO.)

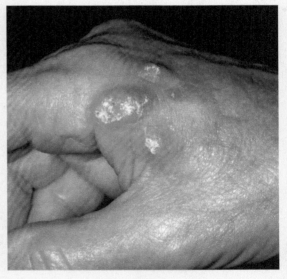

Fig. 29.13. Patient with multiple keratoacanthomas of the hand that have recurred following surgery. The patient also had multiple keratoacanthomas at other sites. (From the Fitzsimons Army Medical Center Collection, Aurora, CO.)

Pathogenesis

Benign lichenoid keratosis (BLK), also known as lichen planus–like keratosis, is a common neoplasm with a vigorous inflammatory infiltrate. In a study of 59 patients, which happened to have clinical photographs taken of the area before the development of BLKs, more than 47% of patients had a preexisting solar lentigo. Under the microscope, a contiguous solar lentigo is identified in over one-third of BLKs. Alternatively, it has been proposed that BLK represents a form of a lichenoid actinic keratosis, because from 5% to 10% of BLKs are contiguous with an actinic keratosis. Finally, it has also been proposed that BLKs are unique neoplasms. In summary, the reason for the lichenoid inflammation is poorly understood.

Clinical Features

- Typically, BLK appears suddenly on the sun-exposed skin of older patients with solar damage.
- BLK is more common in women than men.
- BLK is usually observed on the face, upper chest, and upper extremities.
- BLK is usually solitary, but occasional patients may present with two or more lesions.
- BLK presents as a discrete polygonal papule or nodule, of variable scale. The size ranges from 3 to 10 mm, and the color varies, but admixed hues of pink, red, violet, and brown (Figs. 29.14–29.16) may be seen.

- In some cases, a solar lentigo may be contiguous with the BLK.
- Rare BLK cases manifest Wickham striae, the white reticulate appearance seen in lichen planus.
- About half of BLKs are asymptomatic, with some patients experiencing pruritus or a burning sensation in the lesions.

Diagnosis

- The presentation of a thin scaly lesion, in contiguity with a solar lentigo, suggests the diagnosis.
- In most cases, the clinical assessment is established and malignancy is more optimally excluded by performing a shave biopsy. In rare cases, especially if there is concern for a pigmented lesion, an excision can be performed.

Treatment

- BLK requires no treatment.
- Most lesions are treated with surgical removal, shave biopsy, or excision.
- Cryotherapy is useful, particularly if there is a residual process after biopsy.

Clinical Course

There have been few studies on the clinical course of BLK. Lesions may resolve spontaneously over weeks to months, but some lesions have also been documented to persist for more than 2 years.

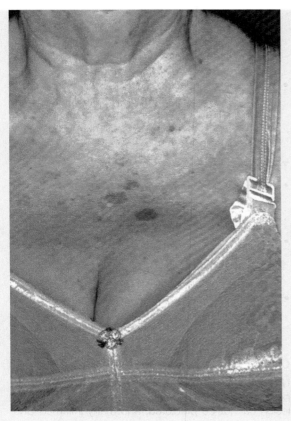

Fig. 29.14. Benign lichenoid keratosis of the upper chest of a woman acutely presenting as a round red lesion. Note the presence of several background solar lentigines. (From the Fitzsimons Army Medical Center Collection, Aurora, CO.)

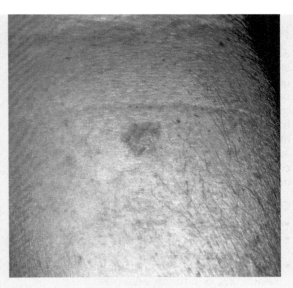

Fig. 29.15. Patient with benign lichenoid keratosis of the upper extremity presenting a scaling indurated lesion. Note that it is arising in a solar lentigo that is clearly present on the superior pole of the lesion. (From the Fitzsimons Army Medical Center Collection, Aurora, CO.)

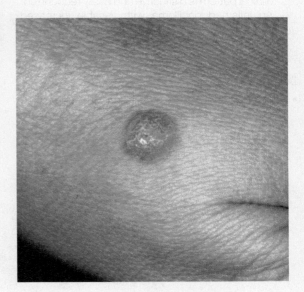

Fig. 29.16. Patient with exophytic benign lichenoid keratosis of the hand (lower left) that is clinically difficult to differentiate from an inflamed seborrheic keratosis or squamous cell carcinoma. (From the Fitzsimons Army Medical Center Collection, Aurora, CO.)

Pathogenesis

Seborrheic keratoses (SKs) are ubiquitous epithelial skin tumors that likely arise from the follicular infundibulum. Most SKs are tan to brown to black exophytic papillomas that appear as if they could be scraped off the skin (see Chapter 28). For unclear reasons, some SKs may become suddenly inflamed, which may alter the clinical appearance. The history of a sudden change and altered appearance may make it difficult to differentiate SKs from SCCs or from other malignancies.

Clinical Features

- Patients often have multiple SKs.
- SKs may have a history of recent or sudden change in a preexisting lesion.
- Most inflamed SKs are located on the head and neck, trunk, or proximal extremities.
- Many SKs may be associated with pruritus.
- Inflamed seborrheic keratoses may be single or multiple and occur in two distinct clinical patterns:
  - An inflamed papilloma with variable scale, surrounded by a rim of erythema (Fig. 29.17). This clinical pattern is distinctive and easily recognized.
  - An inflamed papilloma with variable increased scale but without a rim of erythema (Fig. 29.18). This clinical pattern can be difficult to differentiate from SCC.

Diagnosis

- Sudden changes in a preexisting SK suggest an inflamed SK, and, in many cases, this diagnosis can be made clinically, especially if the patient has a background of numerous SKs. This impression is substantiated by observation of a "stuck-on" papule or plaque with surrounding erythema.
- When suspicion includes an SCC or melanoma, a biopsy should be performed. In most cases, the histologic features are diagnostic of an SK, and a malignant process may be more confidently excluded.

Treatment

- SKs and inflamed SKs are benign, and no treatment is required. If a lesion is symptomatic, or if there is concern for malignancy, simple deep shave or saucerization removal may be the best option.
- Although SKs can be excised, a shave removal can be performed quickly, and there is no need for sutured removal. The specimen can still be examined histologically, confirming the diagnosis.
- Cryotherapy is also useful for symptomatic inflamed SKs if the diagnosis can be made with certitude, but if there is any doubt, the lesion should be biopsied to enable histologic confirmation of the diagnosis.

Clinical Course

Untreated, some but not all inflamed SKs will spontaneously resolve. However, the behavior of any singular lesion cannot be predicted, and many inflamed SKs will persist.

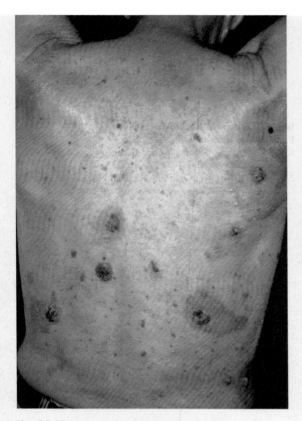

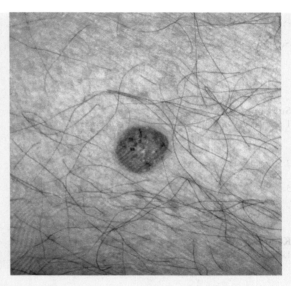

Fig. 29.18. Patient with inflamed seborrheic keratosis without a rim of erythema demonstrating an exophytic lesion with scale and an admixture of red, tan, brown, and black colors. The differential diagnosis could include squamous cell carcinoma and melanoma; this lesion should be biopsied for histologic confirmation of the diagnosis. (From the Fitzsimons Army Medical Center Collection, Aurora, CO.)

Fig. 29.17. Elderly man with numerous seborrheic keratoses (SKs) on his back, with several inflamed SKs demonstrating a prominent rim of erythema and scale. (From the Fitzsimons Army Medical Center Collection, Aurora, CO.)

References

Squamous Cell Carcinoma in Situ (Bowen Disease)

1. Patel GK, Goodwin R, Chawla M, et al. Imiquimod 5% cream monotherapy for cutaneous squamous cell carcinoma in situ (Bowen disease): a randomized, double-blind, placebo-controlled trial. *J Am Acad Dermatol.* 2006;54:1025-1052.

Squamous Cell Carcinoma

1. Carter JB, Johnson MM, Chua TL, et al. Outcomes of primary cutaneous squamous cell carcinoma with perineural invasion. An 11-year cohort study. *JAMA Dermatol.* 2013;149:35-41.
2. Clayman GL, Lee JJ, Holsinger FC, et al. Mortality risk from squamous cell skin cancer. *J Clin Oncol.* 2005;23:759-765.
3. Schmults CD, Karia PS, Carter JB, et al. Factors predictive of recurrence and death from cutaneous squamous cell carcinoma. A 10-year, single-institution cohort study. *JAMA Dermatol.* 2013;149:541-547.

Keratoacanthoma

1. Karaa A, Khachemoune A. Keratoacanthoma: a tumor in search of a classification. *Int J Dermatol.* 2007;46:671-678.

2. Ko CJ, McNiff JM, Bosenberg M, Choate KA. Keratoacanthoma: clinical and histopathologic features of regression. *J Am Acad Dermatol.* 2012;67:1008-1012.
3. Melton JL, Nelson BR, Stough DB, et al. Treatment of keratoacanthomas with intralesional methotrexate. *J Am Acad Dermatol.* 1991;25:1017-1023.

Benign Lichenoid Keratosis (Lichen Planus–like Keratosis)

1. Laur WE, Posey RE, Waller JD. Lichen planus–like keratosis. *J Am Acad Dermatol.* 1981;4:329-336.
2. Morgan MB, Stevens GL. Switlyk S: Benign lichenoid keratosis: a clinical and pathologic reappraisal of 1040 cases. *Am J Dermatopathol.* 2005;27:387-392.

Chapter 30
Papular and Nodular Growths Without Scale

Key Terms

Spitz Nevus
  Atypical Spitz nevus
  Atypical Spitzoid tumor
  Desmoplastic Spitz nevi

Dermatofibroma
  Cutaneous fibrous histiocytoma
  Bednar tumor

Papular and nodular neoplasms without scale comprise many important and potentially deadly tumors of the skin. Although this group of lesions is usually without scale, it is important to recognize that any lesion with significant trauma or inflammation may demonstrate some scale. Moreover, the malignant tumors in this group can attain a large size, may become large indurated plaques, or may outgrow a blood supply to become ulcerated. A partial listing of papular and nodular growths is provided in the box.

> **Papular and Nodular Growths: Differential Diagnosis**
> **Benign**
> - Benign sweat gland neoplasms
> - Dermatofibroma
> - Intradermal nevus
> - Keloid
> - Neurofibroma
> - Spitz nevus
>
> **Malignant**
> - Basal cell carcinoma
> - Dermatofibrosarcoma protuberans
> - Lymphomas
> - Malignant sweat gland carcinomas
> - Metastatic tumors

IMPORTANT HISTORY QUESTIONS

How long has this lesion(s) been present?

This is an important question because some of the entities in this group, such as dermatofibroma and intradermal nevus, tend to be stable over time, whereas other serious conditions, such as lymphomas and metastatic tumors, may be of recent onset or have rapid growth. Exceptions to this rule exist, such as dermatofibrosarcoma protuberans (DFSP) and some basal cell carcinomas, which can demonstrate slow progressive growth, despite being malignant.

Has the lesion changed?

This question is pertinent when evaluating whether a neoplasm lesion is benign or malignant. An affirmative answer to this question should result in a reduced threshold for performing a diagnostic biopsy.

Have you or any member of your family had similar lesions or a history of cancer?

The answer to this question could suggest a potential genodermatosis, such as neurofibromatosis type 1 (NF-1). Also, if the patient has a history of malignancy, the differential diagnosis should be expanded to include a potential metastasis, with a reduced threshold for performing a diagnostic biopsy.

IMPORTANT PHYSICAL FINDINGS

How old is the patient?

Some lesions, such as Spitz nevi, are more likely to occur in children or young adolescents, whereas dermatofibroma and neurofibromas are more common in postpubertal adolescents and young adults. Malignant tumors, including metastases, are more likely to occur in older adults.

How many lesions are present?

This is a critical finding because some lesions, like Spitz nevi, keloids, or dermatofibromas, are more likely to be solitary, whereas metastases and neurofibromas in NF-1 are more likely to present as multiple lesions.

What is the distribution of the lesions?

Some papular and nodular lesions have characteristic anatomic locations. For example, syringomas (small benign sweat gland tumors) are frequently located in the periocular or genital areas. Dermatofibromas often occur on the lower extremities of young adults, particularly women who shave their legs. Basal cell carcinoma and Merkel cell carcinoma are more likely to occur on sun-damaged skin.

Are any of the lesions ulcerated or necrotic?

Although trauma can cause ulceration in any exophytic process, benign or malignant, ulceration is more common with malignant processes, such as basal cell carcinoma, Merkel cell carcinoma, and metastatic tumors. Metastases in particular may ulcerate due to growth that outstrips the blood supply.

Pathogenesis

Basal cell carcinoma (BCC) is the most common cutaneous malignancy in the United States, with more than 4 million new cases occurring each year. BCC is derived from basaloid epithelial cells. For white persons older than 65 years, there is a 40% lifetime chance of developing a BCC. BCCs are caused by mutations in one or more genes of the hedgehog signaling pathway, with the most common mutation occurring in *PTCH1*. The major cause of BCC is long-term ultraviolet (UV) light exposure, punctuated by intense overexposure (sunburns). Less often, BCC may occur from genetic disorders (e.g., basal cell nevus syndrome), excessive arsenic ingestion, or radiation or chronic trauma (e.g., vaccination scars, tattoos).

Clinical Features

- Most BCCs occur in adults and elderly persons, especially those with a history of excess sun exposure.
- Most BCCs develop on sun-exposed skin, but occasionally it may occur on non–sun-exposed skin.
- BCC is usually a solitary process, but because of the degree of solar damage that is present in some persons, multiple separate lesions are not uncommon.
- Subtypes of BCC include the following:
  - Nodular (Fig. 30.1): BCC presenting as a translucent (pearly) papule or nodule, often with central ulceration (Fig. 30.2), variable telangiectasias, and possible pigmentation (particularly in persons with darker skin and eyes). Pigmented BCC may be difficult to differentiate from melanoma (Fig. 30.3). This is the most common BCC subtype in the head and neck area.
  - Superficial spreading BCC: plaque-like lesions with translucent papules at the periphery and a pattern of chiefly horizontal growth. This variant is most common on the trunk, especially the back (Fig. 30.4).
  - Infiltrative, desmoplastic, and morpheaform BCC: morphologic growth types that often yield smaller

or invasive basaloid islands admixed in a variable collagenous or even keloidal stroma. Clinically, these types of BCCs may be deceptive in appearance, resembling an otherwise unexplained scar.

Diagnosis

- BCC is often suspected based upon the clinical appearance, but final assessment and treatment require a biopsy to prove the diagnosis. Management is affected by the histologic growth pattern observed.
- The biopsy technique is determined by the clinical appearance and characteristics of the lesion, but a shave, punch, incisional, or excisional biopsy may be employed.

Treatment

- BCC is a malignant process, and complete surgical extirpation is the treatment modality most often utilized.
- Electrodessication and curettage is a therapeutic option for cases of superficial or nodular BCC, but this technique does not allow for histologic confirmation of uninvolved surgical margins.
- Mohs (micrographically controlled) surgery is the treatment of choice of large BCCs of the face, for tumors with infiltrative, desmoplastic, and/or morpheaform histology, and for many recurrent BCCs.
- Less often, radiation (primarily for large tumors in elderly patients), photodynamic therapy (PDT), cryosurgery, or topical imiquimod and 5-fluorouracil (superficial forms only) may be used.
- Vismodegib and sonidegib represent hedgehog pathway inhibitors used for locally aggressive or rare metastatic BCC or documented basal cell nevus syndrome, but this is the domain of experts.

Clinical Course

BCC represents a malignant process that can destroy normal structures, and it may even extend into bone. Metastatic BCC is a rare event, but it can occur, with more than 350 cases reported in the medical literature.

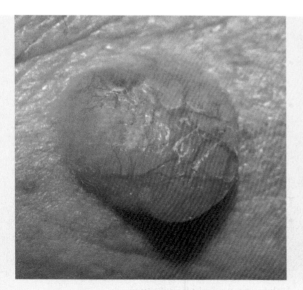

Fig. 30.1. Patient with nodular basal cell carcinoma, with a translucent quality, and telangiectasia. (From the Fitzsimons Army Medical Center Collection, Aurora, CO.)

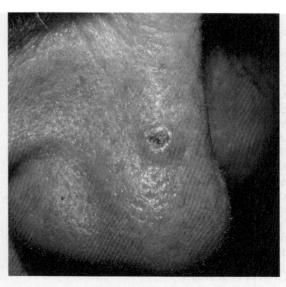

Fig. 30.2. Patient with small, ulcerated, papular basal cell carcinoma. (From the John Aeling Collection, Aurora, CO.)

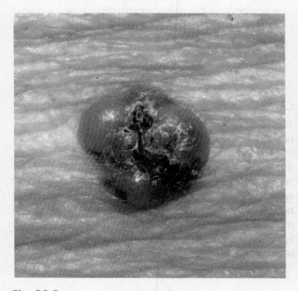

Fig. 30.3. Patient with ulcerated basal cell carcinoma composed of an admixture of translucent and pigmented areas. (From the Fitzsimons Army Medical Center Collection, Aurora, CO.)

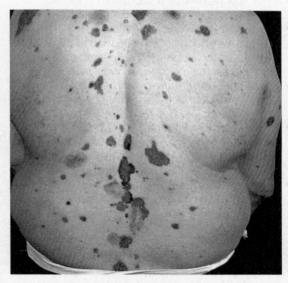

Fig. 30.4. Patient with basal cell nevus syndrome with nodular and superficial basal cell carcinomas, including some that are focally pigmented. (From the Fitzsimons Army Medical Center Collection, Aurora, CO.)

Pathogenesis

Spitz nevi are benign melanocytic neoplasms that are tumors difficult to differentiate from melanoma. The original cases, described by Dr. Sophie Spitz, were called *benign juvenile melanoma*, because of histologic similarities to melanoma, but a generally indolent course. Most Spitz nevi are skin-colored, pink, or red and are nondescript in clinical appearance. The terms *atypical Spitz nevus* and *atypical Spitzoid tumor* (AST) are more recent terms used to describe lesions of uncertain biologic potential that are difficult to differentiate from spitzoid melanoma, even using light microscopy, immunostains, and genetic analysis. Desmoplastic Spitz nevi are lesions characterized by increased stroma, including activated fibroblasts and dense collagen.

Clinical Features

- Spitz nevi occur mostly in whites, of any age, but often in children and adolescents.
- Spitz nevi are typically solitary, but multiple lesions, or even agminated lesions, may occur.
- Spitz nevi present as a papule or nodule that may be dome shaped or even pedunculated.
- Most Spitz nevi are skin-colored, pink, or red, perhaps with telangiectasia (Figs. 30.5 and 30.6). Less often, the lesions are pigmented or resemble other pigmented melanocytic neoplasms.
- Spitz nevi may have overlying scale and/or small keratinous globules that appear white (see Fig. 30.5).
- Historically, most Spitz nevi are of stable size. Rapid growth can occur but is a concerning feature for an atypical Spitz tumor or spitzoid melanoma, and the threshold of biopsy is greatly reduced.
- Spitz nevi may arise on normal skin or in other lesions, including junctional nevi, compound nevi (Fig. 30.7), intradermal nevi, and nevus spilus (Fig. 30.8).

Diagnosis

- Some Spitz nevi are suspected chiefly on clinical grounds. The occurrence of a pink or red papule on the skin of a young white child raises the possibility of a Spitz nevus.
- Spitz nevi with a marked red color may be confused with vascular tumors, such as pyogenic granulomas.
- A final diagnosis is established by shave, punch, or excisional biopsy. The histologic diagnosis is problematic, and it is wise to have any potential Spitz nevus evaluated by an expert dermatopathologist, because some cases are difficult to differentiate from melanoma, especially in adults.

Treatment

- The treatment of Spitz nevi is not standardized. Although some pediatric dermatologists do not re-excise classic Spitz nevi in a child, even when the surgical margin is involved, a 2002 study showed that most dermatologists prefer conservative complete removal of all Spitz nevi.
- The management of atypical Spitz nevi and ASTs is also not standardized, but these lesions are widely considered to have uncertain biologic potential. Nearly all experts recommend complete surgical extirpation, with some authorities even recommending a 1cm clinical margin. The value of a sentinel lymph node (SLN) sampling in an atypical Spitz nevus or AST is unknown. Some series have shown SLN involvement in up to one-third of cases but with dubious prognostic significance.

Clinical Course

The clinical course of Spitz nevi that are not biopsied has never been studied, and never will be studied. The prevalence of Spitz nevi in children and adolescents, relative to that of adults and geriatric patients, suggests that such lesions involute or evolve into conventional nevi. A longitudinal study of suspected Spitz nevi by dermoscopy, with a mean follow-up of 25 months, has revealed dermoscopic features of involution in 80% of the lesions, with the remaining 20% stable or enlarging.

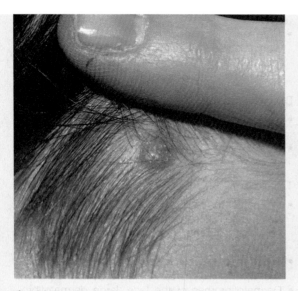

Fig. 30.5. Patient with slightly red papule, with white globules representing aggregates of keratin. (From the William Weston Collection, Aurora, CO.)

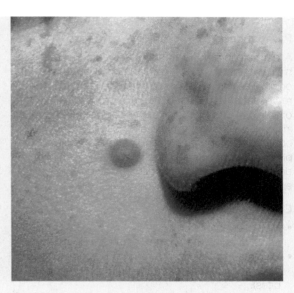

Fig. 30.6. Patient with Spitz nevus presenting as a red papule with focal telangiectasia. (From the Fitzsimons Army Medical Center Collection, Aurora, CO.)

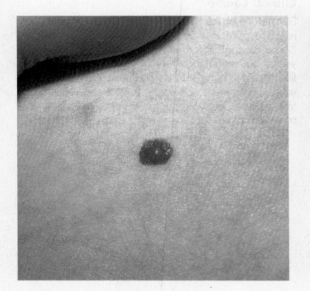

Fig. 30.7. Patient with Spitz nevus arising in a compound nevus. (From the William Weston Collection, Aurora, CO.)

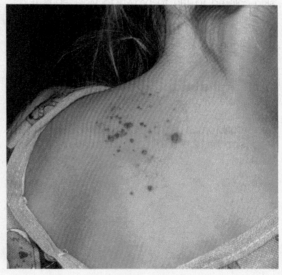

Fig. 30.8. Patient with multiple red Spitz nevi occurring within a nevus spilus. The smaller brown lesions are compound and junctional nevi.

Pathogenesis

A dermatofibroma, also known as cutaneous fibrous histiocytoma, is a common tumor of fibrohistiocytic origin. There is debate as to whether dermatofibromas represent a neoplastic or reactive process. In support of the former is the development of lesions at sites of injury (e.g., shaving trauma on the legs, insect bites), but studies of the methylation pattern of the polymorphic X chromosome–linked androgen receptor have demonstrated that dermatofibromas are clonal proliferations, and are probably neoplastic.

Clinical Features

- Most dermatofibromas occur in persons 20 to 50 years of age, with a slight female predominance.
- Patients may report a history of preceding trauma (e.g., shaving trauma on the legs of women, insect bites).
- Most dermatofibromas occur on the lower extremities but also on the trunk, head, and neck.
- Most dermatofibromas are round to oval, firm, painless papules or nodules. The lesion may be exophytic, dimpled, or flat, with a color that varies from skin-colored to tan to brown to violaceous (Figs. 30.9 and 30.10).
- Rare cases with lipidization may have yellow tones. Occasional cases with abundant hemosiderin may appear dark purple (Fig. 30.11) or black (hemosiderotic dermatofibroma).
- With lateral compression, many dermatofibromas will dimple (Fig. 30.12; dimple sign or Fitzpatrick sign).
- Dermatofibromas usually lack overlying scale unless the lesion has been irritated, inflamed, or traumatized.

- Rare patients with a history of immunosuppression, such as systemic lupus erythematosus or HIV infection, may demonstrate the explosive onset of multiple dermatofibromas.

Diagnosis

- The diagnosis is usually made based on the clinical presentation and clinical appearance.
- A deep shave, punch, incisional, or excisional biopsy may be performed on problematic lesions.

Treatment

- Dermatofibromas are benign and do not require treatment, but some cases are subject to minor continued trauma, particularly on lesions of the lower legs of women (from shaving).
- For problematic lesions, extirpation is usually curative. Smaller lesions can be removed with a punch.
- Dermatofibromas of the face, large dermatofibromas (>2 cm), and dermatofibromas in children are more likely to be locally aggressive and should be completely excised, if surgically feasible.

Clinical Course

Dermatofibromas will often grow slowly until they reach a particular size and then will remain stable. Some dermatofibromas will regress, typically over years, but sometimes rapidly. Some large dermatofibromas will behave in an aggressive fashion. A few so-called "metastatic" cases have been reported in the literature, but whether these cases represent dermatofibromas or unrecognized sarcomas is debated.

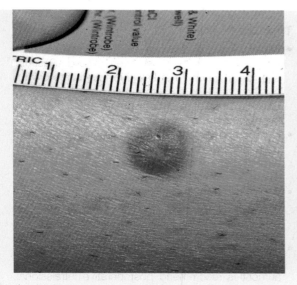

Fig. 30.9. Brownish-violaceous nodule on the leg of a woman. (From the William Weston Collection, Aurora, CO.)

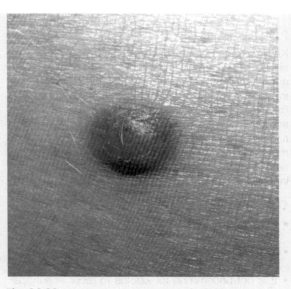

Fig. 30.10. Patient with exophytic brownish-violaceous nodule with evidence of minor superficial trauma. (From the Fitzsimons Army Medical Center Collection, Aurora, CO.)

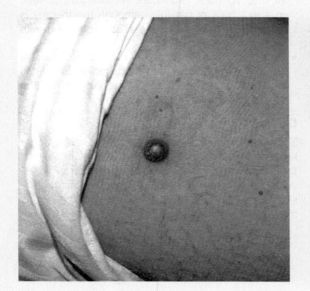

Fig. 30.11. Patient with hemosiderotic dermatofibroma with purple color. (From the Fitzsimons Army Medical Center Collection, Aurora, CO.)

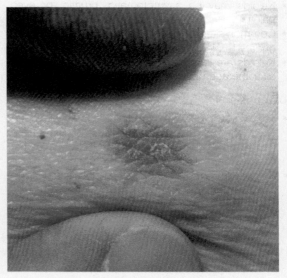

Fig. 30.12. Positive Fitzpatrick sign. Most dermatofibromas dimple with lateral pressure. (From the Fitzsimons Army Medical Center Collection, Aurora, CO.)

Keloid

Pathogenesis

Keloids are benign hyperproliferative growths of abnormal collagen. It is thought that keloids represent an aberrant reparative process that follows cutaneous injuries such as lacerations, piercings, or burns. On the anterior chest, keloids are often associated with acne vulgaris. Less often, keloids may arise without a known (or recognized) traumatic event. Keloids are more common in dark-skinned persons, who are 15 times more likely to develop keloids than light-skinned individuals.

Clinical Features

- Keloids are most common in the second and third decades of life, but keloids can occur at any age.
- Keloids usually develop within weeks to months of a cutaneous injury.
- It is not uncommon for keloids to recur in surgical sites, even after attempts at extirpation.
- Keloids present as firm nodules, and a multinodular appearance is possible (Figs. 30.13–30.15).
- Most keloids are skin-colored or hyperpigmented in comparison to the surrounding unaffected skin.
- Keloids may be asymptomatic, pruritic, or even painful.
- Common sites for keloids include the earlobes (secondary to piercing) and the anterior chest (acne).
- Keloids are less common in later life and are rare after the age of 60 years (Fig. 30.16).

Diagnosis

- The clinical presentation of keloids is usually diagnostic. Some keloids can be difficult to differentiate from hypertrophic scars or from other neoplasms, such as dermatofibrosarcoma protuberans.
- Some keloids require a biopsy for definitive diagnosis. Exophytic keloids, with narrow bases, can be shaved, whereas larger lesions are often sampled with a punch (3–6 mm). In most cases, the histologic findings are diagnostic.

Treatment

- Intralesional triamcinolone acetonide (10–40 mg/mL) is the therapy most often utilized. Patients should be warned that keloid injections are painful but become less so with subsequent treatments. Patients should also be warned about potential hypopigmentation or skin atrophy.
- Flurandrenolide tape (Cordran tape) can be applied overnight, for 2 to 6 weeks, but produces skin atrophy in some cases, and at present, it is difficult to obtain.
- Pentoxifylline (400 mg PO tid) has been used with anecdotal success in preventing recurrence; it is hypothesized that this may be due to inhibited collagen production.
- Small keloids may be excised, but recurrence is a problem in about 40% to 60% of cases. Most authorities recommend postoperative intralesional steroid injection and/or oral pentoxifylline to reduce this rate of recurrence.
- Cryosurgery (two 15- to 20-second freeze-thaw cycles) can be performed every 3 weeks for a total of 6 to 10 visits. Significant improvement is seen in about 50% of patients, although the therapy is painful. Cryosurgery can also be combined with intralesional triamcinolone.
- Radiation therapy is effective, but it is not routinely used, chiefly because of the substantially increased risk of squamous cell carcinoma later in life (the typical patient with keloids is young).

Clinical Course

The clinical course of keloids is highly variable. Some keloids quickly achieve a stable size and are asymptomatic, whereas others continue to enlarge for years, or cause pain and discomfort. Spontaneous regression is uncommon, but some flattening of the lesions may be seen in later life.

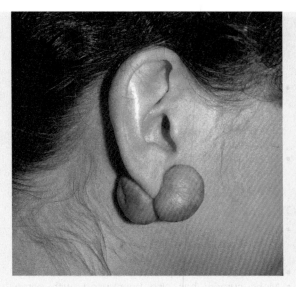

Fig. 30.13. Dumbbell keloid after ear piercing in a person with light skin. Any skin type can develop keloids. (From the Fitzsimons Army Medical Center Collection, Aurora, CO.)

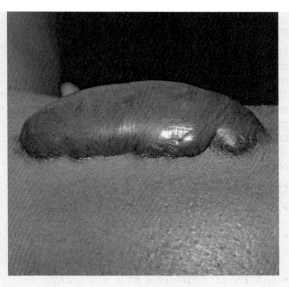

Fig. 30.14. Keloid of the upper shoulder in a young black man. There was no history of previous trauma. (From the Fitzsimons Army Medical Center Collection, Aurora, CO.)

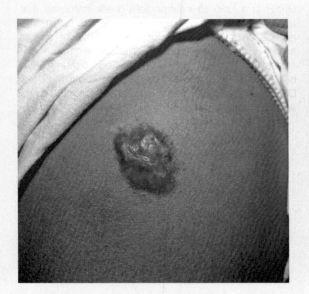

Fig. 30.15. Keloid at vaccination site on the upper arm of a Hispanic man. (From the William Weston Collection, Aurora, CO.)

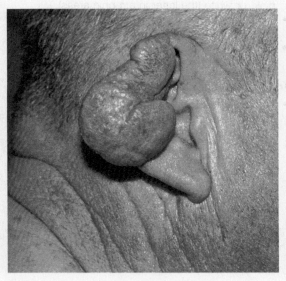

Fig. 30.16. Keloid developing in a graft site in an older patient after Mohs surgery. (From the Fitzsimons Army Medical Center Collection, Aurora, CO.)

Dermatofibrosarcoma Protuberans

Pathogenesis

DFSP, although a rare neoplasm overall, is the most common cutaneous sarcoma. The incidence is estimated to be about 4.2 cases/million persons per year. The cause of the neoplasm is debated, but the tumor is likely derived from $CD34^+$ dendrocytes normally found in the dermis. Most DFSPs possess a reciprocal translocation of chromosomes 17 and 22 or, less often, a supernumerary ring chromosome comprised of portions of chromosomes 17 and 22.

Clinical Features

- DFSP is most common in 20- to 59-year-olds, but can even be present at birth, or in older adults.
- The most common location for DFSP is the trunk, but it may also occur on the arms, legs, or head and neck.
- Typically, DFSP presents as a slow-growing exophytic papule that enlarges to produce additional papules and nodules of various sizes, which protrude above the skin surface (Figs. 30.17–30.20). However, atrophic plaque-like forms, without a protuberant appearance, are not uncommon.
- DFSP is typically skin-colored but it can be red, pink, or white (the latter in atrophic areas).
- DFSP is usually asymptomatic but 10% to 20% of patients with a DFSP report local pain or discomfort.
- Bednar tumor is an uncommon type of DFSP that is pigmented because of admixed melanocytes.

Diagnosis

- The differential diagnosis includes a dermatofibroma, hypertrophic scar, keloid, or any other soft tissue tumor. Often, the diagnosis of a DFSP is suspected because of the clinical history of a slow-growing tumor, with a protuberant papulonodular quality.
- The diagnosis may be established by performing a large deep punch biopsy (6 or 8 mm) or an incisional or excisional biopsy. A shave biopsy should not be performed if DFSP is a serious diagnostic consideration.
- Nearly all DFSPs mark with a CD34 immunohistochemical stain, which is an important part of the overall histologic evaluation.

Treatment

- Complete surgical extirpation of the tumor with 2- to 4-cm margins is the most commonly used treatment.
- Select cases may require adjuvant radiation therapy.
- Mohs surgery has also been used, with some degree of success.
- For patients with unresectable tumors or with metastatic disease, imatinib is the treatment of choice.

Clinical Course

DFSP is a low- to intermediate-grade sarcoma that usually produces damage by local extension into normal structures. In about 5% to 10% of cases, a DFSP contains a fibrosarcomatous element. This subset of DFSP with fibrosarcomatous change often behave in a more aggressive fashion. About 5% of all DFSPs will produce metastatic disease, with the lungs and lymph nodes most often involved.

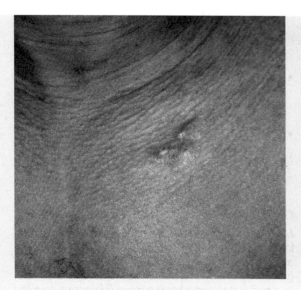

Fig. 30.17. Patient with early dermatofibrosarcoma protuberans on the anterior chest presenting as an enlarging plaque with several papules.

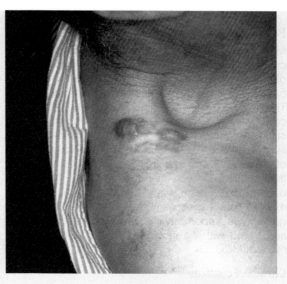

Fig. 30.18. Patient with dermatofibrosarcoma protuberans on the shoulder demonstrating atrophic areas and nodular growth. (From the Fitzsimons Army Medical Center Collection, Aurora, CO.)

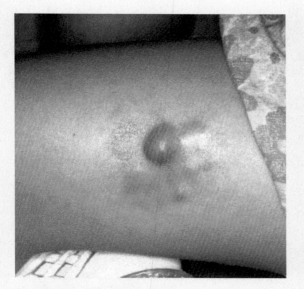

Fig. 30.19. Large dermatofibrosarcoma protuberans with atrophic areas, papules, and a large nodule. This child is 8 years old. (From the Fitzsimons Army Medical Center Collection, Aurora, CO.)

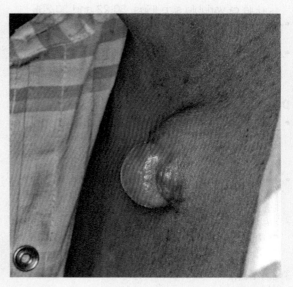

Fig. 30.20. Neglected dermatofibrosarcoma protuberans in an institutionalized patient presenting as a large mass composed of multiple nodules.

Pathogenesis

Merkel cell carcinoma (MCC) is an aggressive, primary cutaneous neuroendocrine carcinoma that is most often comprised of cords, sheets, or strands of small basaloid cells, with minimal cytoplasm (Fig. 30.21). The disputed cell of origin is thought to be the Merkel cell, which is associated with nerve endings found in the basal layer of the epidermis. The oncogenic events are not fully understood, but recent discovery of Merkel cell polyomavirus in MCC has suggested that this virus is involved in tumorigenesis. Moreover, because MCC occurs in elderly persons, in areas of marked solar exposure, it is also believed that solar damage is important. Immunosuppression is also associated with an increased risk for the development of MCC.

Clinical Features

- MCC is most common in white men and typically develops after the age of 50 years. Most cases occur in those 70 years of age or older.
- MCC occurs most often on sun-exposed skin (>80%), with the head and neck particularly affected.
- MCC usually presents as a pink or red papule or nodule of variable size (Figs. 30.22 and 30.23).
- Ulceration of MCC is common (Fig. 30.24), probably due to a high proliferative rate.
- Metastatic MCC is clinically indistinguishable from a primary tumor, but multiple lesions should strongly suggest metastatic disease (Fig. 30.25).

Diagnosis

- MCC does not have a singular diagnostic appearance, and all cases require an adequate biopsy (≥4-mm punch biopsy or incisional or excisional biopsy that extends into the subcutaneous fat).
- The pathologist or dermatopathologist can usually make a specific diagnosis using immunohistochemical stains. Some cases may be difficult to differentiate from metastatic small cell carcinoma of the lung or metastatic neuroendocrine carcinoma that is not of cutaneous origin.

Treatment

- MCC is an aggressive malignancy, and patients should be referred to an appropriate specialty care

environment. Treatment options will depend on the location, general health of the patient, and clinical stage.

- Imaging studies (e.g., computed tomography [CT], magnetic resonance imaging [MRI], positron emission tomography [PET] scan) and sentinel lymph node biopsy are often used to aid staging.
- Treatment uses surgical excision, perhaps micrographic surgery, sentinel node sampling, and post-surgical radiation to local and regional lymph nodes. Immunotherapy and chemotherapy may be used for patients with advanced disease.

Clinical Course

MCC is an aggressive malignancy with a high risk of local recurrence (40%), regional metastases (55%), and distant metastases (36%). Studies have suggested that men and those with tumors of the head and neck often experience a more aggressive course. Women, younger persons, and those with tumors of the extremities may have a generally more favorable course. The 5-year, disease-specific survival rate in one study of 251 patients from a single institution was just 64%, a rate lower than that of melanoma.

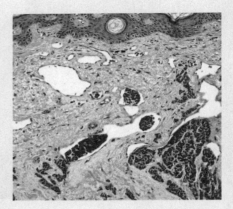

Fig. 30.21. Patient with cords and strands of basaloid cells in the dermis with lymphatic invasion.

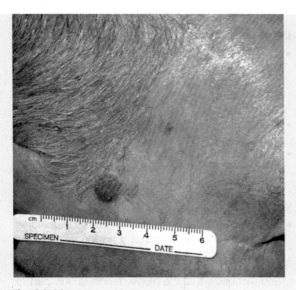

Fig. 30.22. Patient with Merkel cell carcinoma, a small red nodule on sun-damaged skin. (From the Fitzsimons Army Medical Center Collection, Aurora, CO.)

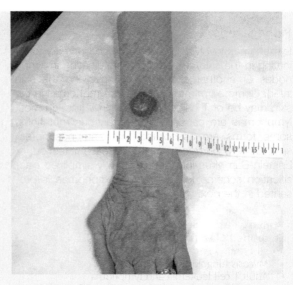

Fig. 30.23. Patient with Merkel cell carcinoma, a large pinkish-red nodule on sun-damaged acral skin.

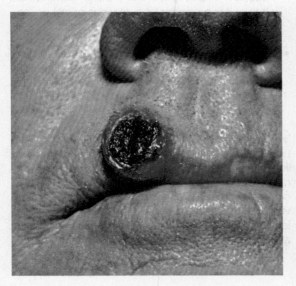

Fig. 30.24. Patient with Merkel cell carcinoma, an ulcerated red nodule on sun-damaged skin. (From the Fitzsimons Army Medical Center Collection, Aurora, CO.)

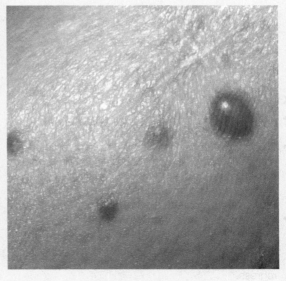

Fig. 30.25. Patient with metastatic Merkel cell carcinoma presenting as multiple red papules and small nodules. (From the Fitzsimons Army Medical Center Collection, Aurora, CO.)

Pathogenesis

Lymphomas involving the skin may be primary (originating in the skin) or secondary (originating in lymph nodes or another site and only involving the skin later). Common primary cutaneous lymphomas in the skin may be of T cell or B cell origin. Although most lymphomas are caused by spontaneous mutations, some forms are associated with immunosuppression, *Borrelia burgdorferi* (Lyme disease) infection, or Epstein-Barr virus infection. A greatly simplified classification scheme for cutaneous lymphomas is presented in the box.

Primary Cutaneous Lymphomas: Simplified Classification

T Cell Lymphomas
- Mycosis fungoides and variants
- Adult T cell leukemia and lymphoma
- Primary cutaneous CD30+ lymphoproliferative disorders
- Subcutaneous panniculitis–like T cell lymphomas
- Extranodal natural killer (NK) and T cell lymphoma, nasal type
- Primary cutaneous peripheral T cell lymphoma, unspecified

B Cell Lymphomas
- Primary marginal zone B cell lymphoma
- Primary cutaneous follicle center B cell lymphoma
- Primary cutaneous diffuse large B cell lymphoma, leg type

Clinical Features

- Lymphomas in the skin may present as a single lesion (Fig. 30.26) or multiple lesions.
- Some cutaneous lymphomas have characteristic distributions. For example, B cell lymphoma often presents on the head and neck or trunk, whereas mycosis fungoides often presents in doubly protected areas, beneath clothing and undergarments.
- Lymphomas presenting in the skin usually present as red or violaceous papules, plaques, tumors, or nodules (Fig. 30.27–30.29). Some lymphomas may produce ulcerative or fungating nodules or may regress.

Diagnosis

- The clinical features of lymphoma are not specific enough for clinical diagnosis, and an adequate biopsy is required (e.g., large punch biopsy, incisional or excisional biopsy that includes the subcutis).
- If palpable lymph nodes are present, they should also be surgically biopsied for histologic evaluation.
- A pathologist, hematopathologist, or dermatopathologist may use immunohistochemical staining, flow cytometry, and polymerase chain reaction (PCR)–based gene rearrangement studies, which are necessary to arrive at a full assessment.
- Once biopsy results are finalized, clinicopathologic correlation and clinical staging are necessary. It is important to stress the limitations of the pathologist, hematopathologist, and dermatopathologist and recognize that the biopsy report is only part of the final assessment. No diagnosis is considered final until the patient has been staged and totality of the circumstances assessed.

Treatment

- Treatment of a lymphoma in the skin depends on whether it is a primary (of cutaneous origin) or secondary lymphoma (originating from another site, such as the lymph node).
- Treatment ranges from excision or local radiation for most primary cutaneous B cell lymphomas of low grade, to topical medicaments or UV therapy for lower stage mycosis fungoides (MF-CTCL), to advanced therapy for higher grade disease.

Clinical Course

Low-grade primary cutaneous B cell lymphoma (follicle center cell, marginal zone) has a 5-year survival rate in excess of 95%. Most patients with lower stage cutaneous T cell lymphoma have an excellent survival rate, but the disease can advance or progress, for unclear reasons. Clearly, the overall prognosis is affected by the specific diagnosis and circumstances.

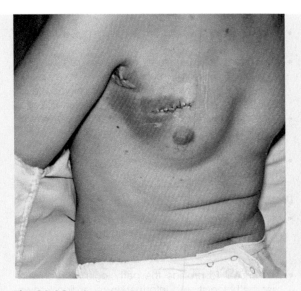

Fig. 30.26. Patient with large red tumor due to peripheral T cell lymphoma, unspecified. (From the Fitzsimons Army Medical Center Collection, Aurora, CO.)

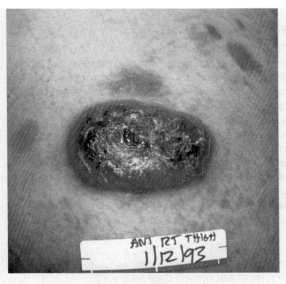

Fig. 30.27. Patient with large partially necrotic tumor diagnoses as primary cutaneous anaplastic large cell lymphoma. (From the Fitzsimons Army Medical Center Collection, Aurora, CO.)

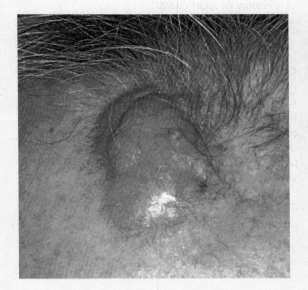

Fig. 30.28. Patient with large red nodule on the forehead, a primary cutaneous follicle center lymphoma. (From the William Weston Collection, Aurora, CO.)

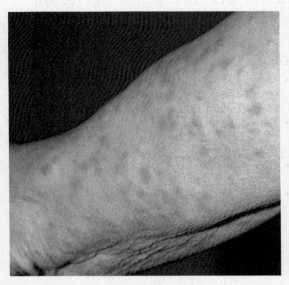

Fig. 30.29. Patient with numerous papules and small nodules in primary cutaneous marginal zone lymphoma. (From the Fitzsimons Army Medical Center Collection, Aurora, CO.)

⚠ Metastatic Tumors ICD10 code C49

MALIGNANT NEOPLASM

Pathogenesis

The incidence of malignancies becoming metastatic to involve the skin has varied in studies, but about 1% to 9% of persons with an internal malignancy will develop skin metastases. In most cases, skin metastases occur in later stages of disease. However, for some patients, it may be the presenting feature of a malignancy. Although most metastatic deposits involve the dermis, a subset of patients may present with deep subcutaneous nodules (see Chapter 35). Malignancies may arrive in the skin by lymphatic or vascular distribution, by surgical implantation, or by local extension. Certain cancers have a varying propensity to involve certain areas of the skin (see box).

Tumors Metastatic to Skin: Common Distribution Patterns
- Breast carcinoma—chest wall, scalp
- Cervical carcinoma—perineum
- Colon carcinoma—abdomen, umbilicus
- Gastric carcinoma—abdomen, umbilicus
- Lung carcinoma—chest wall, scalp
- Pancreatic carcinoma—umbilicus, scalp
- Ovarian carcinoma—umbilicus
- Prostate carcinoma—lower abdomen, perineum
- Renal carcinoma—scalp
- SCC, oropharyngeal—head, neck, shoulders

Clinical Features

- Metastatic deposits in the skin occur more often in elderly persons, simply because they are more likely to have internal malignancies.
- Cutaneous metastatic tumors may affect any region of the body, but different malignancies may have a special affinity for certain anatomic sites.
- Skin metastases may be solitary (Fig. 30.30) or numerous (Fig. 30.31).
- Skin metastases are usually asymptomatic, but pain may occur with nerve impingement or ulceration.

- Primary lesions vary from small papules to large nodules.
- Although most metastatic lesions are red or violaceous in color, some malignancies, such as melanoma, may demonstrate blue-black pigmentation (Fig. 30.32); others may simply appear skin-colored.
- Metastatic lesions may demonstrate an unremarkable overlying surface or may manifest ulceration or necrosis (Fig. 30.33; see Fig. 30.32).
- The patient may be cachectic due to the overall metastatic burden.

Diagnosis

- Metastatic tumors do not have a characteristic appearance, but the definitive diagnosis is established by deep punch, incisional, or excisional biopsy.
- It is critical to provide the pathologist and/or dermatopathologist with information regarding known internal malignancies so that a rapid, economical, accurate histologic diagnosis can be rendered.
- Findings that should arouse suspicion for a metastatic nodule to the skin include the following:
  - History of a known internal malignancy
  - History of rapid growth
  - History of rapid onset of multiple lesions
  - History of recent unexplained or involuntary weight loss

Clinical Course

Clearly, the clinical course of metastatic disease that secondarily involves the skin depends on the primary tumor and systemic treatment options available. In general, once a patient develops multiple metastatic deposits in the skin, the prognosis is poor, and most patients die from the primary malignancy within 2 years.

504

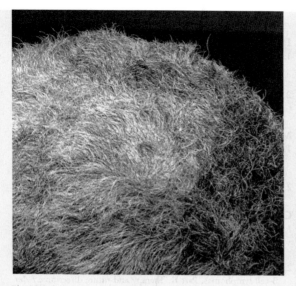

Fig. 30.30. Solitary, nondiagnostic violaceous papule on the scalp in a patient with adenocarcinoma of the lung. This is a common site for lung metastasis. (From the Fitzsimons Army Medical Center Collection, Aurora, CO.)

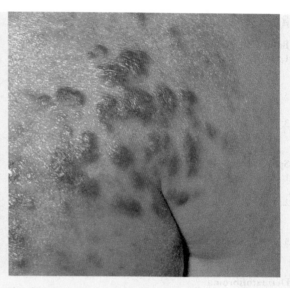

Fig. 30.31. Patient with numerous red papules and nodules of metastatic breast carcinoma of the chest wall and upper arm. (From the Fitzsimons Army Medical Center Collection, Aurora, CO.)

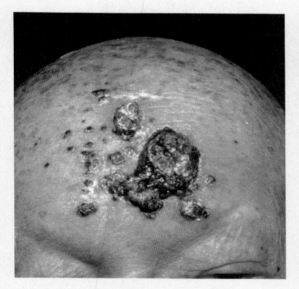

Fig. 30.32. Patient with metastatic melanoma demonstrating blue-black papules and nodules with variable necrosis. (From the Fitzsimons Army Medical Center Collection, Aurora, CO.)

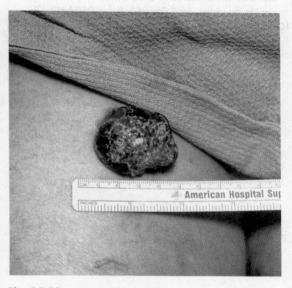

Fig. 30.33. Patient with a solitary, nondiagnostic necrotic tumor of the upper thigh, an atypical location for metastatic small cell carcinoma of the lung. (From the Walter Reed Army Medical Center Collection, Washington, DC.)

References

Basal Cell Carcinoma

1. Newlands C, Currie R, Memon A, et al. Non-melanoma skin cancer: United Kingdom National Multidisciplinary Guidelines. *J Laryngol Otol.* 2016;130(suppl 2):S125-S132.
2. Spates ST, Mellette JM Jr, Fitzpatrick JE. Metastatic basal cell carcinoma. *Dermatol Surg.* 2003;29:650-652.
3. Von Hoff DD, LoRusso PM, Rudin CM, et al. Inhibition of the hedgehog pathway in advanced basal cell carcinoma. *N Engl J Med.* 2009;361:1164-1172.

Spitz Nevus

1. Argenziano G, Agozzion M, Bonifazi E, et al. Natural evolution of Spitz nevi. *Dermatology.* 2011;222:256-260.
2. Luo S, Sepehr A, Tsao H. Spitz nevi and other Spitzoid lesions. Part I. Background and diagnosis. *J Am Acad Dermatol.* 2011;65:1073-1084.
3. Luo S, Sepehr A, Tsao H. Spitz nevi and other Spitzoid lesions. Part II. Natural history and management. *J Am Acad Dermatol.* 2011;65:1087-1092.

Dermatofibroma

1. Hui P, Glusac EJ, Sinard JH, Perkins AS. Clonal analysis of cutaneous fibrous histiocytoma (dermatofibroma). *J Cutan Pathol.* 2002;29:385-389.
2. Mentzel T, Jutzner H, Rütten A, Hügel H. Benign fibrous histiocytoma (dermatofibroma) of the face. Clinicopathologic and immunohistochemical study of 34 cases associated with aggressive clinical course. *Am J Dermatopathol.* 2001;23:419-426.

Keloid

1. Chike-Obi C, Cole PD, Brissett AE. Keloids: pathogenesis, clinical features, and management. *Semin Plast Surg.* 2009;23:174-184.

Dermatofibrosarcoma Protuberans

1. Han A, Chen EH, Niedt G, et al. Neoadjuvant imatinib therapy for dermatofibrosarcoma protuberans. *Arch Dermatol.* 2009;145:792-796.
2. Kalllini JR, Khachemoune A. Dermatofibrosarcoma protuberans: is Mohs surgery truly superior? And the success of tyrosinase kinase inhibitors. *J Drugs Dermatol.* 2014;13:1474-1477.

Merkel Cell Carcinoma

1. Heath M, Jaimes N, Lemos B, et al. Clinical characteristics of Merkel cell carcinoma at diagnosis in 195 patients: the AEIOU features. *J Am Acad Dermatol.* 2008;58:375-381.
2. Oram CW, Bartus CL, Purcell SM. Merkel cell carcinoma: a review. *Cutis.* 2016;97:290-295.

Cutaneous Lymphomas

1. Suárez AL, Pulitzer M, Horwitz S, et al. Primary cutaneous B-cell lymphomas. Part I. Clinical features, diagnosis, and classification. *J Am Acad Dermatol.* 2013;69:329-340.
2. Suárez AL, Querfeld C, Horwitz S, et al. Primary cutaneous B-cell lymphomas. Part II. Therapy and future directions. *J Am Acad Dermatol.* 2013;69:343-354.

Cutaneous Metastasis

1. Beachkofsky TM, Wisco OJ, Osswals SS, et al. Pulmonary cutaneous metastasis: a case report and review of common cutaneous metastases. *Cutis.* 2009;84:315-322.

Chapter 31
Pigmented Lesions

Key Terms

Solar Lentigo
  Lentigo senilis
  Lentigo solaris
Simple Lentigo
  Labial melanotic
    macules
  Lentigo simplex

Melanonychia striata
Simple lentigo
Acquired Melanocytic Nevus
  Acquired moles
  Acquired nevi
  Compound nevus
  Intradermal nevus
  Junctional nevus

Nevus Spilus
  Speckled lentiginous nevus
Atypical (Dysplastic) Nevus
  Atypical nevi
  Clark nevi
  Dysplastic nevi
Lentigo Maligna
  Hutchinson freckle

Pigmented lesions include not only melanocytic neoplasms, such as nevi and melanoma, but also some pigmented keratinocytic processes, such as pigmented seborrheic keratoses, and some hamartomas, such as a Becker nevus. The evaluation of pigmented lesions and hence, this chapter, is especially important because a delayed or missed diagnosis of melanoma may lead to morbidity, or even mortality, in a patient.

IMPORTANT HISTORY QUESTIONS

How long has this lesion been present?

This is an obvious but often overlooked inquiry. The patient's response may range from useful to uncertain to flat-out misleading. Moreover, the development of a "new" lesion is not indicative of only melanoma but it should prompt further inquiry and a more detailed examination of the lesion.

Has the lesion changed?

Any change in a melanocytic lesion should also prompt a more detailed and careful physical examination.

Has the lesion bled?

Benign lesions can be traumatized, with resultant bleeding, but an affirmative response should raise the index of suspicion with regard to cancer.

Do you have a history of an atypical dysplastic nevus or melanoma?

Persons with atypical nevi and/or past melanoma are at increased risk for melanoma.

Is there a family history of atypical nevi or melanoma?

There is a familial tendency to develop atypical moles, which increases one's personal risk of melanoma. Also, a first-degree relative with melanoma increases one's own risk of developing melanoma.

Do you have a history of indoor tanning bed use?

Tanning bed use is associated with an increased risk for melanoma, especially in less common areas, like the buttocks.

Have you ever had sunburn that produced blisters, and, if so, when did you burn?

Persons with multiple blistering sunburns, particularly in youth, are more likely to develop melanoma.

IMPORTANT PHYSICAL FINDINGS

What is the patient's skin type?

Persons with fair skin, blue eyes, and light-colored hair are more likely to develop melanoma. Persons with red hair have an elevated risk of melanoma, and melanoma in this population may be amelanotic.

How many moles does the patient have on his or her body?

A large number of nevi, whether atypical or dysplastic in appearance, or not, are at increased risk for melanoma. Most patients with an atypical/dysplastic nevus syndrome usually have more than 100 nevi.

Do any of the pigmented lesions on a patient's body look different from the rest?

Sometimes called the *ugly duckling sign*, it is always useful to identify any pigmented lesion that looks remarkably different from the patient's other pigmented lesions.

Do any of the pigmented lesions on a patient's body violate the ABCDEs of melanoma?

These are: *A,* asymmetry, *B,* border irregularity, *C,* color variegation (multiple colors), *D,* diameter more than 6 mm (about the size of a pencil eraser), and *E,* evolutionary behavior (e.g., growing, bleeding, itching, burning). This does not mean that anything that violates a component of the ABCDEs is melanoma, but it does indicate that such a lesion must be carefully evaluated, and possibly biopsied, to exclude melanoma.

Solar Lentigo ICD10 code L81.4

Pathogenesis

A solar lentigo, also referred to as *lentigo solaris* and *lentigo senilis*, results from hyperpigmentation of keratinocytes, with a slightly increased number of singular melanocytes. Lentigines are caused by increased cumulative ultraviolet (UV) light exposure. This latter characteristic explains the photodistribution of lentigines and the appearance of lentigines in later life. Although the term *liver spot* is occasionally used by laypersons, it is a term that should be discouraged because lentigines have nothing to do with liver disease.

Clinical Features

- Most solar lentigines occur in persons with fair skin.
- Solar lentigines occur on photoexposed skin, such as the head and neck, upper anterior chest, forearms, and dorsal hands.
- Solar lentigines are usually multiple and are associated with dermatoheliosis (sun-damaged skin).
- Solar lentigines are highly variable in size, ranging from 1 mm to larger than 1 cm.
- Solar lentigines exist as a round or oval macule or patch, which is tan to dark brown. Rare lesions may be black (Figs. 31.1–31.3).
- Solar lentigines are usually symmetric, but some irregularities may be present on occasion.

Diagnosis

- The occurrence of multiple, uniform, tan to brown macules and small patches on the sun-exposed skin of a fair-skinned person with sun damage is usually diagnostic.
- The differential diagnosis includes melanoma in situ (lentigo maligna type), which also occurs in older persons and on sun-damaged skin. In general, melanoma in situ (lentigo maligna type) is larger, with greater irregularity and with more variegated color.
- In problematic cases, a biopsy can be done to exclude melanoma in situ (lentigo maligna type).

Treatment

- No treatment is required for lentigines.
- Broad-spectrum sunscreen and other sun protective measures will lessen melanin production and prevent further sun damage.
- If ablation is desired, one can use liquid nitrogen cryotherapy, usually with only about a 5-second freeze to avoid overtreatment. Destructive therapy of pigmented lesions should be avoided unless the assessment of a benign condition is rendered with the utmost confidence.
- Lasers targeting melanin can be used in select cases, but this is generally done by a specialist.
- Chemical peels and topical bleaching formulations, such as 2% to 6% hydroquinone or 2% mequinol and 0.01% tretinoin (Solage) can be used, but, again, the assessment of benign lentigo must be made with the utmost confidence. Often bleaching from topical agents is incomplete.

Clinical Course

Solar lentigines, when confidently assessed, are benign and require no treatment. Lentigines can be difficult to differentiate from melanoma in situ (lentigo maligna type). Lentigines usually persist and may even increase in number over time with continued sun exposure.

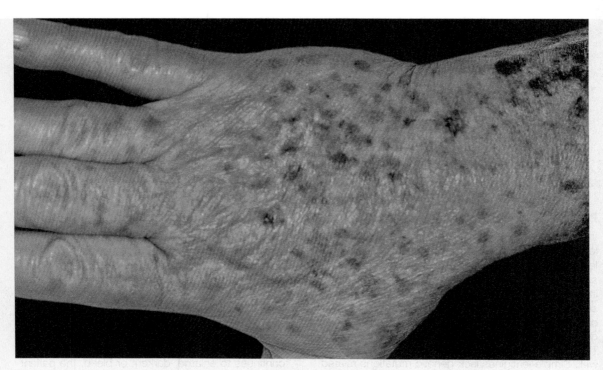

Fig. 31.1. Sun-damaged atrophic skin on the back of a patient's hand with numerous solar lentigines that vary in color from tan to brown to almost black. The area of more proximal discoloration represents solar purpura.

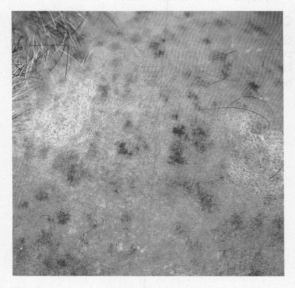

Fig. 31.2. Patient with sun-damaged atrophic skin on the scalp, with numerous solar lentigines that vary in color from tan to brown. The area of yellowish discoloration represents solar elastosis, and the inflamed scaly lesion is an actinic keratosis.

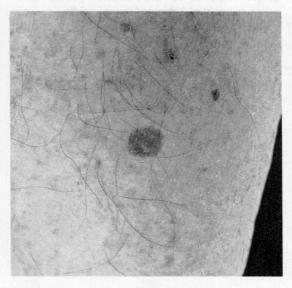

Fig. 31.3. Patient with mildly sun-damaged skin on the leg, with one brown, slightly scaly solar lentigo and a smaller solar lentigo.

Syndromes With Multiple Lentigines
- Carney complex: blue nevi, atrial myxomas, and endocrinopathies
- Centrofacial lentiginosis syndrome: lentigines, spina bifida, mental and learning disorders
- Leopard syndrome: electrocardiographic abnormalities, ocular hypertelorism, pulmonary stenosis, abnormalities of the genitalia, retardation of growth, deafness
- Peutz-Jeghers syndrome: intestinal polyposis

Pathogenesis

In contrast to a solar lentigo, a simple lentigo, or lentigo simplex, is unrelated to sun exposure. Simple lentigines are genetically predetermined and may be seen in some syndromes (see box). Simple lentigines, in contrast to solar lentigines, may occur on mucosal surfaces, such as the lips and genitalia, and are caused by increased melanocytes at the dermoepidermal junction, with increased production of melanin. There is often elongation of epidermal rete ridges as well. Simple lentigines lack genetic mutations related to UV light exposure.

Clinical Features
- Simple lentigines can arise at any age, but most cases occur in children and young adults.
- Simple lentigines can be solitary (Fig. 31.4) or multiple. When lesions are numerous, consider evaluation for a syndrome (Figs. 31.5–31.7).
- Simple lentigines can occur on any site, but the palms, soles, genitalia, and lips are common sites.

- Simple lentigines are usually uniform, round to oval macules, brown to black in color, about 1 to 4 mm in size. Rarely, larger lentigines exist.
- Oral mucosal lentigines are often called *labial melanotic macules*. Genital lentigines may occur as well. In the nail unit, a pigmented streak caused by a lentigo is referred to as *melanonychia striata*.

Diagnosis
- The homogeneous and banal character of simple lentigines is usually diagnostic.
- The differential diagnosis of simple lentigines includes junctional nevi and solar lentigines; the latter occurs on sun-damaged skin and in older persons.
- The diagnosis of a simple lentigo, particularly as distinguished from a junctional nevus or malignant melanocytic process, can be established by biopsy.

Treatment
- Simple lentigines, when confidently assessed, require no treatment and are benign entities.
- As with all pigmented proliferations, if the lesion continues to enlarge, darken, or bleed, the patient should return for re-evaluation considering the changing nature of the process.
- If removal is desired, a shave, punch, or excision biopsy is often the treatment of choice.

Clinical Course

Simple lentigines, like all melanocytic processes, could, in theory, progress to malignant melanoma, but the risk is extremely small. Simple lentigines are not considered premalignant.

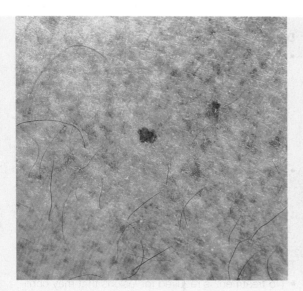

Fig. 31.4. Patient with slightly irregular simplex lentigo on sun-damaged skin. Simple lentigines can arise on sun-exposed skin or non–sun-exposed skin. This one was removed for histologic diagnosis.

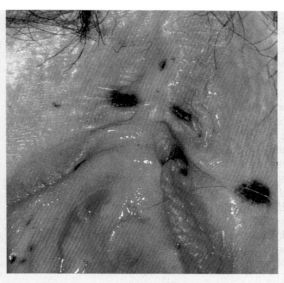

Fig. 31.5. Multiple genital lentigines in a woman with Carney complex. (From the Fitzsimons Army Medical Center Collection, Aurora, CO.)

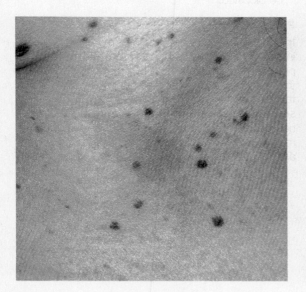

Fig. 31.6. Patient with centrofacial lentiginosis syndrome. Also present is a *café au lait* macule.

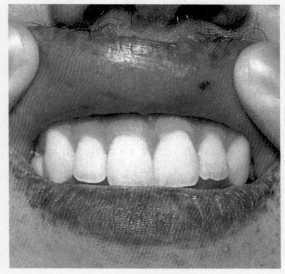

Fig. 31.7. Multiple lentigines on the lip and oral mucosa in a patient with Peutz-Jeghers syndrome. (From the Fitzsimons Army Medical Center Collection, Aurora, CO.)

Acquired Melanocytic Nevus ICD10 code D22 (site dependent)

Pathogenesis

Acquired melanocytic nevi, also known as *acquired nevi*, or acquired *"moles,"* are the most common of benign melanocytic neoplasms. Acquired nevi develop in early childhood and increase in number until adulthood, only to then regress, and decrease in number, in later adulthood. Several factors, including a family history of numerous nevi, light skin, light hair and eye color, and greater sun exposure in youth, are associated with increased nevi. In a longitudinal study of children in Colorado, at 8 years of age, boys had about 30 melanocytic nevi, whereas girls had about 25 melanocytic nevi. Pigmented melanocytic nevi may exhibit nests of cells only at the dermoepidermal junction (junctional nevus), only in the dermis (intradermal nevus), or in both locations (compound nevus). Intradermal nevi are not usually pigmented.

Clinical Features

- Acquired melanocytic nevi appear first in early childhood and increase in number until adulthood.
- Most junctional or compound nevi occur on skin that is intermittently or chronically sun-exposed.
- Junctional nevi are usually tan to black in color, 1 to 6 mm in size, and with a round or oval shape and sharp circumscription.
- Compound nevi are usually raised papules, tan to dark brown in color, with sharp circumscription and regular margins (Figs. 31.8–31.10). Their size is variable, with most compound nevi being between 2 and 8 mm in size, but larger compound nevi are not uncommon (see Fig. 31.10).
- Acral nevi tend to be junctional in nature and are often heavily pigmented (Fig. 31.11).
- Thickened dark hairs may be prominent in larger compound nevi.
- Melanocytic nevi may darken during pregnancy in response to elevated estrogen levels.

Diagnosis

- Most benign melanocytic nevi may be diagnosed based upon the clinical appearance, but sometimes it can be difficult to distinguish benign nevi from pigmented seborrheic keratoses or melanoma. When patients have multiple nevi, most tend to be roughly similar in appearance and size, and outliers should be treated with greater suspicion (the so-called "ugly duckling sign").
- If there is concern regarding a pigmented lesion, a deep shave, punch, or excisional biopsy should be performed. A punch biopsy or excision that removes the pigmented lesion completely allows the pathologist or dermatopathologist to examine the lesion in its entirety and prevents recurrences.

Treatment

- No treatment is required for lesions that may confidently be assessed as benign nevi.
- New or changing lesions, particularly those occurring after 40 years of age, unusually large lesions, irregular or inflamed lesions, and/or lesions substantially different from others on the body should be biopsied.

Prognosis

It is thought that melanocytic nevi regress or involute in the elderly. One study reported that by age 70 patients had an average of two melanocytic nevi on their bodies, although one author (WAH), who maintains a textbook on geriatric dermatology, and routinely sees older patients, believes this is exaggerated. It has been estimated that the rate of development of melanoma in a wholly benign nevus may be as low as 1:100,000/year.

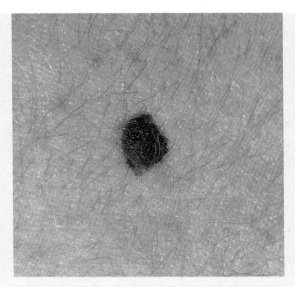

Fig. 31.8. Patient with a dark brown, relatively symmetric compound nevus. (From the Joanna Burch Collection, Aurora, CO.)

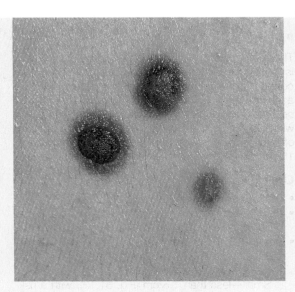

Fig. 31.9. Patient with two compound nevi with a fried egg appearance and a flat macular junctional nevus. (From the Joanna Burch Collection, Aurora, CO.)

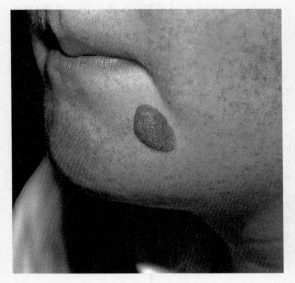

Fig. 31.10. Unusually large acquired, light brown, symmetric compound nevus. The patient also has numerous freckles. (From the Joanna Burch Collection, Aurora, CO.)

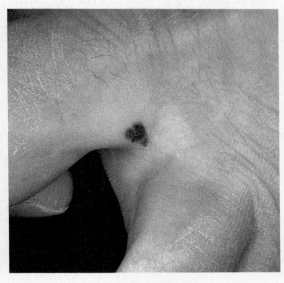

Fig. 31.11. Acquired acral junctional nevus in an adult, with an irregular outline. This lesion was removed for histologic examination. (From the Fitzsimons Army Medical Center Collection, Aurora, CO.)

Pathogenesis

The pathogenesis of congenital melanocytic nevi is poorly understood, but studies have suggested congenital melanocytic nevi behave differently from acquired melanocytic nevi. For example, acquired nevi are monoclonal populations of nevomelanocytes, whereas congenital melanocytic nevi are comprised of multiple clones. It has been estimated that about 1% to 5% of the population has a congenital nevus.

Clinical Features

- Congenital nevi are present at birth.
- Nevi that develop in the first 2 years of life may be called *congenital nevus–like* melanocytic nevi.
- A new classification system was proposed in 2013, but the former classification system is still the most widely used by most dermatologists:
  - Small—less than 1.5 cm (Fig. 31.12), with a risk of malignant degeneration equal to acquired nevi.
  - Medium—less than 1.5 to 19.9 cm (Fig. 31.13), with an elevated but imprecisely known risk of malignant degeneration.
  - Large (giant)—larger than 19.9 cm (Figs. 31.14 and 31.15), with an estimated rate of malignant degeneration of about 5% to 10%/lifetime.
- Large congenital nevi may demonstrate one or more smaller satellite lesions (see Fig. 31.15).
- Congenital nevi with satellite lesions, or those overlying the spine, are more likely to be associated with neurocutaneous melanosis, with hydrocephalus in two-thirds of patients, and with possible seizures.

Diagnosis

- The diagnosis of a congenital nevus is usually established on clinical and historical grounds.
- In some cases, a punch or incisional biopsy can be done for histologic examination, particularly if there is concern for malignant degeneration in a particular area.
- Some authorities recommend that brain or spinal magnetic resonance imaging (MRI) be performed in the setting of large congenital nevi because of the risk of central nervous system (CNS) involvement (neurocutaneous melanosis), but other authorities reasonably question the value of such imaging because there is no adequate treatment for neurocutaneous melanosis.

Treatment

- If any congenital nevus demonstrates changes in size, color, or shape, or if there is a new nodule, ulceration, or features of regression, the lesion must be examined by an expert. It is likely that a biopsy will be performed, which should be examined by a dermatopathologist with expertise in this area.
- There is no standardized management for congenital melanocytic nevi that are stable.
- For small and medium-sized lesions, it is often reasonable to adopt a wait and watch approach, instructing patients and family members to monitor lesions, in cooperation with a health care provider.
- Large or giant congenital nevi are problematic because of the definitive increased risk of malignant degeneration, yet prophylactic excision may be surgically problematic. Ultimately, the risks of general anesthesia in any surgical intervention(s) must be balanced against the risk for melanoma arising in the lesion.

Clinical Course

The risk of malignant melanoma arising in a congenital melanocytic nevus is difficult to calculate with certitude for any individual lesion. Older classification schemes fostered this imprecision due to wide ranges in category sizes, but in general, the larger the lesion, the higher the risk of malignant degeneration. The lifetime risk for malignant melanoma developing in a giant congenital nevus may be as high as 5% to 10%. The risk for medium-sized congenital nevi, and even small congenital nevi, is clearly lower, but studies have reported conflicting data.

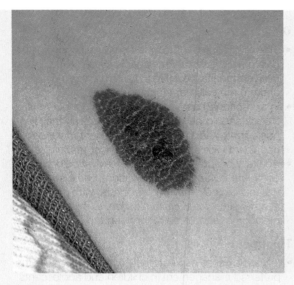

Fig. 31.12. Small oval congenital nevus on the upper thigh of an infant. The smaller, darker papule should be carefully monitored for change.

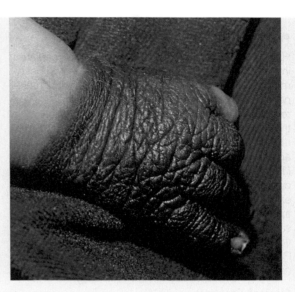

Fig. 31.13. Patient with a medium-sized congenital nevus of the hand. (From the Fitzsimons Army Medical Center Collection, Aurora, CO.)

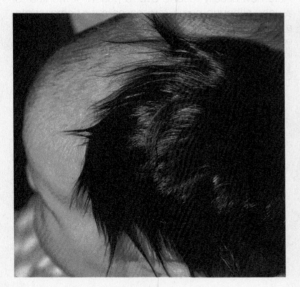

Fig. 31.14. Patient with a giant congenital nevus of the scalp, with enlarged dark hairs. (From the Joanna Burch Collection, Aurora, CO.)

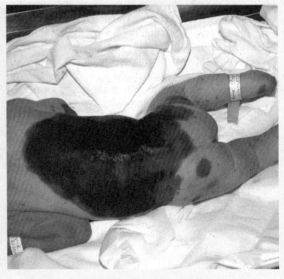

Fig. 31.15. Patient with a giant congenital nevus, with numerous smaller satellite congenital nevi. (From the William Weston Collection, Aurora, CO.)

Pathogenesis

Halo nevi (Sutton nevi) are caused by a cell-mediated inflammatory response directed against nested nevomelanocytes and adjacent junctional epidermal melanocytes. Microscopic examination of a halo nevus reveals a dense infiltrate of lymphocytes surrounding these nests, with a loss of melanocytes at the dermoepidermal junction in the clinically depigmented areas. Research completed by two of the authors (JEF, WAH) showed that normal acquired melanocytic nevi are "immunologically invisible" and do not express human leukocyte antigen (HLA) markers that trigger a host response. For reasons unknown, these same HLA markers are expressed in halo nevi, and this engenders an immunologic response in the host. Patients with vitiligo are more likely to develop halo nevi.

Clinical Features

- Halo nevi usually develop in children and adolescents, although adults may also develop them. There is no predilection for sex or ethnic background.
- Halo nevi are most common on the back (Fig. 31.16).
- Halo nevi usually develop in acquired melanocytic nevi and may be solitary or multiple.
- Early halo nevi consists of skin-colored, tan, or brown papules (Fig. 31.17), with a sharply demarcated area that is depigmented (white skin).
- Mature halo nevi demonstrate loss of the central nevus and replacement with a discrete, round to oval area of depigmentation (white skin).

Diagnosis

- The clinical presentation is usually diagnostic of a halo nevus, but other melanocytic lesions (e.g., blue nevi, congenital nevi [Fig. 31.18], atypical nevi, melanoma) may also demonstrate a halo.
- In exceptional cases, particularly in older persons, a biopsy should be performed to establish the diagnosis firmly and to exclude a malignant melanocytic neoplasm with an inflammatory host response.
- Adults who present with halo nevi should have a complete cutaneous examination, because in rare cases, halo nevi may be associated with melanoma at other sites. An eye examination, to exclude ocular melanoma, should be recommended.

Treatment

- In classic cases no treatment is necessary and is the preferred management in children and adolescents.
- Atypical-appearing halo nevi can be surgically removed. The biopsy only needs to include the central papule and not the entire halo.

Clinical Course

Halo nevi usually resolve over a period of months to a year, although some rare cases may demonstrate a halo that persists for more than a decade. Some cases demonstrate a recurrence of the nevus that incited the halo phenomenon.

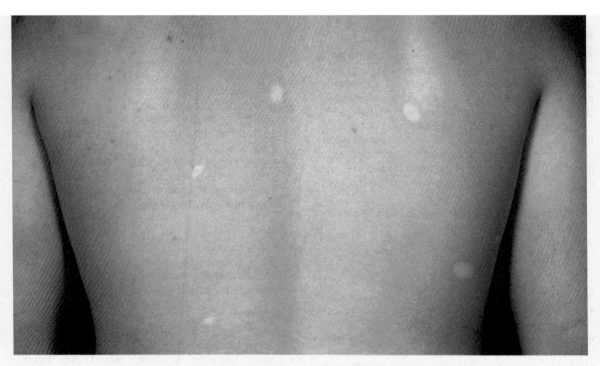

Fig. 31.16. Multiple halo nevi on the back of an adolescent. The back is the most common location of halo nevi. (From the Fitzsimons Army Medical Center Collection, Aurora, CO.)

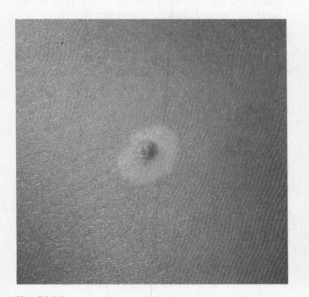

Fig. 31.17. Close-up of a halo nevus demonstrating a slightly pink halo. Pink or reddish tints are more commonly seen in new lesions. (From the Fitzsimons Army Medical Center Collection, Aurora, CO.)

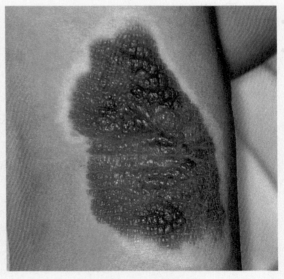

Fig. 31.18. Patient with a congenital halo nevus. (From the William Weston Collection, Aurora, CO.)

Café au Lait Spot ICD10 code L81.4

Pathogenesis

A *café au lait* macule (CALM) is a sharply demarcated area of uniform hyperpigmentation that is present at birth or develops in early childhood. Despite the analogy to coffee with milk, the color can be even darker brown, particularly in persons with darker skin. CALMs are common and are seen in about 10% of the population. The pathogenesis of CALMs is poorly understood. Histologically, CALMs are characterized by a normal number of melanocytes but with increased and abnormally packaged melanosomes.

Syndromes With Multiple *Café au Lait* Spots
- McCune-Albright syndrome
- Neurofibromatosis type I
- Watson syndrome

Clinical Features
- CALMs are present as birth or develop during early childhood.
- CALMs may be solitary or multiple and are most common on the trunk and pelvic girdle.
- CALMs vary in size from less than 1 mm to more than 40 cm in size.
- Smaller CALMs are usually ovoid, whereas larger CALMs often have more irregular borders.
- CALMs vary in color from light tan (Fig. 31.19) to brown (Fig. 31.20).
- CALMs do not have surface changes, color variegation, or increased or enlarged hairs.
- CALMs are associated with three important syndromes:
  - McCune-Albright syndrome: one or more CALMs are present, often unilaterally, and the lesions often possess irregular borders (so-called coast of Maine). Patients may also have unilateral polyostotic fibrous dysplasia or endocrinopathies.
  - Neurofibromatosis type I: typically six or more CALMs with smooth borders (so-called coast of California) that are more than 5 mm in size (Fig. 31.21) or small CALMs in the axillae (incorrectly called *freckling*). This latter finding is called *Crowe sign* (Fig. 31.22).
  - Watson syndrome: CALMs associated with pulmonary valve stenosis, short stature, and low intelligence. Patients with Watson syndrome may also manifest Crowe sign.

Diagnosis
- The diagnosis of a CALM is established by the clinical appearance.
- Biopsies are not usually performed because the histologic findings are not easily recognized.

Treatment
- CALMs require no intervention unless treatment is desired for cosmetic purposes.
- Lasers targeting pigment: pulsed dye lasers, frequency-doubled Nd:YAG lasers, and Q-switched alexandrite lasers may be used to lighten CALMs. There is typically a varied response to laser treatment, and also there is potential for scarring, undesired pigmentary alteration, and recurrence.

Clinical Course

Once present, CALMs persist indefinitely, but do not have any known malignant potential.

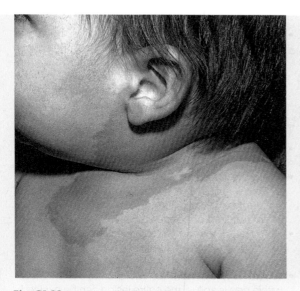

Fig. 31.19. Patient with a large *café au lait* spot of the ear, face, neck, and chest. (From the William Weston Collection, Aurora, CO.)

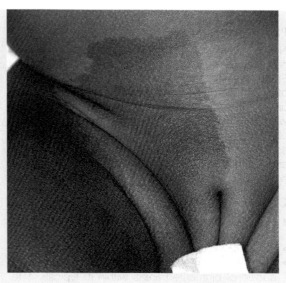

Fig. 31.20. Despite the name, *café au lait* spots can be brown, especially in patients with darker skin color or in McCune-Albright syndrome. (From the Joanna Burch Collection, Aurora, CO.)

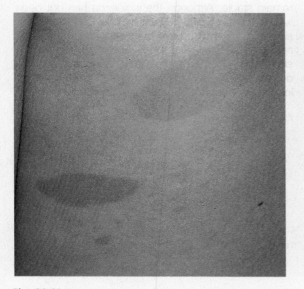

Fig. 31.21. Patient with two *café au lait* spots larger than 5 mm. Note that there are also two smaller lesions that would not meet the criteria for establishing a diagnosis of neurofibromatosis type I.

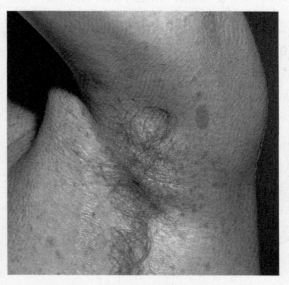

Fig. 31.22. Crowe sign in a patient with neurofibromatosis type I. (From the Fitzsimons Army Medical Center Collection, Aurora, CO.)

Nevus Spilus

Pathogenesis

Nevus spilus, also known as a speckled lentiginous nevus, is a relatively common melanocytic lesion. Epidemiologic studies have reported a prevalence of 1.3% and 2.1% among all persons. Nevus spilus usually presents as a tan macule, similar to a CALM, with other multiple, more intense accumulations of pigmentation. Most cases of nevus spilus present first as a CALM that gradually develops more pigmented areas over time. The pathogenesis of nevus spilus is not well understood.

Clinical Features

- Nevus spilus may be present at birth, usually as a CALM, but may not be evident until childhood.
- Nevus spilus may involve any site of the body.
- Months to years after birth, the CALM will develop additional pigmented areas within it, typically 1 to 3 mm in size (Figs. 31.23–31.25). The speckles may be flat macular or may be elevated, indicative of a junctional or compound nevus. Less often, other types of melanocytic leisons arise within the nevus spilus, including Spitz nevi and atypical nevi.
- The size of lesions can vary from less than 1 cm to more than 30 cm, and lesions may even have a zosteriform pattern (Fig. 31.26).

Diagnosis

- The clinical presentation of nevus spilus, with a tan macule and speckled hyperpigmentation, is rather distinctive. This same pattern may be mimicked by some congenital nevi, but the distinction is somewhat moot because some dermatologists consider nevus spilus to be a subset of congenital nevi.

- Rare cases may require a biopsy, but it is imperative that the clinician doing the biopsy convey the clinical impression of nevus spilus, by description or by an attached photograph, so that the pathologist or dermatopathologist is better prepared to recognize the asymmetric and sometimes subtle findings.

Treatment

- Nevus spilus is a benign lesion, and no treatment is required.
- There are cases of a malignant melanoma arising in nevus spilus, but this is a rare event, and the occurrence is no different from melanoma arising in an acquired or congenital nevus.
- Removal of the darker speckled areas, by punch excision, may render the lesion less obvious, but it can also lead to scarring or surgical complications.
- Where atypical nevi (or melanoma) have arisen within nevus spilus, the entire lesion can be excised.
- Anecdotally, other treatment options have included laser therapy or intense pulsed light therapy.

Clinical Course

Once well established, nearly all nevus spilus lesions remain stable. Although the incidence has not been well studied, atypical (dysplastic) nevi, melanoma in situ, and melanoma have been reported to occur in select cases of nevus spilus. Therefore, the patient should be educated to note any changes in a previously stable nevus spilus and report these changes immediately so that a biopsy can be considered.

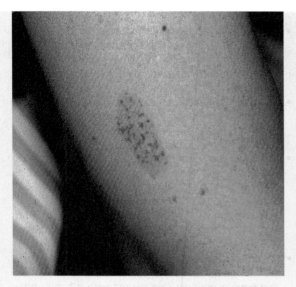

Fig. 31.23. Patient with nevus spilus demonstrating a sharply circumscribed *café au lait* macule, with numerous areas of speckled pigmentation. (From the Joanna Burch Collection, Aurora, CO.)

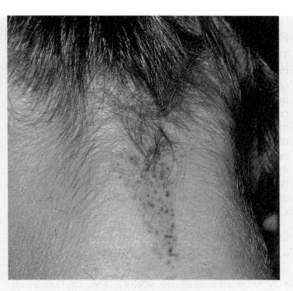

Fig. 31.24. Patient with nevus spilus of the neck demonstrating a sharply circumscribed *café au lait* macule, with numerous areas of speckled pigmentation. (From the William Weston Collection, Aurora, CO.)

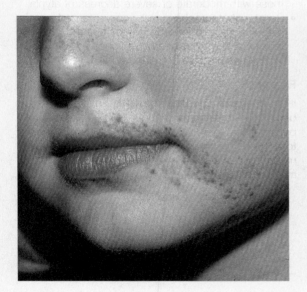

Fig. 31.25. Patient with a larger nevus spilus of the face involving cutaneous surface of the upper and lower lips. (From the William Weston Collection, Aurora, CO.)

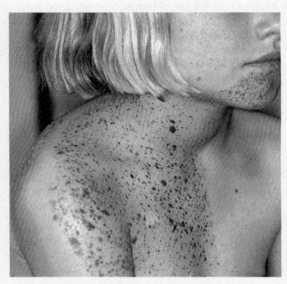

Fig. 31.26. Patient with a giant nevus spilus, with a zosteriform distribution. (From the William Weston Collection, Aurora, CO.)

Atypical (Dysplastic) Nevus ICD10 code D48.5

Pathogenesis

The terminology surrounding atypical nevi is not standardized. Alternative nosology includes dysplastic nevi, Clark nevi, and nevi with cytologic atypia and architectural disorder. The pathogenesis of atypical nevi is poorly understood. It is likely that the development of atypical nevi involves a complex interaction of genetic factors and sunlight exposure. In about one-third of patients with familial atypical moles and melanoma syndrome (FAMMM syndrome), there are germline *CDKN2A* mutations. The pathogenesis of other forms of familial atypical nevi and sporadic atypical nevi is poorly established.

Clinical Features

- Atypical nevi usually appear first in adolescence or early adulthood.
- Atypical nevi may be solitary, few, or numerous (>200).
- The trunk is usually affected by atypical nevi, especially the back (Fig. 31.27). The chest, abdomen, and proximal extremities may also be involved. Sun-protected sites, such as the buttocks, often have fewer atypical nevi.
- Atypical nevi are usually larger than common banal nevi, with most of them being more than 5 mm in diameter (Figs. 31.28–31.30).
- Atypical nevi are highly variable in appearance. The same ABCDE criteria used to distinguish melanoma from banal nevi also characterize atypical nevi:
  - A—asymmetry
  - B—border irregularity
  - C—color variegation
  - D—diameter greater than 6 mm
  - E—evolutionary behavior (e.g., changing, itching)

Diagnosis

- Assessment of any particular nevus as clinically atypical is established by the physical examination.

- Familial atypical nevus syndromes are established through physical exam and queries regarding a personal and/or family history of melanoma. Melanoma in a first-degree relative (parent, sibling, child) is considered significant.
- Histologic assessement of an atypical nevus, and exclusion of melanoma, occurs by biopsy.

Treatment

- The treatment of atypical nevi is not standardized. In persons with numerous clinically atypical nevi, a dermatologist may biopsy only those with a history of change, or only those with an appearance considerably different from others (the "ugly duckling sign"). The biopsy technique used may vary based on the clinical situation.
- Patients with sporadic or familial atypical nevus syndromes need to be educated in self-examination and have a periodic skin exams with a health professional (usually every 6–12 months).
- The management of biopsy-proven atypical nevi with involved surgical margins is not standardized. Some dermatologists remove all atypical nevi completely, whereas others completely remove only those with moderate or severe degrees of atypia.
- Serial photographs and computerized mole mapping have been advocated, but the utility of these measures has been questioned by some. The techniques are also not standardized.

Prognosis

It has been estimated that the risk of an atypical nevus becoming a melanoma is about 1:10,000 per year. In patients with sporadic atypical nevi, there may be up to a 15-fold elevated lifetime increased risk of melanoma. In patients with FAMMM syndrome, the risk may be increased 200- to 1200-fold.

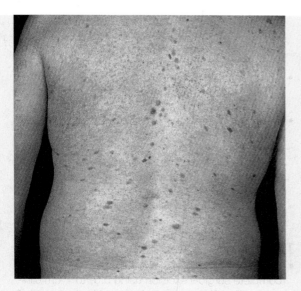

Fig. 31.27. Patient with familial atypical moles and melanoma syndrome demonstrating numerous atypical nevi on the back. (From the Fitzsimons Army Medical Center Collection, Aurora, CO.)

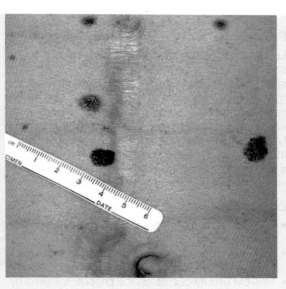

Fig. 31.28. Patient with multiple atypical nevi, with many of them being more than 6 mm. Some of the lesions are concerning for melanoma.

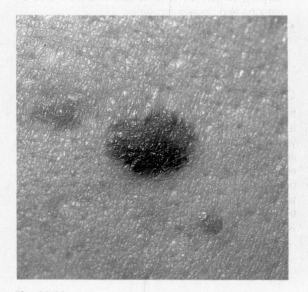

Fig. 31.29. Patient with an atypical nevus demonstrating asymmetric distribution of pigment. This lesion was removed and diagnosed as a "compound nevus with mild cytologic atypia and architectural disorder." (From the Fitzsimons Army Medical Center Collection, Aurora, CO.)

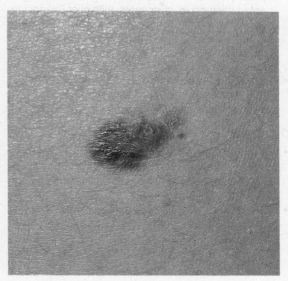

Fig. 31.30. Patient with a severely atypical nevus that is large and asymmetric, with irregular contours, and multiple colors, including shades of brown, tan, and red. (From the Joanna Burch Collection, Aurora, CO.)

☝ Lentigo Maligna   ICD10 code D03 (site dependent)

Pathogenesis

Lentigo maligna, eponymously known as a *Hutchinson freckle*, is a form of melanoma in situ that is strongly associated with cumulative exposure to UV light. Some dermatopathologists eschew use of the term *lentigo maligna* and refer to all cases as melanoma in situ or melanoma in situ, lentigo maligna type (MIS-LM), simply to convey the seriousness of the diagnosis and avoid confusion with a solar lentigo, a benign condition. Epidemiologic evidence demonstrates that the incidence of MIS-LM is increasing.

Clinical Features

- MIS-LM occurs in late middle-aged and elderly patients (most patients are >60 years).
- MIS-LM occurs chiefly in light-skinned individuals with a strong history of outside work (e.g., farmers).
- MIS-LM usually occurs on the cheeks, followed by other areas of the head and neck, upper chest, forearms, and dorsal hands.
- Early MIS-LM appears as a small tan to brown to black macule that may be difficult to distinguish from a solar lentigo (Fig. 31.31).
- Typically, MIS-LM involves slow progressive enlargement of the macule, over years, with ever-increasing irregularities in margin (irregular or notched borders) and in color variegation (Figs. 31.32 and 31.33). Even black (Fig. 31.34), gray, or white (regression) colors may be present over time.
- It is not uncommon for MIS-LM to darken progressively over time, often with an asymmetric growth pattern also identified.

Diagnosis

- A progressively enlarging pigmented macule, with irregular pigment and an irregular margin, occurring on sun-exposed skin in an elderly patient suggests MIS-LM.
- It is important to remember that early MIS-LM may be difficult to distinguish from a solar lentigo, but,

with time, and with serial examination, MIS-LM may become the so-called "ugly duckling" when compared to other solar lentigines.
- The presence of a papule or nodule in suspected MIS-LM should raise concern for invasion (lentigo maligna melanoma).
- The biopsy technique used to establish the diagnosis should vary based upon the clinical situation. In general, if there is concern for invasion, a large punch biopsy (encompassing all or most of the lesion) or an incision or excision should be performed. If the lesion is flat, a deeper shave biopsy might also be considered, especially if a large swath can be encaptured.

Treatment

- For biopsy-proven MIS-LM, the standard of care is complete surgical excision using 0.5- to 1-cm clinical margins. Removal by micrographically controlled (Mohs) surgery is also an option.
- Topical imiquimod has been used in case reports and small series, but generally this is used only in select situations, such as when the patient refuses surgery, surgery is not an option, or there are other reasons (e.g., age, infirmity).
- Select cases can be treated with cryotherapy for many of the same reasons that topical imiquimod might be employed, but this should be done only by physicians with expertise in the technique.

Clinical Course

It is speculated that MIS-LM usually demonstrates a prolonged radial growth phase, perhaps 10 to 20 years or longer, before becoming invasive. A definitive study will never be performed, but it has been estimated that perhaps 50% to 95% of cases will not become invasive in an elderly person's remaining lifetime. However, once extension into the dermis occurs, the prognosis is similar to other types of melanoma when adjusted for Breslow depth.

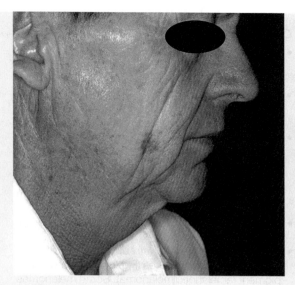

Fig. 31.31. Early tan-brown irregular pigmented macule on sun-damaged skin that was found to be a lentigo maligna by biopsy. (From the Fitzsimons Army Medical Center Collection, Aurora, CO.)

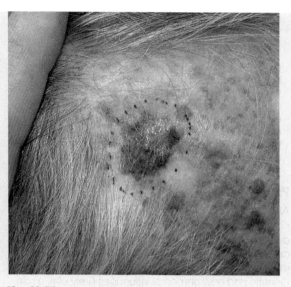

Fig. 31.32. Lentigo maligna at the scalp margin in severely sun-damaged skin. Note that the patient has numerous solar lentigines for comparison.

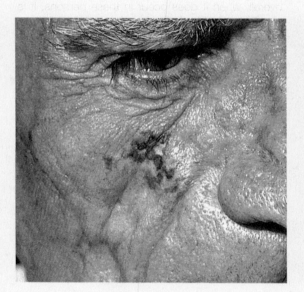

Fig. 31.33. Patient with lentigo maligna demonstrating several areas of spontaneous regression. (From the Fitzsimons Army Medical Center Collection, Aurora, CO.)

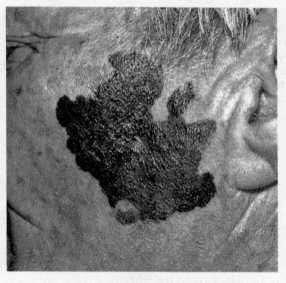

Fig. 31.34. Patient with a neglected lentigo maligna demonstrating a large size and variegation in color. (From the Fitzsimons Army Medical Center Collection, Aurora, CO.)

Are Tanning Beds Safe?

This question is impossible to assess with a randomized prospective trial. An epidemiologic study in the United Kingdom estimated that 370 of the 6000 melanomas seen each year could be attributed to tanning bed exposure. Thus, about 100 patients in the UK die every year due to tanning bed use. Although sun exposure likely remains a main contributory factor for melanoma, tanning bed use increases one's risk of melanoma.

Pathogenesis

Although it is not the most common form of skin cancer, melanoma accounts for 80% of skin cancer deaths. Missed melanoma is among the most common causes of malpractice litigation. The pathogenesis of melanoma is complex and incompletely characterized. Genetic and environmental influences likely play a role, with UV light being an important determinant. Studies have suggested that intermittent exposure to sunlight, and in particular severe (blistering) sunburns in childhood, are associated with melanoma. Most cases of melanoma are sporadic, but about 8% of patients with melanoma will have a first-degree relative with melanoma. The most important genes linked to familial melanoma are *CDKN2A*, *CDK4*, *POT1*, and *TERT*. Heritable mutations in *CDKN2A* are also involved in an increased risk for pancreatic cancer. Melanoma is seen with increased frequency in xeroderma pigmentosum and in patients with the hereditary breast cancer gene, *BRCA2*.

Who Gets Melanoma?

Risk factors for the development of melanoma include the following:

- History of frequent sunburns, particularly blistering sunburns
- History of sunburns as an infant or child
- Multiple nevi (the more nevi, the higher the risk)
- Personal history of atypical nevi
- Personal history of melanoma
- Family history of melanoma (may indicate familial atypical mole syndrome)
- Fair skin, freckling, and light hair
- Immunocompromised patients (less important than the aforementioned factors)

Clinical Features

- Melanoma can arise on normal skin or mucosa, on sun-exposed skin, or within benign nevi, congenital nevi, nevi spilus, blue nevi, or atypical nevi.
- In comparison to common nevi, melanomas are usually larger, with irregular borders, asymmetry, color variegation, and a history of growth or change.
- It is thought that early melanoma usually manifests with horizontal growth (Figs. 31.35 and 31.36), and later there is transition to invasive vertical growth (Figs. 31.37 and 31.38). However, some melanomas can begin with nodular or vertical growth from inception.
- Regression is often a feature of melanoma (see Fig. 31.37).
- Melanoma can present with ulceration and bleeding, papillomatous features (Fig. 31.39), or no visible pigment (amelanotic melanoma). Some melanomas may resemble a scar (desmoplastic melanoma).
- Melanomas can arise on acral surfaces (Fig. 31.40), beneath the nail plate (Fig. 31.41), in the oral cavity (Fig. 31.42), or in periocular or perianal locations. Although blacks are less likely to develop melanoma overall, when it does occur in these persons, it is usually located in the oral cavity, on acral skin, or beneath the nail plate.

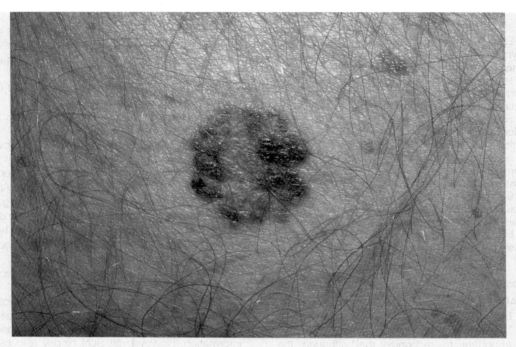

Fig. 31.35. Patient with an early, superficial, spreading melanoma. (From the Fitzsimons Army Medical Center Collection, Aurora, CO.)

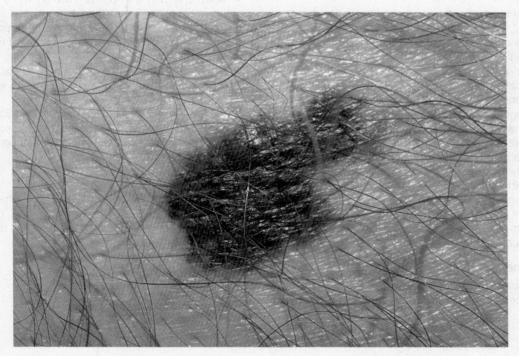

Fig. 31.36. Patient with a superficial spreading melanoma, with an abnormal notch. (From the Fitzsimons Army Medical Center Collection, Aurora, CO.)

ABCDEs of Melanoma

- **A**symmetry
  When a line is drawn through the center of the lesion, the two halves are not symmetric.
- **B**order irregularity
  Melanoma usually demonstrates an irregular or notched border.
- **C**olor variegation
  Multiple colors, or great variations in shades, are a disconcerting finding.
- **D**iameter
  Most (but not all) melanomas are more than 6 mm in diameter.
- **E**volutionary behavior
  Changing lesions (e.g., changing colors and/or size, bleeding, itching) are a point of concern and should prompt more careful evaluation.

Diagnosis

- The ABCDEs of melanoma are useful for assessment by health care providers and by patients (see box).
- It is important to recognize that although the ABCDEs will help identify many melanomas, not all melanomas will be identified with these criteria. Moreover, the criteria overlap with those of atypical nevi.
- A useful diagnostic concept is the "ugly duckling sign." When examining the patient holistically, a melanoma may stand out as different from the patient's other nevi. This should prompt consideration of a biopsy.
- If a patient reports change in a melanocytic lesion, this should be taken seriously, and consideration of a biopsy should transpire.
- A shave, punch, or incisional biopsy does not adversely affect the metastatic potential of melanoma. If concern for melanoma is high, and if surgically feasible, the entirety of the pigmented lesion should be sampled. This affords the pathologist or dermatopathologist with the best opportunity to make an accurate diagnosis. Partial capture of a lesion by biopsy may make it difficult to stage a melanoma accurately.

Treatment

- Surgical excision of melanoma is the treatment of choice, and it is dependent on the depth of invasion.

Whereas anatomic considerations sometimes affect surgery, typically the following margins are utilized:
- Melanoma in situ—0.5- to 1.0-cm clinical margins should be employed.
- Melanoma 1.0 mm or less in depth—a 1.0-cm clinical margin should be employed.
- Melanoma 1.01 to 2.0 mm in depth—a 1- to 2-cm clinical margin should be employed.
- Melanoma 2.0 mm or larger—a 2-cm clinical margin should be employed.
- Clinical and histologic features are used to stage melanoma patients according to American Joint Commission on Cancer (AJCC) guidelines. Staging information can be found at the American Cancer Society website: http://www.cancer.org/cancer/skincancer-melanoma/detailedguide/melanoma-skin-cancer-stages. New AJCC guidelines (8th edition) will take effect on January 1, 2018.
- Sentinel lymph node (SLN) biopsy has not yet been proven to afford a therapeutic advantage, but the procedure can provide important prognostic information. However, an SLN biopsy also carries normal surgical risks with it (e.g., complications of anesthesia, infection, lymphedema), so it is generally considered only in some situations:
  - Melanoma with a depth of invasion more than 1 mm but typically less than 4 mm,
  - Melanoma of 0.76 to 1.00 mm in depth, particularly if there are dermal mitotic figures (pT1b) or other concerning features.
  - Use of SLN biopsy may be affected by the new 8th edition of the AJCC, which will take effect January 1, 2018.
  - The MSLT-II trial, released in June 2017, indicated no survival advantage for complete lymph node detection in patients with an involved sentinel lymph node.

Clinical Course

The American Cancer Society has estimated that for 2017, there will be 87,110 new melanomas diagnosed, and about 9,730 people will die from melanoma ($\approx$6380 men and 3350 women).

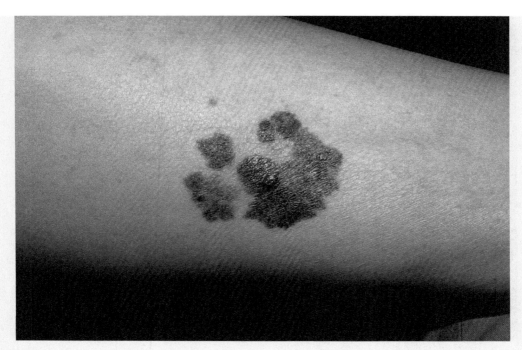

Fig. 31.37. Patient with a superficial spreading melanoma, with regression and an early nodule. (From the Fitzsimons Army Medical Center Collection, Aurora, CO.)

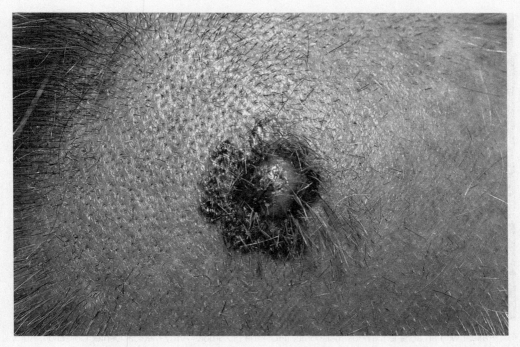

Fig. 31.38. Patient with a superficial spreading melanoma of the scalp that has developed a large nodular component. (From the Fitzsimons Army Medical Center Collection, Aurora, CO.)

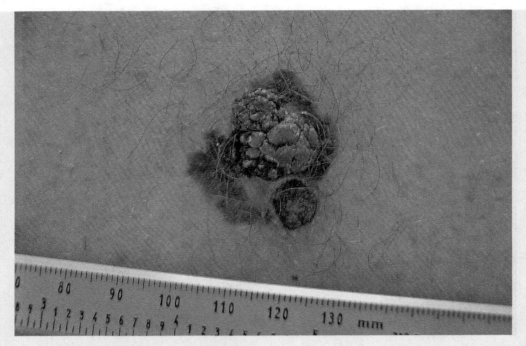

Fig. 31.39. Patient with a superficial spreading melanoma with friable exophytic papillomatous nodule arising in patient with multiple atypical nevi. Note the presence of multiple colors.

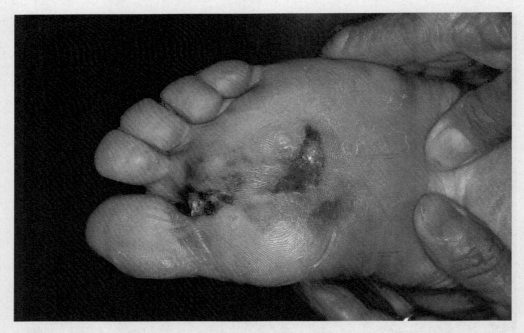

Fig. 31.40. Patient with an acral lentiginous melanoma. (From the Fitzsimons Army Medical Center Collection, Aurora, CO.)

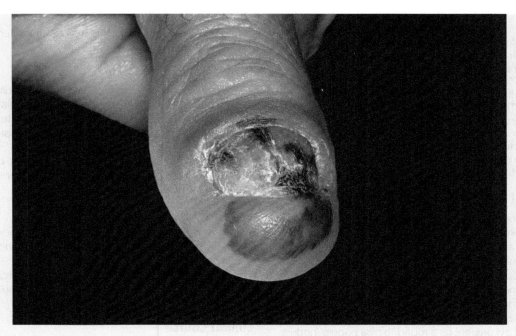

Fig. 31.41. Patient with a subungual melanoma demonstrating pigmentation of the nail plate (Hutchinson sign), nail dystrophy, and extension onto the skin of the thumb. (From the Fitzsimons Army Medical Center Collection, Aurora, CO.)

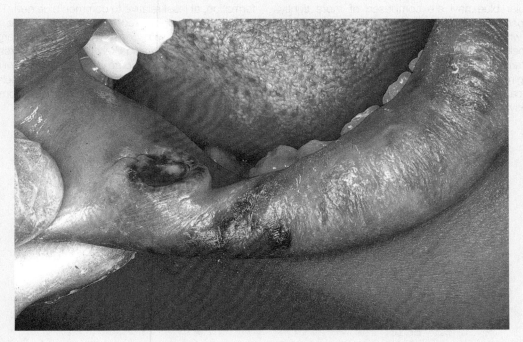

Fig. 31.42. Fatal oral melanoma of the lip and buccal mucosa in a black patient. (From the Fitzsimons Army Medical Center Collection, Aurora, CO.)

Why Are Blue Nevi Blue?

Many have asked, "How does melanin, a brown pigment, create the distinct blue hue of a blue nevus?" The answer lies in the incoherent scattering, also called *Rayleigh scattering* or the *Tyndall effect*. The depositions of small agglomerations of melanin between collagen bundles in the dermis lead to incoherent scattering of reflected light, with production of definite blue hues from these dermal melanocytic processes, such as blue nevi. The sky and the ocean appear blue for similar reasons.

Clinical Features

- Blue nevi may be congenital or acquired.
- Acquired blue nevi usually appear in childhood or in early adulthood.
- Blue nevi are more common in women and in individuals with a darker skin type.
- Blue nevi are usually solitary but may be multiple.
- Blue nevi are most common on the dorsal hands and feet, followed by the face and trunk.
- Blue nevi present as a round to oval papule, nodule, or plaque, of varied size, with a blue to blue-black hue, although some variants may demonstrate shades of gray, brown, or white (Figs. 31.43–31.45).
- Cellular blue nevi are composed of more tightly apposed fusiform melanocytes with lesser melanin, whereas epithelioid blue nevi are composed of epithelioid-appearing melanocytes. The latter is seen in Carney complex, a disorder that also includes lentigines, atrial myxomas, and endocrinopathies.
- Clinical variants of blue nevi include agminated or eruptive blue nevi (Fig. 31.46), giant blue nevi, and targetoid blue nevi, targetoid lesions that alternate blue and white colors.

Diagnosis

- The clinical appearance of blue nevi is usually diagnostic, although the differential diagnosis can include a traumatic (graphite or carbon) tattoo, malignant melanoma, and pigmented basal cell carcinoma.
- Problematic lesions can be removed and/or biopsied with a punch or incisional/excisional biopsy to establish the diagnosis.

Treatment

- Blue nevi are benign, and no treatment is required when the diagnosis is rendered with confidence.
- Surgical removal using an appropriately sized punch or scalpel excision is possible, if desired. Shave biopsies are not advised because blue nevi are often deeply situated.

Clinical Course

Common blue nevi do not manifest an increased risk for malignant degeneration. However, cellular blue nevi may harbor an increased risk of malignant transformation, at least relative to common blue nevi. Thus, many dermatologists recommend that cellular blue nevi be excised with conservative surgical margins. Epithelioid blue nevi also likely possess an increased risk of melanoma, and some epithelioid blue nevi may overlap with so-called "pigmented epithelioid melanocytoma," a controversial entity considered by some to be a low-grade form of melanoma.

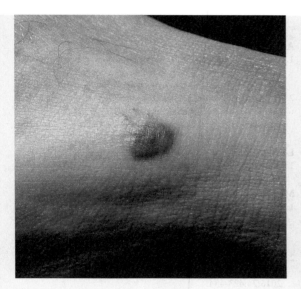

Fig. 31.43. Patient with a common blue nevus demonstrating a characteristic blue color. (From the Fitzsimons Army Medical Center Collection, Aurora, CO.)

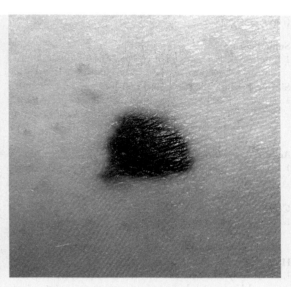

Fig. 31.44. Patient with a common blue nevus, with shades of blue and black. (From the Fitzsimons Army Medical Center Collection, Aurora, CO.)

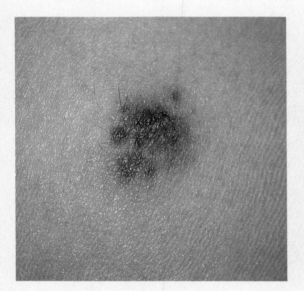

Fig. 31.45. Patient with a large speckled blue nevus, with shades of gray, blue, and black.

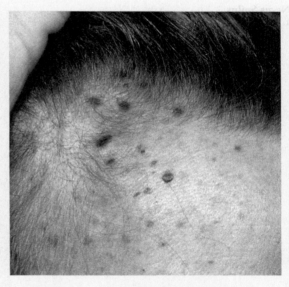

Fig. 31.46. Patient with an unusual case of eruptive blue nevi of the scalp and forehead. (From the Fitzsimons Army Medical Center Collection, Aurora, CO.)

References

Solar Lentigo

1. Ortonne JP, Pandya AG, Lui H, Hexsel D. Treatment of solar lentigines. *J Am Acad Dermatol.* 2006;54:S262-S271.

Simple Lentigo (Lentigo Simplex)

1. Hafner C, Stoehr R, van Oers JMM, et al. The absence of *BRAF, FGFR#,* and *PIK3CA* mutations differentiates lentigo simplex from melanocytic nevus and solar lentigo. *J Invest Dermatol.* 2009;129:2730-2735.

Acquired Melanocytic Nevus

1. Crane LA, Mokrohisky ST, Dellavalle RP, et al. Melanocytic nevus development in Colorado children born in 1998. *Arch Dermatol.* 2009;145:148-156.

Congenital Nevus

1. Vourc'h-Joudain M, Martin L, Barbarot S. Large congenital nevi: therapeutic management and melanoma risk. *J Am Acad Dermatol.* 2013;68:493-498.

Halo Nevus

1. Aouthmany M, Weinstein M, Zirwas MJ, Brodell RT. The natural history of halo nevi: a retrospective series. *J Am Acad Dermatol.* 2012;67:582-586.

Café au Lait Spots

1. Nunley KS, Gao F, Albers AC, et al. Predictive value of café au lait macules at initial consultation in the diagnosis of neurofibromatosis type 1. *Arch Dermatol.* 2009;145:883-887.

Nevus Spilus

1. Vaidya DC, Schwartz RA, Janniger CK. Nevus spilus. *Cutis.* 2007;80:465-468.

Atypical (Dysplastic) Nevus

1. Duffy K, Grossman D. The dysplastic nevus: from historical perspective to management in the modern era. Part I. Historical, histologic, clinical aspects. *J Am Acad Dermatol.* 2012;67:1-16.
2. Duffy K, Grossman D. The dysplastic nevus: from historical perspective to management in the modern era. Part I. Molecular aspects and clinical management. *J Am Acad Dermatol.* 2012;67:19-30.

Lentigo Maligna

1. Smalberger GJ, Siegel Khachemoune A. Lentigo maligna. *Dermatologic Ther.* 2008;21:439-446.

Melanoma

1. Mir M, Chan SC, Khan F, et al. The rate of melanoma transection with various biopsy techniques and the influence of tumor transection on patient survival. *J Am Acad Dermatol.* 2013;68:452-458.
2. Ransohoff KJ, Jaju PD, Tang JY, et al. Familial skin cancer syndromes. Increased melanoma risk. *J Am Acad Dermatol.* 2016;74:423-434.

Blue Nevus

1. Murali R, McCarthy SW, Scolyer RA. Blue nevi and related lesions. A review highlighting atypical and newly described variants, distinguishing features and diagnostic pitfalls. *Adv Anat Pathol.* 2009;16:365-382.

Chapter 32
Vascular Tumors

Key Terms

Infantile (Juvenile) Hemangioma
   Diffuse neonatal hemangiomatosis

Kasabach-Merritt Syndrome
   Hemangioma thrombocytopenia
     syndrome
   Hemangioma with
     thrombocytopenia

Pyogenic Granuloma
   Lobular capillary hemangioma

Vascular tumors include all neoplasms that demonstrate endothelium-lined channels and contain red blood cells (erythrocytes). This chapter is organized so that congenital vascular lesions are discussed first, followed by benign acquired vascular lesions and, finally, malignant vascular tumors. Also included are superficial lymphangiomas with hemorrhage, which may be clinically confused with vascular tumors.

Differential Diagnosis of Vascular Tumors of the Skin

Common
- Cherry angiomas (most common)
- Pyogenic granulomas
- Spider angioma
- Venous lake

Uncommon
- Angiosarcoma
- Angiokeratoma
- Infantile hemangioma
- Kaposi sarcoma
- Port wine stain
- Vascular malformation

IMPORTANT HISTORY QUESTIONS

How long has this lesion(s) been present?

Vascular tumors may be congenital or acquired. This is an important distinction, because some vascular tumors tend to occur in younger individuals (e.g., pyogenic granuloma) and some occur in older adults (e.g., cherry angiomata). Similarly, in general, lesions that are present for many years are less likely to be malignant.

Has the lesion changed?

A history of change or growth can be important in suggesting a malignancy. For example, early angiosarcoma of the scalp might appear initially to be flat and difficult to distinguish from a port wine stain. However, history of recent and/or rapid growth may warrant a biopsy to exclude angiosarcoma.

Have you ever been treated with radiation?

Because angiosarcomas can occur in radiation ports, even years after treatment, this is an important historical factor to ascertain and consider.

IMPORTANT PHYSICAL FINDINGS

How many vascular lesions are present?

Some vascular neoplasms usually occur as multiple lesions on the body (e.g., cherry angiomata, angiokeratomata), whereas other vascular neoplasms usually occur as solitary lesions (e.g., pyogenic granuloma, angiosarcoma).

What is the distribution of the lesions?

Most vascular neoplasms have characteristic patterns of distribution. For example, cherry angiomata often occur on the trunk. Angiosarcoma usually occurs on the head and neck, or in past radiation fields. Pyogenic granulomas usually occur on mucosal surfaces and the digits.

Are the lesions macular or palpable?

Vascular lesions can be flat (e.g., macules, patches) or demonstrate an elevated character. For example, nevus flammeus nuchae (so-called stork bite) is usually macular, whereas pyogenic granulomas and cherry angiomata are nearly always palpable. Some vascular tumors evolve from a flat to a palpable lesion. For example, infantile and juvenile hemangiomas may be flat at birth but rapidly evolve into larger palpable vascular tumors. The presence or absence of ulceration is also an important physical finding.

Are the lesions pulsatile?

Some vascular tumors, such as spider angiomata and pyogenic granulomas, are pulsatile and may demonstrate a feeder vessel on diascopy. Sometimes, the pulsatile nature of a lesion is not evident until the biopsy is performed. For example, pyogenic granulomas may manifest with pulsatile and rapid arterial bleeding when a shave biopsy is performed.

Infantile (Juvenile) Hemangioma ICD10 code D18.0

Pathogenesis

The pathogenesis of infantile hemangioma (IH), also called juvenile hemangioma or strawberry hemangioma, is not well understood. Expression of placental vascular isotopes and an increased incidence of placental abnormalities in mothers of affected children suggest a causal relationship. Infantile hemangiomas usually manifest a period of rapid growth, followed by involution, often occurring over years. IH usually reaches maximum size after 3 to 6 months of growth. A general rule of thumb is that 30% of IH involute by age 3 years, 50% by 5 years, and 70% by 7 years.

Clinical Features

- IH may be present at birth or may appear during the neonatal period.
- IH may present first as telangiectasias, pink macules, or patches or bruise-like lesions. Early lesions can mimic a port wine stain (Fig. 32.1A). Rarely, neonates present with well-developed lesions.
- Well-developed IH manifests with a red lobulated appearance, likened to a strawberry (see Fig. 32.1B).
- Ulceration and hemorrhage can be identified in IH.
- Involution of IH manifests as decreasing size. A gray color may develop. Fully involuted IH can manifests as a white scar because telangiectasias or even atrophy may develop (Fig. 32.2).
- IH varies in size. Lesions may be singular or multiple.
- IH usually affects the skin and mucosa, but internal organs may be involved on occasion (e.g., liver, gastrointestinal tract, lungs).
- Patients with numerous cutaneous lesions (diffuse neonatal hemangiomatosis) are at increased risk for involvement of internal organs (Fig. 32.3).
- IH can obstruct or partially obstruct the oral cavity or respiratory tract, or it may impair vision.

Diagnosis

- Early IH (macular phase) may be difficult to distinguish from port wine stains. It is often the clinical course, with rapid growth, followed by involution, that best establishes the diagnosis of IH.
- A punch or incisional biopsy may be needed in cases that manifest in an unusual way.
- Diffuse neonatal hemangiomatosis can be life-threatening, with mortality rates of 29% to 80%. In this circumstance, ultrasonography, computed tomography (CT), or magnetic resonance imaging (MRI) may be used to evaluate for systemic disease.

Treatment

- Treatment of IH is controversial and depends on the site involved and degree of involvement. If possible, patients should be referred to an expert in congenital vascular lesions.
- Small IH are not often treated. When treatment is desired, flashlamp-pumped pulsed-dye laser, targeting the vasculature, may be used.
- Systemic therapies include intralesional or systemic corticosteroids, recombinant interferon-α, or, more recently, a beta blocker (e.g., propranolol). Systemic corticosteroids may be used in life-threatening or vision-threatening IHs. Since 2008, beta blockers, especially propranolol, have been used off-label as treatment of complicated IH. Use of this drug represents a major development in the area. However, this medication should be used by those with experience in treating pediatric patients.
- Surgical removal is generally limited to smaller and exophytic lesions amenable to extirpation.
- Kasabach-Merritt syndrome requires immediate hospitalization, but treatment is not standardized.

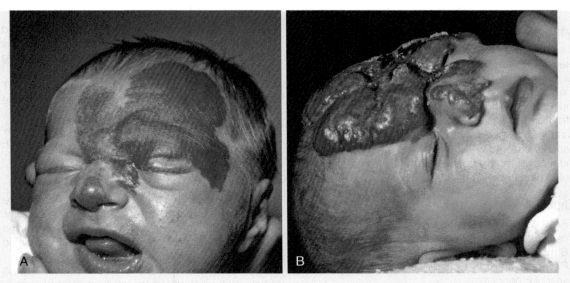

Fig. 32.1. A, Infantile hemangioma at the time of presentation. B, Fully evolved infantile hemangioma (same infant as seen in A), with partial ocular and nasal obstruction. (Both images from the Fitzsimons Army Medical Center Collection, Aurora, CO.)

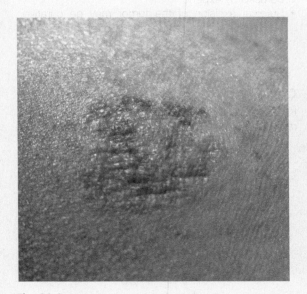

Fig. 32.2. Patient with an involuted infantile hemangioma, with residual telangiectasia, scar, and atrophy. (From the Fitzsimons Army Medical Center Collection, Aurora, CO.)

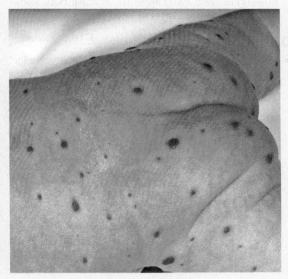

Fig. 32.3. Diffuse neonatal hemangiomatosis. The patient also had numerous lesions in the liver. (From the Fitzsimons Army Medical Center Collection, Aurora, CO.)

Pathogenesis

Kasabach-Merritt syndrome (KMS), occasionally referred to as *hemangioma with thrombocytopenia or hemangioma thrombocytopenia syndrome,* is a rare complication of hemangiomas in neonates and infants. Kaposiform hemangioendothelioma and tufted angioma are the two forms of vascular neoplasms usually associated with KMS. For unknown reasons, patients with KMS develop platelet trapping and a consumptive coagulopathy. Resultant bleeding problems can be life-threatening.

Clinical Features

- KMS usually presents at birth or in the neonatal or early infancy period. Almost all cases occur before 6 months of age.
- Patients with KMS typically have a large congenital vascular neoplasm.
- The vascular neoplasm often demonstrates an abrupt change in size, color, or firmness (Figs. 32.4 and 32.5).
- Affected infants often develop hemorrhage and bruising at sites away from the vascular neoplasm, which include the skin and internal organs.

Diagnosis

- The presentation of a large congenital vascular neoplasm with abrupt change suggests concern for KMS, and this concern is augmented by hemorrhage or bruising of skin away from the vascular neoplasm.

- A complete blood count (CBC), with attention paid to platelet count, is important. Clotting studies should be performed emergently because clotting factors (fibrinogen) are rapidly depleted.
- Imaging studies such as ultrasound, MRI, or CT should be considered to investigate hemorrhage beyond the skin.
- In select cases, a biopsy of the vascular tumor may be considered. Thrombosis in the vascular neoplasm supports the diagnosis.

Treatment

- Immediate admission to a pediatric intensive care unit (ICU), preferably at a tertiary children's facility, is important, because management often requires a multidisciplinary approach, and skilled pediatric nursing is preferred.
- The management of KMS is not standardized and is beyond the scope of this text. Typically, care is supportive and focuses on transfusions of fresh-frozen plasma and platelets. In select cases, treatment with anticoagulant and antithrombotic drugs may be used by experts.
- Surgical excision of the tumor may be curative, but urgent surgical extirpation is often made more difficult because of the bleeding diathesis. This must also be assessed by a pediatric surgeon on a case-by-case basis.

Clinical Course

KMS is a life-threatening emergency, with a mortality rate that approaches 30%.

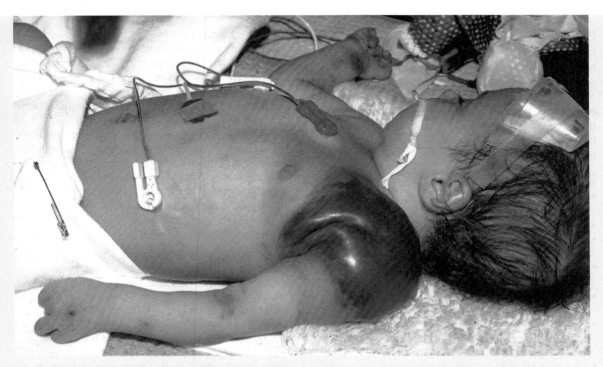

Fig. 32.4. Thrombosed tufted angioma in a patient who developed Kasabach-Merritt syndrome. (From the William Weston Collection, Aurora, CO.)

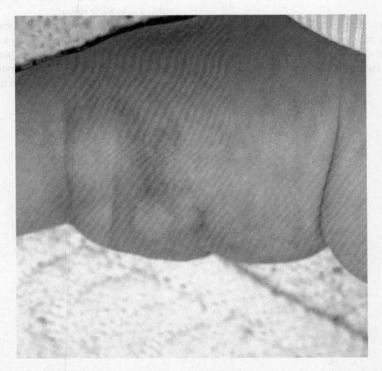

Fig. 32.5. Thrombosed deep hemangioma in a neonate who developed Kasabach-Merritt syndrome.

Pyogenic Granuloma ICD10 code L98.0

Pathogenesis

Pyogenic granuloma, also known as *lobular capillary hemangioma,* is a common vascular neoplasm of unknown pathogenesis. Many cases occur at sites of trauma, and there is an increased incidence during pregnancy, suggesting a hormonal influence. Some drugs, such as oral retinoids, used in severe acne, may be associated with the development of pyogenic granulomas.

Clinical Features

- Pyogenic granulomas usually affect children, adolescents, and young adults.
- Pyogenic granulomas often evolve rapidly.
- Pyogenic granulomas are usually singular, but multiple lesions can develop.
- Although the distribution is highly variable, the face, fingers, lips, and gingivae represent common sites.
- Pyogenic granulomas may develop in preexisting hemangiomas or port wine stains.
- Pyogenic granulomas usually present as red to violaceous exophytic papules that may be pedunculated (Figs. 32.6–32.9).
- Pyogenic granulomas vary in size, but most lesions are about 5 mm in diameter.
- Secondary features of pyogenic granulomas may include ulceration, hemorrhage, and crusting.

Diagnosis

- The clinical presentation of a rapidly growing vascular lesion, often with episodic bleeding, is characteristic of pyogenic granulomas, and, in the right clinical setting, a diagnosis can often be made with confidence.

- In some cases, the differential diagnosis includes a traumatized or inflamed cherry angioma, Spitz nevus, early xanthogranuloma, Kaposi sarcoma, and another ulcerated cutaneous malignancy, such as basal cell carcinoma, squamous cell carcinoma, or melanoma. In these situations, a biopsy is recommended to facilitate a final diagnosis.
- Often, a shave biopsy can be used, but considerable bleeding may occur at the base. This is indicative of an arterial feeding vessel that may require electrocautery. A punch or excision biopsy may also be performed. In most cases, an unequivocal histologic diagnosis may be rendered.

Treatment

- Because pyogenic granulomas often bleed, ulcerate, and otherwise persist, treatment is generally recommended. One exception is a pyogenic granuloma associated with pregnancy, because often such lesions will resolve after delivery.
- A shave biopsy followed by electrodessication or cauterization of the base or use of a styptic agent (e.g., Monsel solution, silver nitrate stick) is the treatment most often used. Occasional patients may demonstrate recurrence, with one or even multiple lesions growing at the site of the original lesion.
- Removal by punch biopsy or conservative excision is often more time-consuming, but the recurrence rate is generally lower.
- Early and small pyogenic granulomas may respond to treatment with a pulsed dye laser that targets the vasculature, although multiple (two to six) treatments are necessary. Liquid nitrogen destruction may also be used with variable success.

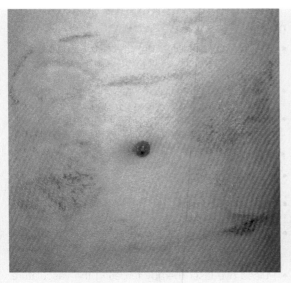

Fig. 32.6. Patient with a bleeding pyogenic granuloma, with a positive Band-Aid sign.

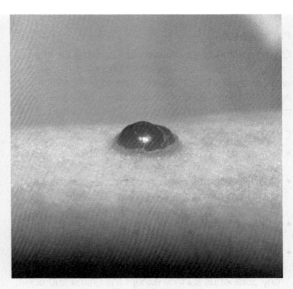

Fig. 32.7. Patient with a classic pyogenic granuloma, with a typical collarette of keratin. (From the Fitzsimons Army Medical Center Collection, Aurora, CO.)

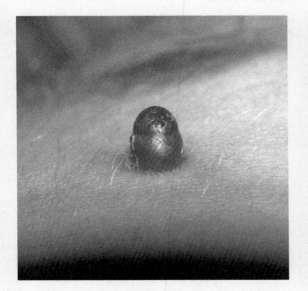

Fig. 32.8. Patient with an unusually exophytic pyogenic granuloma. (From the Fitzsimons Army Medical Center Collection, Aurora, CO.)

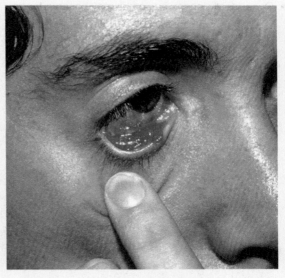

Fig. 32.9. Patient with a pyogenic granuloma of the ocular mucosa. (From the Fitzsimons Army Medical Center Collection, Aurora, CO.)

Cherry Angioma (Hemangioma) ICD10 code D18.00

Pathogenesis

Cherry angiomas, also known as *Campbell De Morgan spots,* are ubiquitous lesions of uncertain cause. It is well recognized that cherry angiomas increase with age. More than 90% of all individuals will have one or more cherry hemangiomas by 70 years of age.

Clinical Features

- Cherry angiomas show no racial or sexual predilection.
- Cherry angiomas begin in late adolescence or early adulthood and continue to appear and/or enlarge until late older age, when the lesions may involute.
- Cherry angiomas may be solitary or numerous (>100).
- Most cherry angiomas are located on the trunk and proximal extremities, but the lesions may occur on any cutaneous surface except the palms and soles.
- Cherry angiomas present as 1- to 4-mm red to red-purple sessile or slightly pedunculated papules (Figs. 32.10 and 32.11).
- Diascopy may produce slight blanching, without pulsation, but complete blanching does not occur.
- Occasionally, cherry angiomas may become tender or change color due to thrombosis (Fig. 32.12).

Diagnosis

- The clinical presentation of cherry angiomas is usually diagnostic, although early lesions can resemble petechiae.
- Inflamed or traumatized cherry angiomas may be difficult to differentiate from pyogenic granulomas.
- In rare cases, a thrombosed cherry angioma may resemble a melanoma and will need to be biopsied.

Treatment

- Cherry angiomas are benign and require no treatment.
- Light electrodessication can be used to destroy lesions if symptomatic or if desired.
- Liquid nitrogen cryotherapy, or the use of another refrigerant spray, followed by curettage, is more effective than cryotherapy alone.
- Pulsed dye laser therapy targeting the vasculature is also effective.
- A superficial shave biopsy can be used for inflamed or traumatized lesions.

Clinical Course

Cherry angiomas continue to increase in number with age but do not have any malignant potential.

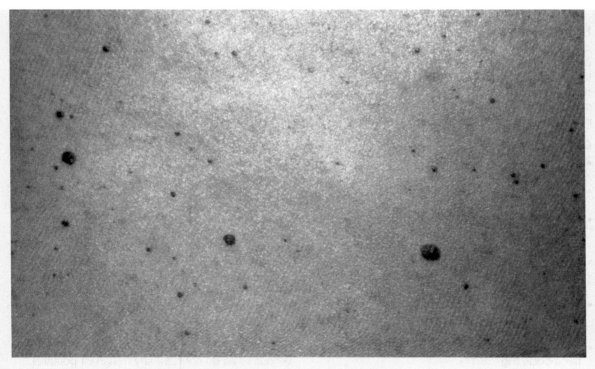

Fig. 32.10. Adult patient with multiple truncal cherry angiomas of different sizes.

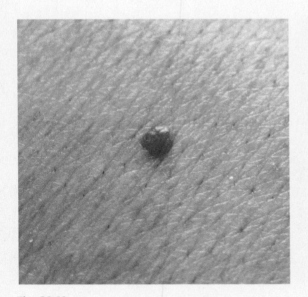

Fig. 32.11. Close-up of a typical cherry angioma.

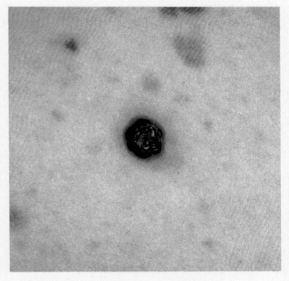

Fig. 32.12. Patient with a thrombosed cherry angioma that could be mistaken for melanoma. (From the Fitzsimons Army Medical Center Collection, Aurora, CO.)

Venous Lake ICD10 code D18.01

Pathogenesis

A venous lake, less often referred to as a *venous varix*, is most likely due to aging and weakening of the supporting structures of blood vessels, leading to dilation. Venous lakes are most prevalent on heavily sun-damaged skin, suggesting that ultraviolet light–induced stromal changes are important.

Clinical Features

- Venous lakes often affect older adults with dermatoheliosis.
- Venous lakes are often solitary, but multiple lesions can occur.
- Venous lakes occur on the sun-damaged skin of the head and neck, including the ears and lips, particularly the lower lip.
- Venous lakes present as soft, compressible, dark blue to purple papules of 1 to 4 mm in size (Fig. 32.13).
- Venous lakes will often largely disappear with compression, slowly filling back to their original size over several seconds.
- Venous lakes may occasionally be firm due to thrombosis (Fig. 32.14).

Diagnosis

- The presentation and clinical appearance are often diagnostic. Occasionally, venous lakes may be confused with blue nevi, but, in this situation, palpation is useful. Blue nevi are firm and do not blanch with compression.
- Rare cases may require a deep shave or punch biopsy for diagnosis. The histologic findings of a dilated and telangiectatic blood vessel, with a thin and unremarkable endothelium and surrounding solar damage, are diagnostic.

Treatment

- Venous lakes are entirely benign and require no treatment.
- If desired, for cosmetic reasons, a venous lake can be removed by a deep shave or punch biopsy or removed if the lesion has caused recurrent bleeding.
- Less often, electrocautery, carbon dioxide laser, tunable dye laser therapy, and other lasers may be used in treatment.

Clinical Course

Venous lakes do not have any malignant potential.

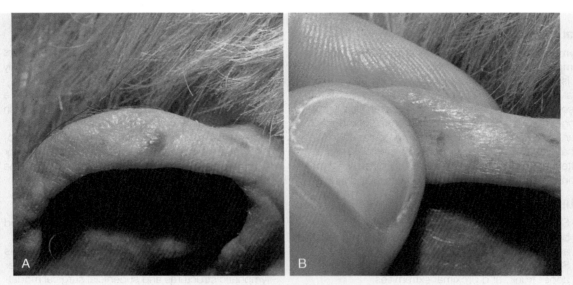

Fig. 32.13 A, Venous lake of the ear on sun-damaged skin. B, Compression produces collapsed venous lakes. (From the Fitzsimons Army Medical Center Collection, Aurora, CO.)

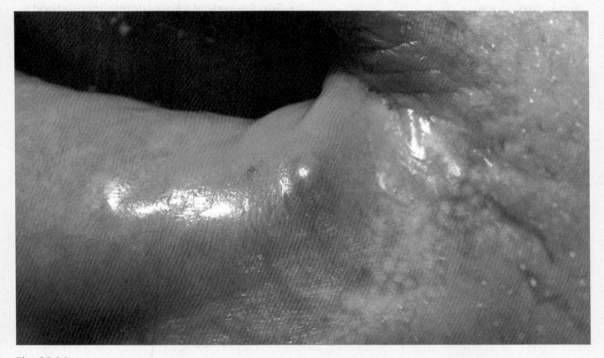

Fig. 32.14. Patient with a thrombosed venous lake of the lip. (From the Fitzsimons Army Medical Center Collection, Aurora, CO.)

Pathogenesis

Lymphangiomas are congenital malformations of lymphatics that may develop anywhere on the skin. It is common to divide lymphangiomas into superficial forms (e.g., lymphangioma circumscriptum) and deep forms (e.g., cystic hygroma, cavernous lymphangioma). Mixed vascular and lymphatic components can exist in a single lesion. Although cutaneous lymphangiomas may clinically appear superficial in nature, often at the microscopic level, the processes may connect to deeper lymphatic and vascular channels.

Clinical Features

- Superficial lymphangiomas are usually present at birth but may not be noticed until childhood or adolescence.
- Superficial lymphangiomas usually affect the neck, upper trunk, and proximal extremities.
- The primary lesion exists as grouped, clear papules, 1 to 3 mm in size, which appear to sit on the surface of the skin and are likened to frog spawn (Fig. 32.15).
- Superficial lymphangiomas can overlie deep cavernous lymphangiomas.
- Most lymphangiomas demonstrate focal hemorrhage into the lymphatic papules and thus resemble a vascular neoplasm (Figs. 32.16–32.18). In some cases, this can suddenly occur, yielding concern by the patient or the parent of a child.

Diagnosis

- Grouped superficial clear papules, present for years and resembling frog spawn on the skin, is generally diagnostic, and a biopsy is not typically required.
- A small clear papule may also be punctured with a no. 11 scalpel blade, and the contents should drain clear watery fluid consistent with lymph.
- Cases with extensive hemorrhage or focal thrombosis may be diagnostically challenging, and a 3- or 4-mm punch biopsy may be performed to clarify the situation.

Treatment

- Cutaneous lymphangiomas are benign lesions, and no treatment is required.
- Surgical treatment of superficial lymphangiomas is often imperfect because a connection to deeper lymphatic structures and superficial surgical modalities may result in recurrence.
- Wider and deeper surgical margins to contend with these connections may result in a significant scar or other surgical sequelae. Moreover, recurrences can still transpire.
- Select superficial lymphangiomas may respond to hypertonic saline injections into the dilated superficial lymphangiomas. This should only be done by individuals with experience in this treatment modality.

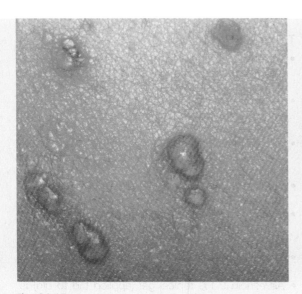

Fig. 32.15. Patient with a superficial lymphangioma resembling frog spawn. (From the Fitzsimons Army Medical Center Collection, Aurora, CO.)

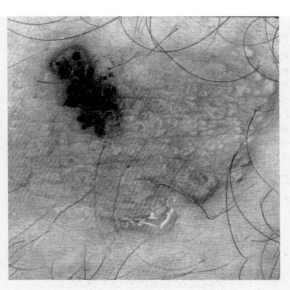

Fig. 32.16. Patient with a superficial lymphangioma with focal thrombosis. The clear yellowish liquid is lymph.

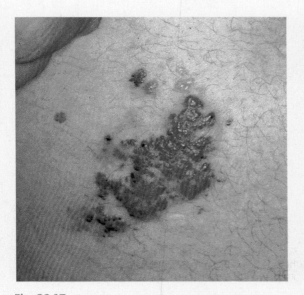

Fig. 32.17. Patient with a superficial lymphangioma with hemorrhage resembling a vascular neoplasm. Note several residual clear papules that are the clinical clue to the diagnosis.

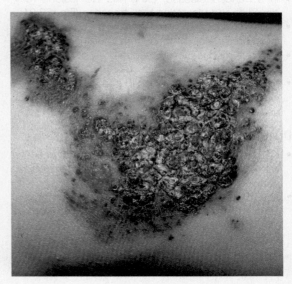

Fig. 32.18. Patient with a large superficial lymphangioma, with hemorrhage and thrombosis. Note the telltale clear papules. (From the William Weston Collection, Aurora, CO.)

Kaposi Sarcoma

Pathogenesis

Kaposi sarcoma (KS) is a condition caused by infection of endothelial cells with human herpesvirus 8 (HHV-8) (Fig. 32.19). Although the condition is technically a malignancy, in immunocompetent persons ("classic" Kaposi sarcoma) the disease usually has an indolent course. In immunocompromised persons (e.g., AIDS patients, transplant patients) KS can have a more aggressive course.

Clinical Features

- Historically, KS occurred in older persons of Mediterranean or Jewish ancestry ("classic" KS). More recently, aggressive forms were observed in immunosuppressed persons, particularly in AIDS patients.
- Classic KS often involves the lower extremities. In immunocompromised persons, the trunk or face may be involved, or even the oral mucosa.
- Early KS presents as round to oval red to violaceous macules ("patch stage" KS).
- Some lesions progress to red-blue or violaceous plaques or tumors (Fig. 32.20).
- In advanced disease, exophytic KS lesions may develop, and ulceration may transpire (Fig. 32.21).
- Patients with extensive disease of the lower extremities can develop lymphedema.
- The oral mucosa is involved in 30% of cases, with the hard palate usually affected (Fig. 32.22).
- Internal organs are involved in about 10% of cases, with lymph nodes and the gastrointestinal tract usually being affected.

Diagnosis

- KS is always in the differential diagnosis of patients with multiple unexplained violaceous macules, papules, nodules, or tumors.
- The diagnosis of KS is established via a punch biopsy or incisional biopsy. The histologic findings of early patch stage lesions can be problematic, but immunohistochemical staining for HHV-8 can be performed, which facilitates the diagnosis in many cases.

Treatment

- Patients are often referred to a tertiary care center or other specialists because treatment is not standardized.
- In HIV-infected persons, antiretroviral therapy is a cornerstone of care and may produce partial or complete remission.
- In transplant patients, the degree of immunosuppression can be reduced, clearly in cooperation with the transplant team.
- In patients with "classic" KS (older patients), usually radiation therapy or excision is used.
- Various single-agent regimens (vinblastine is most often used) or combined chemotherapeutic agent regimens are used, with varied success.
- Intralesional vincristine, vinblastine, and interleukin-2 (IL-2) can be used to manage singular lesions.
- Alitretinoin 0.1% topical gel (applied bid to qid) is U.S. Food and Drug Administration (FDA)-approved for the treatment of KS; in some series, a 36% response rate was demonstrated.

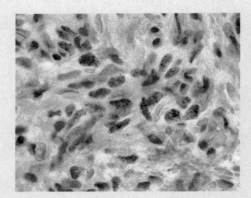

Fig. 32.19. Kaposi sarcoma demonstrating human herpesvirus 8 brown particulates in the nuclei by immunoperoxidase (100×).

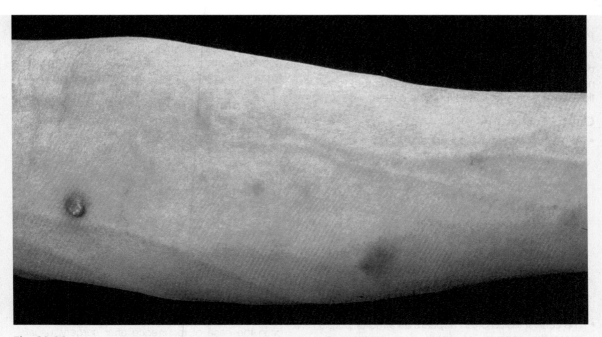

Fig. 32.20. Patch, plaque, and early tumor stage Kaposi sarcoma on the forearm in an HIV-infected individual. (From the Fitzsimons Army Medical Center Collection, Aurora, CO.)

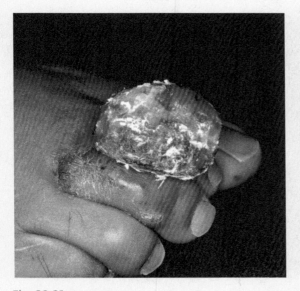

Fig. 32.21. Ulcerated tumor stage Kaposi sarcoma arising in a plaque stage lesion.

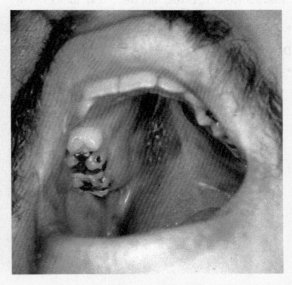

Fig. 32.22. Kaposi sarcoma of the hard palate in an HIV-infected man.

Pathogenesis

Angiosarcoma (AS) is a malignant vascular tumor derived from endothelial cells. Although its cause is not fully understood, chronic lymphedema and radiation therapy are implicated in some cases.

Clinical Features

- Angiosarcoma may occur anywhere, including organ systems other than the skin. Cutaneous angiosarcoma typically presents in one of three clinical situations:
  - Scalp-face AS (Figs. 32.23 and 32.24) is most common in geriatric patients.
  - Radiation-associated AS (Fig. 32.25) occurs in the field of prior radiation therapy.
  - Lymphedema-associated KS (Stewart-Treves syndrome; Fig. 32.26) occurs on the extremities of persons with chronic lymphedema, such as that occurring in the arm after axillary lymph node dissection for breast carcinoma.
- The earliest lesion of AS appears as a red or purple bruise-like macule or patch that progressively enlarges. There is often an ill-defined margin that merges with adjacent normal skin.
- As the condition worsens, red, purple, or even skin-colored papules, nodules, and tumors may develop.
- Advanced lesions of AS frequently bleed or ulcerate.

Diagnosis

- The diagnosis of AS requires a high index of suspicion, and early lesions may be misinterpreted as a bruise or benign vascular condition. AS should be suspected in any older patient, particularly someone with a history of radiation and/or chronic lymphedema and a new, vascular-appearing lesion.
- The diagnosis of AS must be established by biopsy. Usually, a large and deep punch or incisional biopsy, to include subcutaneous fat, is recommended. It must be understood that AS may be difficult or impossible to diagnose on superficial biopsies because the vascular changes in the shallow dermis may be subtle. When AS is a serious clinical consideration, a shave biopsy should not be performed.

Treatment

- If surgery is possible, excision with generous margins is the treatment of choice. AS is notoriously difficult to excise because the margins are difficult to determine, clinically and histologically. Micrographically controlled surgery (Mohs surgery) has no role in the management of AS.
- In large lesions that are not amenable to surgery, or in the case of recurrence after surgery, usually radiation therapy is employed. Radiation therapy may also be used in conjunction with surgery.
- Chemotherapy, primarily doxorubicin, has been used with limited success.

Clinical Course

Angiosarcomas are aggressive soft tissue tumors, with multiple series reporting a 5-year survival rate of 12% to 33%. Most persons with AS die within 9 to 12 months of diagnosis.

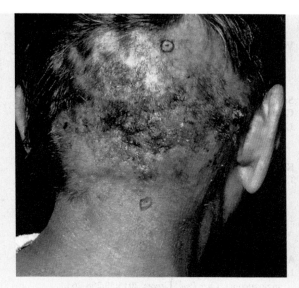

Fig. 32.23. Patient with a fatal, large, ulcerated angiosarcoma of the posterior scalp. Punch biopsy sites are marked for tumor mapping.

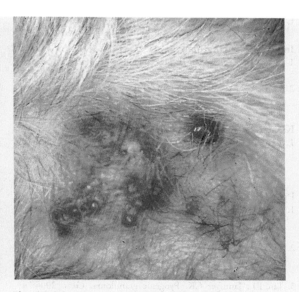

Fig. 32.24. Close-up of angiosarcoma of the scalp. (From the Fitzsimons Army Medical Center Collection, Aurora, CO.)

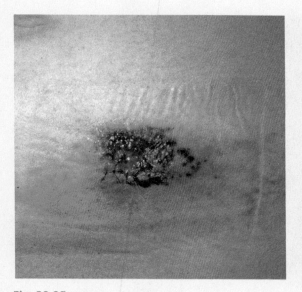

Fig. 32.25. Patient with an ulcerated angiosarcoma of the lower abdomen at the site of radiation. (From the Fitzsimons Army Medical Center Collection, Aurora, CO.)

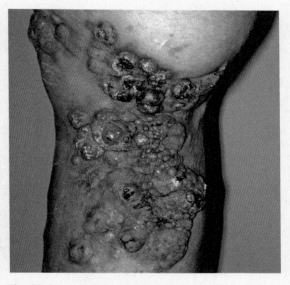

Fig. 32.26. Patient with an angiosarcoma arising in a lymphedematous leg. (From the Fitzsimons Army Medical Center Collection, Aurora, CO.)

References

Infantile Hemangioma

1. Bruckner AL, Frieden IJ. Hemangiomas of infancy. *J Am Acad Dermatol.* 2003;48:477-493.
2. Gutiérrez JCL, Avila L, Sosa G, Patron M. Placental abnormalities in children with infantile hemangioma. *Pediatr Dermatol.* 2007;24:353-355.

Kasabach-Merritt Syndrome

1. Croteau SE, Liang MG, Kozakewich HP, et al. Kaposiform hemangioendothelioma: atypical features and risks of Kasabach-Merritt phenomenon in 107 referrals. *J Pediatr.* 2013;162:142-147. (free online article).

Pyogenic Granuloma

1. Blickenstaff RD, Roenigk RK, Peters MS, Goellner JR. Recurrent pyogenic granuloma with satellitosis. *J Am Acad Dermatol.* 1989;21:1241-1244.
2. Hölbe HC, Frosch PJ, Herbst RA. Surgical pearl: ligation of the base of pyogenic granuloma – an atraumatic, simple, and cost-effective procedure. *J Am Acad Dermatol.* 2003;49:509-510.
3. Lin RL, Janniger CK. Pyogenic granuloma. *Cutis.* 2004;74: 229-233.

Cherry Angioma

1. Aversa AJ, Miller OF. Cryo-curettage of cherry angiomas. *J Dermatol Surg Oncol.* 1983;9:930-932.

Venous Lake

1. Mlacker S, Shar VV, Aldahan AS, et al. Laser and light-based treatments of venous lakes: a literature review. *Lasers Med Sci.* 2016;31:1511-1519.

Superficial Lymphangioma (Lymphangioma Circumscriptum)

1. Bikowski JB, Dumont AMG. Lymphangioma circumscriptum: treatment with hypertonic saline sclerotherapy. *J Am Acad Dermatol.* 2005;53:442-444.

Kaposi Sarcoma

1. Geraminejad P, Memar O, Aronson I, et al. Kaposi's sarcoma and other manifestations of human herpesvirus 8. *J Am Acad Dermatol.* 2002;47:641-655.
2. Schwartz RA, Micali G, Nasca MR, Scuderi L. Kaposi's sarcoma: a continuing conundrum. *J Am Acad Dermatol.* 2008;59:179-206.

Angiosarcoma

1. Dossett LA, Harrington M, Cruse W, Gonzalez RJ. Cutaneous angiosarcoma. *Curr Probl Cancer.* 2015;39:258-263.

Chapter 33
Yellow Lesions

Key Terms

Xanthelasma
Xanthelasma palpebrarum

Nevus Sebaceus
Nevus syndrome
Organoid nevus

Yellow lesions of various shades—yellow, yellow-white, yellow-orange, yellow-red—include an admixture of neoplastic and inflammatory skin disorders. Usually, yellow tints are due to the accumulation of lipid or elastic fibers.

IMPORTANT HISTORY QUESTIONS

How long has the lesion(s) been present?

This question is important because some of disorders in this group, such as xanthogranulomas, tend to be stable over time, whereas other conditions, such as eruptive xanthomas, are more likely to have an explosive onset. Nevus sebaceus is often present at birth, but it then becomes rather quiescent until puberty.

Has the lesion changed?

This question is important because some malignant lesions, including sebaceous gland carcinomas and a small subset of atypical fibroxanthomas (a low-grade malignancy) may also demonstrate a yellow color or yellow hue.

Do you have any known medical problems?

This query is important because some conditions, such as eruptive xanthomas, are associated with uncontrolled diabetes and primary biliary cirrhosis.

Have you or any member of your family had cancer?

Patients with numerous sebaceous gland neoplasms could suffer from Muir-Torre syndrome. This is a heritable condition that predisposes a person to gastrointestinal (GI) and renal cancers. In patients with planar xanthoma, a history of a lymphoid or myeloid malignancy, particularly multiple myeloma, would be important.

Do you take any medications?

Some medications, such as retinoids or corticosteroids, can aggravate or precipitate eruptive xanthomas.

IMPORTANT PHYSICAL FINDINGS

How old is the patient?

Nevus sebaceous can be seen in the neonatal period, but then the condition becomes largely quiescent until puberty. Xanthogranulomas are most often seen in young children. However, most other yellow skin lesions develop during adulthood.

How many lesions are present?

This is a critical finding because metabolic disorders, such as eruptive xanthomas, are characterized by numerous lesions, whereas other neoplastic disorders, such as xanthogranulomas, are typically solitary.

What is the distribution of the lesions?

Many disorders discussed in this chapter have characteristic locations. For example, tuberous xanthomas have a marked predilection for the elbows and knees, whereas xanthelasma, by definition, involves the eyelids. Sebaceous gland carcinoma also frequently involves the eyelid margin.

If multiple lesions are present, is there evidence of a Koebner phenomenon?

Only eruptive xanthomas are characterized by yellow lesions that appear with Koebner phenomena, occurring at sites of skin trauma, often in lines.

Differential Diagnosis of Yellow Lesions

Metabolic
- Eruptive xanthoma
- Normolipemic plane xanthoma
- Tuberous xanthoma
- Verruciform xanthoma
- Xanthelasma
- Xanthoma striatum

Neoplastic
- Sebaceous gland hyperplasia
- Sebaceoma
- Sebaceous adenoma
- Sebaceous gland carcinoma
- Xanthogranuloma

Hamartomatous
- Nevus sebaceous

Eruptive Xanthomata

Pathogenesis

Eruptive xanthomas are caused by an abrupt accumulation of low-density lipids, chiefly triglycerides, in the dermis (Fig. 33.1). Eruptive xanthomas are seen in many hyperlipidemia syndromes, but the most common cause is uncontrolled or poorly controlled diabetes mellitus. Depressed insulin levels result in decreased lipoprotein lipase activity, and elevated blood glucose levels lead to elevated very-low-density lipoprotein (VLDL) levels. The net result is hypertriglyceridemia, which can lead to eruptive xanthomas in the skin. Eruptive xanthomas may also be precipitated by alcohol, oral retinoids, corticosteroids, and estrogens.

Clinical Features

- Eruptive xanthomas typically appear as numerous lesions, sometimes more than 100.
- Early lesions demonstrate variable erythema and can be pruritic or even tender.
- Lesions are often located on the extremities and buttocks but may appear on any cutaneous surface, including mucocutaneous junctions, such as the eyelid margins and near the vermillion border of the lips.
- Lesions are strikingly uniform papules, which may be folliculocentric, and are typically 2 to 5 mm in size. Color varies from red (Fig. 33.2) to yellow-red (Fig. 33.3) to yellow-orange (Fig. 33.4) to yellow.
- The Koebner phenomenon may be present in areas of superficial trauma (see Fig. 33.3).
- Patients who present with eruptive xanthomata are also at risk for acute pancreatitis due to elevated triglyceride levels.

Diagnosis

- A careful clinical history, including medications and a review of systems (history of diabetes), is usually diagnostic when the clinical presentation is also supportive.
- At a minimum, all patients should have a complete serum lipid profile (Fig. 33.5), blood glucose level, routine chemistries, and pancreatic enzymes studies performed.
- A 3- or 4-mm punch biopsy can be done in problematic cases. The histologic findings can be specific or consistent with eruptive xanthoma.

Treatment

- Treatment focuses on the management of the underlying hyperlipidemia through diet, exercise, and lipid-lowering drugs (e.g., fibrates, statins, niacin).
- Remove any potentially complicating or contributing drugs, including alcohol.
- There is no specific treatment of the skin lesions.

Clinical Course

Eruptive xanthomas usually resolve spontaneously, over a period of 2 to 4 weeks. In most cases, there are no residual sequelae, but occasional cases may result in focal but permanent atrophy.

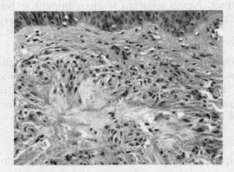

Fig. 33.1. Biopsy of eruptive xanthoma demonstrating free dermal lipid surrounded by lipid-laden macrophages (H&E stain; 200×).

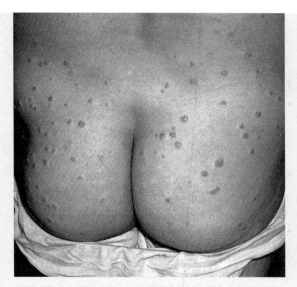

Fig. 33.2. Patient with uniform red papules on the buttocks, a common site for eruptive xanthomata. (From the Fitzsimons Army Medical Center Collection, Aurora, CO.)

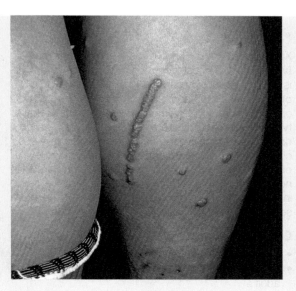

Fig. 33.3. Patient with eruptive xanthomas of the calf demonstrating the Koebner phenomenon. (From the Fitzsimons Army Medical Center Collection, Aurora, CO.)

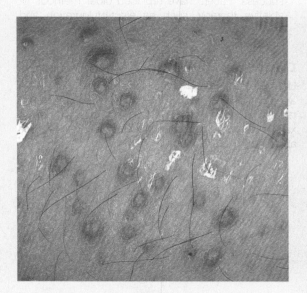

Fig. 33.4. Patient with characteristic yellow-orange papular lesions of eruptive xanthomata, with some being folliculocentric. The white color is due to application of cantharidin in the emergency room for what was thought to have been warts.

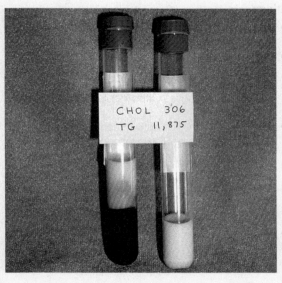

Fig. 33.5. Blood from a patient with eruptive xanthomata. The blood was placed in the refrigerator to accelerate separation of the lipids. (From the Fitzsimons Army Medical Center Collection, Aurora, CO.)

Xanthelasma

Pathogenesis

Xanthelasma, also known as *xanthelasma palpebrarum*, is the most common type of xanthoma. It is estimated to occur in 1.1% of women and 0.3% of men. The pathogenesis of xanthelasma is not entirely understood. Although some patients have type II hypercholesterolemia or type III dysbetalipoproteinemia, many patients have elevated levels of cholesterol, triglycerides, and VLDL and lower levels of high-density lipoprotein (HDL) when compared to normal individuals. Similar lesions can also be seen in diffuse, normolipemic, plane xanthoma (see next section).

Clinical Features

- Xanthelasma is more common in women.
- Typically, the condition appears first in middle-aged adults.
- The condition may be unilateral or bilateral and may affect the upper eyelid, lower eyelid, or both.
- The lesions present as flat, soft, yellow-white or yellow papules or small plaques of varied size (Figs. 33.6 and 33.7) on the periocular skin.

Diagnosis

- The clinical appearance, when combined with the characteristic location, is usually diagnostic.
- A serum lipid profile should be determined in all patients because patients with xanthelasma and lipid abnormalities are more likely to develop atherosclerotic disease. Often no lipid abnormality is detected.
- A shave or snip skin biopsy can be performed in problematic cases. The presence of a superficial band of lipid-laden macrophages (lipophages) is a pattern usually seen in planar xanthomas and xanthelasma.

Treatment

- The treatment of choice is management of the lipid abnormality, if one is present. Usually lipid-lowering drugs, such as statins (atorvastatin) and niacin, are employed. Often, however, no lipid disorder is apparent.
- Surgical removal of small lesions can be accomplished by elevation with tweezers and snipping of the lesion with sharp curved surgical scissors. Larger lesions can be excised and sutured closed.
- Topical ablative therapy includes 70% trichloroacetic acid, left on for 30 to 60 seconds and then neutralized with alcohol. This yields a good or excellent result in about 80% of patients, with some patients requiring a second treatment. Care around the eye is requisite.
- Other options include laser ablation. Various carbon dioxide lasers, Nd:YAG lasers, or potassium titanyl phosphate (KTP) lasers have been used with success. Lasers have replaced older methods of ablative therapy, such as electrofulguration and cryosurgery, which yielded mixed and unpredictable cosmetic results.

Clinical Course

Untreated, xanthelasma may persist indefinitely. Management of lipid levels with drugs, although important to systemic health, does not typically affect xanthelasma. Lesions that are surgically removed or ablated, using any modality, can recur.

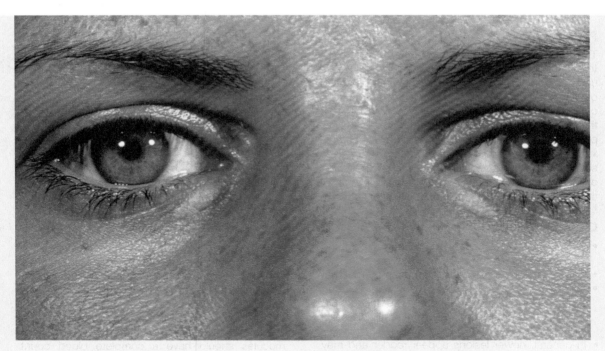

Fig. 33.6. Patient with a bilateral xanthelasma of the lower eyelids demonstrating a characteristic oval yellow-white color.

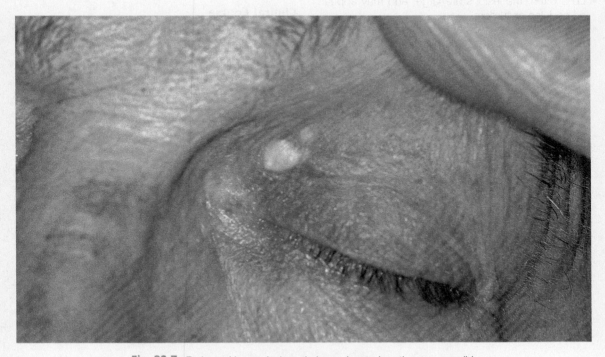

Fig. 33.7. Patient with a typical xanthelasma located on the upper eyelid.

(Juvenile) Xanthogranuloma ICD10 code D76.3

Pathogenesis

The pathogenesis of xanthogranulomas (XGs), referred to as juvenile xanthogranulomas in children, is poorly understood. Histologically, the lesions are comprised of macrophages, xanthomatous cells (macrophages containing lipid), multinucleated histiocytes with lipid at the periphery (Touton giant cells), and scattered lymphocytes and eosinophils. The increased incidence of xanthogranulomas in children with neurofibromatosis suggests a genetic basis. Despite the accumulation of lipid in tissue macrophages (xanthomatous cells) of the lesions, serum lipid studies are invariably normal.

Clinical Features

- Xanthogranulomas usually are seen in infants and children, although they may occur at any age.
- The lesions are usually solitary but can be multiple.
- The primary lesion is usually a red to yellow-red to orange-red papule, without scale (Figs. 33.8 and 33.9). Some lesions may have negligible scale (Fig. 33.10).
- In general, newer lesions appear redder and may resemble a pyogenic granuloma or other vascular lesion (Fig. 33.11).
- Less often, the lesions are larger and may appear as nodules or tumors.
- Ocular xanthogranulomas may also be present in about 0.4% of cases. Complications of ocular XG may include glaucoma, hyphema, and blindness.

- Less often, xanthogranulomas may be present in other organs, including the lung, liver, and pericardium.

Diagnosis

- The clinical presentation of a solitary (or multiple) yellow, yellow-red, yellow-orange, or yellow-brown papule(s) in a child is suspicious for a xanthogranuloma. In most cases. the diagnosis is based solely on the clinical appearance and presentation.
- A shave or punch biopsy is nearly always diagnostic because of the characteristic agglomeration of various cell types and increased lipid in macrophages.

Treatment

- Because xanthogranulomas usually resolve spontaneously over time, no treatment is required.
- An ophthalmic examination may be performed to detect ocular lesions, particularly in infants 2 years old or younger.
- Patients with xanthogranulomas and café au lait macules should have a complete blood count (CBC) performed to exclude myelogenous leukemia because there is a reported association.

Clinical Course

In children, most cases spontaneously resolve within 5 years. Occasionally, lesions will persist into adulthood, or will even first develop in adulthood.

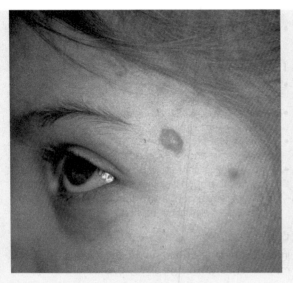

Fig. 33.8. Patient with a typical yellow papular xanthogranuloma. (From the Fitzsimons Army Medical Center Collection, Aurora, CO.)

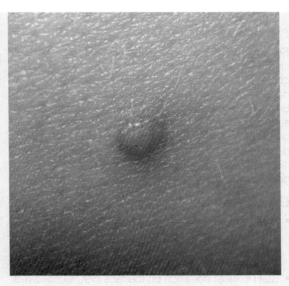

Fig. 33.9. Close-up of a xanthogranuloma demonstrating a yellowish-orange color.

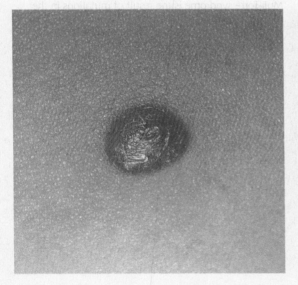

Fig. 33.10. Close-up of a scaly xanthogranuloma with an admixture of red and orange hues. (From the Fitzsimons Army Medical Center Collection, Aurora, CO.)

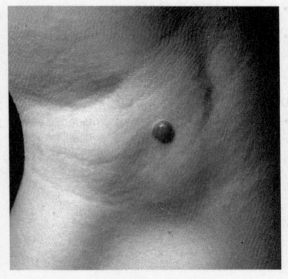

Fig. 33.11. Xanthogranuloma of the axilla in a child that is red, with subtle brownish and orange tints. Xanthogranulomas in which red is the predominant color can be impossible to differentiate from vascular lesions. (From the Fitzsimons Army Medical Center Collection, Aurora, CO.)

Pathogenesis

Sebaceous gland hyperplasia (SGH), also known simply as *sebaceous hyperplasia*, is a benign sebaceous gland neoplasm. It is the most common sebaceous neoplasm. Histologically, SGH is characterized by a central follicular opening, surrounded by enlarged sebaceous glands composed of peripheral basaloid germinative cells and central sebocytes. The pathogenesis is not well understood, but there have been reported examples of familial SGH, supporting a genetic basis.

Clinical Features

- SGH can occur at any age after puberty, but the condition becomes more common in the fourth decade of life and, by the eighth decade, about 25% of individuals have SGH.
- SGH is most common on the face (>90%), followed by the trunk.
- SGH may be solitary or numerous.
- The typical lesion is a yellowish-white to yellow papule, 2–5 mm in size, with central depression (Figs. 33.12 and 33.13).
- Rare variants of giant SGH, which may reach up to 5 cm in diameter, have been reported.
- SGH may be associated with Muir-Torre syndrome, but there are so many cases of SGH unassociated with this syndrome that a detailed workup for Muir-Torre is not encouraged for SGH alone.

Diagnosis

- The diagnosis of SGH is usually made based on the clinical appearance of a yellow or yellow-white papule, located on the face, with a central dell that corresponds to the follicular opening.

- Some cases may resemble basal cell carcinoma, with a rolled border. A shave biopsy is diagnostic.

Treatment

- No treatment is necessary; any treatment performed will be for cosmesis.
- Surgical options include a shave biopsy or punch biopsy for removal.
- Destructive topical treatment options include bichloroacetic acid and trichloroacetic acid.
- Other ablative therapeutic options include photodynamic therapy, laser destruction (e.g., carbon dioxide laser, argon laser, pulsed dye laser), cryosurgery, and electrofulguration.

Clinical Course

Individual lesions of SGH will persist indefinitely and may continue to enlarge slowly over time.

Muir-Torre Syndrome

Muir-Torre syndrome is the result of mutations in the mismatch repair genes *MLH1, MSH2,* and *MSH6* or, rarely, *PMS*. It is inherited in an autosomal fashion, with about 20% of cases being the result of sporadic mutations. Persons with this syndrome manifest a variety of sebaceous neoplasms, including SGH, sebaceous adenomas, sebaceomas, sebaceous gland carcinoma, and internal malignancies. Less often, patients with Muir-Torre syndrome may also have keratoacanthomas. The most common internal malignancies associated with Muir-Torre syndrome are colorectal carcinomas, genitourinary malignancies, and breast carcinomas.

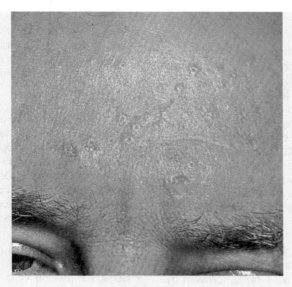

Fig. 33.12. Patient with numerous sebaceous gland hyperplasia neoplasms of the forehead demonstrating characteristic central dells. (From the Fitzsimons Army Medical Center Collection, Aurora, CO.)

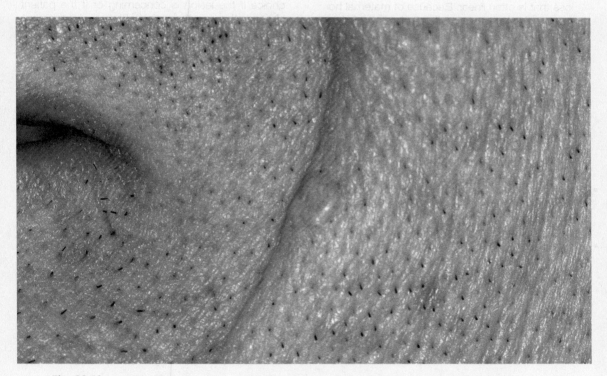

Fig. 33.13. Sebaceous gland hyperplasia. Shown is a close-up of a typical yellow papule with a central dell.

Nevus Sebaceus ICD10 code Q85.9

Pathogenesis

Nevus sebaceus (of Jadassohn), also known as *organoid nevus*, is a common hamartomatous malformation of unknown cause. As a hamartoma, the normal structures of the skin (epidermis, dermis, hair, sweat glands, and sebaceous glands) are present but with abnormal hypertrophy, hyperplasia, and organization. Nevus sebaceus (NS) occurs sporadically; the condition is found in about 0.3% of the population. Histologically, NS is composed of an acanthotic epidermis with papillomatosis, with abnormal and disorderly growth of the sebaceous glands, hair follicles, eccrine sweat glands, and apocrine sweat glands.

Clinical Features

- NS affects all ethnic backgrounds with equal frequency. Men and women are equally affected.
- Most NS occurs on the scalp (~50%), followed by the face (~40%) and neck (~6%), but NS can occur just about anywhere on the body.
- Typically, NS proceeds through three stages:
  - Neonatal phase—presents as a patch of hair loss that is often linear. Because of maternal hormones, the lesions are often indurated, variably papillomatous, and yellowish in color because of the hypertrophy of the sebaceous glands (Figs. 33.14 and 33.15).
  - Childhood phase—maternal hormone levels diminish, the sebaceous gland component involutes, and the lesion flattens, leaving a linear patch of hair loss with a slightly yellow color.
  - Adolescent and adult phase—as the androgen levels rise after puberty, the sebaceous glands again accumulate lipid, and the lesions become more yellow and papillomatous (Fig. 33.16).
- Patients with large and extensive NS may have **epidermal nevus syndrome**, which includes seizures, mental retardation, various structural abnormalities, and ophthalmologic abnormalities (see Fig. 33.15).
- A complication of NS that occurs in later life is the development of a secondary neoplasia, such as basal cell carcinoma, within the lesion. The lifetime risk for the development of secondary neoplasms in NS is probably less than 10%, but some dermatologists prefer complete removal for this reason.

Diagnosis

- The diagnosis of NS is usually made based on the congenital nature of the lesion, history, anatomic location, and clinical appearance.
- Occasional cases of NS may be difficult to distinguish from simple epidermal nevi. In problematic cases, a punch biopsy or incision biopsy should be performed. Histologic examination is usually diagnostic. Shave biopsies are rarely diagnostic and are discouraged.

Treatment

- Serial surveillance is an option unless there is a history of recent growth in the lesion. If there is concern for a secondary malignant neoplasm in the lesion, biopsy and/or removal are necessary.
- Surgical excision is the consensus treatment of choice if the lesion is concerning or if the patient chooses this, but the timing of any excision procedure is controversial and is not standardized.

Clinical Course

Numerous secondary neoplasms have been reported to occur in NS, including syringocystadenoma papilliferum (benign sweat gland tumor), trichoblastoma (benign hair follicle tumor), trichilemmoma (benign hair follicle tumor), and sebaceoma (benign sebaceous gland tumor). A relatively recent 18-year review in Detroit found basal cell carcinoma arose in about 1% of excised cases. The true incidence of basal cell carcinoma in NS is difficult to estimate because many cases in the literature probably represent benign trichoblastomas that are histologically similar to basal cell carcinoma.

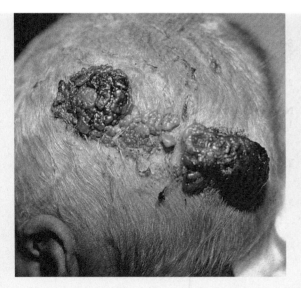

Fig. 33.14. Remarkably papillomatous nevus sebaceus with focal hemorrhage sebaceus in a neonate. (From the Fitzsimons Army Medical Center Collection, Aurora, CO.)

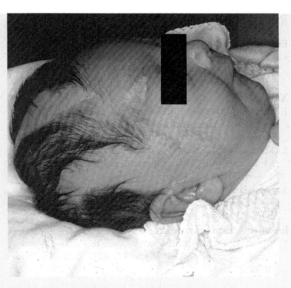

Fig. 33.15. Extensive nevus sebaceus of the scalp and face. This infant is at risk for epidermal nevus syndrome. (From the Fitzsimons Army Medical Center Collection, Aurora, CO.)

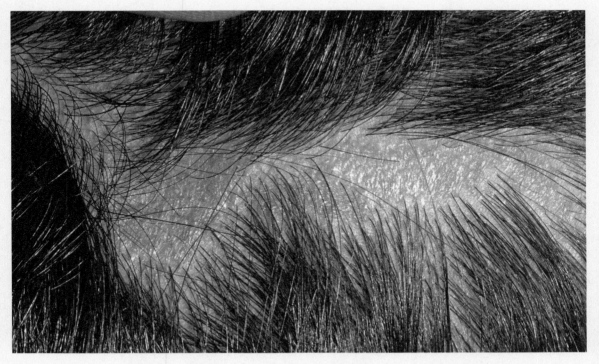

Fig. 33.16. Linear patch of alopecia in an adolescent caused by nevus sebaceus that has become subtly papillomatous and increasingly yellow after puberty. (From the Fitzsimons Army Medical Center Collection, Aurora, CO.)

References

Eruptive Xanthoma

1. Ladizinski B, Lee KC. Eruptive xanthomas in a patient with severe hypertriglyceridemia and type 2 diabetes. *CMAJ*. 2013; 185:1600.

Xanthelasma (Palpebrarum)

1. Kavoussi H, Ebrahimi A, Rezaei M, et al. Serum lipid profile and clinical characteristics of patients with xanthelasma palpebrarum. *An Bras Dermatol*. 2016;91:468-471.
2. Naha TR, Marques JC, Nicoletti A, et al. Treatment of eyelid xanthelasma with 70% trichloroacetic acid. *Ophthal Plast Reconstr Surg*. 2009;25:280-283.
3. Pathania V, Chatterjee M. Ultrapulse carbon dioxide laser ablation of xanthelasma palpebrarum: a case series. *J Cutan Aesthet Surg*. 2015;8:46-49.

Juvenile Xanthogranuloma

1. Pajaziti L, Hapçiu R, Pajaziti A. Juvenile xanthogranuloma: a case report and review of the literature. *BMC Res Notes*. 2014;7:174.

Sebaceous Gland Hyperplasia

1. Eisen DB, Michael DJ. Sebaceous lesions and their associated syndromes: part I. *J Am Acad Dermatol*. 2009;61:549-560.
2. Eisen DB, Michael DJ. Sebaceous lesions and their associated syndromes: part II. *J Am Acad Dermatol*. 2009;61:563-578.

Nevus Sebaceus (of Jadassohn)

1. Altaykan A, Ersoy-Evans S, Erkin G, Özkaya O. Basal cell carcinoma arising in a nevus sebaceous during childhood. *Pediatr Dermatol*. 2008;6:6116-6619.
2. Cribier B, Scrivener Y, Grosshans E. Tumors arising in nevus sebaceus: a study of 596 cases. *J Am Acad Dermatol*. 2000;42:263-268.
3. Rosen H, Schmidt B, Lam HP, et al. Management of nevus sebaceous and the risk of basal cell carcinoma: an 18-year review. *Pediatr Dermatol*. 2009;676-681.

Chapter 34
Cysts and Sinuses

Key Terms

Epidermoid Cyst
  Epidermal inclusion cyst
  Milium
  Ruptured epidermoid cysts

Apocrine Cystadenoma
  Apocrine hidrocystomas
Cutaneous Odontogenic Sinus Tract
  Cutaneous dental sinus tract
  Dentocutaneous sinus tract

True cysts of the skin represent epithelium-lined structures and may be caused by epidermis driven into the dermis (e.g., epidermal inclusion cysts), or they can arise from a variety of normal skin structures, such as hair follicles (e.g., epidermoid cysts, trichilemmal cysts), sebaceous duct (e.g., steatocystomas), apocrine glands and ducts (e.g., apocrine cystadenoma), and eccrine glands and ducts (e.g., eccrine hidrocystoma). Cutaneous sinuses represent epithelium-lined channels that communicate with a deeper process, such as a dental abscess. Finally, there are cyst-like structures of the skin that are not lined by an epithelium but arise from deeper structures, such as tendon-sheath (ganglion) and joint spaces (digital mucous cyst).

Differential Diagnosis of Cystic Lesions of the Skin

Common	Uncommon or Rare
• Epidermoid cyst (most common)	• Cutaneous ciliated cyst
• Trichilemmal (pilar) cyst	• Dermoid cyst
• Apocrine cystadenoma	• Eccrine hidrocystoma
• Digital mucous cyst	• Epidermal inclusion cysts
	• Eruptive vellus hair cysts
	• Median raphe cyst
	• Steatocystoma

IMPORTANT HISTORY QUESTIONS

How long has the lesion(s) been present?

Most cystic structures of the skin are acquired, but dermoid cysts are congenital. Therefore questioning is important when evaluating a potential cyst around the eyes or posterior axial skeleton of a child, because congenital lesions in these areas may connect to deeper structures and are often not amenable to outpatient surgery.

Has the lesion changed?

Malignant tumors may be indistinguishable from cysts, and malignancy may arise in long-standing cysts; thus, change is important to identify. On rare occasion, a squamous cell carcinoma may even develop in common epidermoid cysts, so any change in behavior is a noteworthy event.

IMPORTANT PHYSICAL FINDINGS

How are the lesion(s) distributed?

Some cysts have characteristic locations. For example, trichilemmal cysts are most common on the scalp, whereas apocrine cystadenomas are most common on the eyelid margins.

How many lesions are there?

Some cystic lesions are characteristically solitary (e.g., digital mucous cyst), whereas others are often multiple (e.g., steatocystomas, eruptive vellus hair cysts).

Does the cyst demonstrate transillumination?

Some cysts are filled with clear or translucent material (e.g., apocrine cystadenoma; Fig. 34.1), which can be demonstrated via transillumination. Cysts that contain keratin (e.g., epidermoid cysts) do not transilluminate in the same brilliant manner.

Does the cyst have a punctum?

Epidermoid inclusion cysts nearly always demonstrate a punctum that can be visualized with the unaided eye, whereas other types of cysts, such as a trichilemmal cyst, often do not manifest a punctum.

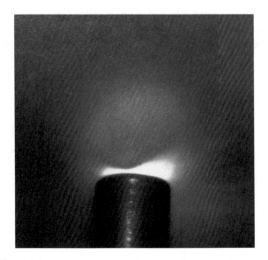

Fig. 34.1. Transillumination of an apocrine cystadenoma.

Epidermoid Cyst ICD10 code L72.0

Pathogenesis

An epidermoid cyst, also called an *epidermal cyst* or *sebaceous cyst* (the latter is inaccurate and is disfavored) is the most common cyst of the skin. Epidermoid cysts are derived from the infundibulum (upper portion) of the hair follicle and are filled with keratin rather than sebaceous material. Some epidermoid cysts may be induced by trauma or follicular inflammation, especially acne (Fig. 34.2). An epidermal inclusion cyst is a closely related entity caused by inclusion of a fragment of epidermis into the dermis, without an attachment to a hair follicle (Fig. 34.3), and it is nearly always related to trauma. A milium (plural milia) is simply a small epidermoid cyst (≤2 mm in diameter).

Clinical Features

- Epidermoid cysts can occur at any age but are most common in adolescents and young adults.
- Epidermoid cysts can be solitary or multiple.
- The face, neck, upper trunk, and scrotum are preferentially affected by epidermoid cysts.
- Epidermoid cysts exist as skin-colored dermal nodules that may extend into the subcutis (see Fig. 34.2).
- A punctum or keratin-filled follicular, comedone-like opening may be present on the skin surface.
- If the punctum is large enough, white, foul-smelling, cheese-like keratin debris may be expressed.
- The size of epidermoid cysts varies, but most are 0.4 to 4 cm in diameter.
- Ruptured epidermoid cysts may engender inflammation, with acute pain, erythema, and dramatic enlargement (Figs. 34.4 and 34.5). Drainage of pus and cystic contents may occur.

Diagnosis

- The clinical presentation of a flesh-colored cystic nodule, located in the dermis and/or subcutis, often with an identifiable punctum, is diagnostic.
- In some cases, foul-smelling keratin debris can be expressed through the punctum or through a small incision with a no. 11 scalpel blade, further establishing the diagnosis.
- Rare cases may require surgical extirpation, with histopathologic assessment for diagnosis.

Treatment

- Epidermoid cysts are benign and do not require treatment unless they are symptomatic or unless there is concern for a commingled malignancy.
- Excision of the entire cyst is often utilized to ensure complete removal.
- An alternative procedure is incision with a no. 11 scalpel blade, or 3- or 4-mm punch, followed by careful removal of the entire the cyst wall with forceps and scissors. Use of this technique is more tedious and requires greater surgical expertise, but it results in a smaller scar.
- Ruptured or inflamed epidermoid cysts can be injected with intralesional triamcinolone (2–5 mg/mL). Cysts that are ripe or have already begun to drain should be incised with a no. 11 scalpel blade, with the contents evacuated, followed by intralesional triamcinolone (2–5 mg/mL). Although erythema may be interpreted as an infected cyst, in most cases the reaction is due to a foreign body response to the keratin, and oral antibiotics are not usually required.

Clinical Course

Once present, epidermoid cysts usually persist. In about one-third of cases, where there is spontaneous rupture of the cyst wall, the cyst is completely destroyed by the inflammatory response, leading to resolution.

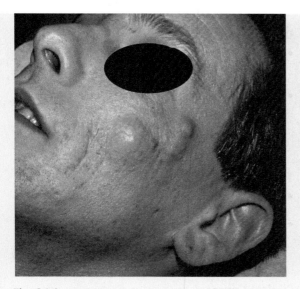

Fig. 34.2. Epidermoid cysts in sites of old acne, a common reason for the development of these cysts. (From the Fitzsimons Army Medical Center Collection, Aurora, CO.)

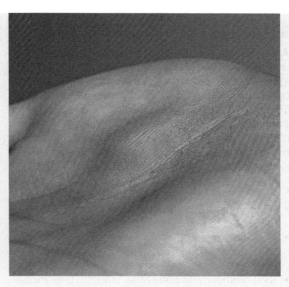

Fig. 34.3. True epidermal inclusion cyst, with no punctum at site of trauma. (From the Fitzsimons Army Medical Center Collection, Aurora, CO.)

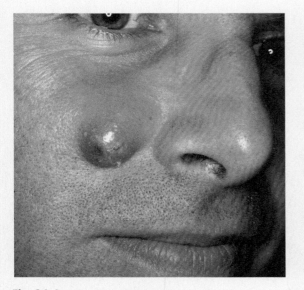

Fig. 34.4. Inflamed epidermoid cyst due to rupture of cyst wall. The inflammation is due to a foreign body reaction and not infection. (From the Fitzsimons Army Medical Center Collection, Aurora, CO.)

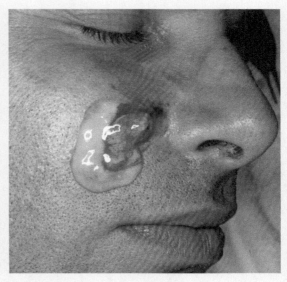

Fig. 34.5. Incision with a no. 11 scalpel blade allows drainage of pus and keratin. (From the Fitzsimons Army Medical Center Collection, Aurora, CO.)

Pathogenesis

A trichilemmal cyst, also known as a *pilar cyst* or *wen,* is the second most common form of follicular cyst. In contrast to epidermoid cysts, which arise from the upper third of the hair follicle, trichilemmal cysts arise from the middle third of the hair follicle, a region called the *isthmus.* The pathogenesis of solitary trichilemmal cysts is unknown, but when multiple trichilemmal cysts are present, a familial autosomal dominant pattern of inheritance has been observed.

Clinical Features

- Trichilemmal cysts develop in adults, with women being affected more often than men.
- The vast majority of trichilemmal cysts involve the scalp, although any area of the body can be affected.
- Trichilemmal cysts present as smooth, firm, mobile subcutaneous nodules (Figs. 34.6 and 34.7).
- The overlying skin is typically normal, although larger lesions on the scalp may produce hair loss.
- No punctum is present in trichilemmal cysts, and inflammation is uncommon.

Diagnosis

- The clinical presentation of a firm, mobile nodule on the scalp of an adult strongly suggests the diagnosis.
- The differential diagnosis often includes an epidermoid cyst, which has a punctum, or a metastatic event on the scalp, which may be suggested by the history and physical examination. In general, trichilemmal cysts are firmer than epidermoid cysts.

Treatment

- Trichilemmal cysts are benign, and no treatment is required.
- Surgical excision is usually easy to perform. Often trichilemmal cysts can be enucleated intact, simply because of a thicker epithelial wall and more compacted keratin.

Clinical Course

Trichilemmal cysts may rarely progress to malignancy (so-called proliferating trichilemmal tumors or trichilemmal carcinomas). Because of this, unusually large or enlarging and changing cysts should be removed.

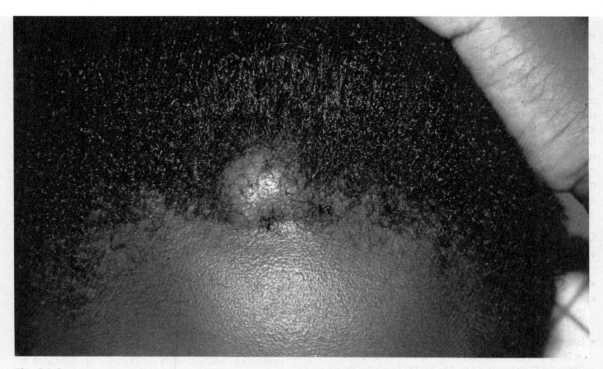

Fig. 34.6. Trichilemmal cyst of the scalp. These are typically firm and do not demonstrate an identifiable punctum. (From the William Weston Collection, Aurora, CO.)

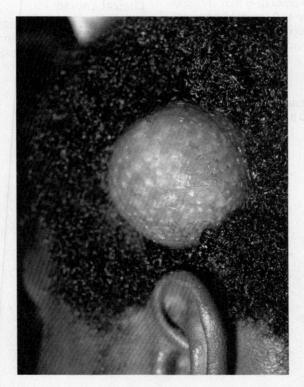

Fig. 34.7. Unusually large trichilemmal cyst of the left parietal scalp. Changing or very large trichilemmal cysts should raise the possibility of malignancy arising within the cyst. (From the Fitzsimons Army Medical Center Collection, Aurora, CO.)

Steatocystoma

Pathogenesis

A steatocystoma is a type of cyst that arises from the sebaceous duct, which connects the sebaceous gland to the hair follicle. Because sebaceous glands are included in the wall of the cyst, the cyst is filled mainly with sebum. *Steatocystoma simplex* is the term applied to a solitary lesion, whereas *steatocystoma multiplex* is the term utilized when a single patient has numerous such cysts. Sometimes multiple lesions are caused by a condition inherited in an autosomal dominant fashion. Steatocystoma multiplex may also occur as part of pachyonychia congenita, a genodermatosis resulting in numerous cutaneous abnormalities.

Clinical Features

- Steatocystomas usually develop in adolescence or adulthood.
- Men and women are equally affected.
- Steatocystomas may be singular (simplex) or multiple (multiplex), with some patients having hundreds of steatocystomas (Fig. 34.8).
- Steatocystomas present as mobile, soft, skin-colored or slightly yellowish cysts, without overlying epidermal changes or puncta. Some lesions demonstrate a translucent quality, with blue or green hues present (Fig. 34.9).
- Most steatocystomas are small (2–6 mm in diameter), but larger lesions of up to 2 cm can be present.
- Most steatocystomas occur on the chest, but the scalp, neck, proximal extremities, and genitalia may also be involved.

Diagnosis

- The diagnosis should be suspected in patients with multiple, soft, skin-colored to slightly yellowish cysts on the chest area. If a family history of similar lesions exists, the diagnosis is nearly certain.
- The diagnosis can also be established by puncturing the cyst wall with a no. 11 scalpel blade, with release of a clear to milky yellow and oily liquid. The contents are usually odorless, in contrast to the contents of epidermoid cysts, which are white in color and foul-smelling.
- In solitary or difficult presentations, the diagnosis is established by removing the cyst with a punch or excisional biopsy and submitting it for examination.

Treatment

- Steatocystomas are benign, and no treatment is required.
- Where desired, individual lesions can be removed by a punch or small excision.
- In patients with numerous cysts, individual cysts can be drained with a needle or a small incision made with a no. 11 scalpel blade. This produces only a temporary improvement but is useful on facial lesions for cosmetic purposes.
- Isotretinoin has been used in some patients with numerous lesions, with moderate improvement in the size of the lesions, but the lesions return slowly once the oral isotretinoin is withdrawn.

Clinical Course

Once present, steatocystomas persist indefinitely unless surgical intervention transpires, but no significant malignant potential exists.

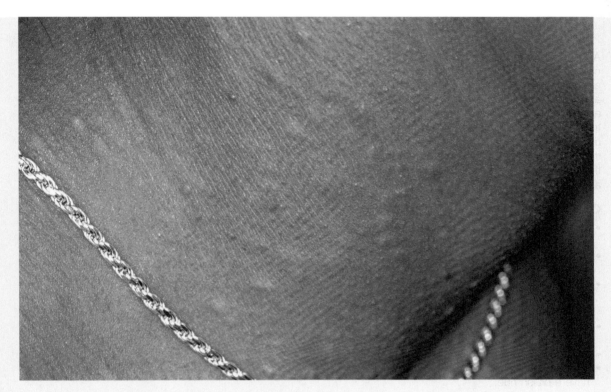

Fig. 34.8. Multiple small, skin-colored to slightly yellowish cystic lesions of steatocystoma multiplex. (From the Fitzsimons Army Medical Center Collection, Aurora, CO.)

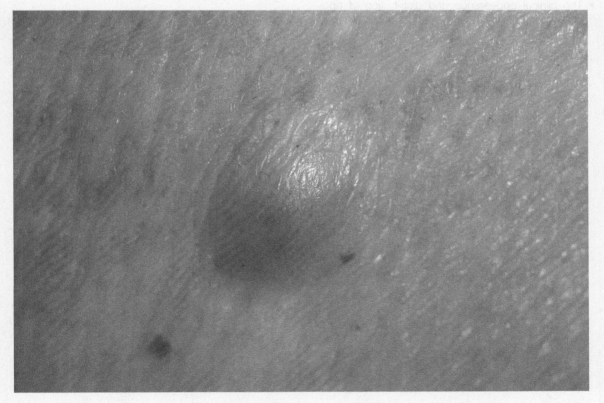

Fig. 34.9. Slightly exophytic steatocystoma, with a green-blue translucent appearance. (From the Fitzsimons Army Medical Center Collection, Aurora, CO.)

Apocrine Cystadenoma ICD10 code D23.9

Pathogenesis

As the name implies, apocrine cystadenomas, also called *apocrine hidrocystomas*, are cystic lesions of apocrine origin. The cysts are usually composed of apocrine ductal and glandular elements. Although any apocrine gland may give rise to these cystic structures, the eyelid margin is a common site of involvement. Apocrine cystadenomas at this site arise from the Moll glands, which are specialized apocrine glands that are found at the eyelid margin. The cause of apocrine cystadenomas is unknown.

Clinical Features

- Apocrine cystadenomas arise in older adults and geriatric patients.
- Usually, apocrine cystadenomas are solitary, but multiple lesions can occur.
- Most cystadenomas are located on the face, especially around the eyelid margins (Figs. 34.10 and 34.11).
- Apocrine cystadenomas present as smooth, dome-shaped papules, which may be compressible.
- Apocrine cystadenomas are usually asymptomatic.
- Apocrine cystadenomas may be translucent or have a bluish hue.

Diagnosis

- The clinical appearance and distribution of apocrine cystadenomas are rather characteristic, although occasional cases may resemble basal cell carcinoma.
- The cystic nature can often be confirmed by compression or via transillumination (see Fig. 34.1).
- The diagnosis can be confirmed by making a small incision with a no. 11 scalpel blade, with the expression of a clear watery fluid.
- Rare cases may require a shave or punch biopsy for diagnosis. The histologic findings are diagnostic.

Treatment

- Apocrine cystadenomas are benign, and no treatment is necessary.
- Shave removal of the apocrine cystadenomas will yield resolution in most cases, but larger lesions may require a punch or small excision biopsy.
- Carbon dioxide laser ablation is curative, but this modality is rarely used due to issues of safety and availability.

Clinical Course

Apocrine cystadenomas are benign sweat gland neoplasms that will persist indefinitely, unless surgical intervention transpires. Slow growth, over a period of years, is common.

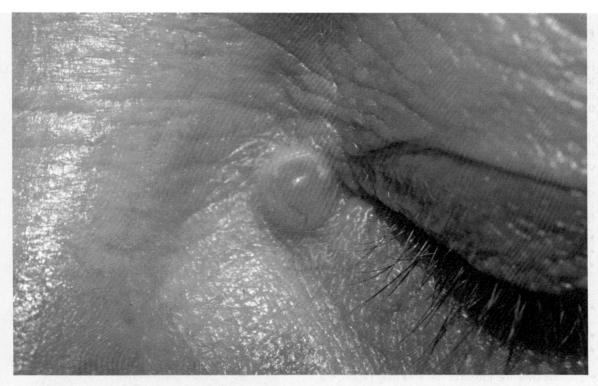

Fig. 34.10. Typical dome-shaped superficial cystic appearance of an apocrine cystadenoma. The medial and lateral aspects of the of the area around the eyes is the classic location. (From the Fitzsimons Army Medical Center Collection, Aurora, CO.)

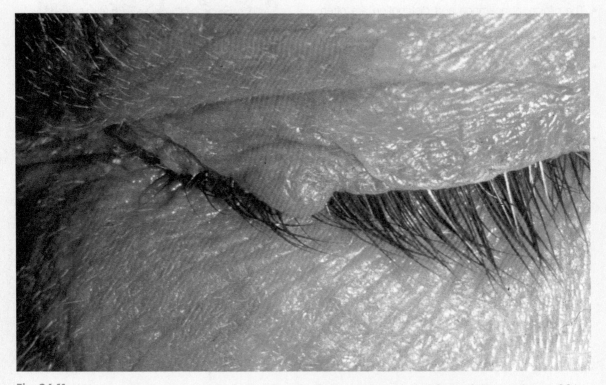

Fig. 34.11. Apocrine cystadenoma on eyelid margin. (From the Fitzsimons Army Medical Center Collection, Aurora, CO.)

Digital Mucous Cyst ICD10 code M71.349

Pathogenesis

The pathogenesis of digital mucous cysts (DMCs) is not fully understood. Evidence suggests they are not true neoplasms but instead are the result of degenerative changes of trauma and aging (e.g., osteoarthritis) at the distal interphalangeal joint. This theory is supported by studies (e.g., surgical dissections and dye studies) that show connections between the joint space and digital mucous cysts. The material in the cysts, like fluid in joints, is composed chiefly of hyaluronic acid that appears clear, with a jelly-like consistency (Fig. 34.12).

Clinical Features

- DMCs usually arise in older adults.
- DMCs are usually asymptomatic but can be tender.
- DMCs are usually located on the dorsal fingers, near the proximal nail fold. Less often, DMCs occur on the toes.
- DMCs present as smooth dome-shaped papules, which may be compressible (Figs. 34.13–34.15).
- DMCs may be skin-colored or translucent.
- Less common variants may be ulcerated, inflamed, or verrucous.
- Lesions over the proximal nail fold may produce a linear depression or groove in the nail plate (Fig. 34.14).

Diagnosis

- The clinical appearance and distribution are often characteristic of DMCs.
- The cystic nature of DMCs can often be confirmed by compression or via transillumination.
- The diagnosis of DMCs can be confirmed by making a small incision with a no. 11 scalpel blade, with expression of a clear, viscous, and gelatinous fluid. However, care should be taken to ensure the joint space does not become infected.
- Rare cases require a shave or punch biopsy for diagnosis. The histologic findings are diagnostic. Again, care should be taken to ensure the joint space does not become infected.

Treatment

- DMCs are benign, and no treatment is required.
- Intralesional triamcinolone can be used but with variable success.
- Surgical excision of the cyst is often used, but ablation of the connection to the joint space is required.
- Shave removal of the cyst, with cauterization of the base by electrodessication, or with use of a chemical agent, such as phenol, may be used.
- DMCs can also be treated by supplying the patient with sterile, 27-gauge needles and with instructions to puncture the cyst and forcibly express the contents. This action may be repeated as often as necessary.
- Less common treatment modalities include carbon dioxide laser ablation and cryosurgery.

Clinical Course

DMCs usually persist indefinitely, but spontaneous resolution can transpire.

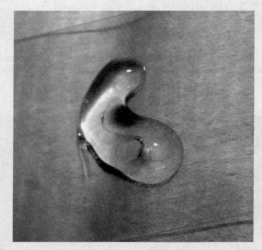

Fig. 34.12. Clear, jelly-like contents of a digital mucous cyst. (From the Fitzsimons Army Medical Center Collection, Aurora, CO.)

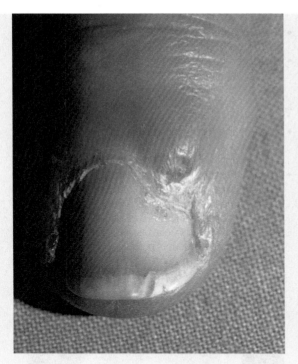

Fig. 34.13. Digital mucous cyst with adjacent scale. (From the Fitzsimons Army Medical Center Collection, Aurora, CO.)

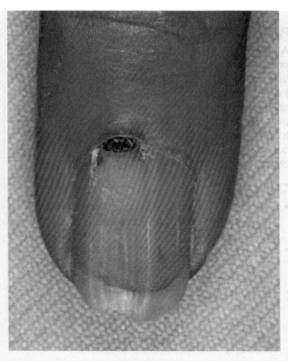

Fig. 34.14. Hemorrhagic digital mucous cyst with nail deformity.

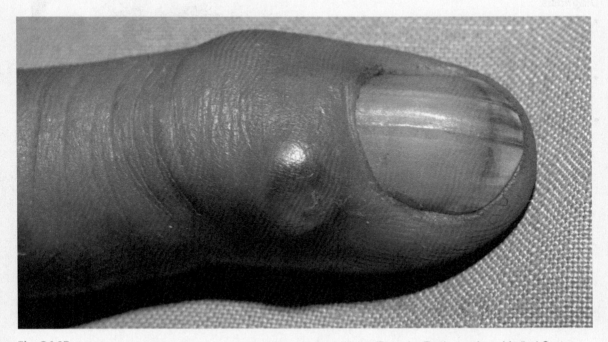

Fig. 34.15. Translucent digital mucous cyst over distal interphalangeal joint. (From the Fitzsimons Army Medical Center Collection, Aurora, CO.)

Cutaneous Odontogenic Sinus Tract ICD10 code K04.6

Pathogenesis

A cutaneous odontogenic sinus tract (COST), also called a *cutaneous dental sinus tract* and *dentocutaneous sinus tract*, is a result of neglected carious teeth that develop a bacterial infection and a periapical abscess. The periapical abscess extends along the periosteum and, ultimately, erodes through the skin to produce an oral or cutaneous sinus tract. Less common causes include dental implants (Fig. 34.16), dental cysts, and unerupted teeth.

Clinical Features

- Typically, COST arises in older adults with poor dental hygiene and carious teeth (Fig. 34.17). In occasional cases, the teeth may appear normal.
- The overwhelming majority of odontogenic sinus tracts (~80%) occur around the mandible, particularly around the chin and submental region.
- The sinus tract may appear as an opening that is often subtly depressed and intermittently discharges purulent material and blood (Fig. 34.18), or it may appear as an opening, with granulation tissue (Fig. 34.19).
- Palpation may demonstrate a variable soft induration.
- Some patients may have systemic evidence of infection, such as malaise and fever.

Diagnosis

- The clinical appearance of a sinus, particularly one that discharges purulent debris in the region of the face and neck and in proximity to the teeth, should raise suspicion of a COST.
- The oral cavity and teeth should be examined for poor oral hygiene and potentially carious teeth or evidence of extensive and failing restorative work.
- Radiographic studies, usually a panoramic (Fig. 34.20) or periapical x-ray, will identify the apical abscess.

- The drainage can be cultured, but most infections will be polymicrobial.
- Biopsies are sometimes used to exclude malignancy. Whereas the histological findings can support the diagnosis, they are not specific.

Treatment

- The treatment of choice is referral to a dentist or oral surgeon for a root canal, removal of teeth, and/or dental implants, as necessary.
- Empiric therapy with antibiotics, in addition to surgery, is often performed if the patient demonstrates systemic signs of infection or is immunocompromised. Treatment options include oral penicillin VK (500 mg PO tid), amoxicillin-clavulanate (500 mg/125 mg PO tid), and clindamycin (300–450 mg PO tid or qid, or 600–900 mg IV q6–8h).

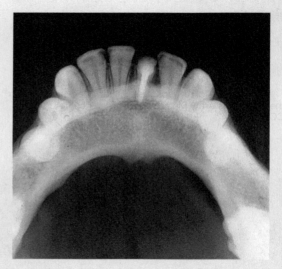

Fig. 34.16. X-ray demonstrating a small apical abscess beneath a dental implant. (From the Fitzsimons Army Medical Center Collection, Aurora, CO.)

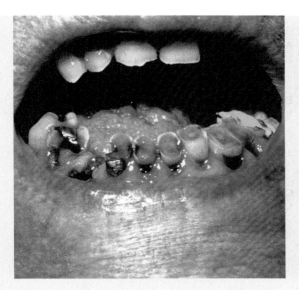

Fig. 34.17. Poor oral hygiene and numerous carious teeth was the source of a cutaneous odontogenic sinus tract in the submental region. (From the Fitzsimons Army Medical Center Collection, Aurora, CO.)

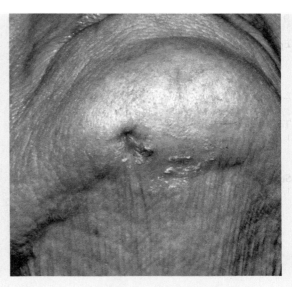

Fig. 34.18. Chronic sinus tract along the anterior mandible. (From the Fitzsimons Army Medical Center Collection, Aurora, CO.)

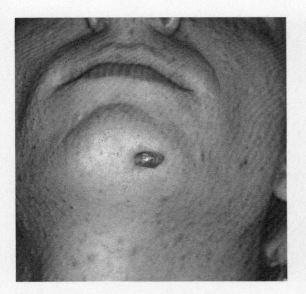

Fig. 34.19. Chronic sinus tract of the chin, with granulation tissue due to an odontogenic sinus tract. (From the Fitzsimons Army Medical Center Collection, Aurora, CO.)

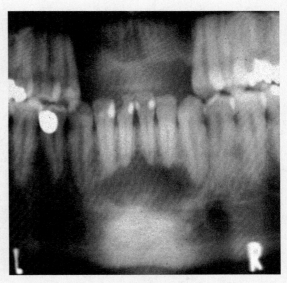

Fig. 34.20. Panoramic dental x-ray demonstrating a massive apical abscess beneath the mandibular incisors. (From the Fitzsimons Army Medical Center Collection, Aurora, CO.)

References

Epidermoid Cyst

1. Moore RB, Fagan EB, Hulkower S, et al. Clinical inquiries. What's the best treatment for sebaceous cysts? *J Fam Pract.* 2007;56:315-316.
2. Zuber TJ. Minimal excision for epidermoid (sebaceous) cysts. *Am Fam Physician.* 2002;65:1409-1412, 1417-1418.

Trichilemmal (Pilar) Cyst

1. Mehrabi D, Leonhardt JM, Brodell RT. Removal of keratinous and pilar cysts with the punch incision technique: analysis of surgical outcomes. *Dermatol Surg.* 2002;28:673-677.

Steatocystoma

1. Duzova AN, Senturk GB. Suggestion for treatment of steatocystoma multiplex located exclusively on the face. *Int J Dermatol.* 2004;43:60-62.

Apocrine Cystadenoma

1. del Pozo J, García-Silva J, Peña-Penabad C, Fonseca E. Multiple apocrine hidrocystomas: treatment with carbon dioxide laser vaporization. *J Dermatolog Treat.* 2001;12:97-100.

Digital Mucous Cyst

1. Bohler-Sommeregger K, Kutsdchera-Hienart G. Cryosurgical management of myxoid cysts. *J Dermatol Surg Oncol.* 1988;14:1405-1408.
2. Karrer S, Hohenleutner U, Szeimies RM, Landthaler M. Treatment of digital mucous cysts with carbon dioxide laser. *Acta Derm Venereol.* 1999;79:224-225.

Cutaneous Odontogenic Sinus Tract

1. Sheehan DJ, Potter BJ, Davis LS. Cutaneous draining sinus tract of odontogenic origin. *South Med J.* 2005;98:250-252.

Chapter 35
Subcutaneous Lumps

Subcutaneous lumps represent a heterogeneous category of cutaneous disorders that usually present as palpable nodules in the deeper extents of the skin and soft tissue. Angiolipomas and lipomas, comprised of vessels and benign adipose, or adipose alone, represent the most common entities in this category of disease. Other neoplasms in this category include metastatic, neural, and fibrohistiocytic tumors.

> **Differential Diagnosis of Subcutaneous Lumps**
> Common
> - Angiolipoma
> - Lipoma
>
> Uncommon (Selected Examples)
> - Hibernoma
> - Lipoblastoma
> - Liposarcoma
> - Malignant fibrous histiocytoma
> - Metastatic solid tumors
> - Metastatic tumors of lymphoid origin
> - Metastatic tumors of myeloid origin
> - Nodular fasciitis
> - Schwannoma
> - Spindle cell lipoma

IMPORTANT HISTORY QUESTIONS

How long has the lesion(s) been present?

Benign tumors, such as angiolipomas and lipomas, typically grow slowly and have been present for years at the time of presentation. A new or rapidly growing subcutaneous growth should raise concern for a more aggressive neoplasm.

Has the lesion changed?

Benign neoplasms typically grow slowly, whereas malignant neoplasms (e.g., liposarcoma, malignant fibrous histiocytoma, metastatic tumors), and some select benign neoplasms (e.g., nodular fasciitis), often demonstrate rapid growth.

Is there a family history of similar lesions?

Angiolipomas and lipomas can both be familial (e.g., benign familial lipomatosis). Therefore, an affirmative answer could indicate an inherited disorder. However, it is important to realize that a negative response to this question does not exclude multiple lipomas or angiolipomas because most cases are sporadic.

IMPORTANT PHYSICAL FINDINGS

How many lesions are present?

Multiple lesions occurring in a person could indicate multiple lipomas, angiolipomas, or even a metastatic process. Other types of tumors, such as liposarcoma, malignant fibrous histiocytoma, or spindle cell lipoma, nearly always occur as a singular process.

How large is the tumor?

In general, small tumors are more likely to be benign, whereas larger tumors are more likely to be malignant. For example, most benign lipomas are less than 5 cm in diameter; most liposarcomas are over 10 cm in size at the time of presentation.

What does the tumor feel like on palpation?

Most lipomas are soft and compressible, whereas most fibrohistiocytic tumors and metastatic tumors often feel firm. Some invasive malignant processes may even seem tethered to underlying structures.

Does the lesion appear to be sharply circumscribed?

Most lipomas and angiolipomas, as well as rare lipomatous tumors, are usually sharply delineated from the surrounding fat. Some can even be moved laterally, whereas metastatic lesions and most fibrohistiocytic tumors usually do not have well delineated margins and infiltrate into the adjacent subcutis.

Where are the lesions located?

The distribution of the lesions can be important. Multiple lipomas and angiolipomas often affect the forearms, thighs, and lateral thorax. Spindle cell lipoma often involves the head and neck.

Pathogenesis

A lipoma is benign tumor of fat. It is a common condition and the most common neoplasm of the subcutis. There is evidence that lipomas, although benign, are often the result of one or more genetic abnormalities. Translocations and other gene rearrangements of the chromosome 12q15 area are among those most often observed. In many cases, multiple lipomas are inherited as an autosomal dominant condition (benign familial lipomatosis).

Clinical Features

- Lipomas usually develop during adulthood but may also present in younger or older patients.
- Rarely, lipomas are present at birth.
- Lipomas may appear anywhere on the body but the upper trunk and extremity are most often affected.
- Lipomas deeper than the subcutaneous tissue (e.g., intramuscular lipomas) can occur.
- Lipomas present as a skin-colored subcutaneous lesion that is soft and circumscribed on palpation (Fig. 35.1). Some lipomas are slightly mobile on palpation.
- Lipomas are often asymptomatic but can be tender or painful, especially when compressed.
- Large lipomas may cause dilation of overlying blood vessels (Fig. 35.2).
- Rare lipomas may compress nerves to produce a peripheral neuropathy.

Diagnosis

- Lipomas often can be diagnosed simply based on the history and clinical presentation of a long-standing, slow-growing, soft, and well-circumscribed subcutaneous nodule, with a fatty consistency.
- If the diagnosis is in question, a biopsy may be performed. It must be remembered that the findings of interest exist deep in the soft tissue, and an incisional or excisional biopsy may be necessary.
- Rare cases potentially associated with a peripheral neuropathy may require magnetic resonance imaging (MRI) for assessment.

Treatment

- Lipomas are benign and do not require treatment.
- For symptomatic lesions, surgical excision may be performed. Many lipomas can be removed by shelling (or squishing) out the lipoma through a small opening, such as a punch biopsy, but this does not work in all cases. Large lipomas (Fig. 35.3), or those located on the forehead or posterior neck, may lie beneath the galea or may be admixed with collagen (fibrolipomas), complicating removal. Liposuction can be done in select cases.

Clinical Course

Untreated, most lipomas reach a stable size and persist indefinitely. Transformation of a benign lipoma to liposarcoma has been described but is rare. Interestingly, lipomas are metabolically independent of the rest of the body and will not usually change in volume, even if a patient gains or loses weight.

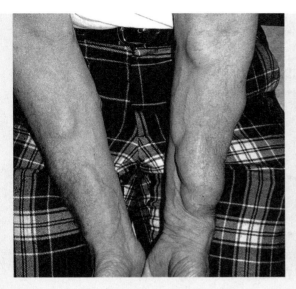

Fig. 35.1. Multiple lipomas. (From the Fitzsimons Army Medical Center Collection, Aurora, CO.)

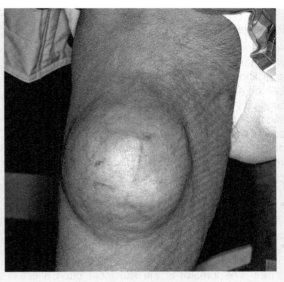

Fig. 35.2. Large lipoma with numerous vessels. (From the Fitzsimons Army Medical Center Collection, Aurora, CO.)

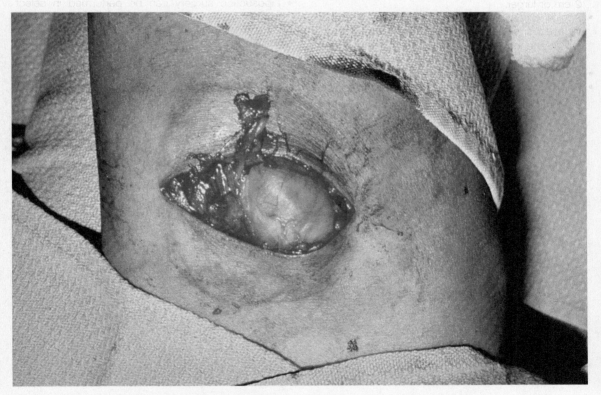

Fig. 35.3. Intraoperative view of intramuscular lipoma demonstrating demarcation. (From the Fitzsimons Army Medical Center Collection, Aurora, CO.)

Angiolipoma ICD10 code D17 (site dependent)

Pathogenesis

Angiolipomas represent the second most common subcutaneous tumor. In about 5% of cases, multiple angiolipomas can be inherited in autosomal dominant fashion (e.g., benign familial angiolipomatosis), which suggests a genetic anomaly that has not been identified. In contrast to lipomas, which are composed only of mature lipocytes, angiolipomas are comprised of mature lipocytes and numerous, thin-walled blood vessels that are often thrombosed.

Clinical Features

- Angiolipomas usually develop in adulthood (20–40 years), but they can also present in younger or older patients. Angiolipomas are rare in children.
- Angiolipomas may appear anywhere on the body. Most occur on the upper trunk and upper extremities. The forearm is the site most often affected (Figs. 35.4 and 35.5).
- Angiolipomas are often asymptomatic but can be tender or painful, especially when compressed.
- More than 90% of cutaneous angiolipomas are 2 cm or larger.
- Angiolipomas present as skin-colored or slightly violaceous, soft to slightly firm, well-circumscribed, subcutaneous lesions. When multiple lesions are present, there is often general symmetry.
- Most cases are slightly mobile with palpation.
- Rare cases can compress adjacent nerves, yielding a peripheral neuropathy.
- Rare cases can develop a locally aggressive growth pattern, with infiltration into skeletal muscle.

Diagnosis

- Angiolipomas are often diagnosed based upon the history and clinical presentation of a long-standing, slow-growing, soft, and well-circumscribed subcutaneous nodule, with a fatty consistency. Angiolipomas are more likely to be painful, in comparison to common lipomas.
- If the diagnosis is in question, a biopsy may be performed. It must be remembered that the findings of interest exist deep in the soft tissue, and an incisional or excisional biopsy may be necessary.
- Rare cases potentially associated with a peripheral neuropathy may require MRI for assessment.

Treatment

- Angiolipomas are benign. No treatment is required.
- Lesions that are painful, or for which removal is otherwise desired, can be treated with surgical extirpation, in a manner similar to that for lipomas.
- Liposuction surgery can be performed in select cases.

Clinical Course

Untreated, angiolipomas usually reach a stable size and persist indefinitely. Malignant transformation to liposarcoma has not been observed in angiolipomas.

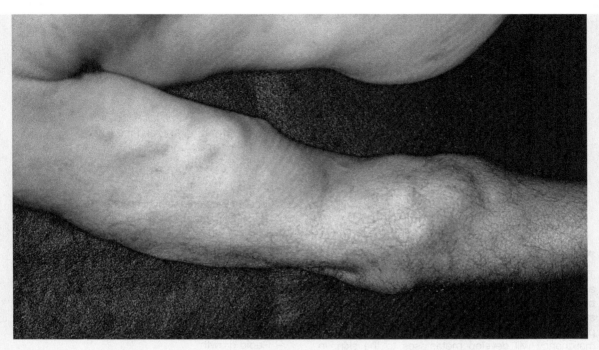

Fig. 35.4. Numerous large angiolipomas of the extremities and trunk. (From the Fitzsimons Army Medical Center Collection, Aurora, CO.)

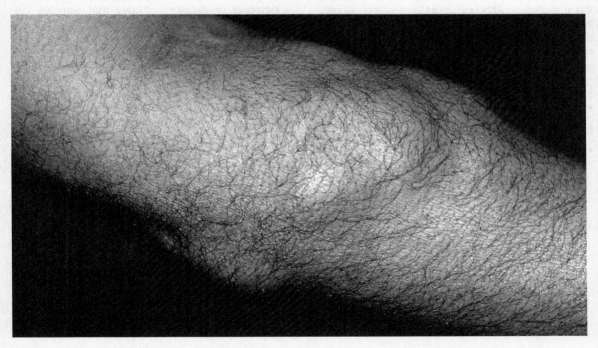

Fig. 35.5. Multiple large cutaneous angiolipomas, with normal overlying skin. (From the Fitzsimons Army Medical Center Collection, Aurora, CO.)

Solid Tumors That Frequently Metastasize to the Skin
- Breast carcinoma
- Colon and rectum adenocarcinoma
- Melanoma
- Oral mucosal malignancies
- Renal carcinoma
- Stomach carcinoma
- Squamous cell carcinoma of the lung

Hematologic Malignancies That Frequently Metastasize to the Skin
- Myeloid leukemias
- Monocytic leukemias
- Non–Hodgkin B cell lymphomas
- T cell lymphomas

Pathogenesis

The incidence of certain malignancies becoming metastatic and involving the skin has varied in studies because of unique aspects of the population under study or for other reasons of methodology. Overall, perhaps 1% to 9% of persons with an internal malignancy will develop metastases to the skin. In most cases, skin metastases occur in later stages of disease. In about 5% of cases, multiple cutaneous metastases may be the presenting feature of the malignancy. Although most metastatic deposits involve the dermis, a subset may present with subcutaneous nodules that mimic fatty neoplasms. The most common malignancies to involve the skin are listed in the box.

Clinical Features

- Metastatic deposits in the skin occur more often in elderly persons, probably because this age group is most likely to have internal malignancies.
- Subcutaneous metastatic tumors may affect any region of the body, with different malignancies having affinities for different sites.

- Subcutaneous metastatic deposits may be solitary or numerous.
- Metastatic nodules are typically asymptomatic, unless there is nerve impingement.
- Metastatic nodules vary in size but can become large.
- Metastatic nodules usually demonstrate an unremarkable overlying skin surface (Figs. 35.6–35.8).
- The patient may be cachectic due to the overall metastatic burden.

Diagnosis

- Subcutaneous metastatic lesions do not have a characteristic appearance and can resemble benign soft tissue tumors, such as lipomas and angiolipomas. The patient depicted in Fig. 35.7 was referred from the emergency room to dermatology for excision of an assumed lipoma.
- Findings that should arouse suspicion for a metastatic nodule to the skin include a history of the following:
  - Known internal malignancy
  - Rapid growth
  - Onset of multiple lesions
  - Recent unexplained weight loss
- The diagnosis is established by doing a deep punch incisional or excisional biopsy that samples the process of key diagnostic interest.

Clinical Course

Clearly, the clinical course of metastatic disease involving the skin depends upon the tumor type and the systemic treatment options that are available. In general, once a patient develops multiple metastatic deposits to the skin, the prognosis is poor. Most patients die from the primary malignancy within 2 years.

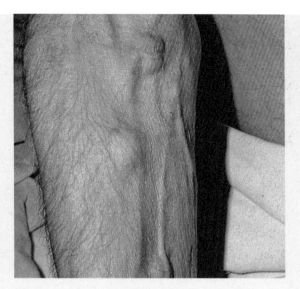

Fig. 35.6. Subcutaneous metastatic acute myeloid leukemia. (From the Fitzsimons Army Medical Center Collection, Aurora, CO.)

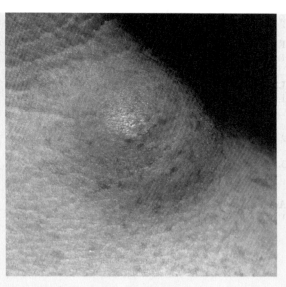

Fig. 35.7. Subcutaneous metastatic melanoma that was clinically thought to be a lipoma. (From the Fitzsimons Army Medical Center Collection, Aurora, CO.)

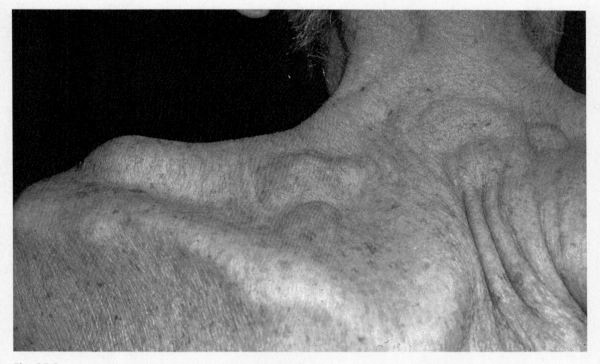

Fig. 35.8. Subcutaneous metastatic adenocarcinoma originating from the stomach in a cachectic patient. (From the Fitzsimons Army Medical Center Collection, Aurora, CO.)

References

Review of Lipomatous Neoplasms

1. Mentzel T. Cutaneous lipomatous neoplasms. *Semin Diagn Pathol.* 2001;18:250-257.

Lipoma

1. Christenson L, Patterson J, Davis D. Surgical pearl: use of the cutaneous punch for the removal of lipomas. *J Am Acad Dermatol.* 2000;42:675-676.
2. Flores LP, Carneiro JZ. Peripheral nerve compression secondary to adjacent lipomas. *Surg Neurol.* 2007;67:258-262.
3. Silistreli OK, Drumus EU, Ulusal BG, et al. What should be the treatment modality in giant cutaneous lipomas? Review of the literature and report of 4 cases. *Br J Plast Surg.* 2005;58:394-398.

Angiolipoma

1. Garib G, Siegal GP, Andea AA. Autosomal-dominant familial angiolipomatosis. *Cutis.* 2015;95:E26-E29.

2. Puig L, Moreno A, de Moragas JM. Infiltrating angiolipomas: report of two cases and review of the literature. *J Dermatol Surg Oncol.* 1986;12:617-619.

Metastatic Tumors

1. Sariya D, Ruth K, Adams-McDonnell R, et al. Clinicopathologic correlation of cutaneous metastases: experience from a cancer center. *Arch Dermatol.* 2007;143:613-620.
2. Schulman JM, Pauli MI, Neuhaus IM, et al. The distribution of cutaneous metastases correlates with local immunologic milieu. *J Am Acad Dermatol.* 2016;74:470-476.

Chapter 36
Cutaneous Diseases of Travelers

A recent study found that skin disease affects up to 8% of travelers. Skin disease is the third most common problem of travelers, after diarrhea and respiratory disorders. It is worthwhile for all health care providers to have a passing familiarity with the major cutaneous diseases that occur in travelers. Although this chapter can only address the issue in a limited fashion, the Centers for Disease Control and Prevention (CDC) has an interactive website where patients and clinicians can enter a travel destination to access country-specific health advisories (https://wwwnc.cdc.gov/travel).

Ten Common Cutaneous Diseases of the Returning Traveler
1. Cutaneous larva migrans
2. Soft tissue bacterial infections
3. Arthropod bites
4. Allergic reaction or urticaria
5. Myiasis
6. Superficial fungal infection
7. Injuries including animal bites
8. Scabies
9. Cutaneous leishmaniasis
10. Tungiasis

IMPORTANT HISTORY QUESTIONS

Where have you traveled recently?

Some diseases are common in certain areas of the world. For example, leishmaniasis is encountered in persons traveling to Central and South America or the Middle East. Myiasis is common in persons traveling to Central and South America or parts of Africa. Even some US territories, such as Puerto Rico, may be affected by diseases, such as Zika virus or chikungunya virus, which can cause a viral exanthem.

Did you develop skin disease before you traveled, while traveling, or after you returned home?

It is important to understand the timeline of disease activity. Some skin disease in the traveler represents aggravation of a preexisting condition, such as atopic dermatitis. Other conditions, such as urticaria and other allergic reactions, can develop during travel simply because of exposure to an allergen. Finally, some conditions such as myiasis and leishmaniasis are notorious for developing in the weeks and months after travel.

Were you outdoors or in a rural area during your travels?

Some diseases, such as leishmaniasis and myiasis, are caused by the bite of flying insects, and determining whether the patient has been outdoors is important (e.g., hiking, camping). Cutaneous larva migrans is a disease associated with exposure to beach sand contaminated with cat or dog feces. Tungiasis, caused by the bite of the sand flea, is also acquired on beaches.

On your trip, did you use preventive measures to avoid disease?

The use of insect repellents, bed netting, and/or sleeping in screened areas with environmental controls are measures that lessen the likelihood of a traveler acquiring some cutaneous diseases. Avoiding direct contact with contaminated beach sand is another measure. For some diseases, such as yellow fever, there is a vaccine for those traveling to endemic areas.

Where and How

Cutaneous larva migrans (CLM) is a parasitic skin infection caused by the hookworms *Ancylostoma braziliense* and *Ancylostoma caninum*, which affect the intestines of cats and dogs. Humans are infected with CLM larvae by placing their bare skin (e.g., feet, hands, buttocks) in contact with sand contaminated by animal feces. The larvae penetrate human skin, but cannot complete a full life cycle. The organism migrates under the skin surface, leading to a so-called creeping eruption. CLM occurs in travelers from sub-Saharan Africa, Asia, Central and South America, and the Caribbean. Some cases occur in the United States, on the Gulf Coast, but use of anthelmintic agents in pets has greatly reduced the rate of endemic acquisition.

Clinical Presentation

CLM causes an erythematous pruritic eruption that migrates (or creeps) under the skin (Fig. 36.1; also see Figs. 17.15 to 17.18). The condition usually begins days or weeks after exposure, but larva can lie dormant for months before migrating. Excoriation can yield ulceration, with secondary infection. The lesions affect skin exposed to sand, such as the hands, feet, and buttocks. The tracks may advance a few millimeters to several centimeters each day.

Diagnosis

The diagnosis of CLM is based on an appropriate travel history and characteristic clinical appearance. Confirmation by biopsy is challenging because the organism is always migrating ahead of the host response.

Prevention and Treatment

Prevention includes wearing shoes in areas of contaminated sand. Many communities ban dogs from beaches for this reason. Oral agents for CLM include albendazole, mebendazole, and ivermectin. Thiabendazole can be used as a topical cream or systemic (oral) agent. Destructive modalities (e.g., liquid nitrogen) are problematic because the organism lies ahead of any visible inflammatory response.

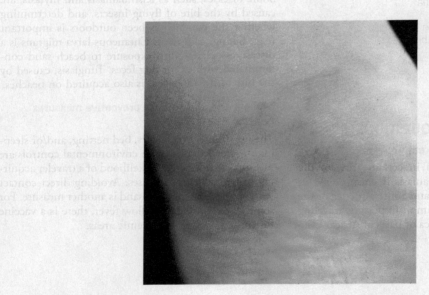

Fig. 36.1. Linear serpiginous lesion on the foot of a child. (From the William Weston Collection, Aurora, CO.)

Myiasis ICD10 Code B87.9

Where and How

Myiasis is a disease caused by the parasitic infestation of the human body with fly larvae. There are different forms of myiasis, but the two types we will concern ourselves herein with are caused by *Dermatobia hominis* (the human bot fly) and *Cordylobia anthropophaga* (the tumbu fly). Bot fly myiasis is seen throughout Central and South America; the fly larva is placed on the skin by mosquitoes in a complex life cycle interplay. Tumbu fly myiasis is seen in Africa (Fig. 36.2); it is caused by clothing and linens hung outdoors, where flies lay eggs on the fabric and that are later in contact with skin.

Clinical Presentation

Myiasis is caused by fly larva burrowing into the skin and maturing there, leading to an expansive nodule. In myiasis, affected persons often complain of a cyst or bump that is associated with a moving sensation. The lesion may grow over weeks or months but, eventually, to complete the life cycle, matured larva must exit the skin to become mature insects. Because the organism must respire, often the nodule is seen to have a central punctum, or breathing hole.

Diagnosis

The diagnosis of myiasis is usually established by a travel history of outdoor exposure at the destination of interest and a clinical situation of a nodule or dermal abscess, often with a central punctum and with the sensation of movement.

Prevention and Treatment

Prevention of bot fly myiasis includes avoiding biting insects in an outdoor environment and the use of bed netting when sleeping outdoors. Prevention of tumbu fly myiasis includes ironing clothing and sheets hung outdoors. Although there are regional treatments for myiasis used by persons in an endemic area, such as bacon fat poultices, excision is the treatment of choice for imported cases of myiasis seen in the United States.

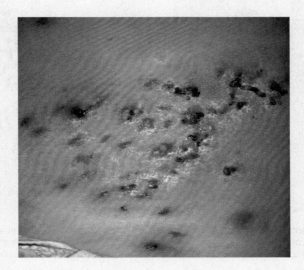

Fig. 36.2. Tumbu fly myiasis. These are numerous abscesses on the abdomen of a traveler who has recently returned from Africa. It is believed that he acquired this from the bed sheets at the hotel where he was staying. (From the Fitzsimons Army Medical Center Collection, Aurora, CO.)

Where and How

All superficial fungal infections can be exacerbated by hot (sweaty) tropical climates, but there are some superficial fungal infections, such as tinea nigra, that occur chiefly in tropical areas outside the United States. Tinea nigra is caused by *Hortaea werneckii,* a pigment-producing fungus.

Clinical Presentation

Tinea nigra often involves the hands and feet and creates a slowly expansive, thin, pigmented patch, with minimal scale (Fig. 36.3), which may be confused with a pigmented lesion, such as acral melanoma.

Diagnosis

Although tinea nigra may mimic a pigmented lesion, a potassium hydroxide (KOH) preparation will demonstrate the pigmented fungus in the same manner in which other superficial fungal infections are recognized (Fig. 36.4). Alternatively, a biopsy can immediately exclude a melanocytic neoplasm and include tinea nigra. Fungal culture yields a pigmented colony with about 1 week of growth.

Prevention and Treatment

Keeping feet dry may aid in prevention. Topical anti-fungal agents, such as ketoconazole, usually lead to resolution of tinea nigra in 2 to 4 weeks. Topical keratolytic agents, such as salicylic acid, can reduce observed pigmentation. Spontaneous resolution is a rare event.

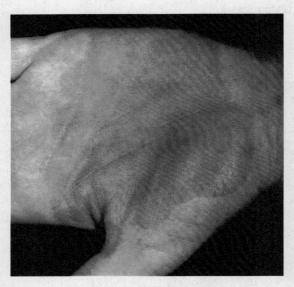

Fig. 36.3. Tan to brown pigmented patch of tinea nigra acquired in Southeast Asia. (From the Fitzsimons Army Medical Center Collection, Aurora, CO.)

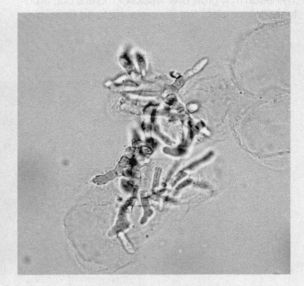

Fig. 36.4. Positive KOH of tinea nigra demonstrating pigmented hyphae (400×). (From the Fitzsimons Army Medical Center Collection, Aurora, CO.)

Where and How

Cutaneous leishmaniasis is a protozoal disease that causes skin ulcers. New World leishmaniasis occurs in extreme South Texas, Mexico, and Central and South America and is caused by the bite of the *Lutzomyia* fly. Old World leishmaniasis is caused by the bite of the *Phlebotomus* fly and is more common in the Middle East, including Israel, parts of south central Asia, and northwest Africa. Flies simply serve as vectors for the protozoal organisms. There are different species of leishmaniasis among New World and Old World categories of disease.

Clinical Presentation

The common denominator in cutaneous leishmaniasis is an ulcer that usually begins weeks, or even a few months, after exposure. Consequently, the disease is often first suspected after the traveler has returned home. The ulcers may have a raised border and are often painless but can be painful, particularly when superinfected. Satellite lesions (Fig. 36.5), regional lymphadenopathy, and nodular lymphangitis (sporotrichoid spread) can be seen.

The ulcers of leishmaniasis usually heal eventually, even without treatment, but result in scarring. A concern with some forms of New World leishmaniasis, particularly that acquired in South America, is mucocutaneous leishmaniasis, which involves the mucosa and can occur years or decades after the cutaneous lesions have resolved. This is one reason why speciation via laboratory testing may be prudent in some cases of New World disease.

Diagnosis

The diagnosis of leishmaniasis should be suspected based on the clinical presentation and an appropriate travel history. A biopsy of the ulcer edge may show characteristic amastigote forms of the parasite in dermal histiocytes, but the number of organisms diminishes over time, and these organisms can be challenging to locate. The CDC offers diagnostic assistance, including a pathology consultation using a commercially unavailable immunohistochemical stain, tissue culture, and/or polymerase chain reaction (PCR)-based speciation. Additional information is available at https://www.cdc.gov/parasites/leishmaniasis/resources/pdf/cdc_diagnosis_guide_leishmaniasis_2016.pdf.

Prevention and Treatment

Lutzomyia and *Phlebotomus* flies bite during the evening hours, and the use of insect repellent and bed netting is necessary to prevent bites. Many forms of leishmaniasis will resolve, even without treatment. Treatment to hasten resolution may include topical paromomycin 15%/gentamicin 0.5% cream, oral fluconazole, itraconazole, or rifampin or intravenous sodium stibogluconate or amphotericin. The only agent approved to treat leishmaniasis in the United States is miltefosine, but it is expensive and it is logistically difficult to use. As noted, because of the risk of mucocutaneous disease with some New World forms (subgenus *Viannia*), advanced testing to determine the species may be prudent in these circumstances to ensure optimal treatment. The CDC and state health department can often assist the clinician.

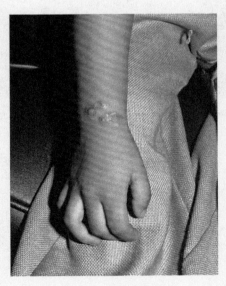

Fig. 36.5. Leishmaniasis in a child returning from Panama. (From the Fitzsimons Army Medical Center Collection, Aurora, CO.)

Where and How

Tungiasis is a disease caused by the sand flea, *Tunga penetrans*. This flea burrows into the skin of humans, usually on the foot, and then lives in parasitic fashion, imbibing blood from the host and laying eggs onto the epithelial surface, where its own hindquarters protrude. It is thought that the disease was acquired by Christopher Columbus, when he made landfall in the Caribbean, but it has spread to parts of Africa, India, Pakistan, and Latin America.

Clinical Presentation

Tungiasis usually affects the feet. The lesion begins as a punctum or ulcer and resembles a discolored nodule, with a central black dot (Fig. 36.6). The flea breathes through an opening in the skin, and the lesion ranges in size from 4 to 10 mm. Lesions can be pruritic, or even painful, although sometimes no symptoms are experienced. In some situations there may be inflammation and swelling. Superinfection is a concern and often is a complicating factor of tungiasis.

Diagnosis

The diagnosis is often suspected based on the travel history and clinical examination. Excision, which is also the treatment of choice, will often provide firm histologic evidence of the infestation.

Prevention and Treatment

Tungiasis can be prevented by avoiding direct contact with infested sand. Tungiasis is often self-limited because the organism dies, and the skin sheds. When treatment is necessary, physical removal is preferred, and often, if the flea is engorged, excision will be necessary. Topical antiparasitic medications such as ivermectin, metrifonate, and thiabendazole have been reported. Also suffocation of the flea using petrolatum jelly or killing the flea with liquid nitrogen is possible. Precautions should be taken to prevent secondary infections and tetanus/gangrene.

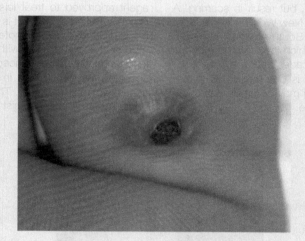

Fig. 36.6. Tungiasis on the toe of a child returning from vacation in Belize. (From the Joanna Burch Collection, Aurora, CO.)

Phytophotodermatitis ICD10 Code L56.2

Where and How

Phytophotodermatitis is a phototoxic reaction that occurs due to the presence of furocoumarins on the skin, typically from plant sources. Citrus fruit, including lime juice, can produce this reaction. Hence, in travel situations it has been given various names, such as Cancun dermatitis and margarita dermatitis because it can occur in lime juice, served with beer or tequila, which leaks on the skin and is then exposed to sunlight. The skin of the mango may also produce phytophotodermatitis.

Clinical Presentation

During the acute stage, there is inflammation, pruritus, and erythematous patches, plaques, or even blisters on the skin. These lesions often assume irregular linear shapes (Fig. 36.7), which suggest an exogenous injury.

The latter stages of phytophotodermatitis consist of hyperpigmentation that is slow to resolve (Fig. 36.8).

Diagnosis

The diagnosis is usually based on the clinical presentation, including unusual or linear configurations of lesions, with a supportive history of sun exposure and exposure to exogenous sources of furocoumarins, including the juice of citrus fruits such as limes.

Prevention and Treatment

Avoiding contact of furocoumarins with the skin, in the presence of sunlight, will prevent phytophotodermatitis. Once the condition has resulted in postinflammatory hyperpigmentation, patience will be necessary because resolution is slow.

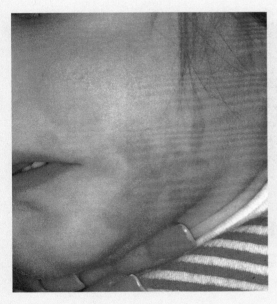

Fig. 36.7. Phytophotodermatitis due to contact with lime in a child demonstrating irregular and strangely linear erythema, with early brownish discoloration. (From the William Weston Collection, Aurora, CO.)

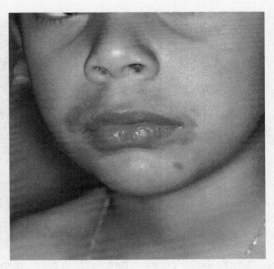

Fig. 36.8. Phytophotodermatitis in a child demonstrating perioral brownish discoloration due to exposure to the skin of a mango. (From the William Weston Collection, Aurora, CO.)

Seabather's Eruption ICD10 Code B65.3

Where and How

Seabather's eruption is a pruritic papular eruption that occurs underneath a swimsuit after exposure to seawater that contains the larval form of the thimble jellyfish, *Linuche unguiculata*. Most cases occur on the eastern Atlantic coast, particularly in Florida and Brazil, from March to August, with a peak incidence in May and June.

Clinical Presentation

Seabather's eruption occurs on skin beneath a bathing suit. A burning or stinging feeling may be experienced on the skin, even while still in the water. As the swimmer gets out of the sea, the nematocyst may release more toxin, resulting in a painful sensation. Showering in fresh water and rubbing with a towel (mechanical stimulation) make the eruption worse. The end result is a rash, consisting of pruritic erythematous papules beneath the bathing suit (Fig. 36.9).

Diagnosis

The diagnosis is established via an appropriate exposure history and the findings of a papular and pruritic rash on skin covered by the bathing suit.

Prevention and Treatment

Prevention includes avoidance of the seawater when *Linuche unguiculata* levels are high. Dilute vinegar or rubbing alcohol can neutralize any toxin that is left on the skin. Topical steroids may be used to treat the rash. Contaminated clothing should be thoroughly washed.

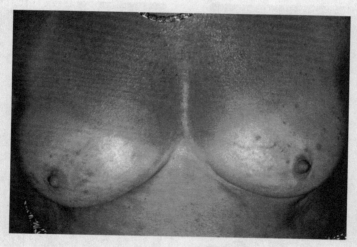

Fig. 36.9. Seabather's eruption demonstrating pruritic erythema papules beneath the bathing suit. (From the Fitzsimons Army Medical Center Collection, Aurora, CO.)

References

Cutaneous Larva Migrans

1. Kincaid L, Klowak M, Klowak S, et al. Management of imported cutaneous larva migrans: a case series and mini-review. *Travel Med Infect Dis.* 2015;13:382-387.

Myiasis

1. Solomon M, Lachish T, Schwartz E. Cutaneous myiasis. *Curr Infect Dis Rep.* 2016;18:28.

Tinea Nigra

1. Nazzaro G, Ponziani A, Cavicchini S. Tinea nigra: a diagnostic pitfall. *J Am Acad Dermatol.* 2016;75:e219-e220.

Leishmaniasis

1. David CV, Craft N. Cutaneous and mucocutaneous leishmaniasis. *Dermatologic Ther.* 2009;491-502.

Tungiasis

1. Feldmeier H1, Keysers A. Tungiasis—a Janus-faced parasitic skin disease. *Travel Med Infect Dis.* 2013;11:357-365.

Phytophotodermatitis

1. Raam R, DeClerck B, Jhun P, Herbert M. Phytophotodermatitis: the other "lime" disease. *Ann Emerg Med.* 2016;67:554-556.

Seabather's Eruption

1. Rossetto AL, Da Silveira FL, Morandini AC, et al. Seabather's eruption: report of fourteen cases. *An Acad Bras Cienc.* 2015;87:431-436.

Chapter 37
Topical Treatment Pearls

INTRODUCTION

Becoming proficient and knowledgeable about skin disease involves the accumulation of experience, but there are certainly pearls that can be shared to expedite the process. For example, even before one writes a single prescription for dermatitis, it is important to consider the patient's bathing habits and overall skin care, because these habits and practices may have caused or perpetuated the skin problem.

> ### Understanding Soap Ingredients
> **Lye-Based**
> - Sodium tallowate
> - Sodium cocoate
> - Sodium palm kernelate
> - Sodium palmate
>
> **Syndet**
> - Sodium lauroyl isethionate
> - Sodium isethionate
> - Sodium cococyl isethionate

BEST SOAPS FOR XEROSIS AND DERMATITIS

Soaps are the most common irritant that people are exposed to each day, yet patients and providers do not always appreciate the differences among various soaps. Normal skin has a slightly acidic pH. The precise pH is site-dependent, but typically the skin pH is between 4.5 and 5.5. The skin has the ability to regulate pH, chiefly via production of lactic acid, with lactate contained in sebum (the so-called lipid mantle).

However, most soaps are lye-based and hence have a high pH in relation to the skin. For example, in one study, Neutrogena soap had a pH of 9.6, and Ivory soap had a pH of 10.1. Although there are other factors that affect the irritancy of a soap, in general, products with a neutral or slightly acidic pH are less irritating (e.g., Dove soap has a pH of 7.3; Cetaphil has a pH of 6.4).

As a general rule, lye-based and so-called natural soaps will often be more irritating than synthetic soaps (termed *syndets* [synesthetic detergents] in the soap industry). The composition of soaps may vary over time, and a brand name may have more than one line containing different components.

The box above lists common lye-based (natural) and synthetic soap ingredients (syndets). Patients do not need to know a long list of ingredients; they only need to know that the primary tensioactive agent of milder soaps has the word *isethionate* in the list of ingredients. All patients with xerosis, dermatitis, or recent dermatitis (within 4 weeks) may benefit from use of a syndet.

GRAM-NEGATIVE TOE WEB INFECTIONS: ANOTHER SOAP ISSUE

Gram-negative toe web infections (GNTWIs) are common in humid climates and in persons with hyperhidrosis. GNTWIs often demonstrate an unpleasant odor and erythema, erosions, and purulence that may be yellow, yellow-green, or green-blue, especially if *Pseudomonas* is a dominant pathogen (Fig. 37.1).

Although prescription antimicrobial therapy is appropriate, a chief goal is to re-establish normal gram-positive commensals (GPCs). Military studies have indicated that use of antibacterial soaps preferentially deplete GPCs and could cause or worsen GNTWIs. This effect is not seen in those using soaps without certain antibacterial agents. Avoidance of over-the-counter (OTC) antibacterial soaps is an important step in the management of GNTWIs. Recently, the US Food and Drug Administration (FDA) asked manufacturers to cease use of 19 antibacterial ingredients in soap, including triclosan and triclocarban.

WHAT IS THE BEST MOISTURIZER?

OTC moisturizers, depilatories, and antiaging products, represent a $121 billion/year industry, often with sophisticated advertising campaigns. Development of

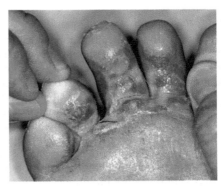

Fig. 37.1. Severe pseudomonal toe web infection. (From the William Weston Collection, Aurora, CO.)

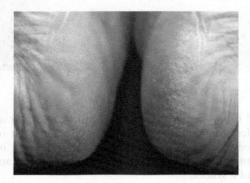

Fig. 37.2. Xerotic heels treated with ammonium lactate *(left)* and an occlusive moisturizer *(right)*.

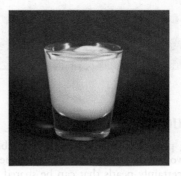

Fig. 37.3. Shot glass rule.

a good moisturizer is a complex issue, but fundamentally, moisturizers have three major components: oils (including petrolatum-based and plant oils) that occlude, humectants that bind water, and biologically active compounds.

Because most moisturizers contain oil, recognizing differences in humectants and biologically active compounds is useful in comparing moisturizers. Common humectants include sugar alcohols (e.g., glycerol, sorbitol), honey, aloe, and urea. Urea is an outstanding humectant. An excellent, cosmetically elegant product suitable for everyday use is Eucerin Intensive Repair, which contains urea (10%) and sodium lactate (5%).

For patients with severe xerosis, products containing 12% ammonium lactate, available in prescription (LacHydrin) and OTC forms (AmLactin) represent excellent products. However, these products are odiferous and may produce a burning sensation when applied, especially if the skin is fissured. Lactic acid and its salt are biologically active and increase the production of hyaluronic acid in the dermis, and normalize keratinization. Hyaluronic acid retains in excess of 1000-fold its weight in water; hence, lactate-containing moisturizers often outperform other products in cases of severe xerosis (Fig. 37.2).

SUNSCREENS

Application of sunscreens

Appropriate counseling regarding sunscreens is rather complex. In general, patients should use sunscreens that are labeled as a *broad-spectrum,* meaning the products provides protection from ultraviolet A (UVA) and ultraviolet B (UVB) light. The label should include the term *water resistant,* which means that it still provides significant coverage after 40 or 80 minutes, as identified on the bottle. The sunscreen protection factor (SPF) indicates protection against UVB only, but products of use should have a rating of 30 or higher. Application is also important. Studies have shown that on average, people apply sunscreen at 50% or less than the concentration at which the SPF was

determined. The so-called shot glass rule of sunscreens (Fig. 37.3) is premised on the idea that shot glasses hold about 1 ounce; this is enough sunscreen to cover the face, arms, torso, and legs once. Sunscreen should be reapplied about every 2 hours and even more often with heavy sweating or water exposure.

When to use sunscreens indoors and under clothing

Most patients and health care providers do not understand that UVA, which is involved in photoaging, photosensitive diseases (e.g., lupus erythematosus, most polymorphous light eruptions), and many photoallergic drug eruptions, passes through window glass and most clothing. Fig. 19.38 illustrates UVA-induced tanning in the shape of a butterfly that occurred through the patient's swimsuit. Patients with photosensitive diseases must use broad-based (UVA, UVB blocking) sunscreens to prevent disease activity. Moreover, use is required whether or not the patient plans to go outdoors. Avobenzone is an excellent UVA blocker and is available in many different products, allowing for the patient's preference. The best sunscreen is one that the patient will use. A leading consumer review magazine has recommended "No-Ad Sport SPF 50 Lotion" as an economical and high-performing sunscreen. For those who desire a spray formulation, Equate Sport Continuous Spray has been recommended.

CORTICOSTEROIDS

How much topical corticosteroid do I need to prescribe?

Topical corticosteroids are available in different strengths and formulations. A common error in prescribing is providing too little medication, to treat the area adequately, for the intended duration. The "fingertip unit" (Fig. 37.4), as measured in adults, is about 0.5 g, and it is enough to treat 2% of the total body surface. Thus, if the patient has 10% of his or her body surface involved, and it is intended for him or her to use a topical corticosteroid twice daily for 10 days, one must prescribe at least 50 g of corticosteroid. Another rule of thumb is that it takes 15 g of material to cover

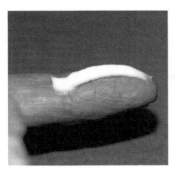

Fig. 37.4. Fingertip unit. (From the John Aeling Collection, Aurora, CO.)

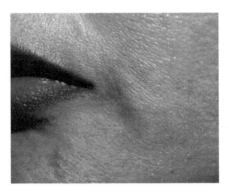

Fig. 37.5. Topical corticosteroid atrophy. (From the William Weston Collection, Aurora, CO.)

the body once, from the neck down. Finally, it is also important to realize that twice-daily use is not twice as effective as once-daily use. It is estimated that a second daily application may provide only 20% to 30% of additional efficacy. In cases of dermatitis or psoriasis that are not severe, once-daily application may have advantages in terms of compliance, lesser risk of overuse, and lower overall cost.

Preventing atrophy from topical corticosteroids

Potent topical corticosteroids can produce atrophy, including epidermal thinning, decreased hyaluronic acid production, reduced collagen fibers, and thinned elastic fibers (striae distensae), after just 1 week of twice-daily use. The patient depicted in Fig. 37.5 developed skin atrophy from prolonged use of betamethasone ointment. An unappreciated prospective study has demonstrated that just 4 weeks' use of topical clobetasol on the forearm, without occlusion, yields a 51% decrease in the thickness of the epidermis and a 47% decrease in hyaluronic acid content. The opposite forearm was treated with topical clobetasol plus twice-daily 12% ammonium lactate. The ammonium lactate-treated site had only a 35% decrease in epidermal thickness and only a 17% decrease in hyaluronic acid content. Moreover, the sites treated with ammonium lactate did not demonstrate decreased melanin production that had been observed in the sites treated with only clobetasol. When anticipating use of potent topical steroids for a skin disorder for a period longer than 2 weeks, concomitant use of 12% ammonium lactate may lessen side effects.

Reference

1. Lavker RM, Kaidbey K, Leyden JL. Effects of topical ammonium lactate on cutaneous atrophy from a potent topical corticosteroid. *J Am Acad Dermatol*. 1992;26:535-544.

Index

Page numbers followed by "*f*" indicate figures, "*t*" indicate tables, "*b*" indicate boxes, and "*e*" indicate online content.

A

ABCDEs of melanoma, 507, 528*b*
Abscesses, 217–230, 217*b*
  dissecting cellulitis of scalp, 224, 225*f*
  furuncle, 218, 219*f*
  hidradenitis suppurativa, 222, 223*f*
  history questions for, 217
  kerion, 228, 228*b*, 229*f*
  mycobacterial furunculosis, 220, 220*f*–221*f*
  physical findings in, 217
  ruptured epidermoid cysts, 226, 227*f*
Acanthosis nigricans, 448, 448*b*, 449*f*
ACD. *see* Allergic contact dermatitis (ACD)
Acetaminophen, for progressive pigmented purpura, 340
Acetic acid, for *Pseudomonas* folliculitis, 382
Ackerman tumor, 461, 474
Acne, 376, 377*f*
Acne vulgaris, in Wood light, 8
Acquired ichthyosis vulgaris, 126, 126*b*, 127*f*
Acquired melanocytic nevus, 512, 513*f*
Acquired moles, 512
Acquired nevi, 512
Acrochordon (soft fibroma), 461, 470, 471*f*
Acrodermatitis continua of Hallopeau, 208, 209*f*
Acropustulosis of infancy, 210, 211*f*
Actinic keratosis, 110, 111*f*
Acute febrile neutrophilic dermatosis, 76
Acute generalized exanthematous pustulosis, 206, 207*f*
Acute hemorrhagic edema (AHE), of infancy, 330, 331*f*
Acute myeloid leukemia, subcutaneous metastatic, 585*f*
Acute paronychia, 404
Acute rheumatic fever, 276
Acute vulgaris, 376, 377*b*, 377*f*
Acyclovir
  for chickenpox, 178
  for herpes simplex virus infection, 182
AD. *see* Atopic dermatitis (AD)
Addison disease, 452, 452*b*, 453*f*
Adenocarcinoma, subcutaneous metastatic, 585*f*
Adrenal insufficiency, 452
Adrenocorticotropic hormone (ACTH), 452
Aeromonas hydrophila, 382
Albendazole, for cutaneous larva migrans, 588
Alcohol consumption, subcutaneous diseases and, 253
Allergic contact dermatitis (ACD), 136, 136*b*–138*b*,
    137*f*–139*f*
  bullous, 174, 175*f*
Alopecia, 385–402
  alopecia areata, 394, 395*f*
  androgenic, 386, 387*f*

Alopecia *(Continued)*
  central centrifugal cicatricial, 400, 401*f*
  classification of, 385*b*
  history questions for, 385
  lupus erythematosus and, 398, 399*f*
  physical findings in, 385
  telogen effluvium, 385, 388, 388*b*, 389*f*
  tinea capitis, 396, 397*f*
  traction, 392, 393*f*
  trichotillomania, 385, 390, 391*f*
Alopecia areata, 394, 395*f*
Aluminum chloride, for erythrasma, 160
△Amino levulinic acid photodynamic therapy, for actinic
    keratosis, 110
Aminoglycoside, antipseudomonal, for ecthyma
    gangrenosum, 234
Ammonium lactate, xerosis treated with, 598*f*
Ammonium lactate-containing moisturizers, for atopic
    dermatitis, 142–144
Amoxicillin-clavulanate, for cutaneous odontogenic sinus
    tract, 576
Amphotericin, of cutaneous leishmaniasis, 591
Amyopathic dermatomyositis, 322
Ancylostoma braziliense, 588
Ancylostoma caninum, 588
Androgenic alopecia, 386, 387*f*
Anesthetic agents, for roseola vaccinatum, 46
Angioedema, 68, 68*b*, 69*f*
Angiolipoma, 582, 583*f*
Angiosarcoma, 550, 551*f*
Animals, exposure to, necrotic and ulcerative skin
    disorders and, 231
Annular and targetoid lesions, 269–288
  differential diagnosis of, 269*b*
  erythema annulare centrifugum, 274, 274*b*, 275*f*
  erythema marginatum, 276, 277*f*
  erythema multiforme, 286, 287*f*
  granuloma annulare, 280, 281*f*
  history questions for, 269
  leprosy (Hansen disease), 284, 285*f*
  Lyme disease, 272, 273*f*
  necrobiosis lipoidica (diabeticorum), 282, 283*f*
  neonatal lupus erythematosus, 278, 279*f*
  physical findings in, 269
  tinea corporis, tinea faciei, and tinea cruris, 270, 271*f*
Annular lesions. *see* Annular and targetoid lesions
Annular lichen planus, 102
Anogenital warts. *see* Condyloma acuminatum
Anti-tumor necrosis factor–α (TNF–α), for pyoderma
    gangrenosum, 246

Antibiotics
  antipseudomonal, for ecthyma gangrenosum, 234
  for atopic dermatitis, 144
  for cutaneous odontogenic sinus tract, 576
  for guttate psoriasis, 98
  for moderate acne, 376
  for necrotizing fasciitis, 232
  for paronychia, 404
Antifibrotic agents, for nephrogenic systemic fibrosis, 364
Antifungal agents, topical
  for seborrheic dermatitis, 158
  for tinea nigra, 590
Antihistamines
  for acropustulosis of infancy, 210
  for allergic contact dermatitis, 136
  for atopic dermatitis, 144
  for bullous allergic contact dermatitis, 174
  for id reactions, 152
  for morbilliform drug eruptions, 32
  for morbilliform viral eruptions, 36
  for pityriasis rosea, 156
  strongest, 64*b*
Antiphosphodiesterase inhibitors, for scleroderma, 356
Antiplatelet drugs, for scleroderma, 356
Antipseudomonal aminoglycoside, for ecthyma
  gangrenosum, 234
Antipseudomonal antibiotic, for ecthyma gangrenosum,
  234
Antipseudomonal β-lactamase penicillin, for ecthyma
  gangrenosum, 234
Antipyretics, for roseola, 38
Antistaphylococcal antibiotics
  for dyshidrosis, 154
  for nummular dermatitis, 150
Antivenin, for necrotic arachnidism, 238
Antiviral therapies, for roseola, 38
Aplasia cutis congenita (APC), 372, 373*f*
Apocrine cystadenoma, 565*f*, 572, 573*f*
Apocrine hidrocystomas. *see* Apocrine cystadenoma
Arachnidism, necrotic, 238, 239*f*
Arterial (ischemic) ulcer, 244, 245*f*
Arthralgias, in purpuric and hemorrhagic disorders
  (P&H), 327
Arthritis, 253
  see also Reactive arthritis; Rheumatoid arthritis
  in plaques with scale, 113
  in purpuric and hemorrhagic disorders (P&H), 327
Arthropod reactions, 429*b*
  bullous, 176, 176*f*–177*f*
  pustular, 212, 213*f*
Arthropods, papular urticaria and, 70*b*
Artificial skin, for stasis ulcers, 242
Ascarine dermatitis, 88, 88*b*, 89*f*
Aspirin
  for cryofibrinogenemia, 346
  for necrotic arachnidism, 238
  for progressive pigmented purpura, 340
Asteatosis. *see* Xerosis

Asthma, papular eruptions and, 83
Asymmetric periflexural exanthem of childhood, 40, 41*f*
Atherosclerotic disease, arterial (ischemic) ulcers and, 244
Athlete's foot. *see* Tinea pedis
Atopic dermatitis (AD), 142–144, 143*f*, 145*f*
Atrophic actinic keratosis, 110
Atrophic disorders, 367–374
  aplasia cutis congenita, 372, 373*f*
  differential diagnosis of, 367*b*
  history questions for, 367
  physical findings in, 367
  postinjection lipoatrophy, 370, 370*b*, 371*f*
  striae, 368, 368*b*, 369*f*
Atrophie blanche (AB), *e*6
Atrophy, from topical corticosteroids, prevention of, 599,
  599*f*
Atypical (dysplastic) nevus, 522, 523*f*
Atypical Spitz nevus. *see* Spitz nevus
Atypical Spitzoid tumor. *see* Spitz nevus
Autoeczematization. *see* Id reactions
Autoinoculation vaccination reaction, 214, 215*f*
Avulsion, surgical, onychomycosis and, 408*b*
Azathioprine
  for cicatricial pemphigoid, *e*2
  for cutaneous polyarteritis nodosa, 266
  for Henoch-Schönlein purpura, 328
  for pemphigus vulgaris, 172
Azelaic acid
  for mild acne, 376
  for rosacea, 380
Azithromycin
  for bullous impetigo, 164
  for chancroid, 248
  for confluent and reticulated papillomatosis, 450

B

B cell lymphomas, 502*b*
Balanitis circinate, in reactive arthritis (Reiter disease),
  116, 117*f*
Balanitis xerotica obliterans, 446
Basal cell carcinoma, 490, 491*f*
Baseline pigmentation, in skin disorders, 3
Bath soaps, in irritant contact dermatitis, 140
BCC. *see* Basal cell carcinoma
Beau lines, 416, 416*b*, 417*f*
Bedbug bites, 90, 90*b*, 91*f*
Bednar tumor, 498
Bees, 436, 436*f*–437*f*
Behavior modification therapy, for trichotillomania, 390
Benign familial angiolipomatosis, 582
Benign juvenile melanoma, 492
Benign lichenoid keratosis, 484, 485*f*
Benign neoplasms, 579
Benzathine penicillin, for primary syphilis, 250
Benzoyl peroxide
  for acne, 376
  for drug-induced acne, 378
Benzyl alcohol, for pediculosis capitis, 430

Betamethasone diproprionate ointment, for dyshidrosis, 154

Bexarotene, for dyshidrosis, 154

Bilirubin, 454

Biologic agents, for rheumatoid nodules, 264

Biopsy
    for acute hemorrhagic edema, 330
    for cicatricial pemphigoid, *e2*
    for cryofibrinogenemia, 346
    for cryoglobulinemia, 344
    for cutaneous larva migrans, 588
    for cutaneous leishmaniasis, 591
    for cutaneous odontogenic sinus tract, 576
    for disseminated gonococcal infection, 334
    for drug-induced acne, 378
    for eosinophilic fasciitis, 360
    excision. *see* Excision biopsy
    for Henoch-Schönlein purpura, 328
    incisional. *see* Incisional biopsy
    for leukocytoclastic vasculitis, 332
    for lichen nitidus, 100
    for limited scleroderma, 358
    of lipoma, 582
    for meningococcemia, 336
    for morbilliform drug eruptions, 32
    for morphea, 354
    for pernio, 348
    for pityriasis lichenoides et varioliformis acuta, 350
    for postinjection lipoatrophy, 370
    for progressive pigmented purpura, 340
    for *Pseudomonas* folliculitis, 382
    punch. *see* Punch biopsy
    for purpura fulminans, 342
    for Rocky Mountain spotted fever, 338
    for roseola, 38
    for scleredema, 362
    for scleroderma, 356
    shave. *see* Shave biopsy

Biotin, for onychoschizia, 414

Bites. *see* Infestations, stings, and bites

Black dot ringworm, 396, 397*f*

Bland emollients, for staphylococcal scalded skin syndrome, 166

Blastomyces dermatitidis, North American blastomycosis from, 472

Blastomycosis, North American, 472, 472*f*–473*f*

Bleach bathes, for atopic dermatitis, 144

Bleomycin, 292

Bleomycin-induced flagellate erythema, hyperpigmentation and, 292, 293*f*

Blistering distal dactylitis, 168, 169*f*

Blisters, 163–204
    in allergic contact dermatitis, 174, 175*f*
    in blistering distal dactylitis, 168, 169*f*
    in bullous impetigo, 164, 165*f*
    in bullous pemphigoid, 194, 195*f*
    in chickenpox, 178, 179*f*
    in dermatitis herpetiformis, 196, 196*f*–197*f*

Blisters (*Continued*)
    in erythema, 51
    in erythema multiforme, 188, 189*f*
    in fixed drug eruption, 186, 186*b*, 187*f*
    fragile, 163*b*
    in hand, foot, and mouth disease, 184, 185*f*
    in herpes gestationis, 198, 198*f*–199*f*
    in herpes simplex virus infection, 182, 183*f*
    in herpes zoster, 180, 181*f*
    history questions for, 163
    in insect and arthropod reactions, 176, 176*f*–177*f*
    in linear IgA bullous dermatosis, 200, 200*b*, 200*f*–201*f*
    in morbilliform eruptions, 31
    in pemphigus foliaceus, 170, 170*b*, 171*f*
    in pemphigus vulgaris, 172, 172*b*, 172*f*–173*f*
    physical findings in, 163
    in porphyria cutanea tarda, 202, 203*f*
    in staphylococcal scalded skin syndrome, 166, 167*f*
    in Stevens-Johnson syndrome, 190, 191*f*
    symptomatic, 163
    tense, 163*b*
    in toxic epidermal necrolysis, 192, 192*b*, 193*f*, 195*f*

BLK. *see* Benign lichenoid keratosis

Blue-grey discoloration, drug-induced, 458, 458*b*, 459*f*

Blue nevus, 532, 532*b*, 533*f*

Borderline leprosy, 284, 285*f*

Borrelia burgdorferi, 354

Bot fly myiasis, 589

Bowen disease. *see* Squamous cell carcinoma in situ

Breathing, difficulty, urticarial eruptions and, 63

Brimonidine, for rosacea, 380

Brouet classification, of cryoglobulinemia, 344

Brown recluse spiders, 238

Brown widow spider, 438*b*

Brunsting-Perry syndrome, *e2*

Bulla, 2*t*–3*t*, 3*f*

Bullous fixed drug eruption, 186, 186*b*, 187*f*

Bullous impetigo, 164, 165*f*

Bullous lichen planus, 102

Bullous morphea, 354

Bullous pemphigoid, 194, 195*f*

Bullous pseudoporphyria, *e4*, *e4b*, *e5f*

Bullous systemic lupus erythematosus, 316

Buschke-Löwenstein tumor, 474

Button hole sign, *e8*

C

Café au lait spot, 518, 518*b*, 519*f*

Calcinosis cutis, 358

Calciphylaxis, 240, 241*f*

Calcipotriene, for morphea, 354

Calcium channel blockers, for scleroderma, 356

Campbell De Morgan spots, 542

Cancer
    in papular and nodular growths without scale, 489
    yellow lesions and, 553

Cancun dermatitis. *see* Phytophotodermatitis

Candida albicans, paronychia and, 404

Candida spp., onychomycosis and, 408
Cantharidin, for molluscum contagiosum, 106
Canthaxanthin, 456*b*
Carbon dioxide laser ablation, for apocrine cystadenoma, 572
Carbuncle, 218
Carney complex, multiple lentigines in, 510*b*, 511*f*
Carotenoderma, 456, 456*b*, 457*f*, 459*f*
Cefepime, for ecthyma gangrenosum, 234
Cefotaxime, for meningococcemia, 336
Ceftazidime, for ecthyma gangrenosum, 234
Ceftizoxime, for disseminated gonococcal infection, 334
Ceftriaxone
    for chancroid, 248
    for disseminated gonococcal infection, 334
    for meningococcemia, 336
    for purpura fulminans, 342
Cefuroxime, for meningococcemia, 336
Cellulitis, 80, 81*f*
    dissecting, of scalp, 224, 225*f*
Central centrifugal cicatricial alopecia, 400, 401*f*
Centrofacial lentiginosis syndrome, multiple lentigines in, 510*b*, 511*f*
Cephalexin, for bullous impetigo, 164
Chancroid, 248, 249*f*
Chemicals, alopecia and, 385
Chemiluminescent enzyme immunosorbent assay (EIA), for morbilliform viral eruptions, 36
Cherry angioma (hemangioma), 542, 543*f*
Cheyletiella blakei, 88, 89*f*
Cheyletiella parasitovorax, 88
Cheyletiella yasgur, 88
Chickenpox, 178, 179*f*
    Tzanck preparation for, 18
Chiggers, 86, 86*b*, 87*f*
Chilblains. *see* Pernio
Childhood eczema. *see* Atopic dermatitis (AD)
Children, anogenital warts in, 466
Chloramphenicol
    for meningococcemia, 336
    for rickettsial infections, 48
    for Rocky Mountain spotted fever, 338
Chlordiazepoxide, for progressive pigmented purpura, 340
Cholinergic urticaria, 66, 67*f*
Chronic bullous disease of childhood. *See* Linear IgA bullous dermatosis
Chronic cutaneous lupus erythematosus, 320, 321*f*
Chronic localized blastomycosis, 472
Chronic paronychia, 404
Chronic venous hypertension, stasis ulcers and, 242
Cicatricial pemphigoid, e2, e3*f*
Cidofovir
    for cutaneous vaccinia infections, 214
    for herpes simplex virus infection, 182
    for orf, 236
Cimex lectularius, 90
Cinacalcet, for calciphylaxis, 240

Ciprofloxacin
    for chancroid, 248
    for *Pseudomonas* folliculitis, 382
Circinate balanitis, in reactive arthritis (Reiter disease), 116, 117*f*
Clarithromycin
    for confluent and reticulated papillomatosis of Gougerot-Carteaud, 450
    for erythrasma, 160
Clark nevi, 522
Clindamycin
    for cutaneous odontogenic sinus tract, 576
    for drug-induced acne, 378
    for erythrasma, 160
Clinical dermatology, 1–6
    color in, 1–3
    configuration and distribution in, 3–5
    dermatologist, 1
    etiologic premises in, 1
    historical information in, 5
    morphology in, 1, 2*t*–4*t*
    palpation and appreciation of texture in, 1
    temporal course in, 5
CLM. *see* Cutaneous larva migrans
Clobetasol ointment, for dyshidrosis, 154
Clomipramine, for trichotillomania, 390
Clotrimazole-betamethasone dipropionate, 128*b*
Clotting disorders, history of, necrotic and ulcerative skin disorders and, 231
Clubbing, nail, 420, 420*b*, 420*f*–421*f*
Cocoa butter, 368*b*
Colchicine
    for leukocytoclastic vasculitis, 332
    for linear IgA bullous dermatosis, 200
Cold urticaria, 66, 67*f*
Collagenase ointment, pyoderma gangrenosum and, 246
Comedones, 378
Complete blood count (CBC)
    for acute hemorrhagic edema, 330
    for disseminated gonococcal infection, 334
    for drug eruption with eosinophilia and systemic symptoms, 34
    for eosinophilic fasciitis, 360
    for Henoch-Schönlein purpura, 328
    for leukocytoclastic vasculitis, 332
    for meningococcemia, 336
    in morbilliform eruptions, 32
    for purpura fulminans, 342
    for scleroderma, 356
Compound nevus, 512
Compression hose, for stasis ulcer, 242
Computed tomography, for pancreatic panniculitis, 258
Condyloma acuminatum, 461, 466, 466*b*, 467*f*
Configuration, in clinical dermatology, 3–5
Confluent and reticulated papillomatosis of Gougerot-Carteaud (CRPGC), 444, 451*f*
Congenital melanocytic nevus, 514, 515*f*
Congenital rubella syndrome, 44

Conjunctival hyperemia, in toxic shock syndrome, 55*f*
Contact dermatitis, bullous allergic, 174, 175*f*
Cordylobia anthropophaga, 589
Corticosteroids
  for acute hemorrhagic edema, 330
  for allergic contact dermatitis, 136
  for alopecia areata, 394
  for atopic dermatitis, 144
  for central centrifugal cicatricial alopecia, 400
  for diaper dermatitis, 146
  for drug eruption with eosinophilia and systemic symptoms, 34
  for dyshidrosis, 154
  for fixed drug eruption, 186
  for guttate psoriasis, 98
  for Henoch-Schönlein purpura, 328
  for irritant contact dermatitis, 140
  for Kawasaki disease, 56
  for lichen nitidus, 100
  for lichen planus, 102
  for limited scleroderma, 358
  for lupus erythematosus, 398
  medium-potency
    for acute generalized exanthematous pustulosis, 206
    for pustular psoriasis, 208
  for morbilliform drug eruptions, 32
  for morbilliform viral eruptions, 36
  for morphea, 354
  for necrotic arachnidism, 238
  for nummular dermatitis, 150
  for pityriasis lichenoides et varioliformis acuta, 350
  for pityriasis rosea, 156
  for plaque psoriasis, 114
  for progressive pigmented purpura, 340
  for pyoderma gangrenosum, 246
  for seborrheic dermatitis, 158
  for stasis ulcer, 242
  for Stevens-Johnson syndrome, 190
  for striae, 368
  for subcutaneous granuloma annulare, 262
  topical, 598–599, 599*f*
    for acropustulosis of infancy, 210
    atrophy from, prevention of, 599, 599*f*
    for pustular arthropod reactions, 212
  for unilateral thoracic exanthem, 40
Corynebacterium minutissimum, in Wood light, 8
Cradle cap, 158
Creeping eruption, 298, 299*f*, 588
CREST syndrome, 353, 358
Crotamiton, for scabies, 84
Crust, 4*f*, 4*t*
Cryofibrinogenemia, 346, 347*f*
Cryoglobulinemia, 344, 344*b*, 345*f*
Cryosurgery, for keloid, 496
Cryotherapy
  for actinic keratosis, 110
  for inflamed seborrheic keratosis, 486

Cryotherapy *(Continued)*
  liquid nitrogen (LN$_2$)
    for verrucae vulgaris, 462
    for verrucous carcinoma, 474
  for molluscum contagiosum, 106
Curettage, for molluscum contagiosum, 106
Cutaneous dental sinus tract. *see* Cutaneous odontogenic sinus tract (COST)
Cutaneous dermoid cyst, *e*10, *e*10*f*–*e*11*f*
Cutaneous diseases, of travelers, 587–595, 587*b*
  cutaneous larva migrans as, 588, 588*f*
  cutaneous leishmaniasis as, 591, 591*f*
  history questions for, 587
  myiasis as, 589, 589*f*
  phytophotodermatitis as, 593, 593*f*
  Seabather's eruption as, 594, 594*f*
  tinea nigra as, 590, 590*f*
  tungiasis as, 592, 592*f*
Cutaneous fibrous histiocytoma. *see* Dermatofibroma
Cutaneous inoculation blastomycosis, primary, 472
Cutaneous larva migrans (CLM), 298, 299*f*, 588, 588*f*
Cutaneous leishmaniasis, 591, 591*f*
Cutaneous lymphomas, 502, 502*b*, 503*f*
Cutaneous odontogenic sinus tract (COST), 576, 576*f*–577*f*
Cutaneous polyarteritis nodosa, 266, 267*f*
Cutaneous vaccinia infections, 214, 214*b*, 215*f*
Cyanoacrylate glue, for habit tic deformity, 422
Cyanosis, in skin, color of, 3
Cyclophosphamide
  for cicatricial pemphigoid, *e*2
  for Henoch-Schönlein purpura, 328
  for pemphigus vulgaris, 172
Cyclosporine
  for cicatricial pemphigoid, *e*2
  for eosinophilic fasciitis, 360
  for pustular psoriasis, 208
  for pyoderma gangrenosum, 246
  for rheumatoid nodules, 264
  for scleroderma, 356
Cyproterone acetate, for androgenic alopecia, 386
Cystic lesions, of skin, differential diagnosis of, 565*b*
Cysts, 565–578
  apocrine cystadenoma, 572, 573*f*
  cutaneous dermoid, *e*10, *e*10*f*–*e*11*f*
  digital mucous, 574, 574*f*–575*f*
  epidermoid, 566, 567*f*
  history questions for, 565
  orbital dermoid, *e*10
  physical findings in, 565
  steatocystoma, 570, 571*f*
  trichilemmal, 568, 569*f*

D

Danazol, for angioedema, 68
Dandruff, 158

Dapsone
  for acropustulosis of infancy, 210
  for bullous pemphigoid, 194
  for leukocytoclastic vasculitis, 332
  for linear IgA bullous dermatosis, 200
  for necrotic arachnidism, 238
  for pustular psoriasis, 208
DD. *see* Diaper dermatitis (DD)
Débridement, surgical, for necrotizing fasciitis, 232
Deep granuloma annulare, 262
Demarcation, 441
Dentocutaneous sinus tract. *see* Cutaneous odontogenic sinus tract (COST)
Depigmented skin, in Wood light, 8
Dermatitis, 135–162
  allergic contact, 136, 136b–138b, 137f–139f
  atopic, 142–144, 143f, 145f
  diaper, 146, 146b, 147f
  dyshidrosis (pompholyx), 154, 155f
  eczematous drug eruptions, 148, 148b, 149f
  erythrasma, 160, 161f
  eyelid, 139b
  in follicular disorders, 375
  history questions for, 135
  id reactions (autoeczematization), 152, 153f
  irritant contact, 140, 141f
  nummular, 150, 150b, 151f
  physical findings in, 135
  pityriasis rosea, 156, 157f
  seborrheic, 158, 159f
  soaps for, 597
Dermatitis herpetiformis, 196, 196f–197f
Dermatobia hominis, 589
Dermatofibroma, 494, 495f
Dermatofibrosarcoma protuberans, 498, 499f
Dermatoglyphs, 462
Dermatographism, 66, 67f
Dermatologists, 1
Dermatology. *see* Clinical dermatology
Dermatomyositis, 322, 323f
Dermatophyte infection, potassium hydroxide preparation for, 10
Dermatosis papulosa nigra (DPN), 461, 468, 469f
Dermoid cysts
  cutaneous, e10, e10f–e11f
  orbital, e10
Dermoids, e10
Desmoplastic Spitz nevi. *see* Spitz nevus
Desquamative gingivitis, e2
DFSP. *see* Dermatofibrosarcoma protuberans
Diabetes mellitus, arterial (ischemic) ulcers and, 244
Diagnostic techniques, 7–30
  equipment for, 7, 7b
  mineral oil preparation, 14, 14f–17f
  potassium hydroxide preparation, 10, 10b, 11f–13f
  punch biopsy, 26, 26b, 27f–29f
  shave biopsy, 22, 23f–25f

Diagnostic techniques *(Continued)*
  Tzanck preparation, 18, 18f–21f
  wood light for, 8, 9f
Diaper dermatitis (DD), 146, 146b, 147f
Diclofenac, for actinic keratosis, 110
Dicloxacillin
  for bullous impetigo, 164
  for staphylococcal scalded skin syndrome, 166
Dietzia papillomatosis, 450
Diffuse erythema, 51–62
Diffuse neonatal hemangiomatosis, 536
Digital mucous cysts (DMCs), 574, 574f–575f
Dimple sign, 494, 495f
Diphenhydramine, for acute generalized exanthematous pustulosis, 206
Diphenhydramine elixir, for cicatricial pemphigoid, e2
Diphenylcyclopropenone (DPCP), for alopecia areata, 394
Direct fluorescent antibody test for *Treponema pallidum* (DFA-TP), 250
Discoid lupus erythematosus, 316, 320, 321f
Discoloration
  in nail, 424, 424b, 425f–427f
  skin. *see* Skin discolorations
Dissecting cellulitis, of scalp, 224, 225f
Disseminated gonococcal infection (DGI), 334, 335f
Distal dactylitis, blistering, 168, 169f
Distribution, in clinical dermatology, 3–5
Doucas-Kapetanakis purpura, 340
Doxycycline
  for acne, 376
  for bullous pemphigoid, 194
  for central centrifugal cicatricial alopecia, 400
  for drug-induced acne, 378
  for pityriasis lichenoides et varioliformis acuta, 350
  for rickettsial infections, 48
  for Rocky Mountain spotted fever, 338
  for rosacea, 380
Drug eruption with eosinophilia and systemic symptoms (DRESS), 34, 34b, 35f
Drug-induced acneiform reactions, 378, 378b, 379f
Drug-induced blue-grey discoloration, 458, 458b, 459f
Drugs
  in bullous pseudoporphyria, e4b
  in guttate psoriasis, 98b
  in photoallergic drug eruption, 310b
  in phototoxic drug eruptions, 312b
  in plaque psoriasis, 114b
  in subacute cutaneous lupus erythematosus, 318b
  in Sweet syndrome, 76b
  in systemic lupus erythematosus, 316b
  urticarial vasculitis caused by, 72b
Dry skin. *see* Xerosis
Dye laser, tunable, for molluscum contagiosum, 106
Dyshidrosis, 154, 155f
Dysphagia, sclerosing and fibrosing disorders and, 353
Dysplastic nevi, 522

E

Ecallantide, for angioedema, 68
Ecthyma gangrenosum, 234, 235f
Eczema
see also Dermatitis
papular eruptions and, 83
Eczema herpeticum, 182, 183f
Eczema vaccinatum, 214
Eczematoid purpura, 340
Eczematoid reactions, 135–162
allergic contact dermatitis, 136, 136b–138b, 137f–139f
atopic dermatitis (childhood eczema), 142–144, 143f, 145f
diaper dermatitis, 146, 146b, 147f
dyshidrosis (pompholyx), 154, 155f
eczematous drug eruptions, 148, 148b, 149f
erythrasma, 160, 161f
eyelid dermatitis, 139b
history questions for, 135
id reactions (autoeczematization), 152, 153f
irritant contact dermatitis, 140, 141f
nummular dermatitis, 150, 150b, 151f
physical findings in, 135
pityriasis rosea, 156, 157f
seborrheic dermatitis, 158, 159f
Eczematous drug eruptions, 148, 148b, 149f
Edema, abscesses and, 217
Efudex, for actinic keratosis, 110
Eggs, mineral oil preparation, 14, 17f
Electron beam therapy, for scleredema, 362
Emollients
for diaper dermatitis, 146
for nummular dermatitis, 150
for roseola vaccinatum, 46
for xerosis, 130
End-stage renal disease (ESRD), calciphylaxis and, 240
Eosinophilic fasciitis (EF), 360, 361f
Epidermodysplasia verruciformis (EV), 464, 465f
Epidermoid cyst, 566, 567f
ruptured, 226, 227f, 566
Epidermoid inclusion cysts, 565
Epidermolysis bullosa, inherited forms of, e4
Epithelioma cuniculatum, 461, 474
Erosion, 4f, 4t
Eruptive xanthomata, 554, 554f–555f
Erysipelas, 78, 79f
Erythema
abscesses and, 217
definition of, 51
differential diagnosis of, 51b
diffuse, 51–62
history questions for, 51
infectiosum, 58, 59f
Kawasaki disease, 56, 56b, 57f
medications for, 51
physical findings in, 51
reticulated, 51–62

Erythema (Continued)
scarlet fever, 52, 53f
toxic shock syndrome, 54, 55f
Erythema ab igne, 60, 61f
Erythema annulare centrifugum, 274, 274b, 275f
Erythema chronicum migrans, 272
Erythema circinatum, 277f
Erythema induratum, 256, 257f
Erythema marginatum, 276, 277f
Erythema multiforme, 286, 287f
bullous, 188, 189f
Erythema nodosum, 254, 255f
drug-induced, 254b
Erythrasma, 160, 161f
in Wood light, 8
Erythromatotelangiectatic rosacea, 380
Erythromycin
for bullous impetigo, 164
for chancroid, 248
for drug-induced acne, 378
for erythrasma, 160
for pityriasis lichenoides et varioliformis acuta, 350
for pityriasis rosea, 156
Erythroplasia of Queyrat, 478, 479f
Esophageal dysmotility, 358
Etretinate, for pityriasis rubra pilaris, 118
Eucerin Plus, for atopic dermatitis, 142–144
Exanthem subitum, 38, 39f
Excision biopsy
for necrotizing fasciitis, 232
for orf, 236
Excoriation, 4f, 4t
Eyelid dermatitis, 139b

F

Fabric softeners, for atopic dermatitis, 142–144
Face washing, 377b
Fairy ring wart, after cryotherapy, 463f
Famciclovir, for herpes simplex virus infection, 182
Female pattern hair loss, 386
Fever
abscesses and, 217
erythema and, 51
in urticarial eruptions, 63
FGFR3 gene, mutations of, epidermal nevus and, 294
Fibroepithelial polyps. see Acrochordon (soft fibroma)
Fibrous histiocytoma, cutaneous. see Dermatofibroma
Finasteride, for androgenic alopecia, 386
Fingernail growth, 416b
Fingertip unit, 599f
Fingertips, desquamation of, 55f
Finkelstein disease, 330
Fire ants, 212, 213f
Fissure, 4f, 4t
Fitzpatrick skin types, 1–3, 3b
Fitzpatrick's sign, 494, 495f
Fixed drug eruption, bullous, 186, 186b, 187f
Flagellate erythema, bleomycin-induced, 292, 293f

Flashlamp-pumped pulsed dye laser, for port wine stain, e12
Flat warts. *see* Verrucae plana
Fluconazole
    for kerion, 228
    for onychomycosis, 408
    oral, for cutaneous leishmaniasis, 591
Fluocinolone ointment, for dyshidrosis, 154
Fluorescent treponemal antibody absorption (FTA-ABS) tests, for primary syphilis, 250
Fluoroplex, for actinic keratosis, 110
5-Fluorouracil
    for actinic keratosis, 110
    for keratoacanthoma, 482
    for squamous cell carcinoma in situ, 478
Fluoxetine, for trichotillomania, 390
Flurandrenolide tape (Cordran tape), for keloid, 496
Flutrimazole shampoo, for tinea (pityriasis) versicolor, 124
Follicular disorders, 375–384, 375*b*
    acute vulgaris, 376, 377*b*, 377*f*
    drug-induced acneiform reactions, 378, 378*b*, 379*f*
    history questions for, 375
    physical findings in, 375
    Pseudomonas folliculitis, 382, 383*f*
    rosacea, 380, 381*f*
Foods
    in atopic dermatitis, 142
    in phototoxic drug eruptions, 312*b*
Formaldehyde, in allergic contact dermatitis, 138*b*
Foscarnet, for herpes simplex virus infection, 182
Fournier gangrene, 232
Fragile blisters, 163*b*
Fragrance-free laundry detergents, for atopic dermatitis, 142–144
Fragrances, in allergic contact dermatitis, 138*b*
Fresh-frozen plasma, for purpura fulminans, 342
Furocoumarins, in skin, 593
Furuncle, 218, 219*f*
Furunculosis, mycobacterial, 220, 220*f*–221*f*
Fusarium spp., 408

G

Gadolinium-enhanced magnetic resonance imaging (MRI) studies, for sclerosing and fibrosing disorders, 353
General anesthesia, for neurofibroma, e8
Generalized morphea, 354
Genital warts, from condyloma acuminatum, 466, 467*f*
Genodermatosis, potential, 489
Gentamicin cream, for cutaneous leishmaniasis, 591
German measles. *see* Rubella
Gianotti-Crosti syndrome, 92, 93*f*
Gilchrist disease. *see* North American blastomycosis
Gingivitis, desquamative, e2
GNTWIs. *see* Gram-negative toe web infections
Goats, direct contact with, 236
Gougerot-Blum purpura, 340
Gram-negative bacteria, erysipelas from, 78
Gram-negative toe web infections (GNTWIs), 597, 597*f*

Gram staining, for ecthyma gangrenosum, 234, 235*f*
Granuloma annulare, 280, 281*f*
    subcutaneous, 262, 263*f*
Griseofulvin
    for kerion, 228
    for lichen planus, 102
    for tinea capitis, 396
Grover disease, 108, 109*f*
Guttate morphea, 354
Guttate psoriasis, 98, 98*b*, 99*f*

H

Habit tic deformity, 422, 423*f*
Haemophilus spp., erysipelas from, 78
Hair pluck, on androgenic alopecia, 386
Hair transplantation, for androgenic alopecia, 386
Halo nevus, 516, 517*f*
Halobetasol ointment, for dyshidrosis, 154
Hand, foot, and mouth disease (HFMD), 184, 185*f*
Hands, baseline x-ray of, for scleroderma, 356
Hansen disease, 284, 285*f*
Hard ticks, 434, 434*f*
Hay fever, 83
Heller disease, 422
Hemangioma
    cherry angioma, 542, 543*f*
    infantile (juvenile), 536, 537*f*
    lobular capillary, 540
    strawberry, 536
Hemangioma thrombocytopenia syndrome, 538
Hemifacial atrophy (coup de sabre), 354
β-Hemolytic streptococci, paronychia and, 404
Hemorrhage
    in morbilliform eruptions, 31
    in urticarial eruptions, 63
Hemorrhagic digital mucous cyst, 575*f*
Henoch-Schönlein purpura (HSP), 328, 328*f*–329*f*
Herpes gestationis, 163, 198, 198*f*–199*f*
Herpes gladiatorum, 182
Herpes progenitalis, 183*f*
Herpes simplex virus (HSV) infection, 182, 183*f*
    erythema multiforme and, 286
    Tzanck preparation for, 18
Herpes zoster, 180, 181*f*
    Tzanck preparation for, 18, 18*f*, 21*f*
Herpes zoster ophthalmicus, 180, 181*f*
Herpetic whitlow, 182
Hidradenitis suppurativa, 222, 223*f*
Histamine-1 (H1), for urticaria, 64
Hives, 63
Hoffman disease, 224
Hormonal therapy, in women, with severe acne, 376
Hortaea werneckii, 590
Hot tub folliculitis, 382
Human herpesvirus-6 (HHV-6), roseola caused by, 38
Human herpesvirus-7 (HHV-7), roseola caused by, 38
Human parvovirus B19 (HPV B19), 58
Hutchinson freckle, 524

Hutchinson sign, 180

Hydration, in rubella, 44

Hydroxychloroquine
   for central centrifugal cicatricial alopecia, 400
   for eosinophilic fasciitis, 360
   for lichen planus, 102
   for lupus erythematosus, 398
   for lupus panniculitis, 260
   for porphyria cutanea tarda, 202
   for rheumatoid nodules, 264

Hyperkeratotic nails, thick, 412, 412*b*, 413*f*

Hyperpigmentation, in skin, in sclerosing and fibrosing disorders, 353

Hypertrophic actinic keratosis, 110, 111*f*

Hypertrophic discoid lupus erythematosus, 320

Hypertrophic lichen planus, 102

Hyphae, in potassium hydroxide preparation, 10, 13*f*

Hypopigmentation, 444

Hypopigmented skin, in Wood light, 8

Hypostome, 434, 434*f*

I

Ibuprofen, for rubella, 44

Icatibant, for angioedema, 68

Ichthyosis
   drug-induced, 126*b*
   systemic causes of, 126*b*

Ichthyosis acquisita, 126, 126*b*, 127*f*

Id reactions (autoeczematization), 152, 153*f*

Idoxuridine, for orf, 236

Imatinib, for neurofibroma, *e*8

Imidazole, topical
   for seborrheic dermatitis, 158
   for tinea pedis and tinea manuum, 128
   for tinea (pityriasis) versicolor, 124

Imipenem
   for ecthyma gangrenosum, 234
   for necrotizing fasciitis, 232

Imiquimod, topical
   for actinic keratosis, 110
   for molluscum contagiosum, 106
   for rosacea, 380
   for squamous cell carcinoma in situ, 478
   for verrucae plana, 464

Immunosuppressive agents
   for nephrogenic systemic fibrosis, 364
   for reactive arthritis (Reiter disease), 116

Immunosuppressive drugs
   for cryofibrinogenemia, 346
   for cryoglobulinemia, 344
   for Henoch-Schönlein purpura, 328

Immunotherapy, for verrucae vulgaris, 462

Impetigo herpetiformis, 208

Incisional biopsy
   for calciphylaxis, 240, 241*f*
   for cutaneous polyarteritis nodosa, 266
   for erythema induratum, 256
   for lupus panniculitis, 260

Incisional biopsy *(Continued)*
   for necrotizing fasciitis, 232
   for pancreatic panniculitis, 258
   for rheumatoid nodules, 264
   for subcutaneous granuloma annulare, 262

Indurated eruptions, 63–82

Infantile acropustulosis, 210

Infantile (juvenile) hemangioma, 536, 537*f*

Infantum, 38, 39*f*

Infections
   see also specific infections
   sclerosing and fibrosing disorders and, 353

Infestations, stings, and bites, 429–440
   bees, 436, 436*f*–437*f*
   history questions for, 429
   pediculosis capitis, 430, 430*f*–431*f*
   pediculosis pubis, 432, 432*f*–433*f*
   physical findings in, 429
   spider bites, 438, 439*f*
   tick bites, 434, 434*f*–435*f*
   wasps, 436, 437*f*
   yellowjackets, 436, 437*f*

Inflamed seborrheic keratosis, 468, 486, 487*f*

Ingrown toenails, 406, 407*f*

Insect reactions, bullous, 176, 176*f*–177*f*

Intradermal nevus, 512

Intralesional therapies
   for keratoacanthoma, 482
   for verrucae vulgaris, 462

Intramuscular lipoma, 581*f*

Intravenous (IV) immunoglobulin, for Henoch-Schönlein purpura, 328

Intravenous immunoglobulin (IVIG), for pemphigus vulgaris, 172

Ionizing radiation therapies
   for mycosis fungoides, 120
   for plaque psoriasis, 114

Irritant contact dermatitis (ICD), 140, 141*f*

Isotretinoin
   for dissecting cellulitis of scalp, 224
   for drug-induced acne, 378
   for pityriasis rubra pilaris, 118
   for severe acne, 376

Itraconazole
   for cutaneous leishmaniasis, 591
   for kerion, 228
   for onychomycosis, 408
   for seborrheic dermatitis, 158
   for sporotrichosis, 302
   for tinea capitis, 396
   for tinea pedis and tinea manuum, 128
   for tinea (pityriasis) versicolor, 124

Ivermectin
   for cutaneous larva migrans, 588
   for pediculosis capitis, 430
   for pediculosis pubis, 432
   for scabies, 84
   for Tungiasis, 592

J

Jaundice, 454, 454b, 455f
Jock itch, in tinea cruris, 270, 271f
Junctional nevus, 512
Juvenile hemangioma. *see* Infantile (juvenile) hemangioma
Juvenile xanthogranuloma, 558, 559f

K

KA. *see* Keratoacanthoma
Kaposi sarcoma, 548, 548f–549f
Kasabach-Merritt syndrome, 538, 539f
Kawasaki disease, 56, 56b, 57f
Keloid, 496, 497f
Keratinocyte, Tzanck preparation and, 18, 21f
Keratoacanthoma, 482, 483f
Keratoacanthoma centrifugum marginatum, 482
Keratodermia blennorrhagica, in reactive arthritis (Reiter disease), 116, 117f
Keratolytic agents, topical, for tinea nigra, 590
Kerion, 228, 228b, 229f, 396, 397f
Ketoconazole, for tinea nigra, 590
Ketoconazole-based shampoo
    for androgenic alopecia, 386
    for tinea (pityriasis) versicolor, 124
Klippel-Trénaunay-Weber syndrome, e12
Koebner phenomenon
    in eruptive xanthomata, 554, 555f
    in guttate psoriasis, 98
    in lichen planus, 102
    in plaques with scale, 113
Koilocytosis, 464
Kraurosis vulvae, 446
Kwashiorkor, 132, 133f

L

Labial melanotic macules, 510
β-Lactamase penicillin, antipseudomonal, for ecthyma gangrenosum, 234
Lamellar dystrophy, 414, 415f
Larva migrans, cutaneous, 588, 588f
Laser ablation, for onychomycosis, 408
Laser therapy, for verrucae vulgaris, 462
Leg ulcers, 242
    chronic, differential diagnosis of, 244b
Leishmaniasis, cutaneous, 591, 591f
Lentigo
    maligna, 524, 525f
    senilis, 508
    simple, 510, 510b, 511f
    simplex, 510
    solar, 508, 509f
    solaris, 508
Leopard syndrome, multiple lentigines in, 510b
Leprosy, 269, 284, 285f
Leukocytoclastic (hypersensitivity) vasculitis, 332, 332b, 333f
Leukonychia mycotica, 408
Lichen aureus, 340

Lichen nitidus, 100, 101f
Lichen planus, 102, 103f
Lichen planus-like keratosis. *see* Benign lichenoid keratosis
Lichen sclerosus, morphea with, 354
Lichen sclerosus et atrophicus, 446, 447f
Lichen striatus, 290, 290b, 291f
Lichenoid purpura, 340
Light therapy
    for alopecia areata, 394
    for guttate psoriasis, 98
Limited scleroderma, 358, 359f
Lindane
    for pediculosis capitis, 430
    for pediculosis pubis, 432
    for scabies, 84
Linear and serpiginous lesions, 289–300
    bleomycin-induced flagellate erythema and hyperpigmentation, 292, 293f
    cutaneous larva migrans, 298, 299f
    history questions for, 289
    lichen striatus, 290, 290b, 291f
    linear epidermal nevus, 294, 294b, 295f
    linear morphea, 296, 297f
    physical findings in, 289
Linear epidermal nevus, 294, 294b, 295f
Linear IgA bullous dermatosis, 200, 200b, 200f–201f
Linear lesions. *see* Linear and serpiginous lesions
Linear morphea, 296, 297f, 354
Lines of Blaschko, 290b
Linuche unguiculata, 594
Lipid mantle, 597
Lipoma, 580, 581f
Liposuction surgery, for lipoma, 582
Liquid nitrogen (LN₂) cryotherapy
    for verrucae vulgaris, 462
    for verrucous carcinoma, 474
Livedoid vasculitis. *see* Livedoid vasculopathy (LV)
Livedoid vasculopathy (LV), e6, e7f
Liver function test (LFT)
    for drug eruption with eosinophilia and systemic symptoms, 34
    for morbilliform drug eruptions, 32
Liver spot, 508
Lobular capillary hemangioma, 540
Localized scleroderma, 296, 297f, 354
Lovibond's angle, 420
Loxoscelism, 238
Lupus erythematosus
    alopecia and, 398, 399f
    bullous systemic, 316
    discoid, 316, 320, 321f
    neonatal, 278, 279f
    subacute cutaneous, 318, 318b, 319f
    systemic, 316, 316b, 317f
Lupus erythematosus panniculitis, 260
Lupus hair, 316
Lupus panniculitis, 260, 261f
Lupus profundus, 260

Lutzomyia fly, 591
Lyme disease, 269, 269*b*, 272, 273*f*
   tick bites and, 434, 435*f*
Lymphadenopathy, in rubella, 44
Lymphangioma, superficial, 546, 547*f*
Lymphangitis, cellulitis and, 80, 81*f*

M

Macule (or patch), 2*f*, 2*t*–3*t*
Magnetic resonance imaging (MRI), for eosinophilic
    fasciitis, 360
Majocchi purpura, 340
Malassezia furfur, in tinea (pityriasis) versicolor, 124
Malathion
   for pediculosis capitis, 430
   for pediculosis pubis, 432
Malignant tumors, cysts *versus*, 565
Margarita dermatitis. *see* Phytophotodermatitis
Marjolin ulcer, 398
MCC. *see* Merkel cell carcinoma
McCune-Albright syndrome, café au lait spots in, 518,
    519*f*
Measles, 42, 43*f*
   vaccination and, 42*b*
Mebendazole, for cutaneous larva migrans, 588
Medications, pellagra-associated, 314
Melanoacanthoma, 468, 469*f*
Melanoma, 526–528, 526*b*, 527*f*, 528*b*, 529*f*–531*f*
   subcutaneous metastatic, 585*f*
Melanonychia striata, 510
Meltzer triad, 344, 344*b*
Meningococcemia, 336, 337*f*
Merkel cell carcinoma, 500, 500*f*–501*f*
Meropenem, for necrotizing fasciitis, 232
Mesotherapy, for striae, 368
Metastatic tumors
   as papular and nodular growths without scale, 504,
    504*b*, 505*f*
   subcutaneous, 584, 584*b*, 585*f*
Metformin, for acanthosis nigricans, 448
Methicillin-resistant *Staphylococcus aureus*, community-
    acquired, 218*b*
Methotrexate
   for bullous pemphigoid, 194
   for central centrifugal cicatricial alopecia, 400
   for cutaneous polyarteritis nodosa, 266
   for keratoacanthoma, 482
   for limited scleroderma, 358
   for pemphigus vulgaris, 172
   for pityriasis lichenoides et varioliformis acuta, 350
   for pityriasis rubra pilaris, 118
   for pustular psoriasis, 208
   for rheumatoid nodules, 264
   for scleroderma, 356
Metrifonate, for tungiasis, 592
Metronidazole, for rosacea, 380
Microdermabrasion, for striae, 368
Miliaria, 94, 95*f*

Milium, 566
Mineral oil preparation, 14, 14*f*–17*f*
Minocycline
   for acne, 376
   for central centrifugal cicatricial alopecia, 400
   for drug-induced acne, 378
   for pyoderma gangrenosum, 246
   for rheumatoid nodules, 264
   for rosacea, 380
   for scleroderma, 356
   for sporotrichoid mycobacterial infection, 304
Minoxidil
   for alopecia areata, 394
   for androgenic alopecia, 386
   for telogen effluvium, 388
Mite, in mineral oil preparation, 14, 14*f*, 17*f*
Mite bites, 88, 88*b*, 89*f*
Mixed connective tissue disease (MCTD), 353
Moisturizers, 597–598, 598*f*
   for dyshidrosis, 154
   for irritant contact dermatitis, 140
Moll glands, 572
Molluscum contagiosum, 106, 107*f*
Mönckeberg arteriosclerosis, 240
Morbilliform drug eruptions, 32, 32*b*, 33*f*
Morbilliform eruptions, 31–50
   differential diagnosis of, 31*b*
   drug, 32, 32*b*, 33*f*
   drug with eosinophilia and systemic symptoms
    (DRESS), 34, 34*b*, 35*f*
   history questions for, 31
   measles, 42, 42*b*, 43*f*
   physical findings in, 31
   rickettsial infections, 48, 48*b*, 49*f*
   roseola, 38, 39*f*
   roseola vaccinatum, 46, 46*b*, 47*f*
   rubella, 44, 45*f*
   unilateral thoracic exanthem, 40, 41*f*
   viral, 36, 36*b*, 37*f*
Morbilliform viral eruptions, 36, 36*b*, 37*f*
Morbillivirus, 42
Morphea, 354, 355*f*
Morphology, definition of, 1
Mucha-Habermann disease. *see* Pityriasis lichenoides et
    varioliformis acuta
Mucocutaneous lymph node syndrome. *see* Kawasaki
    disease
Mucosal lesions, in erythema multiforme, 269
Mucosal membrane pemphigoid. *see* Cicatricial
    pemphigoid
Muir-Torre syndrome, 560*b*
Multiple lipomas, 581*f*
Mupirocin, for bullous impetigo, 164
Mycobacterial furunculosis, 220, 220*f*–221*f*
Mycobacterial infections, sporotrichoid, 304, 305*f*
Mycobacterium chelonae, 221*f*
Mycobacterium leprae, 284
Mycobacterium marinum, 221*f*

Mycophenolate mofetil
    for central centrifugal cicatricial alopecia, 400
    for cicatricial pemphigoid, e2
    for cutaneous polyarteritis nodosa, 266
    for pyoderma gangrenosum, 246
Mycosis fungoides, 120, 120f–121f
Myiasis, 589, 589f
Myrmecia, 462

N

Nagayama spots, 38
Nail disorders, 403–428
    Beau lines as, 416, 416b, 417f
    glossary for, 403b
    habit tic deformity as, 422, 423f
    history questions for, 403
    nail clubbing as, 420, 420b, 420f–421f
    nail discoloration as, 424, 424b, 425f–427f
    onychauxis as, 412, 412b, 413f
    onychocryptosis as, 406, 407f
    onycholysis as, 410, 410b, 411f
    onychomycosis as, 408, 408b, 409f
    onychoschizia as, 414, 415f
    paronychia as, 404, 405f
    physical findings in, 403
    trachyonychia as, 418, 418b, 419f
Nail pitting. *see* Trachyonychia
Nails
    in alopecia, 385
    in guttate psoriasis, 98
    in plaques with scale, 113
    in reactive arthritis (Reiter disease), 116, 117f
    in scaly papular lesions, 97
Naproxen-induced pseudoporphyria, e5f
Naproxen sodium, for bullous pseudoporphyria, e4
Natural soaps, for xerosis and dermatitis, 597
Necrobiosis lipoidica (diabeticorum), 282, 283f
Necrotic and ulcerative skin disorders, 231–252
    arterial (ischemic) ulcer as, 244, 245f
    calciphylaxis as, 240, 241f
    chancroid as, 248, 249f
    differential diagnosis for, 231b
    ecthyma gangrenosum as, 234, 235f
    history questions for, 231
    necrotic arachnidism as, 238, 239f
    necrotizing fasciitis as, 232, 233f
    orf as, 236, 237f
    physical findings in, 231
    primary syphilis as, 250, 251f
    pyoderma gangrenosum as, 246, 247f
    stasis ulcer as, 242, 243f
Necrotic arachnidism, 238, 239f
Necrotic skin disorders. *see* Necrotic and ulcerative skin
    disorders
Necrotizing fasciitis, 232, 233f
Necrotizing soft tissue infections (NSTIs), 232
Neisseria gonorrhoeae, 334
Neisseria meningitides, 336

Neisseria meningitidis, 342
Neomycin, in allergic contact dermatitis, 138b
Neonatal herpes simplex virus infection, 182
Neonatal lupus erythematosus, 278, 279f
Neoplasms, benign, 579
Neoplastic conditions, 1
Nephrogenic systemic fibrosis (NSF), 364, 365f
Neurofibroma, e8, e9f
    plexiform, e8
Neurofibromatosis type I, café au lait spots in, 518, 519f
Neutrogena soap, 597
Nevus
    acquired melanocytic, 512, 513f
    atypical (dysplastic), 522, 523f
    blue, 532, 532b, 533f
    congenital melanocytic, 514, 515f
Nevus flammeus. *see* Port wine stain
Nevus flammeus nuchae, 535
Nevus sebaceus, 562, 563f
Nevus spilus, 520, 521f
Nevus syndrome, 562
Nevus unius lateralis, 294, 295f
Niacin, pellagra and, 314
Nickel, in allergic contact dermatitis, 138b
Nicotinamide, for bullous pemphigoid, 194
Nifedipine, for pernio, 348
Nikolsky sign, 166b
Nodular basal cell carcinoma, 490, 491f
Nodular lymphangitis, 301
Nodular vasculitis, 256
Nodule, 2f, 2t–3t
Nonsteroidal antiinflammatory drugs (NSAIDs)
    for cryoglobulinemia, 344
    for cutaneous polyarteritis nodosa, 266
    for erythema induratum, 256
    for erythema nodosum, 254
    for pernio, 348
    for rheumatoid nodules, 264
North American blastomycosis, 472, 472f–473f
Nummular dermatitis, 150, 150b, 151f

O

Occupation, papular eruptions and, 83
Ocular rosacea, 380
Ointments, for allergic contact dermatitis, 136
Old World leishmaniasis, 591
Omalizumab, for urticaria, 64
Onychauxis, 412, 412b, 413f
Onychocryptosis, 406, 407f
Onycholysis, 410, 410b, 411f
Onychomycosis, 408, 408b, 409f
Onychoschizia, 414, 415f
Onychotillomania, 422, 423f
Oral agents, for cutaneous larva migrans, 588
Oral mucosa
    in blisters, 163
    in linear epidermal nevus, 294, 295f
    in photosensitive disorders, 307

Oral mucosa *(Continued)*
  in plaques with scale, 113
  in scaly papular lesions, 97
Oral mucosal lesions, erythema and, 51
Orbital dermoid cysts, *e*10
Orf, 236, 237*f*
Organoid nevus, 562
Osteoarthritis, 574

P

Pain, subcutaneous diseases and, 253
Palpation
  for linear and serpiginous lesions, 289
  tumor in, 579
  on tumors with scale, 477
Pancreatic panniculitis, 258, 259*f*
Panniculitis
  lupus, 260, 261*f*
  pancreatic, 258, 259*f*
Panorex X-ray, for cutaneous odontogenic sinus tract, 576, 577*f*
Papillomas. *see* Papillomatous and verrucous lesions
Papillomatous and verrucous lesions, 461–476
  acrochordon (soft fibroma) as, 470, 471*f*
  condyloma acuminatum as, 466, 466*b*, 467*f*
  differential diagnosis of, 461*b*
  history questions for, 461
  North American blastomycosis as, 472, 472*f*–473*f*
  physical findings in, 461
  seborrheic keratosis as, 468, 468*b*, 469*f*
  verrucae plana as, 464, 465*f*
  verrucae vulgaris as, 462, 463*f*
  verrucous carcinoma as, 461, 474, 475*f*
Papular acrodermatitis of childhood, 92, 93*f*
Papular and nodular growths without scale, 489–506
  basal cell carcinoma as, 490, 491*f*
  cutaneous lymphomas as, 502, 502*b*, 503*f*
  dermatofibroma as, 494, 495*f*
  dermatofibrosarcoma protuberans as, 498, 499*f*
  differential diagnosis of, 489*b*
  history questions for, 489
  keloid as, 496, 497*f*
  Merkel cell carcinoma as, 500, 500*f*–501*f*
  metastatic tumors as, 504, 504*b*, 505*f*
  physical findings in, 489
  Spitz nevus as, 492, 493*f*
Papular eruptions, 83–96
  bedbug bites, 90, 90*b*, 91*f*
  chiggers, 86, 86*b*, 87*f*
  differential diagnosis of, 83*b*
  Gianotti-Crosti syndrome, 92, 93*f*
  history questions for, 83
  miliaria, 94, 95*f*
  mite bites, 88, 88*b*, 89*f*
  physical findings, 83
  scabies, 84, 85*f*
Papular sarcoidosis, in lichen nitidus, 100
Papular urticaria, 70, 70*b*, 71*f*

Papules, 2*f*, 2*t*–3*t*, 83
Papulopustular rosacea (classic), 380
Paracetamol, for rubella, 44
Parapoxvirus, orf from, 236
Parathyroidectomy, for calciphylaxis, 240
Paromomycin, topical, for cutaneous leishmaniasis, 591
Paronychia, 404, 405*f*
Patch testing, for stasis ulcer, 242
Pediculosis capitis, 430, 430*f*–431*f*
Pediculosis pubis, 432, 432*f*–433*f*
Pediculus humanus var. capitis, 430, 430*f*
Pedicure, sporotrichoid disorders and, 301
Peginterferon alpha-2b, for neurofibroma, *e*8
Pellagra, 314, 314*b*, 315*f*
  medications associated with, 314
Pemphigus foliaceus, 170, 170*b*, 171*f*
Pemphigus vulgaris, 172, 172*b*, 172*f*–173*f*
D-Penicillamine
  for limited scleroderma, 358
  for scleroderma, 356
Penicillin
  for erysipelas, 78
  for meningococcemia, 336
  oral, for cutaneous odontogenic sinus tract, 576
Pentoxifylline
  for keloid, 496
  for pernio, 348
  for progressive pigmented purpura, 340
  for stasis ulcer, 242
Periapical X-ray, for cutaneous odontogenic sinus tract, 576
Perifolliculitis capitis abscedens et suffodiens, 224
Periocular verrucae, 463*f*
Peripheral pulses, in necrotic and ulcerative skin disorders, 231
Periungual telangiectasia, 307
Periungual warts, 463*f*
Permethrin
  for pediculosis capitis, 430
  for pediculosis pubis, 432
  for scabies, 84
Perms, alopecia and, 385
Pernio (chilblains), 348, 349*f*
Peutz-Jeghers syndrome, multiple lentigines in, 510*b*, 511*f*
Pharyngitis, in scarlet fever, 52
Phlebotomus fly, 591
Phlebotomy, for porphyria cutanea tarda, 202
Photoallergic drug eruption, 310, 310*b*, 311*f*
Photodistributed, definition of, 4–5
Photoprotection, for lupus erythematosus, 398
Photosensitive disorders, 307–326
  dermatomyositis as, 322, 323*f*
  differential diagnosis of, 307*b*
  discoid lupus erythematosus as, 320, 321*f*
  history questions for, 307
  pellagra as, 314, 314*b*, 315*f*
  photoallergic drug eruption as, 310, 310*b*, 311*f*
  phototoxic drug eruption as, 312, 312*b*, 313*f*

Photosensitive disorders *(Continued)*
  physical findings in, 307
  polymorphous light eruption as, 308, 308*f*–309*f*
  subacute cutaneous lupus erythematosus as, 318, 318*b*, 319*f*
  sunburn as, 324, 325*f*
  systemic lupus erythematosus as, 316, 316*b*, 317*f*
Phototoxic drug eruptions, 312, 312*b*, 313*f*
Physical urticaria, 66, 66*b*, 67*f*
Phytophotodermatitis, 593, 593*f*
Pigment, in nails, 403, 403*f*
Pigmented actinic keratosis, 110
Pigmented epithelioid melanocytoma, 532
Pigmented lesions, 507–534
  acquired melanocytic nevus, 512, 513*f*
  atypical (dysplastic) nevus, 522, 523*f*
  café au lait spot, 518, 518*b*, 519*f*
  congenital melanocytic nevus, 514, 515*f*
  halo nevus, 516, 517*f*
  history questions for, 507
  lentigo maligna, 524, 525*f*
  melanoma, 526–528, 526*b*, 527*f*, 528*b*, 529*f*–531*f*
  nevus spilus, 520, 521*f*
  physical findings in, 507
  simple lentigo, 510, 510*b*, 511*f*
  solar lentigo, 508, 509*f*
Pilar cyst, 568
Pimecrolimus, topical
  for atopic dermatitis, 144
  for pityriasis alba, 444
  for rosacea, 380
  for vitiligo, 442
Pinch grafts, for stasis ulcers, 242
Piperacillin-tazobactam, for necrotizing fasciitis, 232
Pityriasis alba, 444, 445*f*
Pityriasis lichenoides chronica (PLC), 350
Pityriasis lichenoides et varioliformis acuta (Mucha-Habermann disease), 350, 351*f*
Pityriasis rosea (PR), 156, 157*f*
Pityriasis rubra pilaris (PRP), 118, 119*f*
Pityriasis versicolor. *see* Tinea (pityriasis) versicolor
Plant allergens, in allergic contact dermatitis, 138*b*
Plantar warts, 463*f*
Plaque psoriasis, 114, 114*b*, 115*f*
Plaques, 2*f*, 2*t*–3*t*
  with scale, 113–122
    history questions for, 113
    mycosis fungoides, 120, 120*f*–121*f*
    physical findings in, 113
    pityriasis rubra pilaris, 118, 119*f*
    plaque psoriasis, 114, 114*b*, 115*f*
    predisposition for, 113
    reactive arthritis, 116, 117*f*
Plasmapheresis, for cryoglobulinemia, 344, 345*f*
Plexiform neurofibromas, *e*8
PMS fungal Tzanck stain, in Tzanck preparations, 19*f*
Pneumatic compression, for stasis ulcer, 242
Podophyllotoxin, for molluscum contagiosum, 106

Poison ivy, 136*b*
Polistes dominulus, 437*f*
Polyarteritis nodosa, cutaneous, 266, 267*f*
Polymorphic eruption of pregnancy. *see* Pruritic urticarial papules and plaques of pregnancy
Polymorphous light eruption, 308, 308*f*–309*f*
Pompholyx. *see* Dyshidrosis
Porphyria cutanea tarda, 202, 203*f*
Porphyrins, 8
Port wine stain, *e*12, *e*13*f*
Postinjection lipoatrophy, 370, 370*b*, 371*f*
Potassium hydroxide (KOH) examination
  in tinea capitis, 396
  in tinea (pityriasis) versicolor, 124
Potassium hydroxide (KOH) preparation, 10, 10*b*, 11*f*–13*f*
  for tinea nigra diagnosis, 590, 590*f*
Potassium iodide, oral (SSKI)
  for erythema induratum, 256
  for erythema nodosum, 254
  for sporotrichosis, 302
PR. *see* Pityriasis rosea (PR)
Pramoxine, for roseola vaccinatum, 46
Prednisolone, for leukocytoclastic vasculitis, 332
Prednisone
  for acute generalized exanthematous pustulosis, 206
  for allergic contact dermatitis, 136
  for cicatricial pemphigoid, *e*2
  for cutaneous polyarteritis nodosa, 266
  for eosinophilic fasciitis, 360
  for erythema induratum, 256
  for erythema nodosum, 254
  for herpes gestationis, 198
  for id reactions, 152
  for linear IgA bullous dermatosis, 200
  for lupus panniculitis, 260
  for pemphigus vulgaris, 172
  for pityriasis rosea, 156
  for pyoderma gangrenosum, 246
  for rheumatoid nodules, 264
Prickly heat, 94, 95*f*
Primary cutaneous inoculation blastomycosis, 472
Primary morphologic terms, 1, 2*t*–3*t*
Primary pulmonary blastomycosis, 472
Primary syphilis, 250, 251*f*
Progressive pigmented purpura (PPP), 340, 341*f*
  drug-induced, 340*b*
Progressive systemic sclerosis, 356
Proliferating trichilemmal tumors, 568
Propionibacterium acnes, 376
Pruritic urticarial papules and plaques of pregnancy (PUPPP), 74, 75*f*
Pruritus, in atopic dermatitis, 142
Pseudomonal toe web infection, severe, 597*f*
Pseudomonas spp., 597
  in onycholysis, 410
  in paronychia, 404
  Wood light, 8

Pseudomonas aeruginosa, causing *Pseudomonas* folliculitis, 382
Pseudomonas folliculitis, 375, 382, 383*f*
Pseudoporphyria, bullous, *e*4, *e*4*b*, *e*5*f*
Pseudorheumatoid nodules, 262
Psoralen and ultraviolet A (PUVA)
   for Grover disease, 108
   for lichen planus, 102
Psoriasis
   plaque, 114, 114*b*, 115*f*
   pustular, 208, 208*b*, 209*f*
Pteridine, 8
Pthirus pubis, 432, 432*f*
Pulmonary blastomycosis, primary, 472
Pulse corticosteroids, for pemphigus vulgaris, 172
Pulse methylprednisolone, for Henoch-Schönlein purpura, 328
Pulsed light therapy, for rosacea, 380
Punch biopsy, 26, 26*b*, 27*f*–29*f*
   for actinic keratosis, 110
   for calciphylaxis, 240
   for cicatricial pemphigoid, *e*2
   for cutaneous polyarteritis nodosa, 266
   for drug eruption with eosinophilia and systemic symptoms, 34
   for ecthyma gangrenosum, 234
   for erythema induratum, 256
   of lipoma, 580
   for lupus panniculitis, 260
   for morbilliform viral eruptions, 36
   for necrotizing fasciitis, 232
   for orf, 236
   for pancreatic panniculitis, 258
   for rheumatoid nodules, 264
   for roseola vaccinatum, 46
   for subcutaneous granuloma annulare, 262
   for unilateral thoracic exanthem, 40
Punctate papules, in scarlet fever, 52, 53*f*
Purified protein derivative (PPD) skin test, for erythema induratum, 256
Purpura fulminans, 342, 342*f*–343*f*
Purpuric and hemorrhagic disorders (P&H), 327–352, 327*b*
   acute hemorrhagic edema, 330, 331*f*
   cryofibrinogenemia, 346, 347*f*
   cryoglobulinemia, 344, 344*b*, 345*f*
   disseminated gonococcal infection, 334, 335*f*
   Henoch-Schönlein purpura, 328, 328*f*–329*f*
   history questions for, 327
   leukocytoclastic (hypersensitivity) vasculitis, 332, 332*b*, 333*f*
   meningococcemia, 336, 337*f*
   pernio (chilblains), 348, 349*f*
   physical findings in, 327
   pityriasis lichenoides et varioliformis acuta, 350, 351*f*
   progressive pigmented purpura, 340, 340*b*, 341*f*
   purpura fulminans, 342, 342*f*–343*f*
   Rocky Mountain spotted fever, 338, 338*f*–339*f*

Pustular arthropod reactions, 212, 213*f*
Pustular component, in follicular disorders, 375
Pustular drug eruptions, drug-induced, 206*b*
Pustular eruptions, nonfollicular, 205–216, 205*b*
   acropustulosis of infancy, 210, 211*f*
   acute generalized exanthematous pustulosis, 206, 207*f*
   cutaneous vaccinia infections, 214, 214*b*, 215*f*
   history questions for, 205
   physical findings in, 205
   pustular arthropod reactions, 212, 213*f*
   pustular psoriasis, 208, 208*b*, 209*f*
Pustular psoriasis, 208, 208*b*, 209*f*
Pustules, 2*t*–3*t*, 3*f*
   alopecia and, 385
Pustulosis, of palms and soles, 208, 209*f*
Pyoderma gangrenosum, 246, 247*f*
Pyogenic granuloma, 540, 541*f*
Pyrethrins
   for pediculosis capitis, 430
   for pediculosis pubis, 432
Pyrithione zinc shampoo, for androgenic alopecia, 386

R
Raccoon eyes, in neonatal lupus erythematosus, 278, 279*f*
Radiation therapy
   for keloid, 496
   for squamous cell carcinoma, 480
Ramsey-Hunt syndrome, 180
Rapid plasma reagin (RPR), for primary syphilis, 250
Rash, in papular eruptions, 83
Rayleigh scattering, 532*b*
Raynaud phenomenon, 353, 358
Reactive arthritis (Reiter disease), 116, 117*f*
Red, white, and blue sign, 238
Reiter disease. *see* Reactive arthritis
Repetitive blistering, 163
Reticulated erythema, 51–62
Retinoids
   for acne, 376
   for actinic keratosis, 110
   for pityriasis lichenoides et varioliformis acuta, 350
   for pityriasis rubra pilaris, 118
   for pustular psoriasis, 208
Rheumatoid arthritis, rheumatoid nodules and, 264
Rheumatoid nodules, 264, 265*f*
Rheumatoid nodulosis syndrome, 264
Rhinophyma (phymatous rosacea), 380
RICE therapy, for necrotic arachnidism, 238
Rickettsia rickettsii, 338
Rickettsial infections, 48, 48*b*, 49*f*
Rifampin, for cutaneous leishmaniasis, 591
Ritter disease. *See* Staphylococcal scalded skin syndrome
Rituximab
   for cryoglobulinemia, 344
   for pemphigus vulgaris, 172
Rocky Mountain spotted fever (RMSF), 338, 338*f*–339*f*

Rosacea, 380, 381*f*
Roseola, 38, 39*f*
Roseola vaccinatum, 46, 46*b*, 47*f*
Rough nails. *see* Trachyonychia
Rubber, in allergic contact dermatitis, 138*b*
Rubella, 44, 45*f*
Rubella immunoglobulin G (IgG) antibodies, in
    morbilliform viral eruptions, 36
Rubeola, 42, 42*b*, 43*f*
Rubivirus, 44
"Rule of 78," for poison ivy, 136*b*
Ruptured epidermoid cysts, 226, 227*f*, 566

S

Salicylic acid
    for mild acne, 376
    for tinea nigra, 590
    for verrucae vulgaris, 462
Salicylic acid gel, for molluscum contagiosum, 106
Salmonella spp.
    in acute hemorrhagic edema, 330
    in Henoch-Schönlein purpura, 328
Sarcoidosis, papular, in lichen nitidus, 100
Saucerization biopsy, 22
Scabies, 84, 85*f*
    mineral oil preparation for, 14, 15*f*–17*f*
    pustular, 213*f*
Scaling tumor. *see* Tumors with scale
Scaly disorders, 123–134
    acquired ichthyosis vulgaris (ichthyosis acquisita), 126,
        126*b*, 127*f*
    history questions for, 123
    kwashiorkor, 132, 133*f*
    physical findings in, 123
    tinea manuum, 128, 128*b*, 129*f*
    tinea pedis, 128, 128*b*, 129*f*
    tinea (pityriasis) versicolor, 124, 125*f*
    xerosis (asteatosis, dry skin), 130, 130*b*, 131*f*
Scaly papular lesions, 97–112
    actinic keratosis, 110, 111*f*
    genetic predisposition for, 97
    Grover disease, 108, 109*f*
    guttate psoriasis, 98, 98*b*, 99*f*
    history questions for, 97
    lichen nitidus, 100, 101*f*
    lichen planus, 102, 103*f*
    molluscum contagiosum, 106, 107*f*
    physical findings in, 97
    secondary syphilis, 104, 105*f*
Scarlatina, 52
Scarlet fever, 52, 53*f*
Scarring, in alopecia, 385
SCCIS. *see* Squamous cell carcinoma in situ
Schamberg purpura, 340
Scleredema, 362, 363*f*
Scleredema adultorum, 362
Scleredema of Buschke, 362
Sclerodactyly, 358

Scleroderma, 356, 357*f*
Sclerosing and fibrosing disorders, 353–366
    differential diagnosis of, 353*b*
    eosinophilic fasciitis, 360, 361*f*
    history questions for, 353
    morphea, 354, 355*f*
    nephrogenic systemic fibrosis, 364, 365*f*
    physical findings in, 353
    scleredema, 362, 363*f*
    scleroderma, 356, 357*f*
        limited, 358, 359*f*
Scopulariopsis brevicaulis, 408
Scybala, mineral oil preparation, 14, 17*f*
SD. *see* Seborrheic dermatitis (SD)
Seabather's eruption, 594, 594*f*
Sebaceous cyst, 566
Sebaceous gland hyperplasia, 560, 561*f*
Sebopsoriasis, 158
Seborrhea petaloides, 158
Seborrheic dermatitis (SD), 158, 159*f*
Seborrheic keratosis, 468, 468*b*, 469*f*
    inflamed, 486, 487*f*
Secondary morphologic terms, 1, 4*t*
Secondary syphilis, 104, 105*f*
    in lichen nitidus, 100
Seidlmayer disease, 330
Selective serotonin reuptake inhibitors (SSRIs)
    for habit tic deformity, 422
    for trichotillomania, 390
Selenium sulfide, for tinea (pityriasis) versicolor,
    124
Semipermeable polyurethane membrane, for cutaneous
    vaccinia infections, 214
Sentinel lymph node (SLN) biopsy, 528
Serologic testing
    for neonatal lupus erythematosus, 278
    for North American blastomycosis, 472
    for primary syphilis, 250
    for Rocky Mountain spotted fever, 338
    for secondary syphilis, 104
Serpiginous lesions. *see* Linear and serpiginous lesions
Serum sickness, in morbilliform drug eruptions, 32*b*
Sexual contact, necrotic and ulcerative skin disorders and,
    231
Shampoos, for seborrheic dermatitis, 158
Shave biopsy, 22, 23*f*–25*f*
    for actinic keratosis, 110
    for benign lichenoid keratosis, 484
    for cicatricial pemphigoid, *e*2
    for Grover disease, 108
    for keratoacanthoma, 482
    for pemphigus vulgaris, 172
    for pyogenic granuloma, 540
    for sebaceous gland hyperplasia, 560
    for seborrheic keratosis, 468
    for squamous cell carcinoma, 480
    for squamous cell carcinoma in situ, 478
Sheep, direct contact with, 236

Shigella spp.
    in acute hemorrhagic edema, 330
    in Henoch-Schönlein purpura, 328
Short hyphae, in potassium hydroxide, 13*f*
Shot glass rule, 598, 598*f*
Sign of Leser-Trélat, 468
Simple lentigo, 510, 510*b*, 511*f*
Simple urticaria, 63
Sinuses, 565–578
    cutaneous odontogenic sinus tract, 576, 576*f*–577*f*
    history questions for, 565
    physical findings in, 565
Sirolimus, for neurofibroma, *e8*
Sixth disease, 38, 39*f*
SK. *see* Seborrheic keratosis
Skin barrier creams, for allergic contact dermatitis, 136
Skin biopsy. *see* Biopsy
Skin cancers, 97, 477
Skin color, 1
Skin discolorations, 441–460, 441*b*
    acanthosis nigricans, 448, 448*b*, 449*f*
    Addison disease, 452, 452*b*, 453*f*
    carotenoderma, 456, 456*b*, 457*f*, 459*f*
    confluent and reticulated papillomatosis of Gougerot-Carteaud (CRPGC), 444, 451*f*
    drug-induced blue-grey discoloration, 458, 458*b*, 459*f*
    history questions for, 441
    jaundice, 454, 454*b*, 455*f*
    lichen sclerosus et atrophicus, 446, 447*f*
    physical findings in, 441
    pityriasis alba, 444, 445*f*
    vitiligo, 442, 443*f*
Skin tags. *see* Acrochordon (soft fibroma)
Slapped cheeks, 58, 59*f*
Soaps
    ingredients, 597*b*
    for xerosis and dermatitis, 597
Sodium lactate-containing moisturizers, for atopic dermatitis, 142–144
Sodium stibogluconate, intravenous, for cutaneous leishmaniasis, 591
Sodium sulfacetamide, for rosacea, 380
Sodium thiosulfate, for calciphylaxis, 240
Soft fibroma (acrochordon), 470, 471*f*
Soft tissue x-rays, for calciphylaxis, 240
Solar lentigo, 508, 509*f*
Solar lentigo, benign lichenoid keratosis and, 484
Solar urticaria, 66, 67*f*
Solenopsis invicta, 212, 213*f*
Sonidegib, for basal cell carcinoma, 490
Sorafenib, for neurofibroma, *e8*
Speckled lentiginous nevus, 520
SPF. *see* Sunscreen protection factor
Spider bites, 438, 439*f*
Spironolactone, for androgenic alopecia, 386
Spitz nevus, 492, 493*f*
Split-thickness grafts, for stasis ulcers, 242
Sporothrix schenckii, 302

Sporotrichoid disorders, 301–306
    differential diagnosis of, 301*b*
    history questions for, 301
    mycobacterial infections, 304, 305*f*
    physical findings in, 301
    sporotrichosis, 302, 303*f*
Sporotrichoid mycobacterial infections, 304, 305*f*
Sporotrichosis, 302, 303*f*
Squamous cell carcinoma (SCC), 480, 481*f*
    in actinic keratosis, 110
    suspected, 23*f*
Squamous cell carcinoma in situ, 478, 478*f*–479*f*
Squaric acid dibutyl ester, for alopecia areata, 394
Stanozolol, for cryofibrinogenemia, 346
Staphylococcal scalded skin syndrome, 166, 167*f*
Staphylococcus aureus
    bullous impetigo due to, 164
    erysipelas from, 78
    in Henoch-Schönlein purpura, 328
    in paronychia, 404
    toxic shock syndrome from, 54
Stasis ulcer, 242, 243*f*
Statins, for scleroderma, 356
Steatocystoma, 570, 571*f*
Steatocystoma simplex, 570
Steatocystomas multiplex, 570
Sterile saline, lavage with, for pyoderma gangrenosum, 246
Steroids
    for allergic contact dermatitis, 136
    atrophic disorders and, 367
    for eczematous drug eruptions, 148
    for id reactions, 152
    for Seabather's eruption, 594
Stevens-Johnson syndrome, 190, 191*f*, 286
Stings. *see* Infestations, stings, and bites
Stomatitis, in reactive arthritis (Reiter disease), 116
Stork bite, 535
Strawberry hemangioma, 536
Strawberry tongue
    in Kawasaki disease, 57*f*
    in scarlet fever, 52, 53*f*
Streptococcus spp.
    in acute hemorrhagic edema, 330
    in Henoch-Schönlein purpura, 328
Streptococcus agalactiae, erysipelas from, 78
Streptococcus pneumoniae, in purpura fulminans, 342
Streptococcus pyogenes
    blistering distal dactylitis due to, 168
    erysipelas from, 78
    scarlet fever from, 52
Stretch marks, 368
Striae, 368, 368*b*, 369*f*
Striae alba, 368
Striae distensae, 368
Striae gravidarum, 368
Striae rubra, 368
Stucco keratosis, 468

Sturge-Weber syndrome, *e*12

Subacute cutaneous lupus erythematosus, 318, 318*b*, 319*f*

Subcutaneous diseases, 253–268
  cutaneous polyarteritis nodosa as, 266, 267*f*
  erythema induratum as, 256, 257*f*
  erythema nodosum as, 254, 255*f*
  history questions for, 253
  lupus panniculitis as, 260, 261*f*
  pancreatic panniculitis as, 258, 259*f*
  physical findings in, 253
  rheumatoid nodules as, 264, 265*f*
  subcutaneous granuloma annulare as, 262, 263*f*
  tuberculosis skin test and, 253

Subcutaneous lumps, 579–586
  angiolipoma as, 582, 583*f*
  differential diagnosis of, 579*b*
  history questions for, 579
  lipoma as, 580, 581*f*
  metastatic tumors as, 584, 584*b*, 585*f*
  physical findings in, 579

Sulconazole, for diaper dermatitis, 146

Sulfapyridine, for linear IgA bullous dermatosis, 200

Sulfasalazine, for eosinophilic fasciitis, 360

Sulfur, for scabies, 84

Sunburn, 324, 325*f*
  with goose bumps, 53*f*

Sunscreen protection factor (SPF), 598

Sunscreens, 598, 598*f*
  with broad protection, for eczematous drug eruptions, 148

Superficial lymphangioma, 546, 547*f*

Superficial spreading basal cell carcinoma, 490

Surgery
  for central centrifugal cicatricial alopecia, 400
  for onychocryptosis, 406

Surgical excision, for necrotic arachnidism, 238

Sutton nevi, 516

Sweet syndrome, 76, 76*b*, 77*f*

Syphilis
  primary, 250, 251*f*
  secondary, 104, 105*f*
    in lichen nitidus, 100

Systemic blastomycosis, 472

Systemic disorders, necrotic and ulcerative skin disorders and, 231

Systemic lupus erythematosus, 316, 316*b*, 317*f*

Systemized epidermal nevus, 294

T

T cell lymphomas, 502*b*

Tacrolimus, topical
  for atopic dermatitis, 144
  for rosacea, 380
  for vitiligo, 442

Tanning beds, melanomas and, 526*b*

Tanning pills, 456*b*

Targetoid lesions. *see* Annular and targetoid lesions

Telangiectasia, 358

Telogen effluvium, 385, 388, 388*b*, 389*f*

Temporal course, in clinical dermatology, 5

Tense blisters, 163*b*

Terbinafine
  for kerion, 228
  for onychomycosis, 408
  for sporotrichosis, 302
  for tinea capitis, 396
  for tinea pedis and tinea manuum, 128

Tetracycline
  for acne, 376
  for dissecting cellulitis of scalp, 224

Tetracycline-induced pseudoporphyria, *e*5*f*

Texture, palpation and appreciation of, 1

Thiabendazole
  for cutaneous larva migrans, 588
  for tungiasis, 592

Thoracic dermatome, herpes zoster in, 180, 181*f*

Thymol, for onycholysis, 410

Ticarcillin-clavulanate, for necrotizing fasciitis, 232

Tick bites, 327, 434, 434*f*–435*f*

Tinea capitis
  alopecia and, 396, 397*f*
  in Wood light, 8

Tinea corporis, 270, 271*f*

Tinea cruris, 270, 271*f*

Tinea faciei, 270, 271*f*

Tinea manuum, 128, 129*f*

Tinea nigra, 590, 590*f*

Tinea pedis, 128, 128*b*, 129*f*

Tinea unguium, 408, 408*b*, 409*f*

Tinea (pityriasis) versicolor, 124, 125*f*
  potassium hydroxide preparation for, 10, 13*f*

Toilet seat, condyloma acuminatum and, 466*b*

Tonsillitis, in scarlet fever, 52

Topical heat therapy, for sporotrichosis, 302

Topical therapies
  for condyloma acuminatum, 466
  for verrucae vulgaris, 462

Topical treatment pearls, 597–599, 597*b*
  corticosteroids, 598–599
  gram-negative toe web infections, 597, 597*f*
  moisturizer, 597–598
  soaps for xerosis and dermatitis, 597
  sunscreens, 598, 598*f*

Toxic epidermal necrolysis, 192, 192*b*, 193*f*, 195*f*

Toxic shock-like syndrome (TSLS), 54

Toxic shock syndrome, 54, 55*f*

Trachyonychia, 418, 418*b*, 419*f*

Traction alopecia, 392, 393*f*

Transient acantholytic dermatosis, 108

Translucent digital mucous cyst, 575*f*

Trauma, to nail, 403

Travelers, cutaneous diseases of, 587–595, 587*b*
  cutaneous larva migrans as, 588, 588*f*
  cutaneous leishmaniasis as, 591, 591*f*
  history questions for, 587

Travelers, cutaneous diseases of *(Continued)*
  myiasis as, 589, 589*f*
  phytophotodermatitis as, 593, 593*f*
  Seabather's eruption as, 594, 594*f*
  tinea nigra as, 590, 590*f*
  tungiasis as, 592, 592*f*
Treponema pallidum, 250
Treponema pallidum particle agglutination (TP-PA) tests,
    for primary syphilis, 250
Treponema-specific tests, for primary syphilis, 250
Tretinoin
  for confluent and reticulated papillomatosis of
      Gougerot-Carteaud, 450
  for pityriasis alba, 444
  for rosacea, 380
Tretinoin gel, topical, for verrucae plana, 464
Triamcinolone
  intralesional
    for alopecia areata, 394
    for central centrifugal cicatricial alopecia, 400
    for cicatricial pemphigoid, *e*2
    for digital mucous cysts, 574
    for epidermoid cyst, 566
    for lupus erythematosus, 398
    for rheumatoid nodules, 264
  ointment, for dyshidrosis, 154
Triamcinolone acetonide, intralesional
  for dissecting cellulitis of scalp, 224
  for keloid, 496
Trichilemmal carcinomas, 568
Trichilemmal cysts, 565, 568, 569*f*
Trichobezoar, gastric, 390
Trichogram, on androgenic alopecia, 386
Trichophyton rubrum, in onychomycosis, 408
Trichotillomania, 385, 390, 391*f*
Tricyclic antidepressants, for trichotillomania, 390
Triple antibiotic ointment, for Grover disease, 108
Trombicula alfredduges, 86
Trombiculid mites, 87*f*
Trombiculosis, 86, 86*b*, 87*f*
True cysts, of skin, 565
Tuberculoid leprosy, 284, 285*f*
Tuberculosis, subcutaneous diseases and, 253
Tuberculosis skin test, positive, 253
Tumbu fly myiasis, 589, 589*f*
Tumor necrosis factor-α inhibitors, for dissecting cellulitis
    of scalp, 224
Tumors with scale, 477–488
  benign lichenoid keratosis as, 484, 485*f*
  differential diagnosis of, 477*b*
  history questions for, 477
  inflamed seborrheic keratosis as, 486, 487*f*
  keratoacanthoma as, 482, 483*f*
  location of, 477
  physical findings in, 477
  rapid growth of, 477
  squamous cell carcinoma as, 480, 481*f*
  squamous cell carcinoma in situ as, 478, 478*f*–479*f*

Tunga penetrans, 592
Tungiasis, 592, 592*f*
Twenty-nail dystrophy, 418
Two feet-one hand syndrome, 128, 129*f*
Tyndall effect, 532*b*
Tzanck preparation, 18, 18*f*–21*f*

U
Ugly duckling sign, 507
Ulcerative skin disorders. *see* Necrotic and ulcerative skin
    disorders
Ulcers, 4*f*, 4*t*
  arterial (ischemic), 244, 245*f*
  cutaneous leishmaniasis, 591
  leg, 242
    chronic, differential diagnosis of, 244*b*
  in necrotic and ulcerative skin disorders
    base of, 231
    extent of, 231
    shape of, 231
Ultraviolet B (UVB) light, narrow-band, for Grover
    disease, 108
Ultraviolet B (UVB) therapy, for pityriasis rosea, 156
Ultraviolet (UV) light therapy, for pityriasis lichenoides et
    varioliformis acuta, 350
Unilateral thoracic exanthem, 40, 41*f*
Unna boots, for stasis ulcer, 242
Urinary porphyrins, in Wood light, 8
Urticaria, 64, 64*b*, 65*f*
Urticarial eruptions, 63–82
  angioedema, 68, 68*b*, 69*f*
  cellulitis, 80, 81*f*
  erysipelas, 78, 79*f*
  history questions for, 63
  papular urticaria, 70, 70*b*, 71*f*
  physical findings in, 63
  physical urticarias, 66, 66*b*, 67*f*
  pruritic urticarial papules and plaques of pregnancy, 74,
      75*f*
  Sweet syndrome, 76, 76*b*, 77*f*
Urticarial vasculitis, 72, 73*f*
  drugs causing, 72*b*
UVA1 phototherapy
  for morphea, 354
  for scleredema, 362
  for scleroderma, 356

V
Vaccination, measles and, 42*b*
Vaccinia immune globulin, for cutaneous vaccinia
    infections, 214
Vaccinia infections, cutaneous, 214, 214*b*, 215*f*
Vaccinia necrosum, 214
Valacyclovir, for herpes simplex virus infection, 182
Varicella-zoster immune globulin (VZIG), for chickenpox,
    178
Varicella-zoster virus infections, Tzanck preparation for,
    18

Vascular tumors, 535–552
  angiosarcoma, 550, 551*f*
  cherry angioma (hemangioma), 542, 543*f*
  differential diagnosis of, 535*b*
  history questions for, 535
  infantile (juvenile) hemangioma, 536, 537*f*
  Kaposi sarcoma, 548, 548*f*–549*f*
  Kasabach-Merritt syndrome, 538, 539*f*
  physical findings in, 535
  pyogenic granuloma, 540, 541*f*
  superficial lymphangioma, 546, 547*f*
  venous lake, 544, 545*f*
Vasculitis, urticarial, 72, 72*b*, 73*f*
Vasculopathy, livedoid, *e*6, *e*7*f*
Vasodilators, for scleroderma, 356
Venereal disease research laboratory (VDRL) tests, for
    primary syphilis, 250
Venereal warts. *see* Condyloma acuminatum
Venous lake, 544, 545*f*
Venous varix, 544
Verrucae palmaris, 462
Verrucae plana, 464, 465*f*
Verrucae plantaris, 462, 463*f*
Verrucae vulgaris, 462, 463*f*
Verrucous carcinoma, 461, 474, 475*f*
Verrucous lesions, papillomatous and, 461–476
  acrochordon (soft fibroma) as, 470, 471*f*
  condyloma acuminatum as, 466, 466*b*, 467*f*
  development of, 461
  differential diagnosis of, 461*b*
  history questions for, 461
  North American blastomycosis as, 472, 472*f*–473*f*
  physical findings in, 461
  seborrheic keratosis as, 468, 468*b*, 469*f*
  verrucae plana as, 464, 465*f*
  verrucae vulgaris as, 462, 463*f*
  verrucous carcinoma as, 461, 474, 475*f*
Vesicles, 2*f*, 2*t*–3*t*, 163–204
  in erythema, 51
Vesiculobullous lesions, 289
Vespula pennsylvanica, 437*f*
Viral culture, in rubella, 44
Viral serologic studies, for morbilliform viral eruptions, 36

Vismodegib, for basal cell carcinoma, 490
Vitamin K, for purpura fulminans, 342
Vitiligo, 442, 443*f*

W

Warts. *see* Verrucae vulgaris
Wasps, 436, 437*f*
Water exposure, follicular disorders and, 375
Watson syndrome, café au lait spots in, 518
Wen, 568
Wheal, 2*t*–3*t*, 3*f*
Wickham striae, 102, 103*f*
Wood light, 8, 9*f*
  for skin discoloration, 441
Wright-Giemsa stain, in Tzanck preparation, 19*f*,
    21*f*

X

X-rays
  for cutaneous odontogenic sinus tract, 576, 577*f*
  soft tissue, for calciphylaxis, 240
Xanthelasma, 556, 557*f*
Xanthelasma palpebrarum, 556
Xanthogranuloma, juvenile, 558, 559*f*
Xanthomata, eruptive, 554, 554*f*–555*f*
Xerosis, 130, 130*b*, 131*f*
  drug-induced, 130*b*
  soaps for, 597
  treated with ammonium lactate, 598*f*

Y

Yeast infection, potassium hydroxide preparation for, 10,
    13*f*
Yellow lesions, 553–564
  differential diagnosis of, 553*b*
  eruptive xanthomata, 554, 554*f*–555*f*
  history questions for, 553
  juvenile xanthogranuloma, 558, 559*f*
  nevus sebaceus, 562, 563*f*
  physical findings in, 553
  sebaceous gland hyperplasia, 560, 561*f*
  xanthelasma, 556, 557*f*
Yellowjackets, 436, 437*f*